T0320917

FIFTY YEARS OF
MAGNETOENCEPHALOGRAPHY

FIFTY YEARS OF MAGNETOENCEPHALOGRAPHY

BEGINNINGS, TECHNICAL ADVANCES, AND APPLICATIONS

Edited by Andrew C. Papanicolaou,
Timothy P. L. Roberts, and
James W. Wheless

OXFORD
UNIVERSITY PRESS

OXFORD
UNIVERSITY PRESS

Oxford University Press is a department of the University of Oxford. It furthers
the University's objective of excellence in research, scholarship, and education
by publishing worldwide. Oxford is a registered trade mark of Oxford University
Press in the UK and certain other countries.

Published in the United States of America by Oxford University Press
198 Madison Avenue, New York, NY 10016, United States of America.

Library of Congress Cataloging-in-Publication Data
Names: Papanicolaou, Andrew C., editor. | Roberts, Timothy P. L., editor. |
Wheless, James W., editor.
Title: Fifty years of magnetoencephalography : beginnings, technical advances,
and applications / Andrew C. Papanicolaou, Timothy P. L. Roberts,
James W. Wheless (eds.).
Description: New York, NY : Oxford University Press, [2020] |
Includes bibliographical references and index.
Identifiers: LCCN 2020001420 (print) | LCCN 2020001421 (ebook) |
ISBN 9780190935689 (hardback) | ISBN 9780190935702 (epub) |
ISBN 9780190935719
Subjects: LCSH: Magnetoencephalography—History.
Classification: LCC RC386.6.M36 F54 2020 (print) |
LCC RC386.6.M36 (ebook) | DDC 616.8/047548—dc23
LC record available at https://lccn.loc.gov/2020001420
LC ebook record available at https://lccn.loc.gov/2020001421

1 3 5 7 9 8 6 4 2

Printed by Integrated Books International, United States of America

CONTENTS

SECTION III. APPLICATIONS TO EPILEPSY

SECTION IV. SOMATOSENSORY, MOTOR, AND LANGUAGE MAPPING

PREFACE

HALF A century has gone by since magnetoencephalography (MEG) was invented. For half that time, various clinical and research applications of it were attempted with considerable success, notably in the area of epilepsy and presurgical functional mapping. Yet the best way, out of several, to apply MEG and interpret the findings still remains conjectural. Accordingly, the purpose of this book is, first, to take stock of the current applications and to discuss and facilitate decisions on the part of the users as to how to optimize such applications; second, to assess the new clinical and research applications, especially for markers of neuropsychiatric and other disorders; and third, to evaluate the new instruments and analytic procedures that have been recently developed. This book, therefore, may serve as a standard of clinical practice and as a source of ideas for expanding the applications of MEG. It consists

of five sections. The first, of great historical interest, written by three pioneers in the field, reflects their recollections on how the field was initiated and developed. The second section consists of five technical chapters that deal with the neuronal basis of MEG, the different models of MEG systems currently available and those under development, and the different signal analysis procedures.

The third section consists of six chapters detailing the applications of MEG in the management of epilepsy. Specifically, they provide information about the relative efficacy of MEG in identifying the irritative and ictal onset zones and its contributions to decisions regarding placement of subdural grid and depth electrodes in pediatric and adult epilepsy surgery candidates. The three chapters of the fourth section provide descriptions of the clinical contributions of MEG to the understanding and topography of somatosensory motor and language networks and its use in presurgical evaluation of patients. The fifth section consists of three chapters that detail the contributions of MEG to the elucidations of brain mechanisms of cognition. The sixth and final section consists of five chapters that describe the uses of resting-state as well as task-specific MEG signals in identifying resting-state and function-specific neuronal networks and the application of such data to the diagnosis of neurodegenerative and psychiatric disorders. The book ends with a brief postscript that summarizes the editors' appraisal of the current state of the technological, clinical, and research developments of MEG.

Andrew C. Papanicolaou
Timothy P. L. Roberts
James W. Wheless

ABOUT THE EDITORS

Andrew C. Papanicolaou is Professor Emeritus of the University of Tennessee, College of Medicine, where he served as Founder and Chief of the Division of Clinical Neuroscience; Visiting Professor of Neurology at the National University of Athens, Greece; President of the Advisory Board of the Center of Applied Neuroscience at the University of Cyprus; and Honorary Member of the Hellenic Clinical Neurophysiology and Neuropsychology Societies. He has served on the Board of Regents of the University of Ioannina, Greece; as Director of the Center of Clinical Neuroscience at the University of Texas—Houston Medical Center; and as Professor in the Departments of Neurosurgery, Neurology, and Pediatrics of the same institution. He was also Adjunct Professor of Psychology at the University of Houston and of Linguistics at Rice University. He founded and directed the Summer Institute of the International Neuropsychological Society, and he founded the International Society for the Advancement of Clinical Magnetoencephalography and the postgraduate program in Neuropsychology at the National University of Athens. His publications include technical articles and several books on clinical, theoretical, and philosophical topics.

Timothy P. L. Roberts received his BA (1988) and PhD (1992) from Cambridge University in England, with training in Natural Sciences (Physics) and research in magnetic resonance imaging. He was a postdoctoral fellow in Neuroradiology at the University of California—San Francisco (UCSF) from 1992 to 1994 before joining the faculty as Assistant and Associate Professor. In 1994, he cofounded the UCSF Biomagnetic Imaging Laboratory.

After a period as Professor of Medical Imaging (and Canada Research Chair) at the University of Toronto, since 2005 he has been Professor of Radiology at University of Pennsylvania and Vice-Chair of Radiology, Research at Children's Hospital of Philadelphia, where he holds the Oberkircher Family Endowed Chair in Pediatric Radiology. His research focuses on multimodal imaging and electrophysiology in pediatric disorders such as epilepsy and autism spectrum disorder, and he has published more than 300 manuscripts in the field of advanced imaging and electrophysiology. He is an authority on the use of magnetoencephalography. He is funded by grants from the National Institutes of Health, the US Department of Defense, and the Simons Foundation. He serves as Associate Editor for Frontiers in Integrative Neuroscience and was elected a Distinguished Investigator of the Academy for Radiology Research in 2016.

James W. Wheless is currently Professor and Chief of Pediatric Neurology and Le Bonheur Chair in Pediatric Neurology at the University of Tennessee Health Science Center and Director of the Neuroscience Institute and the Le Bonheur Comprehensive Epilepsy Program, Le Bonheur Children's Hospital, in Memphis, Tennessee. His undergraduate degree in pharmacy and doctorate in medicine were obtained from the University of Oklahoma. His pediatric neurology training was at Northwestern University and the Medical College of Georgia. He then founded the Texas Comprehensive Epilepsy Program in Houston before moving to Tennessee to found the Le Bonheur Comprehensive Epilepsy Program. He has published extensively in the field of epilepsy, authoring three textbooks and more than 250 manuscripts, and he has presented at numerous national and international meetings. His interests have included new drug development for epilepsy, use of dietary therapy to treat epilepsy, epilepsy surgery in children, neurostimulation, and the use of noninvasive imaging techniques in the evaluation of children and adolescents for epilepsy surgery and for functional mapping.

CONTRIBUTORS

Abbas Babajani-Feremi, PhD
Associate Professor
Division of Pediatric Neurology
Department of Pediatrics
Department of Anatomy and Neurobiology
University of Tennessee Health Science Center
Neuroscience Institute
Le Bonheur Children's Hospital

Gareth R. Barnes, PhD
Professor of Neuroimaging
Wellcome Centre for Human Neuroimaging
UCL Institute of Neurology

James Baumgartner, MD
Board-Certified Pediatric Neurosurgeon and
    Surgical Director
Advent Health for Children's Comprehensive
    Epilepsy Center

Elena Boto, PhD
Research Fellow
Sir Peter Mansfield Imaging Centre
University of Nottingham

Richard Bowtell, PhD
Professor of Physics
Sir Peter Mansfield Imaging Centre
University of Nottingham

Susan M. Bowyer, PhD
Department of Neurology
Henry Ford Hospital
Wayne State University

Matthew J. Brookes, PhD
Professor of Physics
Sir Peter Mansfield Imaging Centre
University of Nottingham

Felicha T. Candelaria-Cook, PhD
The Mind Research Network

Eduardo M. Castillo, PhD
Director Magnetoencephalography
  Laboratory
Advent Health for Children

Won Seok Chang, MD, PhD
Associate Professor
Division of Stereotactic and Functional
  Neurosurgery
Yonsei Medical Gamma Knife Center
Department of Neurosurgery
Yonsei University College of Medicine

Chun Kee Chung, MD, PhD
Professor of Neurosurgery
Seoul National University Hospital
Professor of Department of Brain and
  Cognitive Sciences
Seoul National University

David Cohen, PhD
Athinoula A. Martinos Center for Biomedical
  Imaging
Department of Radiology
Massachusetts General Hospital
Charlestown
Harvard Medical School
Boston

Jaisalmer de Frutos-Lucas, MSc
Laboratory of Cognitive and Computational
  Neuroscience
Center for Biomedical Technology
Collaborative Genomics Group
School of Medical and Health Sciences
Edith Cowan University
Biological and Health Psychology
  Department
School of Psychology
Universidad Autonoma de Madrid

Xavier De Tiège, MD, PhD
Laboratoire de Cartographie fonctionnelle du
  Cerveau
UNI—ULB Neuroscience Institute
Université libre de Bruxelles (ULB)
Department of Functional Neuroimaging
Service of Nuclear Medicine
CUB Hôpital Erasme
Université libre de Bruxelles (ULB)
University of Muenster

Benjamin T. Dunkley, PhD
Scientist, Hospital for Sick Children
Assistant Professor, University of Toronto

J. Christopher Edgar, PhD
Associate Professor of Radiology
Department of Radiology
Research Division, The Children's Hospital of
  Philadelphia

A. S. Fokas, MD, PhD
Chair of Nonlinear Mathematical Science
University of Cambridge

William Gaetz, PhD
Associate Professor of Radiology
Children's Hospital of Philadelphia
Perelman School of Medicine
University of Pennsylvania

Joachim Gross, PhD
Professor of Systems Neuroscience
University of Muenster

Matti S. Hämäläinen, PhD
Professor of Radiology
Harvard Medical School
Athinoula A. Martinos Center for Biomedical
  Imaging
Department of Radiology
Massachusetts General Hospital

Parham Hashemzadeh, PhD
Professor
Bryant University
Beijing Institute of Technology-
  Zhuhai-China

Ryan Hill, MSc
Postdoctoral student
Sir Peter Mansfield Imaging Centre
University of Nottingham

Niall Holmes, PhD
Research Fellow
Sir Peter Mansfield Imaging Centre
University of Nottingham

Risto J. Ilmoniemi, PhD
Professor
Department of Neuroscience and Biomedical
    Engineering
Aalto University School of Science

Makoto Ishida, PhD
Research Assistant
Department of Epileptology
Tohoku University

Masaki Iwasaki, MD, PhD
Director
Department of Neurosurgery
National Center Hospital of Neurology and
    Psychiatry

Woorim Jeong, PhD
Postdoctoral Research Fellow of Neuroscience
    Research Institute
Seoul National University

Kazutaka Jin, MD, PhD
Associate Professor
Department of Epileptology
Tohoku University

Veikko Jousmäki, PhD
Aalto NeuroImaging
Department of Neuroscience and Biomedical
    Engineering
Aalto University School of Science
Cognitive Neuroimaging Centre
Nanyang Technological University

Yosuke Kakisaka, MD, PhD
Assistant Professor
Department of Epileptology
Tohoku University

Martin Kaltenhäuser, Dr. rer. nat.
Department of Neurosurgery
University Hospital Erlangen

Kyousuke Kamada, MD, PhD
Department of Neurosurgery
Asahikawa Medical University

Akitake Kanno, PhD
Assistant Professor
Department of Electromagnetic
    Neurophysiology
Tohoku University

Toivo Katila, Dr. Techn
Professor (emer.) of Biomedical Engineering
Helsinki University of Technology

Lloyd Kaufman, PhD, Dsc. (honoris causa)
Professor Emeritus of Psychology and Neural
    Science
New York University

**Tara Kleineschay, R. EEG/EP T.,
CLTM, CMEG**
MEG Laboratory Technologist
Magnetoencephalography Laboratory
Advent Health for Children

Milena Korostenskaja, PhD
Head
Functional Brain Mapping and Brain-
    Computer Interface Lab
Advent Health for Children

Richard M. Leahy, PhD
Professor
Electrical and Computer Engineering
University of Southern California

Ki Hyeong Lee, MD, MS
Medical Director of the Comprehensive
    Pediatric Epilepsy Center
Advent Health for Children

James Leggett, PhD
Research Fellow
Sir Peter Mansfield Imaging Centre
University of Nottingham

David López-Sanz, PhD
Laboratory of Cognitive and Computational
  Neuroscience
Center for Biomedical Technology
Experimental Psychology Department
School of Psychology
Universidad Complutense de Madrid

Fernando Maestú, PhD
Laboratory of Cognitive and Computational
  Neuroscience
Center for Biomedical Technology
Experimental Psychology Department
School of Psychology
Universidad Complutense de Madrid
Department of Civil Engineering and
  Computer Science
University of Rome

Junko Matsuzaki, PhD
Visiting Scholar
Children's Hospital of Philadelphia

Stephanie Mellor, MSc
Postdoctoral student
Wellcome Centre for Human Neuroimaging
UCL Institute of Neurology

Gregory A. Miller, PhD
Professor of Psychology
Departments of Psychology, and Psychiatry
  and Biobehavioral Sciences
University of California

Nobukazu Nakasato, MD, PhD
Professor
Department of Epileptology
Tohoku University

Yoshio Okada, PhD
Professor of Pediatrics
Harvard University

Shin-ichiro Osawa, MD, PhD
Assistant Professor
Department of Neurosurgery
Tohoku University

Hiroshi Otsubo, MD
Director of Clinical Neurophysiology
Division of Neurology
The Hospital for Sick Children
Professor
Department of Paediatrics
University of Toronto

Dimitrios Pantazis, PhD
Principal Research Scientist
Massachusetts Institute of Technology

Christos Papadelis, PhD
Professor of Pediatrics
TCU and UNTHSC
School of Medicine

Andrew C. Papanicolaou, PhD
Professor of Neuroscience Emeritus
University of Tennessee Health Science Center

John F. L. Pinner, PhD
The Mind Research Network and Psychology
  Department
University of New Mexico

Stefan Rampp, PD Dr. med.
Department of Neurosurgery
University Hospital Erlangen and University
  Hospital Halle (Saale)

Roozbeh Rezaie, PhD
Associate Professor
Division of Pediatric Neurology
Department of Pediatrics
University of Tennessee Health Science Center
Neuroscience Institute
Le Bonheur Children's Hospital

Timothy P. L. Roberts, PhD
Oberkircher Family Chair in Pediatric Radiology
Vice Chair Radiology Research
Children's Hospital of Philadelphia

Gillian Roberts, PhD
Postdoctoral Student
Sir Peter Mansfield Imaging Centre
University of Nottingham

Kristina Safar, PhD
Research Fellow
Hospital for Sick Children

Panagiotis G. Simos, PhD
Department of Psychiatry and Behavioral
    Sciences, School of Medicine
University of Crete

Isabel Solis, MS
The Mind Research Network and Psychology
    Department
University of New Mexico

Julia M. Stephen, PhD
The Mind Research Network
Lovelace Biomedical Research Institute

Gianluca Susi, PhD
Laboratory of Cognitive and Computational
    Neuroscience
Center for Biomedical Technology
Experimental Psychology Department, School
    of Psychology
Universidad Complutense de Madrid
Networking Research Center on Bioengineering
Biomaterials and Nanomedicine
    (CIBER-BBN)

Margot J. Taylor, PhD
Director of Functional Neuroimaging
Hospital for Sick Children

Tim M. Tierney, PhD
Research Fellow
Wellcome Centre for Human Neuroimaging
UCL Institute of Neurology

James W. Wheless, MD, FAAP, FAAN
Professor and Chief of Pediatric Neurology
Le Bonheur Chair in Pediatric Neurology
University of Tennessee Health Science Center
Director
Neuroscience Institute
Le Bonheur Comprehensive Epilepsy Program
Le Bonheur Children's Hospital

Tony W. Wilson, PhD
Associate Professor
Department of Neurological Sciences
University of Nebraska Medical Center

SECTION I

THE BEGINNINGS

1

THE FIRST MAGNETOENCEPHALOGRAPHY REPORT: 1968

David Cohen

I AM one of several biomagnetism "old-timers" who have been asked to write something about this special occasion: the 50th anniversary of magnetoencephalography (MEG). The event that occurred 50 years ago was the first MEG publication, of which I was the author (Cohen, 1968), so I will write about that publication; I will tell about some of the ideas and circumstances of that event. This is the first time I have elaborated on that paper, so I may ramble around a bit, and I apologize for the casual style.

The paper we are talking about is shown in Figure 1.1. On publication, it was newsworthy but was actually not a memorable paper because the magnetic method was too difficult for other investigators to reproduce; the paper only served to call attention to the existence of this extremely weak magnetic field, which at that time I believe was the weakest field ever measured. What I will do here is to first show some previously unpublished material, related to the equipment.

Next, I will discuss the following points: the general atmosphere of biomagnetism at that time, the local atmosphere for biomagnetism at the University of Illinois, some of the people around me during the MEG work, the direction of future research, and finally, some random recollections.

1.1. DETAILS OF THE EQUIPMENT

The main items of equipment in the paper were a magnetically shielded room (MSR) and a magnetic detector, which was a million-turn copper coil. The purpose of the MSR was to reduce the external unwanted magnetic fields, and a photo of this MSR is shown in Figure 1.2. The coil detector is shown in Figure 1.3. Figure 1.4 shows the "shaking" coils.

David Cohen, *The First Magnetoencephalography Report: 1968* In: *Fifty Years of Magnetoencephalography*. Edited by:
Andrew C. Papanicolaou, Timothy P. L. Roberts, and James W. Wheless, Oxford University Press (2020). © Oxford University Press.
DOI: 10.1093/oso/9780190935689.003.0001.

SCIENCE

Magnetoencephalography:
Evidence of Magnetic Fields
Produced by Alpha Rhythm

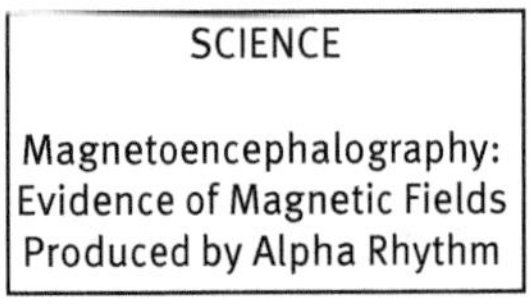

FIGURE 1.1 The essence of the *Science* article of 50 years ago, which is considered the beginning of magnetoencephalography, and apparently the first use of this word. This paper is of no practical value because the technology was too difficult to reproduce (Cohen, D. [1968]. Magnetoencephalography: Evidence of magnetic fields produced by alpha-rhythm currents. *Science, 161,* 784–786.)

1.2. THE GENERAL ATMOSPHERE FOR BIOMAGNETISM

At that time, about 1967, the people who seriously thought about biomagnetism (and bioelectricity) were mostly the electrocardiologists; the electric field of the heart was the focus. Some names that come to mind are Otto Schmitt, Richard McFee, Stanley Rush, David Geselowitz, and Robert Plonsey. Predicting and understanding ischemic hearts and myocardial infarctions were the significant problems in cardiology. However, Rush and Driscoll did shift his

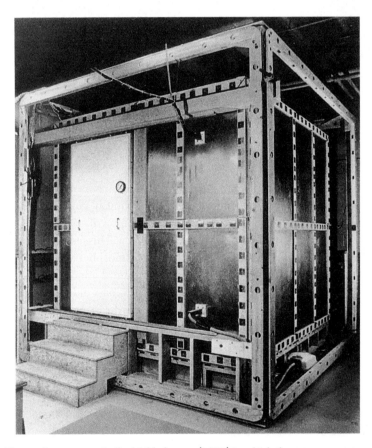

FIGURE 1.2 The two-layer magnetically shielded room (MSR) in which the measurements were made. It consisted of two outer layers of molypermalloy and one inner layer of welded pure aluminum. This was the first MSR used in biomagnetism. Its performance as a shield was not very good but was actually a match to the noisy coil detectors I used. External coils around the room are contained in the wooden frame. These were used to study MSR technology by bucking out the earth's DC magnetic field through the room. There were also coils wound in and around the permalloy layers, used for 60-Hz "shaking," an MSR technology that I had developed and thought promising at that time.

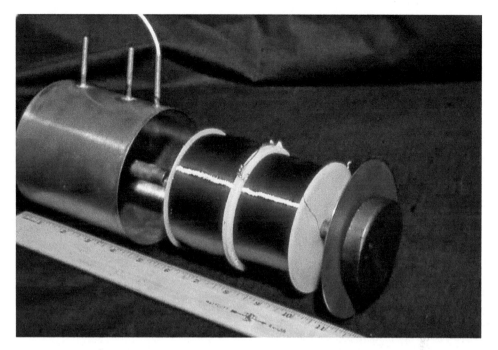

FIGURE 1.3   The one-million-turn copper coil detector, pulled apart for illustration. A ferrite (black) cap and rod increased the signal-to-noise ratio by about a factor of 4. The two copper "chimneys" were used for cooling experiments with liquid nitrogen; with my technology at the time, as I recall, the cooling made more problems than it solved. The physics that went into the coil design was actually quite elaborate, involving noise, frequency response, and resonance calculations. I believe I was involved in months of hard work to optimize the design. I recall no reported prior work to make things easier.

attention to electroencephalography (EEG) for a while, in 1968, with a good paper on current distributions in the head (Rush & Driscoll, 1968). There was no modeling yet of the complex EEG, similar to the clear modeling of the heart's single dipole. EEG modeling appeared later, stimulated by advances in MEG modeling, due to whole-head MEG mapping. Actually, my 1968 MEG paper does assume a single dipole model of the simple alpha-rhythm setup that I used (Cohen, 1968).

1.3. THE LOCAL ATMOSPHERE FOR BIOMAGNETISM

By "local," I mean the atmosphere in the physics department at the new University of Illinois, in downtown Chicago, where I did my initial MEG research. There were basically two groups. The first group centered on physics chairman Professor Lester Winsberg, who brought me on board in 1965 to start biomagnetism (see "stories" on my website: http://davidcohen.mit.edu); they liked new ideas and technologies. On the other hand, there was an opposing group who wanted only traditional physics and disapproved of new unconventional research being done in that department. For several years, Lester's group prevailed, but sometime in 1967 he lost his political power, and the other group seized control. Not good for biomagnetism! So, my MEG research, leading to the 1968 *Science* paper, took place in an unpleasant and hostile atmosphere. The new researchers that Lester brought in, including me, were eventually told by the new regime to clear out and make room for new people who were doing traditional physics.

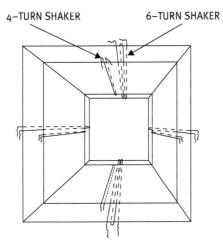

FIGURE 1.4   Coils used for "shaking" in the Illinois room, linked around the outer two permalloy layers. Not shown is the inner layer of pure aluminum. When a steady 60-Hz current is passed through the coils in series, the permeability of the high-mu layers increases by a factor of 2 or more, and the shielding factor of the room rises accordingly. However, one problem prevented this shaking from becoming useful for shielded rooms in general: the large 60-Hz magnetic field that leaked to the inside of the room and "swamped" the detector. I learned to buck it out, but it was difficult and impractical. When working properly, one could throw a simple switch and turn the shielding factor from low to high.

1.4. THE PEOPLE AROUND ME INVOLVED IN MAGNETOENCEPHALOGRAPHY

My EEG colleague and teacher was John R. Hughes, a professor of neurology at Northwestern University. He was an outstanding and versatile expert in the field and quickly taught me everything I needed to know about electrical physics and electrophysiology of the EEG, at least at that time. I have not been in contact with him for some years, and just looked him up online. Apparently, he is still going strong and, according to one website, is the "author of eight books (including one translated into in four languages and that being the most popular book in the EEG world) and 545+ peer-reviewed articles." Somewhat surprisingly, he has also written a popular book on the relationship of the assassinations of John F. Kennedy and mobster Sam Giancana! He believed that the MEG would eventually be important, and his encouragement was a perfect antidote to the unbelievers in the physics department. Indeed, I thank you again John, 50 years later.

Another outstanding scientist who influenced me was Humberto Fernandez-Moran, professor of biophysics at the University of Chicago. His field was electron microscopy, not EEG, but he was a master of academic politics as well as new physics ideas, and on many Sunday afternoon walks around Chicago, he taught me month-to-month survival in the toxic atmosphere in my department. He was a strong supporter of the birth of the 1968 MEG. Alas, he later suffered a tragic ending.

1.5. DIRECTION OF FUTURE RESEARCH

In one sense, the value of this paper was to clarify what was needed, at the time, to turn the MEG into a valid technology. What was needed, I learned quite simply, was a vast improvement of the signal-to-noise ratio of the equipment. What was needed was a much more sensitive magnetic detector and a much better shielded room. And indeed, several years later, at the Massachusetts Institute of Technology (MIT), I pushed in those directions and was fortunate enough to produce the superconducting quantum-interference device (SQUID) low-noise MEG (Cohen, 1972). But the earlier 1968 paper allowed me to move in the right direction and reach that goal.

1.6. SOME RANDOM RECOLLECTIONS

- The thrill of watching, late one night and alone, the first magnetic alpha-rhythm signal growing out of noise, from a subject's brain, after 8 or 10 minutes of signal-averaging . . .

- The fun of later telling Lester Winsberg (the chairman who hired me) that the magnetic field of the brain indeed existed . . .
- The pleasure of showing this phenomenon to John Hughes, my EEG teacher . . .
- My total ignorance, at that time, of the electrical complexity of the human brain— the EEG traces at that time, such as epileptic events, were only cookbook signals . . .
- The fun when the *Science* paper generated publicity, especially when the publicity led to an offer by MIT of a new and friendly home for my biomagnetism work . . .
- The rough guards of the science building at night, who were trained at an Illinois state penitentiary, as rough as the politics at this new street-car state university . . .
- The continuous need for a better lower-noise detector, and the bad behavior of coil detectors in general . . .
- The enjoyment of this work, much more fun compared with the large, rigid, atom-smashing synchrotron, on which I previously worked . . .
- The fun of working on biomagnetism with bright physics student-assistants . . .
- My belief that biomagnetism would one day be an important new window into the human body . . .

REFERENCES

Cohen, D. (1968). Magnetoencephalography: Evidence of magnetic fields produced by alpha-rhythm currents. *Science, 161,* 784–786.

Cohen, D. (1972). Magnetoencephalography: Detection of the brain's electrical activity with a superconducting magnetometer. *Science, 175,* 664–666.

Rush S., & Driscoll, D. A. (1968). Anesthesia & Analgesia. *47*(6), 717–723.

2

THE BEGINNING OF BIOMAGNETISM AND MAGNETOENCEPHALOGRAPHY RESEARCH IN FINLAND IN THE 1970S

Toivo Katila

We tend to overestimate the effect of a technology in the short run and underestimate the effect in the long run. (Amara's Law)

2.1. INTRODUCTION

The interest in studying biomagnetism (BMG) caught fire from the new findings in the United States. The first magnetocardiogram (MCG) results using the superconducting quantum-interference device (SQUID) had just been just published (Cohen, Edelsack, & Zimmerman, 1970). The measurements were conducted using the SQUID magnetometer constructed by Dr. James Zimmerman (National Bureau of Standards, Boulder) in the magnetically shielded room at the Massachusetts Institute of Technology (MIT), built by Dr. David Cohen. For the first time, the real-time MCG recordings were comparable in quality with the ordinary electrocardiograms (ECGs).

In 1970, I was looking for a new research field. Biomagnetism research seemed to combine several familiar themes, such as measurement techniques, signal processing, instrumentation, and low-temperature techniques. Two student colleagues and I had erected the liquid helium-4/helium-3 cryostat in the novel Low Temperature Group, led by Professor Olli Lounasmaa at the Department of Technical Physics of Helsinki University of Technology (HUT; now Aalto University). We had used SQUID in previous experiments as an ultrasensitive magnetic field detector and had prepared point contact SQUIDs ourselves. To gain the necessary medical expertise, we contacted medical specialists at the Helsinki University Central Hospital (HUCH) in 1970. Right away, they showed interest on the new research method, and we decided to set up a research project whose goal would be to "to build a biomagnetism measurement equipment of our own design, perform biomagnetic measurements using the equipment for medical research and clinical applications."

Toivo Katila, *The Beginning of Biomagnetism and Magnetoencephalography Research in Finland in the 1970s* In: *Fifty Years of Magnetoencephalography.* Edited by: Andrew C. Papanicolaou, Timothy P. L. Roberts, and James W. Wheless, Oxford University Press (2020).
© Oxford University Press. DOI: 10.1093/oso/9780190935689.003.0002.

But, how could we finance a new field without evidence from research results? Finally, and luckily, in May 1971 a Finnish research foundation awarded us a grant that enabled one student to work on a Master's thesis and purchase the most important equipment to start the project. The magnetometer we needed to build ourselves. In the beginning, the project crew included just one student and me. However, young minds are often overoptimistic and not afraid of risks.

2.2. THE FIRST PROTOTYPES

2.2.1. Prototype I

The first MSc student, Antti Ahonen, started his work in June 1971. His task was the construction of the ultrasensitive SQUID magnetometer. The contribution of the medical collaborators would start only when the magnetometer was working. The first goal for the new instrument was to be able to record in real time the magnetic field of the human heart. However, it was not that simple. The only benchmark publication was still Cohen's work (Cohen et al., 1970), but our instrument had to work without the magnetically shielded room. At that time in Finland, the cost of such a room would have been much too high. Measurements without a shielded room were thought to be difficult; for example, the earth's magnetic field is about a million times stronger than the required measurement sensitivity. In addition, various human activities were known to cause additional problems, especially in laboratory surroundings.

Ahonen became acquainted with the problem very quickly but also rigorously. The first measurements of a human heart were done at the start of winter. For testing, laboratory surroundings were too noisy, so we carried the magnetometer out onto the ice in the middle of a shallow-water bay close to the laboratory. The frost and freezing cold wind were discouraging, especially because the measurement subject started shaking as soon as he took off his overcoat. The Finnish winter even prevented

many trials. In any case, the first milestone was reached: The prototype of a functional SQUID magnetometer was constructed.

In his thesis work, Ahonen had investigated several problems that needed to be resolved in order to build the next prototype, a magnetometer for practical biomagnetic studies. For that, a completely new construction was required. In summer 1972, Antti left biomagnetism behind, but later on he made valuable contributions to biomagnetic instrumentation and business.

2.2.2. Prototype II

Pekka Karp was our next MSc student, starting his job in August 1972. His task was to build a new SQUID magnetometer, taking into consideration the results obtained by Antti Ahonen. Now, we could also define the goals for Karp's work more precisely: sensitivity of $1pT/Hz^{1/2}$ ($1pT = 10^{-12}$ Tesla) at the band up to 100 Hz. This should be enough for MCG, comparable to good-quality ECGs, but the requirements for brain studies could not yet be defined. The instrument had to allow measurements in reclining position at rest. In addition, there were a number of technical details that will not be discussed here. Magnetometers were suitable for use in magnetically shielded rooms. The other coil configurations could also be asymmetric.

Although Karp was inexperienced in this new field, he was working very efficiently in building the second prototype of the magnetometer. Our medical collaborators were waiting eagerly for its completion—and it was built promptly. Figure 2.1 shows the cross-section of the instrument, a glass cryostat looking like a very special vacuum flask. The SQUID gradiometer is resting at the bottom of the inner space, and it is immersed in liquid helium. The superconducting coils constitute a first-order axial gradiometer (Figure 2.2B). The electronics unit is located outside the cryostat at room temperature. It is connected to the SQUID by an rf-line and is monitoring the state of the SQUID.

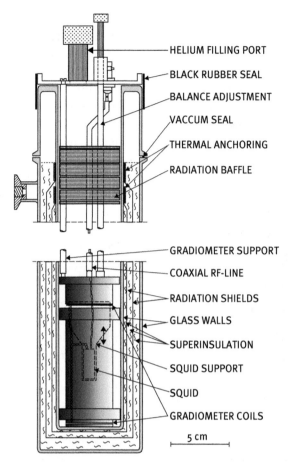

FIGURE 2.1   The second prototype of our SQUID magnetometer. (Used with permission, © Pekka Karp 1973.)

Manufacturing the cryostat involved testing of special materials, calculations, and problems (e.g., in heat conduction, radiation, and finally fabrication). Karp also made a number of improvements to the handling of liquid helium and SQUIDs. He summarized: "After these improvements the reliability of the process improved so much that the same SQUID could be used in consecutive coolings, without SQUID retuning, dozens of times." The deepest sense of this sentence can be understood only by a person who is familiar with

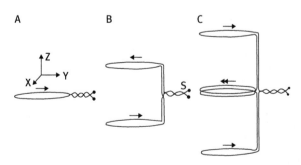

FIGURE 2.2   Some examples of sensing coil configurations used in the 1970s: (A) magnetometer, (B) first-order gradiometer, and (C) second-order gradiometers.

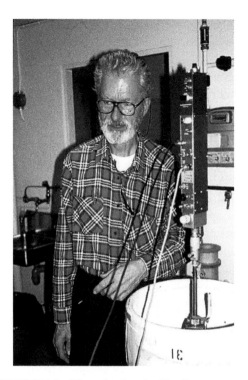

FIGURE 2.3 Photo that I took of Jim Zimmerman measuring the properties of SQUIDs made by him and by us in Otaniemi. The SQUID sensor (not seen in the figure) is at the bottom of the central rod in liquid helium. The SQUID control unit at the upper end of the rod is a commercial product of the SHE company, but greatly designed by Jim.

the unpredictable behavior of the early point-contact SQUIDs.

We got many important tips from the leading researcher in the field, James Zimmerman (Figure 2.3). He visited us several times in the 1970s and became my personal friend. Jim had a good sense of humor. One time, we were testing a new dewar in an open meadow, far from the buildings. In the middle of the measurements, it started to rain, and the measurement subject got drenched. We felt bad about the bad weather, but Jim's friendly comment was: "The weather is always beautiful."

Next, we had to find a suitable measurement site. This time we were lucky. A wooden cottage, which had been used earlier for geomagnetic measurements and constructed without any magnetic materials, became available (Figure 2.4). Furthermore, it was located less than half a mile from our laboratory. The measured rms noise of the biomagnetic recordings there was about 0.4 pT/Hz$^{1/2}$. The quality of the recordings was good, for the time being. Both magnetic and concurrent electric signals were frequency modulated recorded on magnetic tape. The first milestone of our project had been reached: The group had constructed

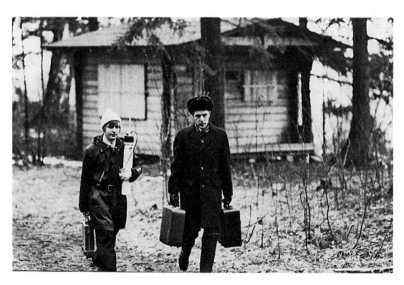

FIGURE 2.4 For measurements, the key parts of the equipment were carried along a footpath to and from the cottage. Note that I am the bag carrier (on the right), and the most precious SQUID instrument is carried by Pekka Karp. (Used with permission by the photographer Hannu Lindroos, ©1973.)

its own biomagnetic measurement facility, whose quality was among the best at that time.

2.3. THE START OF BIOMAGNETIC SQUID MEASUREMENTS

The first BMG measurements were made at the end of 1972. At the same time, the important collaboration with medical people for "the use the equipment for medical research and clinical applications" started. Our first publication forum was the National Meeting on Biophysics and Biotechnology in Finland in January 1973 (Karp & Katila, 1973a). Results of MCG measurements were published. The same topic was also presented also in an international conference (Karp & Katila, 1973b).

Cohen's group had already published in 1972 a preliminary report on the MCG signals in normal subjects (Cohen & McCaughan, 1972). In 1973, together with our important medical collaborators Pentti Siltanen and Matti Saarinen, we did somewhat more extensive MCG mappings of both normal and abnormal subjects, and this report was published in 1974 (Saarinen, Karp, Katila, & Siltanen, 1974).

Do the biomagnetic recordings carry new information of practical benefit compared with bioelectric studies? In 1973, we started biomagnetic studies of fetal MCGs and surface electric recordings (fetal ECGs), together with simultaneously recorded maternal signals (maternal MCGs and maternal ECGs). Our medical collaborator was Veikko Kariniemi, MD. The report of this pioneering work was published in 1973 (Kariniemi, Karp, & Katila, 1973). The size of the fetal MCG signal was only about 5 pT (50 ngauss) (Figure 2.5). The signal of the fetal heart has one very important application, the calculation of the fetal heart rate (FHR). The variation of the FHR was used to follow the oxygenation state of the fetal brain (Kariniemi, Ahopelto, Karp, & Katila, 1974).

However, in an external FECG, especially during the last trimester of gestation, the fetal complexes diminish to become insufficient for calculation of FHR variation. This drawback was mostly excluded in magnetic FHR studies. The ability of the magnetic measurements to examine the degree of oxygenation of the brain was the first result to support our belief that *magnetic studies can bring new information for practical use compared with electric studies.* It is clear that the accurate FHR calculation from the magnetic recording (see the

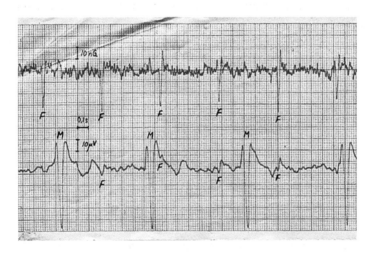

FIGURE 2.5   A sample of ink recording from the pioneering measurements of the fetal magnetocardiogram (*upper curve*) and the simultaneously recorded external fetal electrocardiogram (*lower trace*). The letter F indicates fetal and M maternal heart beats. The traces were used for oxygenation studies of fetal brain. (Reproduced from the original inkjet recording.)

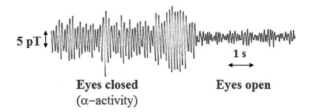

5 pT ↕

1 s

Eyes closed
(α–activity)

Eyes open

FIGURE 2.6   Magnetoencephalography (MEG) α-wave. This measurement of the magnetic α-waves was made without a magnetically shielded room. The signal quality was comparable to electroencephalogram registrations. (Reproduced from the original inkjet recording.)

upper trace in Figure 2.5) is easy, but it is difficult or even impossible in other cases, such as here in the electric recording (lower trace). Note that some 20 years later, studies of fetal MCG became popular again, and even fetal magnetoencephalography (MEG) studies have been made.

2.3.1. α-Wave Recordings

Cohen was first to publish magnetic α-wave recordings worthy of consideration (Cohen, 1972, 1975). Both SQUID studies were carried out in MIT's magnetically shielded room. Meanwhile, in 1974 we also published studies of α-waves, made without magnetic shielding (Ahopelto, Karp, Katila, Lukander, & Mäkipää, 1974). The reproduction of the ink recording in Figure 2.6 depicts the typical feature of the α-wave: The amplitude declines to a small fraction when the relaxed subject first has his eyes closed and then open. Our new MSc students,

Jorma Ahopelto, Ronald Lukander, and Pentti Mäkipää played an important part in the works mentioned previously.

In Figure 2.6, the amplitude of the MEG α-wave was about 5 pT and that of the simultaneously recorded electroencephalogram (EEG) about 30 μV. The sensitivity of the SQUID gradiometer was 0,1 pT/Hz$^{1/2}$ (rms) from 0.05 to 100 Hz. The measurement band was limited to 8 to 13 Hz. A simultaneous MEG/EEG recording is shown in Figure 2.7.

2.3.2. Improving the Measurement Technique

When comparing the first electric and magnetic registrations of the α-waves (see Figure 2.7), we did not see yet any notable benefits of the magnetic studies compared with the EEG. We hoped that more sensitive magnetic instrumentation and more accurate studies would change the situation. The new

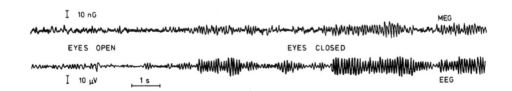

I 10 nG   MEG

EYES OPEN   EYES CLOSED

I 10 μV   1 s   EEG

FIGURE 2.7   Simultaneously recorded magnetoencepalogram and electroencephalogram (EED) signals. The magnetometer was located on the occipital region of the scalp, and the component perpendicular to the scalp was measured. The two EEG electrodes were also located on the occipital region of the other side of the head. (From Ahopelto, J., Karp, P. J., Katila, T. E., Lukander, R., & Mäkipää, P. [1974]. Gradiometric observation of the magnetic brain waves, report TKK-F-A233. Helskinki: Helsinki University of Technology, Figure 1, with the permission of Aalto University.)

UHF-SQUID electronics started working at the beginning of 1975, and it was reported at LT14 conference in August of the same year (Ahopelto, Karp, Katila, Lukander, & Mäkipää, 1975). When the pumping frequency of the SQUID was increased to 450 MHz, the magnetic field sensitivity of the system improved to 0,02 pT/Hz$^{1/2}$ (20 fT/Hz$^{1/2}$). We proclaimed proudly: "This new device with the improved sensitivity will be mainly used for magnetoencephalography." At that time our research group consisted of five technical members and four medical collaborators. Unfortunately, the space available here is not sufficient for detailed introduction of their important contributions.

Another question was how to record wave-type phenomena such as the α-wave. Evidently, that would necessitate *multichannel detection* of the magnetic field. In 1982 our group prepared the first of such instruments, a three-channel magnetometer. Suitable SQUIDs were obtained from Laboratoire d'Electronique des Technologies de l'Information (LETI) in collaboration with Dr. Denis Duret. For clinical applications, a *measurement site in a hospital* would also be required, which we achieved only in the mid-1990s.

2.4. MEASUREMENTS AND MODELING

2.4.1. Studies of the Magneto-oculogram

The head neurologist at HUCH led a new medical collaborator, Pekka Saar, to work with us. He directed our research interest to the head and to further MEG studies. Soon we came across the artifacts caused by signals from human eyes: It was known that eye movements and change of illumination were disturbing factors generating electric signals in the EEG measurements. The mapping of the magnetic field caused by the retinal DC current was one of our pioneering works (Karp, Katila, Mäkipää, & Saar, 1976). The simple measurement scheme is shown in Figure 2.8.

During the measurements, the subject moves his eyes over an angle between two fixation points. The difference of the magnetic fields between the two positions is mapped on the left in Figure 2.9. The diameters of the circles in Figure 2.9 are proportional to the difference. The *open circle* indicates that the field is directed inward. We called this result the magneto-oculogram (MOG), by analogy to the electro-oculogram (EOG). The MOG

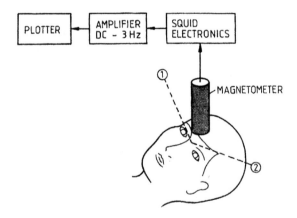

FIGURE 2.8   The measurement of the magneto-oculogram shown schematically. Here the component of the field perpendicular to the frontal plane outside the face is mapped. The subject moves his eyes over an angle of 55 degrees between two fixation points. (From Katila, T., Maniewski, R., Poutanen, T., Varpula, T., & Karp, P. [1981]. Magnetic fields produced by the human eye. *Journal of Applied Physics, 52,* 2565–2571, Figure 4, with the permission of AIP Publishing.)

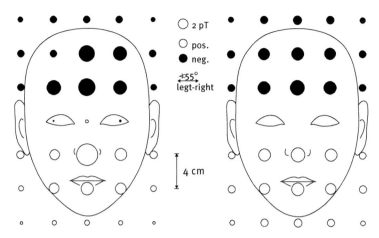

FIGURE 2.9   (*Left*) Measured distribution of the magneto-oculogram field perpendicular to the frontal plane for horizontal movement of the eyes. (*Right*) Calculated field using a model with current dipoles in the eyes, pointing forward at zero angle. (From Katila, T., Maniewski, R., Poutanen, T., Varpula, T., & Karp, P. [1981]. Magnetic fields produced by the human eye. *Journal of Applied Physics, 52*, 2565–2571, Figure 9, with the permission of AIP Publishing.)

measurements were started in 1975 and reported internationally in 1976 (Karp et al., 1976). Compared with the MEG signals, the MOG fields can be higher, and thus possible MOG artifacts have to be carefully eliminated.

2.4.2. Simple Modeling

The right side of Figure 2.9 depicts the calculated MOG field distribution. The measured magnetic field was simulated to be caused by two equal current dipoles, one in each eye. The plotted field values on the right side correspond again to field differences between the two directions in Figure 2.8. The resulting current vector is pointing to the left. This model is, of course, pretty rough (e.g., the complexity of the electric volume currents in the head has been ignored). The eyes themselves are not electrically homogeneous, and the surrounding head contains tissues of very different electrical properties, such as bone and blood. For more accurate calculations, three-dimensional imaging techniques would have been required, but these were not available at that time.

As a first approximation, however, the calculated field agrees rather well with the measured one. Thus, the eyes could be electrically represented by forward-pointing current dipoles in the retina, as expected by anatomy.

2.4.3. Studies of the Magnetoretinogram

Change in illumination of the retina gives rise to a change in the retinal current, resulting in a signal measurable on the skin, the electroretinogram (ERG). In the ERG studies, a light pulse generates a transient stream with components of the pigment epithelium, Müller cells, and photoreceptors. We investigated the corresponding magnetic signal, the magnetoretinogram (MRG), in studies commenced in 1977. The experimental setup is shown in Figure 2.10. The trigger ignites a flashlight pulse with a length of about 1 ms. To eliminate the magnetic interference, the trigger is isolated by optical fiber.

Simultaneously measured ERG (curve a) and MRG (curve b) signals are shown in Figure 2.11. The signals displayed at time point x of

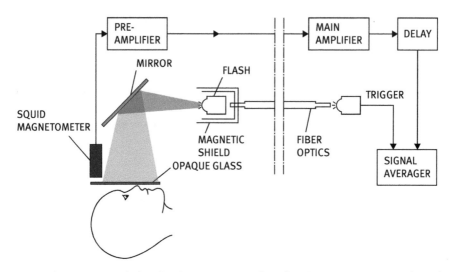

FIGURE 2.10   The experimental setup for electroretinogram (ERG) and magnetoretinogram (MRG) measurements. (From Katila, T., Maniewski, R., Poutanen, T., Varpula, T., & Karp, P. [1981]. Magnetic fields produced by the human eye. *Journal of Applied Physics, 52*, 2565–2571, Figure 5, with the permission of AIP Publishing.)

the curves are the α-wave of the ERG/MRG. The large signal between 100 and 200 ms is due to eye movement. In the MRG study, the component of the magnetic field approximately perpendicular to the skull was measured near the eye. The noise level of the measurement is 20 fT/Hz$^{1/2}$. The α-wave of the MRG is clearly visible, although its size is only about 0.1 pT. Therefore, curve b in Figure 2.11 is an average of 124 signals. The magnitude of the signal also depended heavily on the measuring site. In summary, we had found the MRG wave, but its small size and sensitivity to disturbances (e.g., MOG) did not encourage optimism toward its clinical applications. At least at the time.

2.4.4. Visualization of Research Data and Solving the Inverse Problem

At the beginning of our studies, the measured fields were presented by circles much the same way as in Figure 2.9. The improved data processing of computers made more sophisticated computations possible. The contour line presentation (Figure 2.12) provided a new and more informative perspective of illustrating the data. Still, we were pretty far from the final goal of solving the inverse problem, that is, calculating the sources (source currents) directly from the measured data and showing them visually. Clearly, this would require, in addition to comprehensive measurement data, knowledge of the shape and electromagnetic properties of the source body. Even then, mathematics indicates that there is no unique solution to the general (unrestricted) inverse problem, even if both electric and magnetic fields are known outside the body. Thus, we still have to be satisfied with restricted and approximate solutions of sources.

2.5. EVOKED RESPONSES OF THE BRAIN

Mappings of MOG and MRG were preliminary steps toward our more specific brain studies. The electrically evoked responses of the brain had been studied for a long time and diligently. Our setup in Figure 2.10 was close to what was needed for studies of visually evoked potentials (VEPs) and fields (VEFs) of the brain. In 1977 and 1978, our group did preliminary measurements of visual and auditory evoked responses. The signals were small, even after averaging, and compared with electric

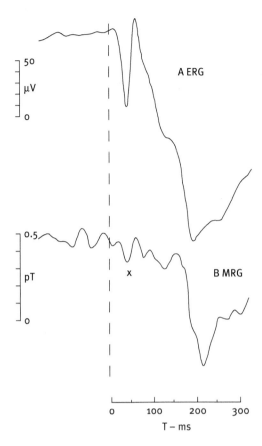

FIGURE 2.11 Simultaneous recordings of the electroretinogram (ERG) and magnetoretinogram (MRG) of a normal subject. The bandwidth is 0.1 to 30 Hz. (A) Reference ERG measurement with skin electrodes from the right eye. The curve is an average of 14 samples. (B) The MRG measured above the right eye, an average of 124 signals. (From Katila, T., Maniewski, R., Poutanen, T., Varpula, T., & Karp, P. [1981]. Magnetic fields produced by the human eye. *Journal of Applied Physics, 52,* 2565–2571, Figure 14, with the permission of AIP Publishing.)

recordings, the new information value seemed modest. Not really encouraging.

Elsewhere, the interest in evoked magnetic responses was on the increase. In his summary on biomagnetic research, Cohen had published preliminary results both on evoked EEG and MEG transient responses of the light flash (Cohen, 1975). Soon thereafter, the New York University group made public their studies on visual stimulation (Brenner, Williamson, & Kaufman, 1975). Their studies were carried out

in the middle of Manhattan without a magnetically shielded room—a respectable achievement in the very noisy surroundings, where the magnetometer noise was also inevitably high. In any case, they found an important result: ". . . in MEG strong responses could be detected only in a 3-cm-long region on the midline of the scalp. This localizability may be contrasted with the classic evoked potential, which is widespread." This was good news for localization of sources by means of magnetic studies. Later on, the localization of signal sources became one of the key applications of biomagnetic research and, at the same time, a matter of controversy.

The interest in magnetic brain measurements was increasing in hospital clinics in Finland as well. In the following discussion, we present two examples of our evoked potential and evoked magnetic field studies. When Saar was leaving our group, researchers at Helsinki University Hospital expressed their wish to continue the collaboration in magnetic brain studies. First, we restarted the auditory evoked response measurements. After Saar, postgraduate student Riitta Hari (medicine) began collaboration with our research group. For her doctoral thesis, she had already measured elsewhere auditory evoked transient and sustained potentials of the human EEG. Our first joint research was a study of auditory evoked magnetic fields. Both transient and sustained evoked magnetic fields and electrical potentials of the human brain were measured. The first results were published nationally in 1979 (Hari, Aittoniemi, Järvinen, Katila, & Varpula, 1979) and were also included in Hari's PhD dissertation. Other important members in the study were Kari Aittoniemi, Marja-Leena Järvinen, and Tero Varpula, all MSc students of HUT. Publishing continued in international forums (Hari, Aittoniemi, Järvinen, Katila, & Varpula, 1980; Aittoniemi, Hari, Järvinen, Katila, & Varpula, 1981).

Figure 2.12 shows some of the results measured in 1979, using our latest magnetometer then available. The binaural stimulus was a 1-kHz square-wave sound that was 800 ms

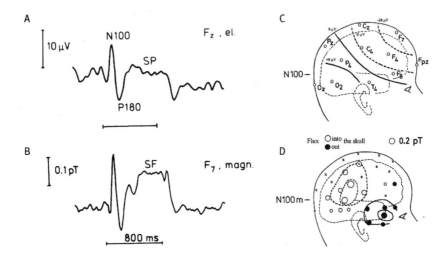

FIGURE 2.12 Auditory evoked responses of one subject: (A) electric potential; (B) magnetic field; (C) contour maps (isopotential lines) of the scalp potential N100; (D) scalp amplitudes (isofield lines) of N100m of the component of the magnetic field perpendicular to the skull. (From Aittoniemi, K., Hari, R., Järvinen, M-L., Katila, T., & Varpula, T. [1981]. Localization of neural generators underlying auditory evoked magnetic fields of the human brain. In S. N. Erné, H. D. Hahlbohm, H. Lübbig (Eds.), *Biomagnetism: Proceedings of the Third International Workshop, Berlin (West)*, May 1980 (pp. 415–422). Berlin, Boston: De Gruyter.)

in duration and repeated once every 4 s. The signal coil of the first-order gradiometer (as in Figure 12.2B, but asymmetric) was a circular loop with a diameter of 2 cm, situated 35 mm above the skin and measuring the component of the magnetic field perpendicular to the scalp. The signals were recorded using a bandwidth of 0.03 to 15 Hz, and 60 to 330 responses per one location were averaged. The number of measurement locations was about 30.

In Figure 2.12, the averaged electric and magnetic responses from the right hemisphere of one of the subjects (S2) are shown at the measurement positions given. Clear similarities existed between the curve shapes of electric and magnetic responses. On the right side, the contour maps of the electric potential N100 and the magnetic field N100m are presented. The components N100, P180, and SP of the electric potential all had corresponding magnetic counterparts of N100m, P180m, and SF.

Our primary task was to estimate the source current distributions in the brain during the main deflections, again a typical source localization problem. It is seen in Figure 2.12C that the potential is widely spread without clear maxima or minima. For N100m in Figure 2.12D, two amplitude extrema of opposite polarities at the estimated ends of the Sylvian fissure are seen clearly. On the fissure, only the component parallel to the skull could be detected. On basis of the magnetic data, it was concluded that the source currents can, as a first approximation, be described by two bilateral current dipole sources, located at the primary auditory cortices and directed downward in the layer. Note that the details of electric N100 data alone were not sufficient for estimating the locations of the source currents. Therefore, the magnetic recording seemed to be superior in localizing the sources compared with the electric potential. One could also interpret that the measured magnetic field is principally due to the source currents, but the electric potential N100 (of course) is due to the volume currents.

2.5.1. Motor Field

In the following discussion, we present another example of the power of studies of the magnetic evoked fields. It was known that the preparation and execution of a self-initiated voluntary movement is associated with neural activity in several brain areas. Motor neurons in the cerebral cortex begin to fire already before the movement. They give rise to motor potentials (MPs), consisting of several distinct components, seen in the scalp recorded EEG. We investigated two earliest of them. First begins the *readiness potential* (N1), a slow negative shift at the precentral areas that may start even more than 1 s before movement. Next appears the *premotion potential* (N2), starting a few hundred milliseconds before the movement. The neural sources of MPs in general could not be uniquely localized on the basis of the scalp EEG recordings alone. Even simple current dipole modeling shows that the source generally is not located directly "below" the potential extremum, as it was often assumed in the past.

The MEG was thought to be more efficient in detecting and localizing the activity of the motor area. At the time of our measurements, MEG changes preceding *hand and finger* movements were about to be published (Zimmerman, 1981). We measured the magnetic counterparts of N1 and N2, the *readiness field* (MF1), and the *premotion field* (MF2), active before a self-paced voluntary *foot* movement. Our task was to localize their neural current sources.

The magnetic field component perpendicular to the skull was measured in locations shown by the grid in Figure 2.13. The distance between adjacent points in the grid was 3 cm. The pick-up coil (ϕ = 2 cm) was situated approximately 2 cm above the scalp, and the intercoil distance of the first-order asymmetric gradiometer was 14 cm. The frequency band was 0.03 to 100 Hz, with a 50-Hz notch filter. Figure 2.13 (right side) shows magnetic field recordings of one subject along the line connecting the amplitude extrema of the signal. The *vertical line* points out the onset of the

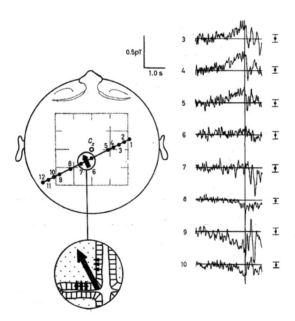

FIGURE 2.13   Magnetic field preceding self-paced plantar flexions of right foot of one of the four subjects, measured with a first-order differential SQUID gradiometer. The signals presented are averages of around 70 flexions. The onset of the electromyographic activity served as a trigger for the signal averaging. (Reprinted by permission from Hari, R., Antervo, A., Katila, T., Poutanen, T., Seppänen, M., Tumomisto, T., & Varpula, T. [1983]. Cerebral magnetic fields associated with voluntary limb movements in man. *Il Nuovo Cimento D, 2,* 484–494.)

electromyogram. Upward signal indicates the magnetic field directed into the skull. The polarities of MF1 and MF2 clearly change along this line (right side).

Analysis of the neural sources of magnetic fields suggested that the MF1 shifts preceding foot movements are largely generated by tangential current sources on the mesial surface of the contralateral hemisphere (see inset at lower left in Figure 2.13). The estimated source depth was 3 cm below the scalp. It was evident that the same sources also contributed strongly to the measured electric MPs. In this study, our new collaborators were psychologist Arja Antervo and MSc students T. Poutanen, M. Seppänen, and T. Tuomisto.

At the Fourth International Workshop on Biomagnetism, in Rome (1982), we presented the results shown in Figure 2.13 (Antervo et al., 1983; Hari et al., 1983). In this conference, Weinberg, Deecke, Brickett, and Boscher (1983) showed MEG studies of fields preceding finger, foot, and toe movements and speech (Weinberg,). Our results were in modest agreement with their study. However, we could not exclude the presence of some other sources that were not well visible in the measurements. Another study had been made by Okada, Williamson, and Kaufman (1982), who used a visual stimulus and flexion of the index finger. Without analyzing the various studies in detail, I will only add Okada's later comment at the NATO Advanced Study Institute on Biomagnetism. In the proceedings of the meeting, Okada made a timely summary of studies of evoked magnetic fields. He wrote: "Within the span of only a few years, rather substantial advances in understanding the functional organization of the human brain have been made through measurements of its evoked magnetic fields" (Okada, 1983, p. 399). Undoubtedly so, but still new instruments and methods were emerging, such as computed tomography, magnetic resonance imaging (MRI), functional MRI, and effective digital image processing. They partly complemented

and partly replaced the MEG studies. However, they could not compete with MEG or EEG in time resolution.

2.6. EPILOGUE

Let me, after 40 years, thank all of you who were involved in our work in 1970s: students, researchers, and collaborators. Better thanks late than too late.

Since the beginning of the 1980s, research in biomagnetism and equipment manufacturing has been particularly intense in Finland. Here are some examples: In 1980, the first magnetically shielded room was completed at HUT. Dr. Risto Ilmoniemi, today professor of biomedical engineering at Aalto University (previously HUT), was involved already in the construction of this room. The site of the room was still as in the original initiative, but the funds for construction were granted to the separate Low Temperature Laboratory. HUT's second biomagnetism research group, focused on brain research, started operations there in 1982, and Dr. R. Hari joined this group. The group has been very well equipped and successful in their work.

Our ambition for a new hospital environment research site was realized when the BioMag research center was established at HUCH in 1995. The center has state-of-the art brain and heart magnetometers in two magnetically shielded rooms and, among other things, two navigated transcranial magnetic stimulators. The instruments are manufactured by Finnish companies operating internationally. Elsewhere in Finland, both biomagnetism research and applications have been productive as well.

A small plant has grown up to a big tree.

REFERENCES

Ahopelto, J., Karp, P. J., Katila, T. E., Lukander, R., & Mäkipää, P. (1974). *Gradiometric observation of the magnetic brain waves.* Report TKK-F-A233. Helsinki: Helsinki University of Technology.

Ahopelto, J., Karp, P. J., Katila, T. E., Lukander, R., & Mäkipää, P. (1975). An UHF SQUID gradiometer for biomagnetic measurements. In M. Krusius & M. Vuorio (Eds.), *Proceedings of the 14th International Conference on Low Temperature Physics* (vol. 4, pp. 262–265). Amsterdam: North-Holland.

Aittoniemi, K., Hari, R., Järvinen, M-L., Katila, T., & Varpula, T. (1981). Localization of neural generators underlying auditory evoked magnetic fields of the human brain. In S. N. Erné, H. D. Hahlbohm, H. Lübbig (Eds.), *Biomagnetism: Proceedings of the Third International Workshop, Berlin (West),* May 1980 (pp. 415–422). Berlin, Boston: De Gruyter.

Aittoniemi, K., Katila, T., Kuusela, M-L., & Varpula, T. (1979). Magnetoretinography: Detection of the transient magnetic field of the eye. In *Digest of the Fifth International Conference on Medical Physics and XII International Conference on Medical and Biological Engineering* (chap. 94.6). Jerusalem, Israel.

Antervo, A., Hari, R., Katila, T., Poutanen, T., Seppänen, M., & Tuomisto, T. (1983). Cerebral magnetic fields preceding self-paced plantar flexions of the foot. *Acta Neurologica Scandinavica, 68,* 213–217.

Brenner, D., Williamson, S. J., & Kaufman, L. (1975). Visually evoked magnetic fields of the human brain. *Science, 190,* 480–482.

Cohen, D. (1972). Magnetoencephalography: Detection of the brain's electrical activity with a superconducting magnetometer. *Science, 175,* 664–666.

Cohen, D. (1975). Measurements of the magnetic fields produced by the human heart, brain, and lungs. *IEEE Transactions on Magnetics, 11,* 694–700.

Cohen, D., Edelsack, E. A., & Zimmerman, J. E. (1970). Magnetocardiograms taken inside a shielded room with a superconducting point-contact magnetometer. *Applied Physics Letters, 16,* 278–280.

Cohen, D., & McCaughan, D. (1972). Magnetocardiograms and their variation over the chest in normal subjects. *American Journal of Cardiology, 29,* 678–685.

Hari, R., Aittoniemi, K., Järvinen, M-L., Katila, T., & T. Varpula. (1979). Auditory evoked transient and sustained magnetic fields of human brain: Localization of neural generators. TKK Report Series TKK-F-A 399.

Hari, R., Aittoniemi, K., Järvinen, M-L., Katila, T., & Varpula, T. (1980). Auditory evoked transient and sustained magnetic fields of the human brain. *Experimental Brain Research, 40,* 237–240.

Hari, R., Antervo, A., Katila, T., Poutanen, T., Seppänen, M., Tuomisto, T., & Varpula, T. (1983). Cerebral magnetic fields associated with voluntary limb movements in man. Fourth International Workshop on Biomagnetism, Rome, Italy. *Il Nuovo Cimento D, 2,* 484–494.

Kariniemi, V., Ahopelto, J., Karp, P. J., & Katila, T. E. (1974). The fetal magnetocardiogram. *Journal of Perinatal Medicine, 2,* 214–216.

Kariniemi, V., Karp, P. J., & Katila, T. E. (1973). The foetal magnetocardiogram. Report TKK-F-A212. Helsinki: Helsinki University of Technology.

Karp, P. J., & Katila, T. E. (1973a). Magnetocardiography using a SQUID. In L. Patomäki & A. Kiuru (Eds.), *Proceedings of the First National Meeting on Biophysics and Biotechnology* (pp. 168–171). Helsinki, Finland.

Karp, P. T., & Katila, T. E. (1973b). Magnetocardiography using a SQUID. In R. Albert, W. Vogt, & W. Helbig (Eds.), *Digest of the 10th International Conference on Medical and Biological Engineering* (p. 250). Germany: Dresden.

Karp, P. J., Katila, T. E., Mäkipää, P., & Saar, P. (1976). Magneto-oculography: Detection of the DC magnetic field of the eye. In *Digest of the 11th International Conference on Medical and Biological Engineering* (pp. 504–505). Ottawa, Canada.

Katila, T., Maniewski, R., Poutanen, T., Varpula, T., & Karp, P. (1981). Magnetic fields produced by the human eye. *Journal of Applied Physics, 52,* 2565–2571.

Okada, Y. Motor field. (1983). In S. J. Williamson (Ed.), *Biomagnetism: An interdisciplinary approach.* NATO Advanced Study Institute on Biomagnetism, Rome, Italy. New York, NY: Plenum Press.

Okada, Y. C., Williamson, S. J., & Kaufman, L. (1982). Magnetic field of the human sensorimotor cortex. *International Journal of Neurosciences, 17,* 33–38.

Saarinen, M., Karp, P. J., Katila, T. E., & Siltanen, P. (1974). The magnetocardiogram in cardiac disorders. *Cardiovascular Research, 8,* 820–834.

Weinberg, H., Deecke, L., Brickett, P., & Boschert, J. (1983). Slow magnetic fields in the brain preceding voluntary movement. Fourth International Workshop on Biomagnetism, Rome, Italy. *Il Nuovo Cimento D, 2,* 495–504.

Zimmerman, J. T. (1981). Magnetic investigations of cortical excitation and inhibition preceding voluntary movement. PhD Thesis, University of Colorado, Boulder.

3

A VIEW FROM THE BEGINNING OF MAGNETOENCEPHALOGRAPHY

AFTER HALF A CENTURY

Lloyd Kaufman

I WAS not yet working on magnetoencephalography (MEG) when David Cohen (1968) discovered that alpha rhythms of the electroencephalography (EEG) are associated with detectable magnetic fields outside the human head, although I had read this first paper. Cohen (1972) took a critical second step when he introduced the point-contact superconducting quantum-interference device (SQUID) to the as yet almost unknown MEG community. Before that, Cohen was busy with building a magnetically shielded room, which was another step forward.

I first arrived on the scene later, probably in 1973. I had already been doing research on vision for 8 or 9 years, using evoked potentials, first at the Sperry Rand Research Center in Sudbury, Massachusetts, and, a bit later, at the Psychology Department of New York University (NYU). Both the physics and psychology departments had received "excellence" grants from the National Science Foundation (NSF), which adjudged both departments to be on the threshold of achieving that status. The awards allowed the departments to enhance lab space and equipment as well as their faculties. This enabled NYU to hire outstanding experienced as well as younger promising research scientists. A new building was constructed for physics adjacent to the psychology building with upgraded new labs. Already in my 40s I had the good fortune to be appointed to NYU with the rank of full professor of experimental psychology. My first office was located in a narrow splinter of a building where I had a tiny room to use as a laboratory. My good fortune was significantly improved by the fact that the new physics and upgraded psychology buildings were connected so that members of the two

Lloyd Kaufman, *A View From the Beginning of Magnetoencephalography: After Half a Century* In: *Fifty Years of Magnetoencephalography.* Edited by: Andrew C. Papanicolaou, Timothy P. L. Roberts, and James W. Wheless, Oxford University Press (2020). © Oxford University Press. DOI: 10.1093/oso/9780190935689.003.0003.

departments were able to meet and talk with each other. This made it possible for me to meet Samuel J. Williamson, a young associate professor in the physics department.

Sam was a condensed matter physicist interested in superconductivity. Evidently, he knew of David Cohen's success in using induction coils to detect the brain's magnetic field as well as David's work with the relatively new SQUID. I had been working on steady-state visually evoked potentials (VEPs), and Sam and I quickly recognized the possibility that we might be able to do some experiments together using a SQUID-based sensor. I already knew that steady-state VEPs are quite weak compared with the more commonly studied and relatively broad-band transient VEPs. In discussing plans for work on VEFs, I assumed these hypothetical steady-state fields were probably similarly weak, perhaps an order of magnitude weaker than the peak amplitude of the transient VEF.

Doug Brenner was a bright and energetic graduate student already studying with Sam. Doug had learned to work with point-contact SQUIDs (manufactured by SHE Inc.) in Sam's lab. We added Doug to our team from the outset, and it was a great decision. My own lab happened to be on the ninth floor of the psychology building. Sam's low-temperature lab was on the same floor, but on the physics side. We could get from one to the other simply by walking up or down a very short staircase.

We made many false starts before starting to record. For example, we began with a stainless steel dewar, which made detecting anything impossible. Normally such dewars are used in well-shielded enclosures. Sam quickly recognized that currents were induced in the stainless steel by fields of external sources. Lacking a magnetically shielded room, we had to procure a fiberglass dewar. I no longer recall how or where we got it, but we might have raided my grant on VEPs to buy one.

Of course, we had to acknowledge that the noise level due to extraneous sources, such as nearby elevators, would overwhelm our SQUID. Sam suggested a second-order gradiometer which Doug wound on a phenolic rod. Together we made an educated guess and used a 3.5-cm baseline between each coil of each pair of coils constituting the gradiometer. We felt it to be a reasonable separation for maximizing signal strength and minimizing noise from distant sources. To gain more flexibility, the design incorporated a set of small trim coils that could be adjusted to yield an overall configuration that would better cancel noise from distant sources. We then got started by setting up electronics to generate visual stimuli suitable for use in Sam's lab that were basically similar to those used in my own VEP studies.

At first, in pilot studies, we used a two-phase lock-in amplifier to detect periodic visual evoked fields (VEFs) at frequencies near the alpha band. This is an excellent way to extract one frequency at a time from a time-varying signal masked by noise. About 7 years previously, I assumed that extremely intense light flashes would be more likely than less intense flashes to produce large-amplitude VEPs. I was very wrong. At first, I used a stroboscope to generate flashes of light. However, it was also prone to exhibit electrical artifacts that could be confused with transient VEPs. So, I stopped using it. I then tried rotating a disk with holes drilled in it to chop light from a 12-V auto lamp seen in a Maxwellian view (where light appears to the viewer to be spread across the surface of a lens). This was created by forming an image of the lamp's filament in the pupil of the subject's eye. Because of the intensity of the resulting illuminance of the subject's retina, we had to filter out long-wavelength light to eliminate potential damage to the eye. However, despite my intuition that more intense stimuli would produce more robust VEPs, this was not true. So, we avoided that approach as well. Instead, we generated patterned stimuli of modest luminance on the surface of an oscilloscope to avoid saturating the visual system. This worked quite well in my VEP lab, so we imported the apparatus to Sam's lab. The stimuli were sinusoidal gratings of specifiable spatial frequencies that could be abruptly and periodically switched to a uniform featureless field of light with an average spatial distribution of luminance equal to that when the pattern of bars was visible on the screen. It is worthwhile to emphasize that there was no net change in average luminance with this stimulus. This average luminance never changed for either patterned or uniform stimuli. Hence, the evoked field was due solely to the periodic change from pattern to no pattern. The response was time-locked to the frequency of switching. Naturally, in the actual experiment, we ran trials with no subject in place in order to rule out artifacts.

3.1. OUR FIRST VISUALLY EVOKED FIELD EXPERIMENT

Our first subjects (usually Sam or Doug) lay face down to look through an aperture cut into the plywood panel on which they lay. This is illustrated in Figure 3.1. The bottom of the tail section of the dewar hanging above the subject's head was positioned tangentially to the occipital scalp. Our pilot experiments looked promising but, despite some strong hints of signals, sometimes we were still overwhelmed by noisy sources at relatively great distances. Ultimately, we came to know our environment and realized

that subway trains zipping by below us at a distance of 40 m were shaking the entire building. Finally, we decided to begin a night shift and do our experiments between 10:00 or 11:00 PM and 4:00 AM. This made it possible to get good results. Our first results on evoked visual fields are described in Figure 3.2. As was confirmed in our second experiment (see later), this particular form of our stimulus elicited VEFs in response to the second harmonic of the fundamental temporal frequency of the stimulus, which I knew signified that the involved neural circuits were essentially nonlinear. Our resulting paper was published in *Science* (Brenner, Williamson, & Kaufman, 1975).

Our main objective in conducting this experiment was simply to establish that it could be done. Our next step was to see if we could learn something about the visual system by conducting such studies. We had a modest goal. In those days, neuroscientists and psychologists had a strong interest in relating Fourier transform concepts to theories of how the visual system works. It was known, for example, that the visual system is not uniformly sensitive in detecting gratings of different spatial frequencies. Rather, gratings of low and high spatial frequencies require more contrast to be detected during psychophysical

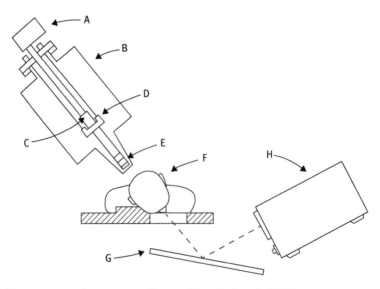

FIGURE 3.1   The experimental arrangement for recording visual evoked fields.

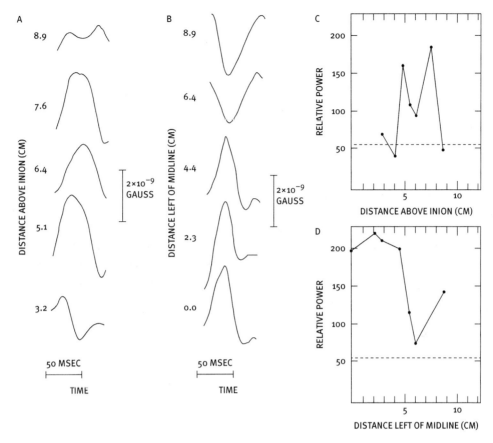

FIGURE 3.2 Examples of visual evoked fields recorded over different locations of the posterior cortex.

experiments than gratings of an intermediate spatial frequency (e.g., ~ 4 c/deg). In fact, the so-called spatial modulation transfer function (MTF) used by optical engineers is applied by visual scientists to describe the relative sensitivity of the eye to patterns of different spatial frequency. We were not seeking to measure the MTF here, but were merely exploring how the visual system as a passive sensory system responded to patterns of different spatial frequencies.

3.2. THE SECOND VISUALLY EVOKED FIELD EXPERIMENT

In this experiment (Williamson, Kaufman, & Brenner, 1978), we employed two basic stimuli. The first was essentially the same as the one we used in the preceding VEF experiment. Typically, we alternated between a uniform field and a sinusoidal grating at a rate of 8 Hz. This was the fundamental temporal frequency of stimulus presentation. The second stimulus was also composed of two alternating images, but this time the grating abruptly changed in spatial phase: It switched periodically from one phase to another (i.e., shifting abruptly 180 degrees in relative spatial phase). We referred to the first type of stimulus as one that flickered, and the second as contrast reversing. I think it would have been more accurate to change the description of the first type of stimulus from "flickering" to one that alternated from one spatial frequency to another, while the second might be better described as switching its spatial phase. In our first experiment using the flickered stimulus, we found no response at the fundamental temporal frequency of 8 Hz. However, strong responses occurred at 16 Hz, the frequency of its second harmonic. With the contrast reversal stimulus, we saw strong responses both at the fundamental stimulus frequency (8 Hz) and at its second harmonic, again a sign of nonlinearity.

Doug and I were watching responses accumulate on the screen of an oscilloscope driven by a primitive analogue-averaging computer. (The instrument was a 100-channel Waveform Eductor produced by Princeton Applied Research.) We watched the average VEF waves grow out of the background noise as we changed the stimulus from one spatial frequency to another while the temporal frequency remained constant. We thought that we had seen the phase of the response change as we went from one spatial frequency to another. So, we started to pay close attention to response phase. After accumulating a large number of responses at different spatial frequencies, it became apparent that there was a systematic shift toward increasing relative

phase with spatial frequency. We finally got Sam up from the subject's prone position and showed him the result. He quickly confirmed our impression and, after examining the data, we realized that the phase changes may well reflect increases in the latency of the VEF, and hence in the brain's response to the stimuli (see Figure 3.3 for results).

We did not realize it when we started this experiment, but Breitmeyer (1975) had already completed a related study. However, although his stimulus range overlapped the gratings we employed, his data were based on the simple reaction time (RT) of subjects to the onset of presentation of gratings. On learning of his paper, we were delighted to see that his data complemented ours. As is evident in Figure 3.3, his curves approximate the trends in our data. Adding a constant amount of time to each data point would produce very similar curves. The difference could be largely eliminated by

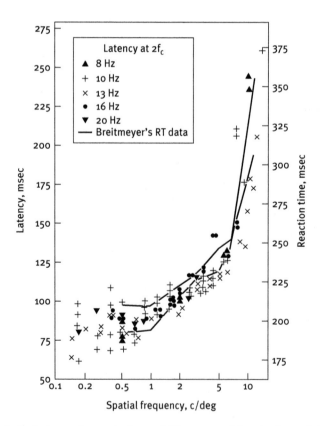

FIGURE 3.3   The relation between changes in the spatial frequency of the stimulus and the visual evoked field latencies.

adding this constant to our data after the phase shift is converted to latency.

Since it was possible that organizing a motor response may well vary with cognitive states, overall alertness, and other nonsensory factors, so could the VEF (and similar VEP) data. This opens the question of what the VEF represents: Could it depend on activity in the motor cortex, the primary sensory pathways before reacting, or even post-reaction cortical activity? Our finding that adding a constant to the latency of the VEF may predict RT is tantalizing. It suggests that the VEF in this case is largely related to processing of signals that had just arrived at the visual cortex through the visual pathways. Such a conclusion could also justify the widespread practice of cognitive scientists to make inferences about factors underlying changes in, say, duration of memory search from using simple RT measures.

Extensive psychophysical data had shown that the human visual system requires more contrast to detect spatial frequencies lower than about 1 c/deg. Our MEG recordings showed that at higher spatial frequencies, the phase of the VEF increases linearly up to about 10 c/deg, but there is no systematic change for frequencies less than 1 c/deg. Also, gratings at about 4 c/deg require the least amount of contrast to be detected, while at higher spatial frequencies, up to well above 10 c/deg, sensitivity progressively diminishes, until it falls to the point when the grating is unresolvable by the human eye, at about 60 c/deg. Thus, the MTF is actually a U-shaped function. We did not find this in our data. It seems likely that it occurred because we used only one level of contrast, and all of our gratings were less than 8 c/deg.

We were aware that research on the visual systems of cats, owls, and some monkeys had led others to the conclusion that low spatial frequency stimuli seemed not to show systematic changes in latency with spatial frequency. This is reflected in the RT data of Figure 3.3 and also in our VEF data. It has also been shown to be present in VEP data. In general, low spatial

frequencies appear to be better stimuli for affecting what came to be called transient or X channels in the visual systems of these animals, while higher spatial frequencies are more effective stimuli for the so-called sustained or Y channels. However, Y and X channels have never been found in the human visual system. Even so, these findings appear to offer support for the emerging concept of treating the visual system as a collection of diverse channels. Despite the evidence that X and Y channels do not exist in humans, such hypothetical processes have been fruitful.

About 2 years later, Yoshio Okada joined our lab as a postdoctoral fellow. He led a number of important projects in our lab. Among these was an experiment in which we measured the MTF using our single-channel system (Okada, Kaufman, Brenner, & Williamson, 1982). In this study, we used five different levels of contrast as well as multiple spatial frequencies in a multifactorial experiment. Our paper explicitly compares the results of the described experiments with pioneering psychophysical experiments that launched our understanding of how the visual system processes Fourier components composing visual patterns. Such studies were ultimately foundational for what may be termed a *multiple-channel hypothesis*. Of course, we mustn't forget that there were already many psychophysical studies, as well as VEP experiments, before the MEG experiments that are of special interest to the readers of this chapter. A good example of the extensive VEP domain is the work of Campbell and Kulikowski (1970), who described how contrast of gratings affect the VEP. Okada et al. (1982) offer an extensive treatment of this as well as the relevant literature from the psychophysical domain.

As emphasized earlier, it is clear that X and Y channels cannot be related to our VEF latency variation with spatial frequency. Perhaps we should consider more recently discovered properties of channels in the human visual pathways. Some years ago, it was recognized that the human lateral geniculate nucleus

(LGN) contains six different layers, two of which contain large neurons. Hence, these layers are referred to as *magnocellular layers,* while another single layer, the *parvocellular layer,* contains smaller neurons. The so-called M cells of the magnocellular layers receive input from particular ganglion cells of the retinas, as do the P cells of the parvocellular layer, which receives input from retinal midget ganglion cells. It must be pointed out that other cell types exist in the other layers of the LGN. Some of the traits of the X cells are similar to those of the M cells, while P cells share some of the nominal traits of Y cells. However, it must also be pointed out that I retired about 25 years ago and lack the knowledge needed for fully informed speculation. I can only point out that M cells have response traits similar to those of transient X cells, as do the retinal ganglion cells that send them signals. Similarly, P cells respond best to higher spatial frequencies and share this trait with the midget cells of the retina. But I am now aware that there are many additional pathways from LGN to superior colliculus and other nuclei of which I have no clear knowledge. I am not conversant with other attempts to deduce the properties of M and P pathways, or of any other relatively recently discovered pathways in the visual system. I urge interested readers to seek out more recent data.

These initial years were a very exciting time for me, as I learned an enormous amount about low-temperature physics as well as properties of magnetic fields and of volume currents as well as how these may be affected by the skull, brain, and other tissues having different conductivities. Not being a trained physicist, I not only relied on Sam for verbal instructions on superconductivity but also found an enormously fascinating book on the history of that field. This was back in 1974. I happened upon it on a shelf in my public library. Its title was *The Quest for Absolute Zero* and was written by K. Mendelssohn (1966). Although now out of print, a few used copies are occasionally available. I found it to be a wonderful introduction to superconductivity

for those who are not trained physicists. It has remained a good book!

3.3. OUR FIRST MAPPING STUDIES

Even during our first VEF study, we observed that the VEF differed in both amplitude and polarity at different locations over the occipital lobe. Figure 3.2 displays traces of VEFs that differ from each other. These differences in amplitude occurred as we moved upward along the midline of the skull from the level of the inion (which is where I used to paste electrodes to pick up VEPs). At positions near the bottom of the skull, VEFs were down in noise. The trace obtained along the midline and 3.2 cm above the inion was indistinguishable from noise. At still higher points on the midline, we saw strong VEFs, only to fall to the noise level again somewhere between positions 8 and 9 cm. VEFs were directed outward from the scalp on one side of the midline, while those of opposite polarity were re-entering the scalp on the opposite side of the midline. I do not recall seeing such dramatic reversals with VEPs. Data such as these are good evidence that detailed mapping of the locations of emerging and re-entering magnetic fields might well make it possible to locate VEF sources. At that time, it was common to assume that an equivalent current dipole was a suitable model for actual sources of VEFs. We saw this as a tantalizing goal and realized that we sorely needed many channels for simultaneous mapping of the field.

After our first VEF experiment, we thought that it may well be possible to use MEG to noninvasively map primary projection areas of several sensory pathways on the cerebral cortex. The importance of such a task lay partly in the fact that an enormous amount of information about these areas already existed. This information was gained in part by studying patients with penetrating wounds of their brains. Other studies applied electric stimuli during brain surgery to exposed brain tissue. These and related results were well known. Even if we could not add anything of value to this knowledge base, we might still be able to verify MEG's ostensible potential for locating specific functional areas noninvasively. Ultimately, this became one of the more valuable potential applications before brain surgery. Hence, our lab set out to map the somatosensory cortex. Our first significant results are described in a paper by Brenner, Lipton, Kaufman, and Williamson (1978). We were limited by our single-channel system because we had to measure the field at many different places to obtain a convincing map of the field normal to the scalp. Related work by Hari, Aitoniemi, Katila, and Varpula (1980) described transient auditory evoked fields (AEFs) in response to stimuli affecting the auditory cortex. I recall that one of my Finnish friends told me that these early experiments were conducted without shielding but in a wooden hut far from any signs of civilization, including subway trains and elevators. The responses shown by Hari et al. demonstrate remarkably clear and well-resolved transient components that seem to have been recorded at or near the field extrema—the places where fields normal to the scalp are centered on places where maximal exiting and re-entering fields were measured. These too were measured using a single channel system, so many repeated and time-consuming measurements appear to have been made. This made it possible for the authors to locate the likely positions of the neural sources of the components, assuming that a single equivalent dipole model describes the source. Our own maps of the steady-state somatosensory evoked field (SEF) also strike me as being a notable accomplishment, especially when one considers that we also were still tied to our single-channel system.

By 1980, I was no longer the main lab member sitting at the experimenter's station. This job was taken for a time by Gian Luca Romani, a visiting scientist from Rome who did most of the planning and running of our experiment. Again, we were lucky in the sense that we were able to limit ourselves to steady-state responses. Our goal was to use stimuli composed of audible frequency carrier waves ranging in five steps from 200 to 5 KHz. These frequencies were selected to ensure that they would cover a wide-enough range to excite neurons tuned to respond to the sounds they created. The one thing each carrier had in common was that all of them were modulated by a 32-Hz sinusoid. We had hypothesized that the neurons responding periodically at the frequency of 32 Hz would be those tuned to respond to the acoustic frequencies of the carriers. I helped with assembling diverse analogue electronics capable of generating these stimuli as well as with setting up the function generators and other devices used to produce the modulated sound waves. Details may be found in the paper by Romani, Williamson, Kaufman, and Brenner (1982). I believe it was the first application of MEG to describe the tonotopic organization of the human auditory cortex. Furthermore, it is a lovely example of Sam's virtuosity as a theorist, which also justifies a close reading of the original paper. A second paper was submitted as a very brief research note to *Science* (Romani, Williamson, & Kaufman, 1982). Although these papers appeared almost 40 years ago, they are probably the best example of what could have been done in the very early days of MEG.

3.4. TIME MARCHES ON

Much of our contribution to the advancement of MEG came in the form of doctoral students, postdocs, and visiting scholars with whom we collaborated. I can't help but think of some of the brilliant people I had the good fortune to work with. I must mention some of them. They came from diverse disciplines, but mostly from physics and psychology. All of the predocs and postdocs remain very young in my mind's eye, but some have reached retirement age. I am especially fond of Jai Zhu Wang, who came all the way from China to earn her doctorate in physics at NYU. She spent substantial time in our lab. Jai Zhu no longer works in MEG, but her contributions are very important. One was her quest for inverse solutions, which is summarized in a chapter she wrote for a book on magnetic source imaging of the human brain (Lu & Kaufman, 2008). Two more of my personal favorites are the late Olli Lounassma and his student Risto Ilmoniemi. Olli literally traveled around the world to end up in New York, where he spent many months working with us on a daily basis. He insisted that we at least pretend that he was only a postdoc. Actually, he was an intellectual powerhouse. I still miss him. Risto spent 2 or 3 years working with us and continues to be my friend and sometime advisor. His work as a major figure in our field and also in other areas of imaging is or should be well known to all of you. Then there is my dear friend Yoshio Okada who came to us as a postdoc from the lab of the late Bill Estes, a famous mathematical psychologist then at Rockefeller University. After his immersion in experimental psychology, Yoshio decided that he wanted to know more about how the brain works. He quickly mastered all he had to know about MEG, which is proven by his many accomplishments in our lab. After completing several important papers such as the VEF paper mentioned already, Yoshio decided that he wanted to get closer to actual brains. So, he jumped ship and moved on to our medical school, where he undertook to learn more about the genesis of magnetic fields at the neuronal level. He worked with turtle cerebellum and neural structures of other subhuman species; thereby illuminating our understanding of the neurogenesis of extracranial magnetic fields. From there, he went on to study infants, so that today he uses a 375-channel system (not the single-channel he started with) of his own design and which he partially built himself. Not bad for a young psychologist! Now, as the Director of Boston Children's Hospital's MEG laboratory, he continues to do research on neonates and to apply his new instrument toward improving infants with epilepsy. Another psychologist who trained with us is Zhong-Lin Lu, who joined us after coming to New York from China to enroll in the doctoral program at

NYU's physics department. He began in physics but confessed that he was always intrigued by cognitive science. Somehow we captured his attention, so he came to our lab and did his dissertation with Sam. We quickly recognized that, despite some initial shyness, Zhong-Lin was extremely bright. As time went by, we had to revise our estimate of Zhong-Lin upward, and then upward again, and again. By the time he finished his doctorate, he wanted to become a postdoc in our lab. After dealing with my temptation to go along with him, I finally concluded that we had taught Zhong-Lin all that we had to offer. So, I reluctantly suggested that he move on to work with my friend George Sperling. George invited Zhong-Lin to be his postdoctoral student in the psychology department at the University of California at Irvine, where they were building a world-class faculty. Later, George thanked me for my suggestion because he found Zhong-Lin to be a truly brilliant and creative collaborator. Zhong-Lin has held several distinguished professorships at Ohio State University, where he directs a MEG lab as well as labs involving many different forms of brain imaging. He is clearly one of our lab's most luminous products. I understand Zhong-Lin is returning to NYU.

I was privileged to work with other very strong people during my time in the NYU Neuromagnetism Laboratory. I am honored to have been so fortunate, but I lack the time and space to go further.

3.5. WHERE I WOULD GO FROM HERE

I thought I would finish my section by suggesting some research projects that may accelerate progress in MEG. Upon thinking about it, I realize that I have not been keeping up with the literature in a systematic manner and therefore may not be qualified to offer meaningful advice to a much more advanced generation. However, I thought there might be some value in my mentioning an area in which I once had a serious interest, but never got around to fully exploiting. If readers know this area, then you are excused if you leave me here.

At one time, I was fascinated by some puzzling auditory phenomena. These included two related illusions. One was the *missing fundamental,* and the other was known as the *combination tones.* If one listens to a complex tone composed of a set of pure tones of, say, one at 1,000 Hz, another at 1,200 Hz, a third at 1,400 Hz, as well as others from the same series, it is likely that when listening to the set, it appears to be accompanied by a tone of 200 Hz, even though it is not physically present. This is known as the missing fundamental. The combination tones may be heard when listening to a pair of harmonically unrelated tones. For example, listening to a tone at, say, 107 Hz and another at 190 Hz, you may also hear a tone of about 297 Hz (the sum frequency) and another at 83 Hz (the difference frequency). I also happened on Helmholtz's classic *Sensations of Tone,* where I encountered his theory that both of these illusions could be explained by nonlinear responses of the ear to these physical sounds.

These and other encounters with effects of nonlinearities led me to my own doubts about some points of view based on the assumption of linearity and the unwitting assumption of some that the superposition principle applies to neural tissue (Kaufman, 1974). I wondered, for example, if we could capitalize on the idea that since neural tissue is essentially nonlinear, the response to two harmonically unrelated signals concurrently applied to a common nonlinear network would interact with each other to produce frequency doubling and, perhaps, frequencies unrelated harmonically to those of the physically applied stimuli (e.g., sum and difference frequencies). These frequencies cannot be detected using conventional signal averaging. The reason is simply that modern averaging computers are effectively comb filters designed to discriminate against frequencies that are harmonically unrelated to the frequencies of the trigger stimuli. This is why the averaging process may well be discarding important information along with

noise. We need knowledge of the nature of the nonlinearity to achieve some measurements of such stimulus-related consequences. Since nonlinearity results in interaction of applied signals with each other, and also with applied signals and ongoing brain activity, the problem is complicated. However, this interaction is reflected by the presence of modulation of each frequency of the ongoing activity of neuronal populations with each frequency of stimulation affecting that same population, so a very rich set of data awaits the work of young and strong researchers. The question remains: What are we discarding along with the noise when we are seeking "clean" responses? It is fairly easy to show that we can detect stimulus-related sum and difference frequencies by multiplying the frequencies precisely at the frequencies of, say, two different stimuli and isolating the resulting sum and difference frequencies. These may be used as triggers for conventional averaging of the MEG to record any significant activity at those frequencies. Another approach I have used is to cancel all activity contained in ongoing MEG activity and then use a rectified band of that activity to determine whether the remaining ongoing MEG was displaying amplitude modulation at the frequency of the applied signal. But this is getting complicated. Of course, frequency doubling is easy to see, as it commonly appears during many experiments. I wonder if anybody has sought to find out if there are reasons why it appears, and why it doesn't.

Another of my interests was binocular vision and stereopsis. In fact, I am currently working on a paper related to this area, but I am limiting myself to psychophysical results I obtained some years ago. I did, however, try to conduct a MEG study involving separate application of different stimuli to the two eyes, but either at a corresponding retinal place or at very widely disparate places. My preliminary results were very promising, but I never completed my experiments. Somewhat later, I discovered that my dear friend David Regan had independently entertained similar ideas, a fact that encouraged me that they were in good hands. Quite a few years later, I invited him and his late wife M. P. Regan to write a chapter for a book on magnetic source imaging (Lu & Kaufman, Eds., 2008). This chapter is rich with ideas and examples of how one might exploit the nonlinearities of neural tissue. One of the great pioneers in this area was Henk van der Tweel, who, with his colleagues, also explored related ideas. Citations of their work, which goes back more than half a century, are provided by Regan and Regan (2008). Much of this work appears to have missed the attention of most MEG researchers. So, my suggestion is that this is a promising area for extensive exploration where the good spatial resolution afforded by the magnetic modality can make it possible to identify and locate networks where signals actually interact with each other, and even pick up signals characterized by apparently superimposable responses. These could be generated in physically independent circuits so close to each other they cannot be resolved by MEG alone.

ACKNOWLEDGMENT

I am deeply indebted to Yoshio Okada, who edited this chapter. He managed to correct several significant errors of omission and of commission, but I am solely responsible for any remaining errors.

REFERENCES

Breitmeyer, B. G. (1975). Simple reaction time as a measure of the temporal response properties of transient and sustained channels. *Vision Research, 15*, 141–412.

Brenner, D., Lipton, J., Kaufman, L., & Williamson, S. J. (1978). Somatically evoked magnetic fields of the human brain. *Science, 199*, 81–83.

Brenner, D., Williamson, S. J., & Kaufman, L. (1975). Visually evoked magnetic fields of the human brain. *Science, 190*, 480–482.

Campbell, F. W., & Kulikowski, J. J. (1970). The visual evoked potential as a function of the contrast of a grating pattern. *Journal of Physiology, 222*, 345–356.

Cohen, D. (1968). Magnetoencephalography: Evidence of magnetic fields produced by alpha-rhythm currents. *Science, 161*, 784–786.

Cohen, D. (1972). Magnetoencephalography: Detection of the brain's electrical activity with a superconducting magnetometer. *Science, 175*, 664–666.

Hari, R., Aitoniemi, L, Järvinen, M.-L., Katila, T., & Varpula, T. (1980). Auditory evoked transient and sustained magnetic fields of the human brain localization of neural generators. *Experimental in Brain Research, 40*, 237–240.

Kaufman, L. (1974). *Sight and mind*. New York, NY: Oxford University Press.

Lu, Z. L., & Kaufman, L. (Eds.). (2008). *Magnetic source imaging of the human brain*. Mahwah, NJ: Lawrence Erlbaum.

Mendelssohn, K. (1966). *The quest for absolute zero: The meaning of low temperature physics*. New York, Toronto: McGraw-Hill World University Library.

Okada, Y. C., Kaufman, L., Brenner, D., & Williamson, S. J. (1982). Modulation transfer functions of the human visual system revealed by magnetic field measurements. *Vision Research, 22*, 319–333.

Regan, D. M., & Regan, M. P. (2008). Techniques for investigating and exploiting nonlinearities in brain processes by recording responses evoked by sensory stimuli. In Lu, Z-L., & Kaufman, L. (Eds.), *Magnetic source imaging of the human brain*. Mahwah, NJ: Lawrence Erlbaum.

Romani, G. L., Williamson, S. J., & Kaufman, L. (1982). Tonotopic organization of the human auditory cortex. *Science, 216*, 1339–1340.

Romani, G. L, Williamson, S. J., Kaufman, L., & Brenner, D. (1982). Characterization of the human auditory cortex. *Experimental Brain Research, 47*, 381–393.

Williamson, S. J., Kaufman, L., & Brenner, D. (1978). Latency of the neuromagnetic response of the human cortex. *Vision Research, 18*, 107–110.

SECTION II

TECHNICAL ADVANCES

4

PHYSIOLOGICAL BASES OF MAGNETOENCEPHALOGRAPHY AND ELECTROENCEPHALOGRAPHY

Yoshio Okada

4.1. THE ORIGIN OF MAGNETOENCEPHALOGRAPHY AND ELECTROENCEPHALOGRAPHY SIGNALS BASED ON THE CLASSIC VIEW OF NEURON ELECTROPHYSIOLOGY

Fifty years ago, magnetoencephalography (MEG) started as a new noninvasive method, an alternative to electroencephalography (EEG), for studying human brain functions (Cohen, 1968). As this technique started to develop, it was clear early on that there is a need for understanding how brain activity, such as spontaneous brain rhythm and event-related neuronal responses, produces the accompanying MEG signal.

The origin of EEG had been investigated by many notable scientists before the emergence of MEG, including Lorente de Nó (1947), Rall (1962a, 1962b) and Ranck (1963a, 1963b). Each neuron had been represented by a core conductor cable with the sodium and potassium channels discovered by Hodgkin and Huxley (1952) and others. These active, voltage-sensitive, time-dependent conductances were localized in the soma and initial segment of the axon of the cables models. The dendrites were represented by passive cables with a fixed-resistance connecting parallel capacitance-resistance circuits in series along the cable. This passive cable model of the dendrites with excitatory or inhibitory postsynaptic receptors and the soma and axon with the active conductances had been used to explain the origins of EEG.

Figure 4.1, taken from a standard textbook on EEG (Niedermeyer & Lopes da Silva, 1987), shows how EEG signals had been thought to be generated by intracellular currents in a neuron. Excitatory input, in this case at a distal terminal of the dendrite (see Figure 4.1, *left*), produces depolarization of the transmembrane potential in the

Yoshio Okada, *Physiological Bases of Magnetoencephalography and Electroencephalography* In: *Fifty Years of Magnetoencephalography*.
Edited by: Andrew C. Papanicolaou, Timothy P. L. Roberts, and James W. Wheless, Oxford University Press (2020). © Oxford University Press.
DOI: 10.1093/oso/9780190935689.003.0004.

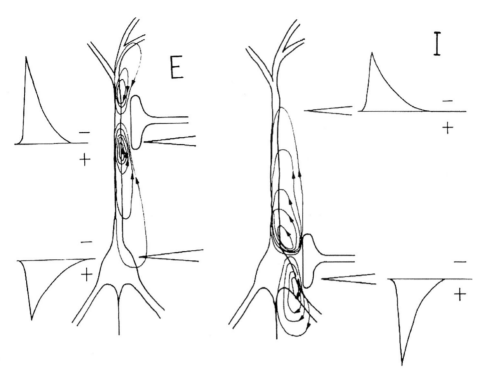

FIGURE 4.1   Schematic illustration of the intracellular current generated by an excitatory (E) synaptic input *(left)* and an inhibitory (I) synaptic input *(right)* onto a pyramidal cell. These intracellular currents in principle can generate scalp electroencephalogram signals. (From Lopes da Silva, F., & Rotterdam, A. [1987]. _____ _____ In E. Niedermeyer & F. Lopes da Silva (Eds.), *Electroencephalography:* Basic principles, *clinical applications, and related fields* [2nd ed., pp. 29–41]. Baltimore, MD: Urban & Schwarzenberg. Reprinted with permission from the publisher.)

synaptic input region and hyperpolarization in the distal dendritic terminals and in the proximal dendrite and soma, according to electrotonic passive membrane potential changes governed by the basic cable model of the neuron (Lopes da Silva & Rotterdam, 1987). An inhibitory synaptic input, in this case in the soma, produces membrane hyperpolarization in the region of the synaptic input and depolarization in the distal dendrites at the distances determined by the electrotonic length of the basal and apical dendrites. This pattern of postsynaptic membrane potential change produces intracellular currents between the current sink and source that serve as the basis for EEG signals on the scalp. Graded postsynaptic potentials (PSPs) were thought to generate the intracellular currents that generate the EEG signals.

In contrast to EEG, very little work had been done on the physiological basis of MEG until the mid-1980s. Possible physiological origins of MEG were considered within the framework of the existing view of physiological origins of EEG (Okada, 1983a, 1983b).

4.2. MODERN CONCEPTS OF ELECTROPHYSIOLOGY OF NEURONS

Since the early years of EEG and MEG research, the concept of electrophysiology of neurons has undergone dramatic changes with discoveries of various types of ionotropic and metabotropic channels (Hille, 1992, 2001). Ionotropic channels include those channels that are directly activated by the ions that cross the membrane with opening of the receptors. This family of channels includes ligand- and voltage-gated channels and calcium-gated channels. Metabotropic channels include those that are opened by a neurotransmitter, which then activate a cascade of intracellular second messengers responsible for starting slow flow of currents across the postsynaptic membrane. The ionotropic active channels are located throughout neurons, in contrast to the classic concept of neurons in which voltage-gated channels are localized in the soma/axon region near the initial segment (Stuart, Spruston, Sakmann, & Häusser M, 1997).

The intrinsic active channels distributed throughout the dendrites and soma are important for understanding the physiological origins of MEG and EEG signals because they determine the intracellular currents generated in the cells (Llinás, 1988; Stuart et al., 1997). For example, a synaptic input onto a distal portion of the apical dendrites can activate the low-threshold sodium conductances in the initial segment, and this in turn can generate sodium and calcium spikes that propagate toward the basal dendrites and back-propagate toward the terminals of the apical dendrites (Stuart et al., 1997). The depolarization of many terminal branches of the apical dendrites can then synchronize the synaptic inputs across many branches of the apical dendrites for increasing the synchrony of postsynaptic response. The dendritic depolarization then can synchronize the action of many presynaptic neurons for enhancing the information processing that can be performed by each neuron in the network. This pattern of postsynaptic activation is quite different from the classic view in which graded PSPs in individual dendrites were considered as generators of EEG signals. The interpretation of MEG as well as EEG signals then must be based on understanding of how the active and passive elements of the neurons jointly govern the population currents and thus the macroscopic signals.

Roger Traub is one of the leading authorities on the development of mathematical models of neurons and neuronal networks based on the modern view of central neuron electrophysiology. He and his colleagues have developed models of single neurons and neuronal networks for the cerebral cortex, hippocampus, and cerebellum that incorporate active channels discovered in the central neurons (Traub, Jefferys, Miles, Whittington, & Toth, 1994; Traub, Middleton, Knopfel, & Whittington, 2008; Traub, Wong, Miles, & Michelson, 1991; Traub et al., 2005). In these models, each neuron is represented by a multicompartmental core-conductor cable with dendritic branches. Figure 4.2 shows a model of a pyramidal cell in the hippocampus with branched dendrites (Traub et al., 1994). Each compartment has one or more active channels, including voltage-gated sodium, calcium, and potassium channels. These neurons are connected to each other through excitatory and inhibitory connections mediated by ligand-gated channels.

4.3. MATHEMATICAL MODELS BASED ON MODERN CONCEPTS OF ELECTROPHYSIOLOGY OF NEURONS FOR UNDERSTANDING PHYSIOLOGICAL BASES OF MAGNETOENCEPHALOGRAPHY AND ELECTROENCEPHALOGRAPHY

Mathematical models based on the modern concept of electrophysiology of neurons have been developed for understanding the physiological origins of MEG and EEG signals. A mathematical neuronal network mode of the CA3 of hippocampus based on the network model of Traub (Traub & Miles, 1991; Traub et al., 1994) and a single realistic neuron model of the principal neurons of the cerebral cortex based on the model of Mainen and Sejnowski (1996) have been described.

4.3.1. Single-Cylinder, Multicompartment Model of CA Neurons

Figure 4.3 shows a network model of pyramidal cells and inhibitory interneurons in the CA3 of hippocampus (Murakami, Zhang, Hirose, &

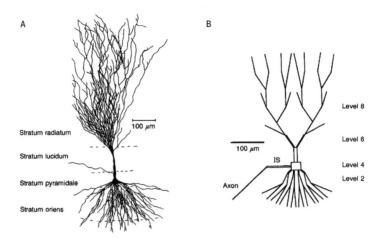

A

Stratum radiatum

Stratum lucidum

Stratum pyramidale

Stratum oriens

100 μm

B

Level 8

Level 6

100 μm

IS

Level 4

Level 2

Axon

FIGURE 4.2   Realistic core-conductor, multicompartment cable model with branched dendrites for the pyramidal cells in hippocampus. (A) Histological image of a pyramidal neuron in hippocampus. (B) A branched dendrite multicompartment core-conductor cable model of the pyramidal cell. IS = initial segment next to a soma. (From Traub, R. D., Jefferys, J. G. R., Miles, R., Whittington, M. A., & Toth K. [1994]. A branching dendritic model of a rodent CA3 pyramidal neurone. *Journal of Physiology, 481*, 79–95.)

Okada, 2002). The pyramidal cells (e-cells) are multicompartment cylindrical core conductors. Each e-cell has excitatory synapses (NMDA: *N*-methyl-D-aspartate receptor; AMPA: α-amino-3-hydroxy-5-methyl-4-isoxazolepropionic   acid receptor) in compartments 3 and 15 (see Figure 4.3A). It also has two types of inhibitory synapses (GABA-A and GABA-B: gamma-aminobutyric acid receptors of fast A type and slower B type, respectively). GABA-A receptors are located in the soma and adjacent compartments 8 and 10. GABA-B receptors are located in compartments 3 and 15. These cells have six types of active channels: gNa—sodium conductance; gK(DR)—potassium conductance of delayed rectifier type; gK(A)—fast potassium conductance of A type; gCa—calcium conductance; gK(C)—calcium-dependent voltage-gated potassium conductance; and gK(AHP)—potassium conductance of after hyperpolarization type). They are distributed across the dendrite with the distributions shown in Figure 4.3A.

The inhibitory cells (i-cells) are also cylindrical with NMDA and AMPA receptors in compartments 3 and 15 and GABA-A receptors in the soma and in the adjacent compartments (8–10), as in the e-cells (see

Figure 4.3B). They have two types of Hodgkin-Huxley active channels [gNa and gK(DR)] located only in the soma, as in the classic neuron models.

These cells are arranged in a rectangular grid (see Figure 4.3C). Since the model was developed to account for experimental data, the model neuronal circuit has a realistic geometry with a bipolar electrode along the longitudinal axis of the pyramidal cells and the magnetic field detectors (SQ2 and SQ4) 2 mm above the model with the dimensions comparable to the experimental situation (see Figure 4.8 later). The e-cells and i-cells are connected as shown in Figure 4.3D. Each e-cell receives synaptic contacts from 20 out of 100 randomly selected e-cells with a synaptic weight that is an exponential function of the distance between the cells divided by a space constant. Each of 20 i-cells receives contacts from 20 out of 100 randomly selected e-cells with a fixed synaptic strength independent of cell-to-cell distance. Each of 100 e-cells receives synaptic contacts from 12 out of 20 randomly selected i-cells with a fixed synaptic weight. As described later, this model proved to be useful in relating three types of data—intracellular potentials from

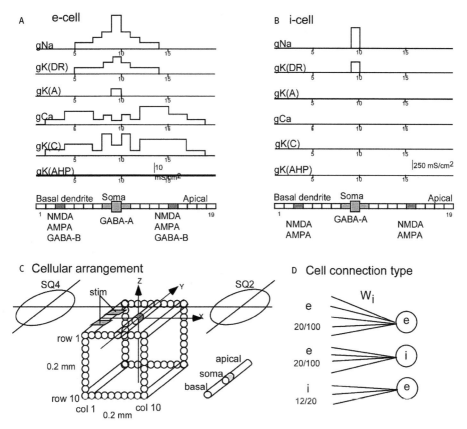

FIGURE 4.3   Neuronal network of cylindrical pyramidal cells in CA3. (A) Distribution of active channels along the cylindrical dendrites and soma in an e-cell. (B) Distribution in an i-cell. (C) Neural network of 100 e-cells and 20 i-cells relative to a bipolar stimulating electrode pair with a four-channel Superconducting QUantum-Interference Device (SQUID) magnetic field detector (SQ2 and SQ4 are shown). (D) Cell connection scheme between e- and i-cells. See the text for abbreviation definitions and explanations. (From Murakami, S., Zhang, T., Hirose, A., & Okada, Y. C. [2002]. Physiological origins of evoked magnetic fields and extracellular field potentials produced by the guinea-pig CA3. *Journal of Physiology, 544,* 237–251.)

the pyramidal cells, extracellular potentials in a CA3 slice, and magnetic fields above the slice. The model provides a quantitatively accurate account of these three types of data within a single theoretical framework, demonstrating that one can use the concepts in this model to understand the physiological origins of MEG and EEG.

4.3.2. Realistic Three-Dimensional Models of Cortical Neurons

A more realistic model of cortical principal neurons was developed for understanding MEG signals from the mammalian cerebral cortex (Murakami & Okada, 2006). Figure 4.4 shows the four principal neurons—Layer V pyramidal cell, Layer III pyramidal cell, Layer IV spiny stellate cell, and Layer III aspiny cell—that were represented in the 1996 Mainen model (Mainen & Sejnowski, 1996). In the Murakami and Okada model, each cell is described by a three-dimensional multicompartment in which each segment of the dendrites, axon, and soma is represented by a cylinder with a maximum length of 50 μm. Each compartment has its own geometrical properties of length and diameter, passive properties including membrane capacitance, membrane resistance and intracellular resistance, and five voltage-dependent

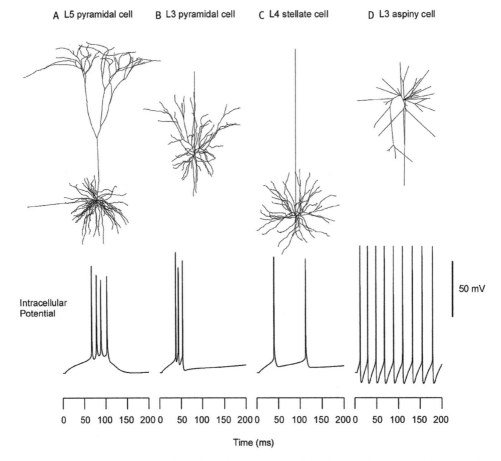

A L5 pyramidal cell   B L3 pyramidal cell   C L4 stellate cell   D L3 aspiny cell

Intracellular Potential

50 mV

0 50 100 150 200 0 50 100 150 200 0 50 100 150 200 0 50 100 150 200

Time (ms)

FIGURE 4.4 Multicompartment realistic three-dimensional models of principal neurons of the cerebral cortex. (Adapted from Murakami S., & Okada Y. [2006]. Contributions of principal neocortical neurons to magnetoencephalography and electroencephalography signals. *Journal of Physiology, 575*, 925–936.)

conductances [gNa, gK(DR), gK(M)—slow non-inactivating potassium conductance of the M type, gCa, and gK(C)]. The channel distributions in the Mainen model were used in the Murakami and Okada model. The transmembrane potentials (see Figure 4.4) produced by a burst input were consistent with empirical data for all four cell types, indicating that the biophysical models were appropriately implemented.

4.3.3. Differences Between the Classic and Modern Neuron Models

Figure 4.5 illustrates how an excitation of one region of the Layer V pyramidal cell, in this case with a constant inward current injection into the soma, produces depolarization and generates

intracellular currents in a classic cell with passive dendrites and in a modern cell with active conductances in the dendrites (Murakami & Okada, 2006). The neuron contained two types of active conductances, gNa and gK(DR), without additional conductances such as gCa and gK(C). The classic cell in Figure 4.5A was created by placing gNa and gK(DR) in the soma and axon. The cell in Figure 4.5B contained these two conductances uniformly distributed in the basal dendrites and the proximal trunk of the apical dendrites up to the first branch. The cells in Figures 4.5C and D had these conductances uniformly distributed throughout the dendrites up to the apical terminals. The channel density was two and a half times higher in the cell in Figure

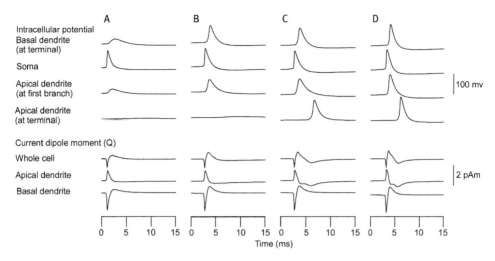

FIGURE 4.5 Comparison of membrane depolarization profile across the dendrites in a classic neuron and modern neurons (various versions of a neuron with active conductances). (A) gNa and gK(DR) only in the soma axon. (B) gNa and gK(DR) uniformly in soma, basal dendrites, and proximal apical dendrites up to the first branch. (C) Both conductances distributed uniformly throughout the dendrites. (D) gNa and gK(DR) 2.5× higher than in C. (From Murakami S., & Okada Y. [2006]. Contributions of principal neocortical neurons to magnetoencephalography and electroencephalography signals. *Journal of Physiology, 575*, 925–936.)

4.5D compared with the cell in Figure 4.5C. The stimulation produced depolarization in the soma, which in turn led to a cascade of activation of the passive and active conductances. The voltage gradient along the longitudinal axis of each compartment produced intracellular current. The net intracellular current was used to compute the current dipole moment Q in the cell. Current injection into the soma of the classic neuron (Figure 4.5A) produced a simple sharp spike in the soma. This potential electrotonically conducted to the apical and basal dendrites with a time delay and a rate of attenuation determined by the space constant. The depolarization did not reach the apical terminals. The cell in Figure 4.5B generated spikes in the basal and proximal apical dendrites with a delay as in model 1, but the amplitudes were larger. The depolarization still did not reach the apical terminals. In the cells in Figure 4.5C and D, the potential propagated toward the basal and apical terminals without the gradual decrease in amplitude. The spikes were similar in amplitude all the way up to the terminals of the apical dendrites. The net Q in the entire cell was biphasic in the classic model cell and in the

cell with active conductances limited to the first apical branch, but it was triphasic in the cells with fully distributed active conductances. The somatic activation produced a fast action current directed toward the basal terminals, and then the current toward the apical dendrites became stronger. The relative strengths of the basally and apically directed current depended on the geometry of each cell type, with the apical current dominating in the Layer III cell. The triphasic waveform is due to a long-lasting backpropagation of the sodium current to apical dendritic terminals.

The full models with gNa and gK(DR) throughout the dendrites support the backpropagation. The low-threshold, high-density gNa in the initial segment of the axon can become activated first even when there is a distal input in the apical dendrites. This sodium spike then produces the back-propagating spikes along the apical dendrites toward their terminals, as in actual neurons (Stuart et al., 1997). Note that the waveform of Q would have been more complex if gCa and gK(C) were present in this model neuron, as will be discussed later.

4.4. PHYSIOLOGICAL BASES OF MAGNETOENCEPHALOGRAPHY AND ELECTROENCEPHALO-GRAPHY: PHYSIOLOGICAL ORIGINS OF MAGNETO-ENCEPHALOGRAPHY AND ELECTROENCEPHALOGRAPHY SIGNALS FROM THE CEREBELLUM

The classic and modern neurons have been used to elucidate the physiological bases of MEG and EEG signals. I will focus on the genesis of population signals synchronized to a stimulation of the cells because it is both theoretically and experimentally simpler than analysis of rhythmic activity of the brain. Insights from studies of evoked activity will be useful for extending the analysis to understanding of brain rhythms (Steriade, 2001, 2003). Most of the work on this issue has been carried out by our group over the past 30 years

since the mid-1980s. Thus, the material will be drawn primarily from this line of work.

The nature of the intracellular currents producing magnetic and electric signals from the cerebellum has been studied using an in vitro preparation of an entire intact cerebellum of turtle because the cellular organization is locally essentially the same as in the human cerebellum, but the entire cerebellum is a flat, smooth, circular tissue with a three-dimensional orthogonal geometry well-suited for experimental analysis (Huang, Nicholson, & Okada, 1990; Lopez, Chan, Okada, & Nicholson, 1991; Okada, Lauritzen, & Nicholson, 1987; Okada & Nicholson, 1988; Okada, Nicholson, & Llinas, 1989). It is a flat spheroid, 1 mm in thickness in vitro (Figure 4.6C), although it is curved like a bowl in situ. It has the molecular layer below the dorsal surface, the Purkinje cell layer in the

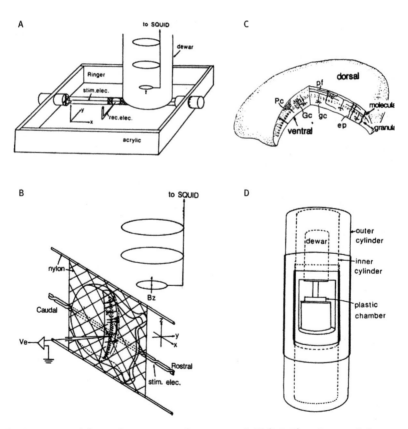

FIGURE 4.6 Experimental design for measuring the magnetic field (MEG) and extracellular potentials (EEG) from an intact cerebellum of turtle in vitro. (From Okada, Y. C., & Nicholson, C. [1988]. Magnetic evoked field associated with transcortical currents in turtle cerebellum. *Biophysical Journal, 53,* 723–731.)

middle, and the ventral granular. The afferents carrying the climbing fibers and mossy fibers enter the cerebellum through a pair of cerebellar peduncles. The climbing fibers make excitatory synaptic contacts around the proximal trunk of the apical dendrites of the Purkinje cells, each cell receiving synaptic input from a single climbing fiber. The mossy fibers make excitatory synaptic contacts onto numerous granule cells. The Purkinje cells send the efferents to the cerebellar nuclei, which then connect the cerebellum to many structures in the brain.

In the series of studies shown in Figure 4.6, an intact cerebellum, after being separated from the rest of the brain, was placed in a bath of physiological solution, suspended with a net just below the bath surface (see Figure 4.6A and B). The midline was stimulated with a pair of insulated wires that were twisted, except over the region of stimulation, where the wires were parallel to each other, and the insulating enamel was removed. The evoked extracellular potentials were measured with a glass micropipette inserted in the cerebellum at a known fixed depth. The evoked magnetic field was measured with a one channel gradiometer with the detection coil above the midline of the cerebellum. The magnetic field measurements were carried out inside a magnetic shield with a rotatable window (see Figure 4.6D). This methodology was developed de novo specifically for measuring the evoked magnetic field from this type of in vitro brain preparation.

Stimulation of the dorsal midline produced an evoked magnetic field outside the bath. The field 17 mm above the cerebellar midline varied systematically along the rostral-caudal axis of the cerebellum (Figure 4.7, left). The stimulus

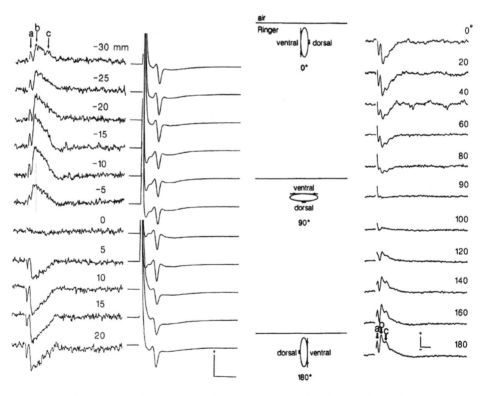

FIGURE 4.7   Evoked magnetic field measured along one axis parallel to the rostral-caudal axis of the cerebellum (*left*) and extracellular field potential measured at a fixed depth in the molecular layer (*right*). Calibration: 1 pT/2mV/10 ms (*left*), 1 pT/5 ms (*right*). (Adapted from Okada, Y. C., & Nicholson, C. [1988]. Magnetic evoked field associated with transcortical currents in turtle cerebellum. *Biophysical Journal, 53,* 723–731.)

artifact was eliminated with a cancellation coil in series with the isolated stimulating circuit. Thus, each trace shows only the field produced by intracellular currents in the cerebellum. The evoked potential simultaneously determined with each field measurement was invariant during all the measurements, showing that the stimulation and preparation were stable. The amplitudes of three components of the evoked field (a—1.0 ms, b—3.4 ms, c—8.4 ms) varied along the rostral-caudal axis according to the Biot-Savart law that governs the relationship between a dipole current source and the magnetic field (see Okada & Nicholson, 1988, for the quantitative analysis). This result showed that the magnetic field was generated by dipolar currents in the cerebellum.

Figure 4.7, right shows that these currents were perpendicular to the cerebellar surface, directed along the depth of the cerebellum, parallel to the longitudinal axis of the Purkinje cells. The figure shows the variation of the magnetic field at the field maximum as the cerebellum was continuously rotated around the cerebellar midline. The magnetic field was maximum when the cerebellum was oriented vertically with the field polarity being opposite at 0 and 180 degrees. The field was virtually zero at 90 degrees. The result is consistent with the theory (Geselowitz, 1970, 1973; Geselowitz & Grynszpan, 1973) and phantom studies (Cohen & Hosaka, 1976) indicating that the magnetic field should be due to the component of the current tangential to the bath surface in our experimental study. Thus, the physiological current was oriented along the longitudinal axis of the Purkinje cells. Other studies have shown that the magnetic field was due to a dipolar current sink and source located in the molecular layer, indicating that the field was produced by intracellular currents in the Purkinje cells (Okada, 1989; Okada et al., 1989). Thus, the Purkinje neurons appear to be the principal neurons capable of producing magnetic fields from the cerebellum. Since the electrophysiology and anatomy of cerebellum are invariant across the evolutionary scale up to the human,

the results suggest that the Purkinje cells in human cerebellum may be capable of producing evoked magnetic fields detectable outside the head. Some reports have claimed detection of activity originating in the human cerebellum recorded with MEG (Hashimoto, Kimura, Tanosaki, Iguchi, & Sekihara, 2003; Ioannides & Fenwick, 2005; Jousmaki, Hamalainen, & Hari, 1996; Tesche & Karhu, 1997).

4.5. PHYSIOLOGICAL BASES OF MAGNETOENCEPHALOGRAPHY AND ELECTRO-ENCEPHALOGRAPHY: PHYSIOLOGICAL ORIGINS OF MAGNETOENCEPHALOGRAPHY AND ELECTROENCEPHALOGRAPHY SIGNALS FROM THE HIPPOCAMPUS

4.5.1. Experimental Analysis

The physiological origins of the magnetic and electrical signals from the hippocampus were studied using in vitro guinea pig hippocampal slice preparations (Kyuhou & Okada 1993; Okada, Wu, & Kyuhou, 1997; Wu & Okada 1998, 1999, 2000). Figure 4.8 shows the experimental arrangement. A transverse hippocampal slice of guinea pig was prepared following the conventional method, by slicing the hippocampus along the plane orthogonal to the longitudinal axis of the intact hippocampus (see Figure 4.8A). Alternatively, a longitudinal slice was prepared by cutting the hippocampus along the plane orthogonal to the conventional transverse plane and then sectioning the slice to prepare a rectangular slice of CA1 or CA3. The resulting longitudinal slices were rectangular, as shown in Figure 4.8C, containing the pyramidal cell layer and the stratum oriens and radiatum. The longitudinal axes of the pyramidal cells, which ran orthogonally to the cell layer, were parallel to each other. Thus, the evoked field from these neurons summated to produce detectable MEG signals above the slice. The slice was placed on a nylon net of the

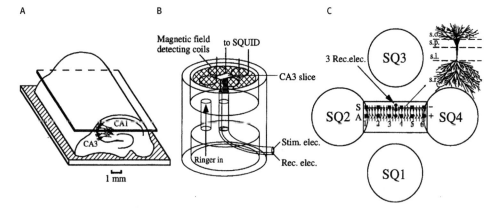

FIGURE 4.8   Experimental method for measuring intracellular potentials, extracellular potentials, and magnetic field just out the slice. (A) The hippocampus of guinea pig was cut conventionally along the transverse plane to prepare transverse slices or cut along the plane perpendicular to the transverse plane to prepare CA1 or CA3 slices. (B) A slice was placed on a nylon net. Oxygenated Ringer solution (physiological saline) flowed around the slice. An array of bipolar stimulating electrodes and extracellular recording electrodes were placed in the slice from below. The magnetic field was measured with a four-channel Superconducting QUantum-Interference Device (SQUID) array 2 mm above. (C) Geometrical arrangement of a rectangular CA1 or CA3 slice with an array of bipolar stimulating electrodes, an array of extracellular recording electrodes, and four magnetic field detection coils (4 mm diameter on a 6-mm square) 2 mm above the slice. *Inset* shows schematic of a pyramidal cell. (From Wu, J., & Okada, Y. C. [1998]. Physiological bases of the synchronized population spikes and slow wave of the magnetic field generated by a guinea pig longitudinal CA3 slice preparation. *Electroencephalography and Clinical Neurophysiology, 107,* 361–373.)

slice chamber (see Figure 4.8B). The pyramidal neurons were horizontal and parallel to the surface of the bath in order to maximize the signals from these neurons. As shown in Figure 4.8C, an array of bipolar electrodes was placed along the pyramidal cell layer, and the pyramidal cells were depolarized in the apical dendrite, soma, or basal dendrite region. The resulting synchronized population activity in the slice was measured with an array of extracellular electrode along the longitudinal axis of the pyramidal cells simultaneously with a four-channel miniature magnetic field detection coil array (each coil 4 mm in diameter separated by 6 mm on a square grid) 2 mm above the slice. In some experiments, intracellular potentials were measured from the same preparation using the same stimulating electrode array or a single bipolar electrode for relating the three types of signals from the slice preparation.

Figure 4.9 shows the spatial distribution of the magnetic field measured above a longitudinal CA1 slice (Okada et al., 1997). It is bipolar with a mirror-image distribution centered over the slice. This dipolar pattern is typical of the field distribution from hippocampal slice preparations. It shows that the field was produced by dipolar currents along the longitudinal axis of the pyramidal cells that were oriented perpendicular to the cell layer.

Figure 4.10 shows the relationship between the evoked magnetic field on two sides of the slice and extracellular potentials along the longitudinal axis of the pyramidal cells orthogonal to the cell layer in a longitudinal CA3 slice (at the locations shown in Figure 4.8C). The relationship between these two types of signals depends on placement and polarity of the bipolar stimulating electrodes. When the soma region of the pyramidal cells was depolarized with the array of bipolar electrodes (see Figure 4.10A), spike component **a** of the magnetic field had the polarity indicating that the underlying intracellular current was directed toward the basal dendrite,

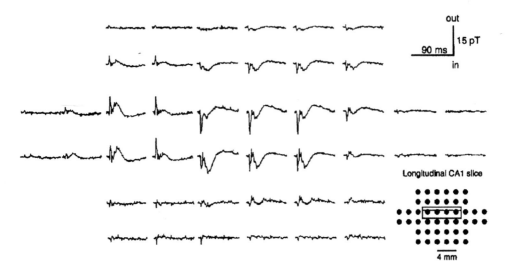

FIGURE 4.9   Spatial distribution of the magnetic field 2 mm above the longitudinal CA1 slice of guinea pig at the locations shown in the *inset* relative to the slice. Stimulus at 10 ms in the traces; artifacts were small and removed. (From Okada, Y. C., Wu, J., & Kyuhou, S. [1997]. Genesis of MEG signals in a mammalian CNS structure. *Electroencephalography and Clinical Neurophysiology, 103,* 474–485.)

whereas components **b, c,** and **d** all had the same polarity indicating that the underlying current was directed toward the apical direction. The polarities were reversed when the apical dendrite area was stimulated with the negative electrode in the apical layer (see Figure 4.10B). The

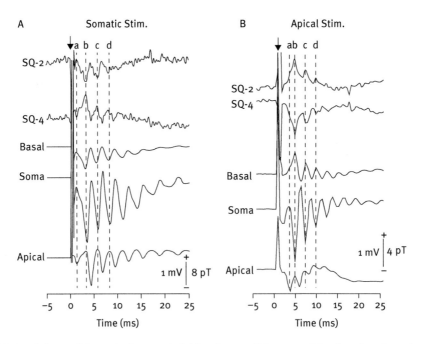

FIGURE 4.10   Polarity of the evoked magnetic field and extracellular potential at three locations along the pyramidal cells for the somatic (A, negative electrode in the soma area) and apical (B, negative electrode in the apical dendrite area) stimulations. (From Wu, J., & Okada, Y. C. [1998]. Physiological bases of the synchronized population spikes and slow wave of the magnetic field generated by a guinea pig longitudinal CA3 slice preparation. *Electroencephalography and Clinical Neurophysiology, 107,* 361–373.)

latencies of these spike peaks matched the peaks of the spikes in the extracellular potentials measured simultaneously at the different locations along the longitudinal axis of the pyramidal cells, indicating that the electrical signal was produced by the same underlying intracellular current. The polarities of the potentials were consistent with the direction of the underlying intracellular currents for the evoked field.

Intracellular potentials in the pyramidal cells were measured in addition to the external magnetic field and extracellular potentials in order to test whether these three diverse types of signals from the slices are produced by common intracellular currents in the preparation. The experimental arrangement shown in Figure 4.8 was used to measure evoked fields at locations SQ-2 and SQ-4 simultaneously with the extracellular potentials at three locations along the longitudinal axis of the pyramidal cells (Figure 4.11, top). In a separate set of experiments, the same preparation was used to measure the extracellular potential (Vex) simultaneously with the intracellular potential (Vin) from a pyramidal cell (see Figure 4.11, bottom). The Vex was used as reference for comparing the evoked field and the intracellular potential. Although the waveforms were related, there were many differences among these signals. It was, therefore, difficult to experimentally identify the exact relationship between these three types of signals.

4.5.2. Theoretical Account of Evoked Magnetic Field, Extracellular Potentials, and Intracellular Potentials

We used the mathematical model of the neuronal networks in the CA3 described earlier (see Figure 4.3) to better understand the relationship among these signals. Our objective was to determine quantitatively whether they were all due to common underlying intracellular currents.

4.5.3. Evoked Magnetic Field

Figure 4.12 shows that the model can account for the measured evoked field under the two conditions of stimulation. The theoretical waveforms matched the measured waveforms in shape, latency, polarity, and amplitude of all the components. Under the somatic stimulation, the evoked field was biphasic for both the empirical and theoretical waveforms. Under the apical stimulation, the waveform was triphasic for both. The time and magnitude scales are common for theory and data. Thus, the spike latencies were nearly identical for both the model and data. The amplitude and shape of the slower variations were also captured by the model. The model, however, could not capture all the features accurately. The first spike in the evoked field under the somatic stimulation was larger in the data than in the model. The latency of the second slow component under the somatic stimulation was slightly shorter for the model than the data. Even though there were some discrepancies between the model and data, it appears that the model was able to capture the essential features of the empirical data.

The model was also able to account for the effects of various specific blockers of active conductances. Figure 4.13 shows the effect of tetraethylammonium (TEA), which enhances the slow wave for the evoked field. The initial component was not affected, but the slow wave increased in amplitude when TEA was added to the bath. The effect could be explained as due to TEA shifting the steady-state activation curve of gK(C) to a more depolarized direction, in the example shown in Figure 4.13 from a depolarization voltage (V) of 10 mV to 12 mV (Murakami et al., 2002). Similarly, the model could explain effects of a specific blocker 4AP, which blocks gK(A) and extends the activation time constant of AMPA receptors, on the evoked field (Murakami et al., 2002).

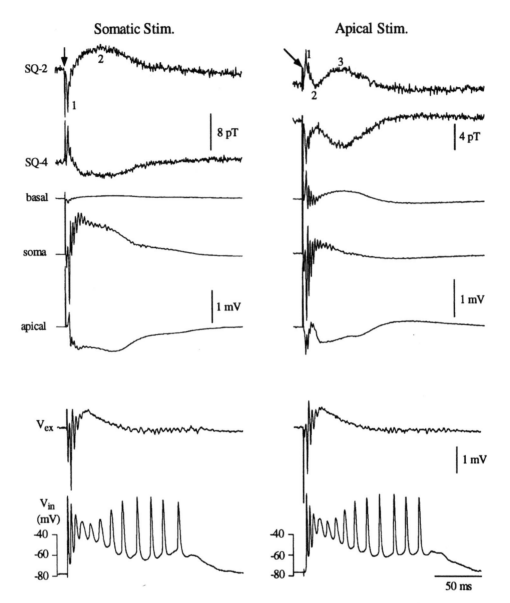

FIGURE 4.11 Evoked magnetic field, extracellular potentials, and intracellular potentials from a pyramidal cell measured in a longitudinal CA3 slice of guinea pig for stimulation of the soma and apical dendrite areas. (From Wu, J., & Okada, Y. C. [1998]. Physiological bases of the synchronized population spikes and slow wave of the magnetic field generated by a guinea pig longitudinal CA3 slice preparation. *Electroencephalography and Clinical Neurophysiology, 107*, 361–373.)

4.5.4. Intracellular Potentials in the Pyramidal Cells

The model could also explain the measured intracellular potentials from a pyramidal cell recorded at different positions relative to a pair of bipolar stimulation electrodes placed along the longitudinal axis of the pyramidal cells (Figures 4.8 and 4.14). The intracellular potential was recorded at four different locations along the pyramidal cell layer relative to a bipolar stimulating electrode under both the somatic and apical stimulation conditions. The model captured the change in latency of the evoked response and the waveform exhibiting a train of spikes superimposed on a burst.

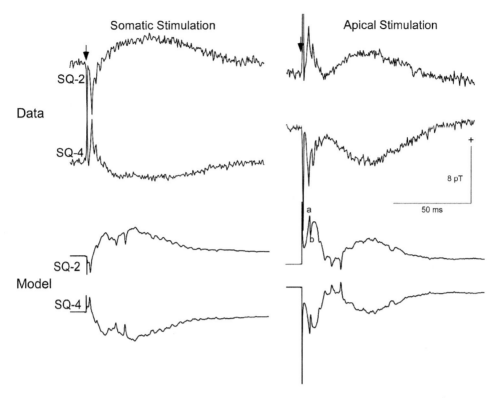

FIGURE 4.12   Theoretical waveform and measured magnetic field for a longitudinal CA3 slice. (From Murakami, S., Zhang, T., Hirose, A., & Okada, Y. C. [2002]. Physiological origins of evoked magnetic fields and extracellular field potentials produced by the guinea-pig CA3. *Journal of Physiology, 544*, 237–251.)

4.5.5. Extracellular Potentials in the Slice

The model could also account for the laminar extracellular field potential profiles obtained with the somatic and apical stimulations. Figure 4.15 shows the results for a somatic stimulation condition. Two laminar profiles of the extracellular potential are shown, one recorded close to a pair of bipolar stimulating electrodes ("Direct stimulation") and another recorded between two pairs of stimulation electrode ("Synaptic stimulation") where the cells are mostly activated synaptically. The recording positions are shown relative to the cell layer. For the Direct stimulation, the model could account for the waveform, polarity, latency, and amplitude of the potentials across three layers of the hippocampus. The model accounted for the latency of the initial component **a** and the variation of its latency with laminar position. The model also correctly showed a positive polarity of the slow wave in the oriens/cell layer

region and a negative polarity in the radiatum. For the Synaptic stimulation, the model similarly provided a quantitatively accurate account of the shape and polarity of the slow wave with a train of spikes superimposed on the wave. The amplitudes of all the components of the theoretical waveforms were comparable to the measured.

In conclusion, the quantitatively accurate account of the three types of data given by a single model indicates that these three diverse types of data were produced by the common underlying intracellular current.

4.5.6. Contributions of Active Conductances to Generation of Magnetoencephalography and Electroencephalography Signals

The contribution of each active conductance separately to the MEG and EEG signals is very difficult to analyze empirically. However, using a mathematical model, this is possible. Murakami, Hirose, & Okada (2003) determined the current dipole moment Q(t) produced by each major conductance in their model as a function of time. Also, they determined the Q(t) due to a combination of conductances. Figure 4.16 shows the Q(t) for a combination of gNa + gK(DR) and the Q(t) for gCa + gK(C). The contributions of gK(A), gK(AHP), and synaptic currents were estimated by computing the Q(t) as each new conductance was activated in the model neurons. The dashed waveforms are the Q's produced by all the conductances combined, for all cells and separately for the directly activated and the synaptically activated populations of neurons. For the directly activated cell, the sum of gNa and gK(DR) accounts for the spikes but does not explain the overall envelope of the waveform. The sum of gCa and gK(C) accounts for the slow variation of the Q(t), but not the spikes. These four conductances together account for most of the Q(t). gK(A) and gK(AHP) have little effect. The synaptic current accounts for the slow component. The synaptically activated cell produced a slowly varying Q with its magnitude comparable to that for the directly activated cell. The Q was mostly due

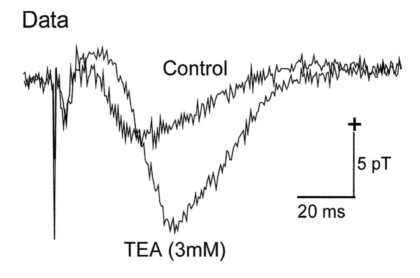

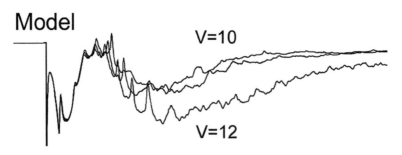

FIGURE 4.13   Effects of tetraethylammonium (TEA) on the evoked field explained by increasing the activation voltage of gK(C). (From Murakami, S., Zhang, T., Hirose, A., & Okada, Y. C. [2002]. Physiological origins of evoked magnetic fields and extracellular field potentials produced by the guinea-pig CA3. *Journal of Physiology, 544*, 237–251.)

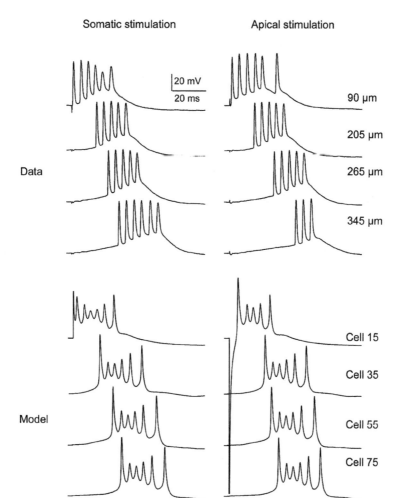

Somatic stimulation   Apical stimulation

20 mV
20 ms

Data

90 μm
205 μm
265 μm
345 μm

Model

Cell 15
Cell 35
Cell 55
Cell 75

FIGURE 4.14   Comparison of the theoretical and experimentally measured intracellular potentials of the pyramidal cell as a function of position of the cell relative to a pair of bipolar stimulation electrode. (From Murakami, S., Zhang, T., Hirose, A., & Okada, Y. C. [2002]. Physiological origins of evoked magnetic fields and extracellular field potentials produced by the guinea-pig CA3. *Journal of Physiology, 544*, 237–251.)

to the combination of gCa and gK(C), with some notable visible contributions of gNa and gK(DR) and the synaptic currents. The delay in the onset of the Q reflects the position of the cell relative to the stimulating electrode and intervening neurons that activate synaptically activated cells.

These results are based on a mathematical model of the neuronal network that has been validated experimentally by comparing theoretical results against empirical results. Thus, they are valuable for inferring the contributions of various types of intracellular currents to MEG and EEG signals. The Q(t) produced

by the underlying population of neurons in Figure 4.16 are proportional to the MEG and EEG signals. Thus, the results can be used to infer the contributions of different types of currents to evoked MEG and EEG signals. We conclude that the slowly varying signals in general mostly reflect intracellular currents produced by calcium spikes and associated potassium conductances, whereas the population spikes are mostly due to the sodium and potassium conductances. This view is quite different from the classic view of MEG and EEG being produced by graded postsynaptic currents produced by synaptic activation.

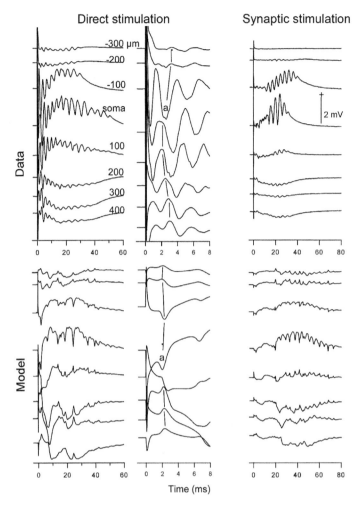

FIGURE 4.15 Laminar extracellular potential profile in a longitudinal CA3 slice measured (Data) and theoretical (Model) for somatic stimulation. (From Murakami, S., Zhang, T., Hirose, A., & Okada, Y. C. [2002]. Physiological origins of evoked magnetic fields and extracellular field potentials produced by the guinea-pig CA3. *Journal of Physiology, 544,* 237–251.)

4.6. PHYSIOLOGICAL BASES OF MAGNETOENCEPHALOGRAPHY AND ELECTROENCEPHALOGRAPHY: PHYSIOLOGICAL ORIGINS OF MAGNETOENCEPHALOGRAPHY AND ELECTROENCEPHALOGRAPHY SIGNALS FROM THE CEREBRAL CORTEX

4.6.1. Evoked Magnetic Fields From the Cerebral Cortex Based on Single-Neuron Models

The realistic single-neuron models of the principal neurons in the cerebral cortex (see

Figure 4.4) provide insights into the roles of these neuronal cell types in producing the MEG and EEG signals from the neocortex. Figure 4.17 shows the $Q(t)$ for each of the four principal neurons with the full array of conductances implemented in the cells. The waveforms are produced by constant current injection into the soma. The Layer 5 pyramidal cell is capable of producing a Q showing a strong burst with a train of spikes riding on the burst. The Layer 3 pyramidal cell produces a similar burst with an overlapping spike train. The magnitude of the burst-related Q is stronger for the Layer 5 cell than for the Layer 3

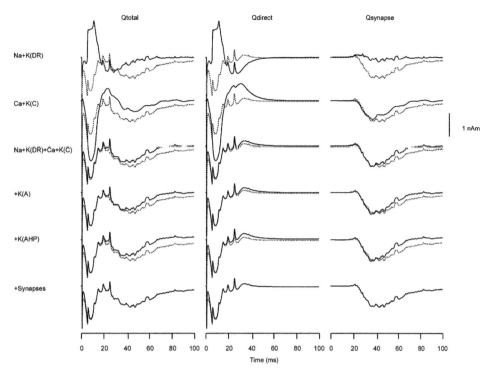

FIGURE 4.16   Relative contributions of the different conductances to the aggregate population current dipole moment Q(t). Apical stimulation condition. Qdirect = Q for the population of neurons directly activated by the stimulation; Qsynapse = Q for the synaptically activated population of cells; Qtotal = Qdirect + Qsynapse. *Dashed curves* = Q(t)'s due to all conductances. (From Murakami S., Hirose A., & Okada Y. C. [2003]. Contribution of ionic currents to magnetoencephalography [MEG] and electroencephalography [EEG] signals generated by guinea-pig CA3 slices. *Journal of Physiology, 553,* 975–985.)

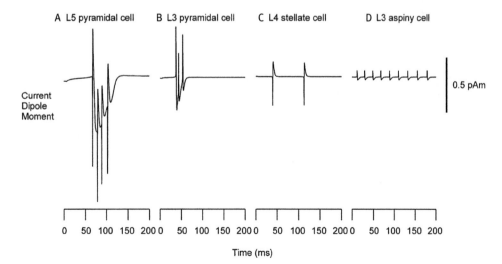

FIGURE 4.17   Net current dipole moment Q(t) in individual principal neurons of the mammalian cerebral cortex. (From Murakami S., & Okada Y. [2006]. Contributions of principal neocortical neurons to magnetoencephalography and electroencephalography signals. *Journal of Physiology, 575,* 925–936.)

cell. The spiny stellate cell in Layer 4 produces a single spike followed by a brief spiky component. The Q of the burst was about 0.46 pAm for the Layer 5 cell and about 0.19 pAm for the Layer 3 cell, whereas the second component of the Q for the spiny stellate cell was about 0.12 pAm. The longitudinal axes of these three types of neurons are perpendicular to the cortical surface. This implies that these three types of cells could produce a magnetic field of about 404 fT, about 168 fT, and about 101 fT when 10,000 such cells are synchronously active at a distance of 2 cm from a sensor array. These levels of magnetic field can be clearly detected with the modern MEG instruments after averaging about 100 responses because their noise levels are typically 5 to 10 fT/$\sqrt{\text{Hz}}$. The aspiny stellate cell in Layer 3 could also produce some Q, but their net current across a population of similar cells is expected to self-cancel because of random orientations of these neurons.

The model also revealed that the spikes could produce a strong net dipolar current. In the classic views, graded postsynaptic currents were considered as the dominant contributor to the macroscopic signals outside the brain. The spikes were believed to produce quadrupolar currents and thus not to produce signals far away from the active neurons. These results from the realistic neuron models indicate it may be possible to detect the spikes with MEG and EEG if a sufficiently large number of neurons are synchronously active. The Q's of the spikes were approximately 0.5 pAm. This means it is necessary to have only 10,000 cells firing synchronously to produce a MEG signal of as much as 400 to 500 fT. This unexpected result is supported by various lines of experimental evidence. Our data, to be described next, from an in vivo swine with a large highly developed gyrencephalic brain strongly support this conclusion. Jones and Barth (1999) have shown that the barrel cortex of the rat, its primary somatosensory cortex representing the vibrissa, is capable of producing highly synchronized high-frequency (>200 Hz) oscillations. Curio, Hashimoto, and their

colleagues have shown that the somatosensory cortex of humans can produce highly synchronized signals around 600 Hz detectable with MEG and EEG (Curio et al., 1994; Hashimoto, Mashiko, & Imada, 1996). Telenczuk, Baker, Herz, & Curio (2011) have shown that the somatosensory cortex of monkey can produce high-frequency spike-related signals detectable with EEG.

4.6.2. Evoked Magnetoencephalography and Electroencephalography Signals From the Cerebral Cortex in Vivo

The physiological origins of evoked MEG and EEG from the cerebral cortex were studied using an in vivo juvenile swine preparation (Ikeda, Leyba, Bartolo, & Okada, 2002; Ikeda, Wang, & Okada, 2005). Figure 4.18 shows the somatosensory evoked field (SEF) measured at 2 mm above the primary somatosensory area (SI) of the swine. The snout is represented around the SI cortex centered at the sulcal naris (Okada, Lähteenmäki, & Xu, 1999). The activity was produced by electrical transcutaneous stimulation of one location of the snout. The spatial distribution in Figure 4.18B is dipolar, as is the case for the isolated turtle cerebellum and guinea pig hippocampal slice preparations. The field reverses polarity at location marked "x," which is on the lateral sulcal edge of the SI. The polarity of the first component shows it was produced by intracellular currents directed toward the cortical surface in the lateral sulcal wall of the SI. Figure 4.18, right shows the wide-band and narrow-band SEFs at four locations centered at "x." The initial component of the SEF contains high-frequency signals centered at 600 Hz (Ikeda et al., 2002). The high-frequency signal reverses its polarity at the same location as for the wideband SEF, indicating that both were generated by the same active tissue.

Figure 4.19 shows the laminar profile of both the wide- and narrow-band somatic evoked potentials (SEPs) measured in the active tissue.

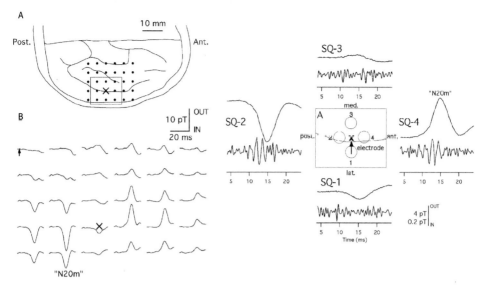

FIGURE 4.18 Somatosensory evoked field (SEF) from the swine. (A) Exposed cerebral cortex of the swine. (B) SEF measured at locations shown in A. (C) Wide-band (1–3,000 Hz) SEF and high-frequency (417–2,083 Hz) SEF at four locations centered at "x." Laminar extracellular potentials were measured from the same preparation after the SEF measurements with a microelectrode inserted perpendicular to the cortical surface in the sulcus at "x." (Adapted from Ikeda, H., Wang, Y., & Okada, Y. C. [2005]. Origins of the somatic N20 and high-frequency oscillations evoked by trigeminal stimulation in the piglets. *Clinical Neurophysiology, 116,* 827–841.)

The wideband SEP showed polarity reversal along the depth. An in vivo application of a nonspecific antagonist of excitatory amino acid receptors, kynurenic acid ("Kyna"), blocked the initial component of the wide-band SEP. Kyna did not affect the initial components of the high-frequency SEP, but it blocked the later components, indicating that the initial component was presynaptic, arising from the ascending axons of the specific thalamic neurons located in Layer IV, whereas the subsequent components were postsynaptic to the first input. The high-frequency signals detectable with MEG are consistent with the theoretical results obtained with the realistic model of the principal neurons (see Figure 4.17).

The relationship between SEF and SEP is shown in Figure 4.20. These signals were measured *simultaneously* from the SI of the swine in vivo in order to compare them under the identical conditions (Ikeda et al., 2005). The time traces are during the presynaptic and postsynaptic periods, leading to the first major wide-band component ("N20"). For the high-frequency component, the current source density (CSD) profile obtained from the laminar depth profile of the SEP shows a quadrupolar component with the sink in Layer IV, the expected location for axonal terminals from the specific thalamic axons, at time **a** (9 ms). This initial event leads to a dipolar current sink-source pattern which moves to Layer II by 16 ms. It produces the second current sink-source pair in Layer V, starting at 11 ms. The timing of the current sink-source pairs corresponds exactly to the high-frequency signals in the SEF. The wide-band N20 emerges starting around 10 ms and reaches the peak at 15 ms. This component is due to a pair of current sink-sources, one in the Layer II/III and the other in Layer V. The presence of these two dipolar generators is consistent with the realistic cortical neuron model of Figure 4.4. The onset and peak latencies of the SEF precisely match the peak of the CSD profile simultaneously recorded with the SEF.

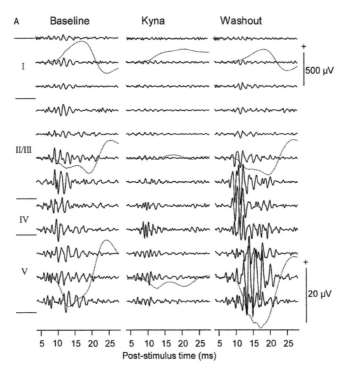

FIGURE 4.19   Somatic evoked potential (SEP) measured along the lamina of the active sulcus of the SI cortex. (A) Wide-band and narrow-band SEP before, during, and after application of a nonspecific antagonist, kynurenic acid ("Kyna"), of excitatory amino acid receptors into the active tissue. (Adapted from Ikeda, H., Leyba, L., Bartolo, A., & Okada, Y. C. [2002]. Synchronized spikes of thalamocortical axonal terminals and cortical neurons are detectable outside the brain of piglet with high-resolution MEG. *Journal of Neurophysiology, 87*, 626–630.)

In conclusion, the evoked MEG and EEG signals from the cerebral cortex appear to be generated by the same intracellular generators, in this case the cells in Layers II/III and V. This conclusion is consistent with the results obtained for the cerebellum and hippocampus.

4.7. INSIGHTS GAINED FROM STUDIES ON PHYSIOLOGICAL BASES OF MAGNETOENCEPHALOGRAPHY AND ELECTROENCEPHALOGRAPHY

The systematic series of studies carried out since the mid-1980s has provided some useful insights into the physiological bases of MEG and EEG signals. The results from the three structures of the brain—cerebellum, hippocampus, and cerebral cortex—that have been accumulated over a 30-year period have provided evidence pointing to a view of physiological origins of evoked MEG and EEG that is different from the classic view. The results also revealed some interesting consistency across all the studies on the nature of the underlying neuronal currents generating MEG and EEG signals.

4.7.1. Magnetoencephalography and Electroencephalography Signals Reflect the Currents Generated by Sodium, Calcium, and Potassium Conductances

The classic view is that MEG and EEG signals reflect graded postsynaptic currents in

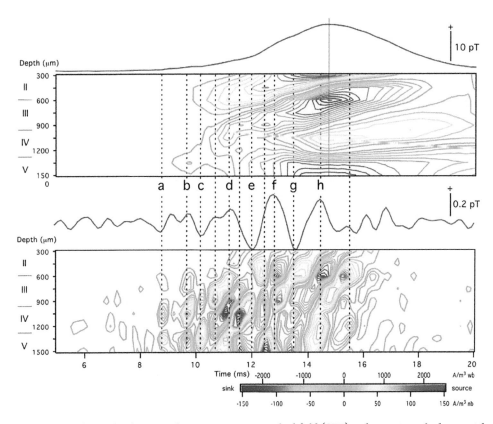

FIGURE 4.20   Relationship between the somatosensory evoked field (SEF) and somatic evoked potential (SEP) in the primary somatosensory cortex of swine for the wide-band "N20" and high-frequency component (400–2,000 Hz). SEF and the laminar profiles of SEP in the active sulcal area of the cortex were recorded simultaneously. The laminar profile was used to compute the current source density (CSD) along the depth. (From Ikeda, H., Wang, Y., & Okada, Y. C. [2005]. Origins of the somatic N20 and high-frequency oscillations evoked by trigeminal stimulation in the piglets. *Clinical Neurophysiology, 116*, 827–841.)

the dendrites (Lopes da Silva & Rotterdam, 1987). According to the modern view incorporated in the mathematical models used to study the genesis from the hippocampus and cerebral cortex (Murakami et al., 2002; Murakami & Okada, 2006), the MEG and EEG signals are produced by four types of currents—postsynaptic currents, passive electrotonically produced currents, dendritic currents produced by gNa/gK(DR) and gCa/gK(C), and spikes generated by gNa and gK(DR). The synaptic and graded passively generated electronic currents contribute relatively little. In the directly activated neurons, spikes are determined by a combination of gNa and gK(DR), whereas the slow envelope is mostly due to a combination of gCa and gK(C). The sum of these four active conductances accounts for most of the MEG and EEG signals from this population of cells. For the synaptically activated neurons, gNa and gK(DR) contribute little to the overall Q because the timing of spike generation is not synchronized; most of the Q is due to the combination of gCa and gK(C), which produces more slowly varying currents and thus less cancellation across the population of this type of cells. Evoked MEG and EEG signals from humans and in vivo animal preparations are expected to be a weighted sum of the activity from the directly activated population of neurons and synaptically activated neurons with the weight depending on the manner of external stimulation.

4.7.2. Synchronization of Neuronal Activity Within Local Neuronal Circuits

The studies of the hippocampus in vitro and cerebral cortex in vivo from mammalian brain preparations revealed that neurons in local circuits can produce highly synchronized activity across a population of neurons. A train of spikes was often seen in the evoked MEG and EEG signals from hippocampal slices. For example, the spike train was clearly seen in the results shown in Figure 4.3 for a longitudinal CA3 slice. In this preparation, the inhibitory circuit was blocked with an antagonist of GABA-A, picrotoxin, added to the bath. However, a synchronized train of spikes was observed in the extracellular potentials averaged across the entire length of the slice and with the magnetic field recording from the same preparation in normal physiological saline without picrotoxin (Okada et al., 1997). In this study, the evoked activity was elicited by an array of bipolar electrodes along the pyramidal cell layer; thus, the synchronization produced by this array could have been responsible for the synchronize spikes. However, synchronized spikes were observed from spontaneously occurring activities in the same preparation in picrotoxin and 4AP (Okada & Xu, 1996), suggesting that the neurons tend to synchronize their activity when the inhibitory circuit is blocked.

There is stronger evidence that the central nervous system produces highly synchronized activity. The trigeminal pathway in the juvenile in vivo produces highly synchronized spikes in the trigeminal nucleus when the snout is electrically stimulated (Kato, Wang, Papuashvili, & Okada, 2003). The presynaptic spikes from the specific trigeminal projection fibers of the thalamus and postsynaptic activity in the primary somatosensory cortex were highly synchronized (Ikeda et al., 2002, 2005). The synchronized activity was evident postsynaptically at the cortical level, as was shown in Figures 4.18 to 4.20 (Ikeda et al., 2002, 2005).

The realistic model of the principal neurons of the cortex showed that the action potentials generated by gNa and gK(DR) are capable of producing strong current dipole moments and therefore should be detectable with MEG or EEG if a population of neurons fire synchronously. Thus, these spikes could be studied with the macrotechniques. Curio, Hashimoto, and their colleagues have shown that high-frequency signals could be detected from the somatosensory cortex of humans and monkeys (Curio et al., 1994; Hashimoto et al., 1996; Telenczuk et al., 2011). Based on our analysis, these signals are most likely produced by spike trains. Therefore, MEG and EEG could be used to study the information carried by the synchronized population activity in humans. We consider, as others have suggested earlier (Jones & Barth, 1999; Telenczuk et al., 2011), that synchronization of activity across a population of neurons is useful for increasing the accuracy, reliability, and information content of the signals processed in the brain.

4.7.3. Invariance in Anatomy and Physiology Generating Magnetoencephalography and Electroencephalography Signals

A meta-analysis of the results obtained from the diverse set of preparations during the last 30 years has revealed interesting invariant properties of MEG and EEG. Figure 4.21 summarizes the current dipole moment density q expressed as current dipole moment Q per unit surface area of the cortex in units of nAm/mm^2 for a wide range of species across the evolutionary scale (Murakami & Okada, 2015). Figure 4.21A shows the values of q obtained from the three different preparations used in our group. The values are shown separately for different experiments. These values have been corrected for distortions produced by the final size of the magnetic field detector and secondary sources present at boundaries

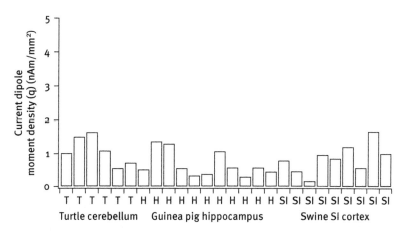

FIGURE 4.21 Current dipole moment density **q** in units of nAm/mm². **q** is the density of Q within the cortex normalized to a unit surface of cortex in mm². (A) **q** from different experiments using three types of preparations used by Okada and his colleagues between 1984 and 2015. (B) **q** estimated for other brain tissues based on estimates of Q and active cortical surface obtained by other investigators in addition to ours. (From Murakami, S., & Okada, Y. [2015]. Invariance in current dipole moment density across brain structures and species: Physiological constraint for neuroimaging. *NeuroImage, 111*, 49–58.)

separating regions of different electrical conductivities. The averaged values of **q** in these three types of preparation are shown together with the values either directly obtained or estimated from values of Q and surface area of the active cortex reported in previous studies by others for a diverse range of species across the evolutionary scale ranging from reptiles to humans. The maximum value of **q** is about 1 nAm/mm² for this range of species, except in the rat, in which the single value of **q** estimated by Riera et al. (2012) is about twice that of this maximum value. It is possible that this anomalously high value may be due to the presence of two pairs of dipoles within the same barrel column, adding to the empirically measured value of **q**.

The mathematical model of pyramidal cells shown in Figure 4.3 was used to find out whether this value of 1 nAm/mm² is consistent with the model (Murakami & Okada, 2015). Figure 4.22A shows the intracellular potential (transmembrane potential) and current dipole moment Q in a cell of the model as a function of cell radius. The time waveform and amplitude of the intracellular potential was virtually invariant of cell radius, even though the peak

voltages were slightly larger for the smaller cells. The Q, on the other hand, depended on cell radius. Figure 4.22B relates the peak value of Q to radius of the cylindrical cell, separately for the first spike and the burst. (Note that the vertical axis of Figure 4.22B is correct. The vertical axis in the original article was erroneously 1/10 of the values shown here.) This dependence is expected because Q is proportional to the cross-sectional area of the cylinder when the current density in the cell is constant. The value of **q**, however, is nearly independent of cell radius, as shown in Figure 4.23. The value is about 2 to 3 nAm/mm² for the first spike and 3 to 0.7 nAm/mm² for the burst. These values were obtained without adjusting any of the parameters of the model used to explain the empirically measured intracellular potential, extracellular potentials, and magnetic field from the hippocampal CA3 preparation. Therefore, the theoretical values are within a factor of two of the empirically determined values across the wide range of species without any adjustment of the model parameters.

The invariance in **q** found from the above theoretical and experimental analysis of MEG data is consistent with the estimate obtained

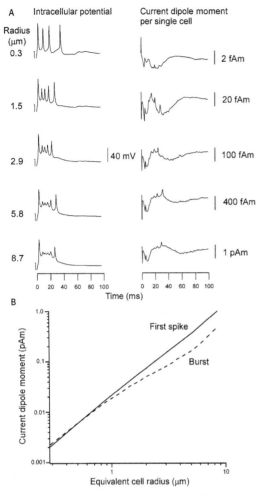

A   Intracellular potential   Current dipole moment
per single cell

Radius
(μm)
0.3

1.5

2.9 |40 mV

5.8

8.7

| 2 fAm

| 20 fAm

| 100 fAm

| 400 fAm

| 1 pAm

0 20 40 60 80 100   0 20 40 60 80 100
Time (ms)

B

FIGURE 4.22   Relationship between intracellular potential and Q versus cell diameter in the cylindrical model neuron. (A) Intracellular potential and Q versus cell radius. (B) Q versus cell radius for the first spike and burst amplitude. (From Murakami, S., & Okada, Y. [2015]. Invariance in current dipole moment density across brain structures and species: Physiological constraint for neuroimaging. *NeuroImage, 111*, 49–58.)

with magnetic resonance imaging (MRI) (Sundaram et al., 2016) (Figure 4.24). These investigators have placed an isolated intact turtle cerebellum (see Figure 4.6C) in a cylindrical chamber inside a 4.7T MRI scanner. Stimulation of one cerebellar peduncle (at the location shown by a *circle* in the peduncle in Figure 4.24A) elicited synchronized metabotropically mediated population activity

in the caudal portion of the tissue ipsilateral to the side of stimulation. The local field potential (LFP) was monitored with a microelectrode placed in the caudal area. The currents oriented along the depth of the cerebellum produced a circular local magnetic field Δ**B** around it. This field was directed along the same direction as the Bo field of the magnet, with the field oriented in the same direction as Bo on the left side and in the opposite direction on the right side of the active tissue. This produced a phase shift Δφ in the precession of protons in the water molecules with Δφ greater than 0 on the left side and Δφ less than 0 on the right side. The phase shift is proportional to the value of Δ**B** for the gradient echo method used. The values of Δ**B** calculated from Δφ were greater than 0 on the left side and less than 0 on the right side (see Figure 4.24A). These values of Δ**B** can be treated just like the MEG data measured outside the brain, instead of inside the brain in this case. Thus, current dipole moment Q was computed for each square millimeter of the active tissue (see Figure 4.24B). Figure 4.24C shows the dynamic statistical parametric map (dSPM) with a probability value of 10-5. Figure 4.24D is the distribution of Q estimated from the LFP measurements of the evoked response. The estimate of q = Q/mm² was 1 to 2 nAm/mm², consistent with the invariant value of q found with the series of MEG studies.

This physiological constant is due to two types of invariance found across the same phylogenetic scale. The dipole moment density **q** is determined by the intracellular current density **J** and intracellular volume fraction. The intracellular volume fraction is 1 − **α**, where **α** is the extracellular volume fraction. These values are found to be invariant across a wide range of species down to reptiles (Sykova & Nicholson, 2008). Thus, the total amount of current within a unit cross-sectional area of the cortex is proportional to **J**, and this value is the same across the species if the value of **J** is constant. The current density **J** is determined by electrophysiological characteristics of neurons. It turns out that the intracellular potentials have comparable

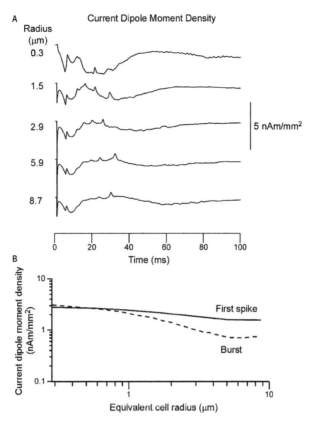

FIGURE 4.23   Invariance of current dipole moment density **q** with model cell size. (A) **q** for the range of individual e-cells varying in radius. (B) **q** versus cell radius for the first spike and burst of the evoked response waveform. (From Murakami, S., & Okada, Y. [2015]. Invariance in current dipole moment density across brain structures and species: Physiological constraint for neuroimaging. *NeuroImage, 111,* 49–58.)

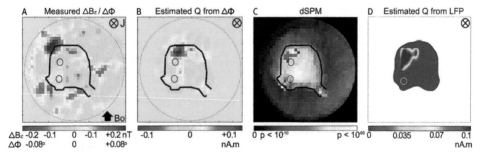

FIGURE 4.24   Spatial map of $\Delta\Phi$ and current density matching the active tissue determined with local field potentials (LFPs). (A) Spatial map of $\Delta\Phi$ during the peak of the LFP averaged across seven animals. (B) Minimal norm estimate of current dipole moment Q (nAm in each voxel) with a maximum of 1.013 nAm/mm² (directed into the page $\otimes$), based on the $\Delta\Phi$ map in A. (C) Statistical significance map of the density estimate in (B). Areas shown are (p < 10-5, log scale), after Bonferroni correction. (D) The density map of the active tissue determined with LFP. Bo is rostral to caudal. (Taken from Figure 14 of Sundaram, P., Nummenmaa, A., Wells, W., Orbach, D., Orringer, D., Mulkern, R., & Okada, Y. (2016). Direct neural current imaging in an intact cerebellum with magnetic resonance imaging. *NeuroImage, 132,* 477–490.)

maximum amplitudes, and the accompanying values of **J** are similar across the species (e.g., Traub et al., 1991, 1994, 2005, 2008). Thus, the invariance in these basic anatomical and physiological parameters constrain the properties of MEG and EEG signals. MEG and EEG signals are not free to vary arbitrarily, but they are governed by the basic anatomical and electrophysiological properties of the central nervous system. The physiological constant **q** of approximately 1 nAm/mm² is governed by a property that has been conserved across the evolution.

This invariance in **q** may be useful for interpreting MEG and EEG signals because their amplitudes indicate the minimal cortical surface of the active tissue producing the signals. For example, Q is quite large for epileptiform signals (137–275 nAm; Oishi et al., 2002) or the evoked responses elicited by painful stimulation (16–153 nAm; Baumgärtner, Vogel, Ohara, Treede, & Lenz, 2011). The invariance in **q** implies that the minimal surface area of the volume of cortex producing such signals must be as much as about 2 to 3 cm.² Physiological constraints have not been used in improving the inverse solutions for MEG or EEG. The **q** might possibly serve as a useful constraint for interpreting these signals.

These new insights that we have gained from a systematic study of physiological bases of evoked MEG and EEG signals provide a solid foundation for expanding applications of these noninvasive techniques for studying human brain functions. As described in the other chapters in this book, the biomagnetic instrumentation is continuing to improve. New methods such as the atomic magnetometer (also called optically pumped magnetometer) are being used to develop new instruments with more flexibility and sensitivity. The advances in analysis software continue with the capability for real-time monitoring and analysis of brain activities, possibly down to single episodes of brain activity. Similarly, new EEG techniques such as dry electrode EEG and wireless EEG are being developed. As these new approaches improve the field of MEG and EEG, we expect that firm understanding of the physiological origins of MEG and EEG signals will serve as an important foundation for advancing our understanding of human brain functions across the entire life span from the fetus in utero to the 100-year-olds.

ACKNOWLEDGMENTS

I wish to thank the National Institutes of Health for the uninterrupted support with grants R01-NS21149 and R01-NS30968 (PI, Okada) that have allowed me to carry out the studies described in this contribution over a 30-year period. I wish to express appreciation to all of my collaborators who are listed in the publications, especially Charles Nicholson and Rodolfo Llinás, who were instrumental in enabling me to start the study of physiological bases of MEG and EEG described here. I decided to study the foundation of MEG and EEG after carrying out some of the initial MEG studies on healthy adult volunteers starting in 1979 in the Neuromagnetism Laboratory of the two pioneers, Professor Lloyd Kaufman, a psychologist, and Professor Samuel Williamson, a low-temperature physicist, at the New York University. This initial human study served as the motivation for the studies described here.

REFERENCES

Baumgärtner, U., Vogel, H., Ohara, S., Treede, R. D., & Lenz, F. (2011). Dipole source analyses of laser evoked potentials obtained from subdural grid recordings from primary somatic sensory cortex. *Journal of Neurophysiology, 106,* 722–730.

Cohen, D. (1968). Evidence of magnetic fields produced by alpha-rhythm currents. *Science, 161,* 784–786.

Cohen D., & Hosaka H. (1976). Magnetic field produced by a current dipole. *Journal of Electrocardiology, 9,* 409–417.

Curio, G., Mackert, B., Burghoff, M., Koetitz, R., Abraham-Fuchs, K., & Haerer, W. (1994). Localization of evoked neuromagnetic 600 Hz activity in the cerebral somatosensory system. *Electroencephalography and Clinical Neurophysiology, 91,* 483–487.

Geselowitz, D. B. (1970). On the magnetic field generated outside an inhomogeneous volume conductor by internal current sources. *IEEE Transactions on Magnetics, 6,* 346–347.

Geselowtitz, D. B. (1973). Electric and magnetic field of the heart. *Annual Review of Biophysics and Bioengineering, 2,* 37–64.

Grynszpan, F., & Geselowitz, D. B. (1973). Model studies of the magnetocardiogram. *Biophysical Journal, 13,* 911–925.

Hashimoto, I., Kimura, T., Tanosaki, M., Iguchi, Y., & Sekihara, K. (2003). Muscle afferent inputs from the hand activate human cerebellum sequentially through parallel and climbing fiber systems. *Clinical Neurophysiology, 114,* 2107–2117.

Hashimoto, I., Mashiko, T., & Imada, T. (1996). Somatic evoked high-frequency magnetic oscillations reflect activity of inhibitory interneurons in the human somatosensory cortex. *Electroencephalography and Clinical Neurophysiology, 100,* 189–203.

Hille, B. (1992, 2001). *Ion channels of excitable membranes* (2nd and 3rd eds.). Sunderland, MA: Sinauer.

Hodgkin, A. L., & Huxley, A. F. (1952). A quantitative description of membrane current and its application to conduction and excitation in nerve. *Journal of Physiology, 117,* 500–544.

Huang, J. C., Nicholson, C., & Okada, Y. C. (1990). Distortion of magnetic evoked fields and surface potentials by conductivity differences at boundaries in brain tissue. *Biophysical Journal, 57,* 1155–1166.

Ikeda, H., Leyba, L., Bartolo, A., & Okada, Y. C. (2002). Synchronized spikes of thalamocortical axonal terminals and cortical neurons are detectable outside the brain of piglet with high-resolution MEG. *Journal of Neurophysiology, 87,* 626–630.

Ikeda, H., Wang, Y., & Okada, Y. C. (2005). Origins of the somatic N20 and high-frequency oscillations evoked by trigeminal stimulation in the piglets. *Clinical Neurophysiology, 116,* 827–841.

Ioannides, A. A., & Fenwick, P. C. (2005). Imaging cerebellum activity in real time with magnetoencephalographic data. *Progress in Brain Research, 148,* 139–150.

Jones, M. S., & Barth, D. S. (1999). Spatiotemporal organization of fast (>200 Hz) electrical oscillations in rat vibrissa/barrel cortex. *Journal of Neurophysiology, 82,* 1599–1609.

Jousmaki, V., Hamalainen, M., & Hari, R. (1996). Magnetic source imaging during a visually guided task. *Neuroreport, 7,* 2961–2964.

Kato, S., Wang, Y., Papuashvili, N., & Okada, Y. C. (2003). Stable synchronized high-frequency signals from the main sensory and spinal nuclei of the pig activated by Aß fibers of the maxillary nerve innervating the snout. *Brain Research, 959,* 1–10.

Kyuhou, S., & Okada Y. C. (1993). Detection of magnetic evoked fields associated with synchronous population activities in the transverse CA1 slice of the guinea pig. *Journal of Neurophysiology, 70,* 2665–2668.

Llinás, R. (1988). The intrinsic electrophysiological properties of mammalian neurons: A new insight into CNS function. *Science, 242,* 1654–1664.

Lopes da Silva, F., & Rotterdam, A. (1987). _____ _____ In E. Niedermeyer & F. Lopes da Silva (Eds.), *Electroencephalography: Basic principles, clinical applications, and related fields* (2nd ed., pp. 29–41). Baltimore, MD: Urban & Schwarzenberg.

Lopez, L., Chan, C. Y., Okada, Y. C., & Nicholson, C. (1991). Multimodal characterization of population responses evoked by applied electric field in vitro: Extracellular potential, magnetic evoked field, transmembrane potential, and current-source density analysis. *Journal of Neuroscience, 11,* 1998–2010.

Lorente de Nó, R. (1947). Action potential of the motoneurons of the hypoglossus nucleus. *Journal of Cellular and Comparative Physiology, 29,* 207–287.

Mainen, Z. F., & Sejnowski, T. J. (1996). Influence of dendritic structure on firing pattern in model neocortical neurons. *Nature, 382,* 363–366.

Murakami S., Hirose A., & Okada Y. C. (2003). Contribution of ionic currents to magnetoencephalography (MEG) and electroencephalography (EEG) signals generated by guinea-pig CA3 slices. *Journal of Physiology, 553,* 975–985.

Murakami S., & Okada Y. (2006). Contributions of principal neocortical neurons to magnetoencephalography and electroencephalography signals. *Journal of Physiology, 575,* 925–936.

Murakami, S., & Okada, Y. (2015). Invariance in current dipole moment density across brain structures and species: Physiological constraint for neuroimaging. *NeuroImage, 111,* 49–58.

Murakami, S., Zhang, T., Hirose, A., & Okada, Y. C. (2002). Physiological origins of evoked magnetic fields and extracellular field potentials produced by the guinea-pig CA3. *Journal of Physiology, 544,* 237–251.

Niedermeyer, E., & Lopes da Silva, F. (1987). *Electroencephalography: Basic principles, clinical applications and related fields* (2nd ed.). Baltimore, MD: Urban & Schwarzenberg.

Oishi, M., Otsubo, H., Kameyama, S., Morota, N., Masuda, H., Kitayama, M., & Tanaka, R. (2002). Epileptic spikes: Magnetoencephalography versus simultaneous electrocorticography. *Epilepsia, 43,* 1390–1395.

Okada, Y. C. (1983a). Inferences concerning anatomy and physiology of the human brain based on its magnetic field. *Il Nuovo Cimento D, 2,* 279–409.

Okada, Y. C. (1983b). Neurogenesis of evoked magnetic fields. In S. J. Williamson, G-L. Romani, L. Kaufman, & I. Modena (Eds.), *Biomagnetism: An interdisciplinary approach* (pp. 399–408). New York, NY: Plenum Press.

Okada, Y. C. (1989). Recent developments on the physiological basis of magnetoencephalography. In S. J. Williamson, M. Manfried Hoke, G. Stroink, & M. Kotani (Eds.), *Advances in biomagnetism* (pp. 273–278). New York, NY: Plenum Press.

Okada, Y. C., Lähteenmäki, A., & Xu, C. (1999). Comparison of MEG and EEG on the basis of somatic evoked responses elicited by stimulation of the snout in the juvenile swine. *Clinical Neurophysiology, 110,* 214–229.

Okada, Y. C., Lauritzen, M., & Nicholson, C. (1987). Magnetic field associated with neural activities in an isolated cerebellum. *Brain Research, 412,* 151–155.

Okada, Y. C., & Nicholson, C. (1988). Magnetic evoked field associated with transcortical currents in turtle cerebellum. *Biophysical Journal, 53,* 723–731.

Okada, Y. C., Nicholson, C., & Llinas, R. (1989). Magnetoencephalography (MEG) as a new tool for non-invasive realtime analysis of normal and abnormal brain activity in humans. In D. Ottoson & W. Rostene (Eds.), *Visualization of brain functions* (pp. 245–266). New York, NY: Stockton Press.

Okada, Y. C., Wu, J., & Kyuhou, S. (1997). Genesis of MEG signals in a mammalian CNS structure. *Electroencephalography and Clinical Neurophysiology, 103,* 474–485.

Okada, Y. C., & Xu, C. (1996). Single-epoch neuromagnetic signals during epileptiform activities in guinea pig longitudinal CA3 slices. *Neuroscience Letters, 211,* 155–158.

Rall, W. (1962a). Theory of physiological properties of dendrites. *Annals of the N Y Academy of Science, 96,* 1071–1092.

Rall, W. (1962b). Electrophysiology of a dendritic neuron model. *Biophysical Journal, 2,* 145–167.

Ranck, J. B. (1963a). Specific impedance of rabbit cerebral cortex. *Experimental Neurology, 7,* 144–152.

Ranck, J. B. (1963b). Analysis of specific impedance of rabbit cerebral cortex. *Experimental Neurology, 7,* 153–174.

Riera, J. J., Ogawa, T., Goto, T., Sumiyoshi, A., Nonaka, H., Evans, A., Miyakawa, H., & Kawashima, R. (2012). Pitfalls in the dipolar model for the neocortical EEG sources. *Journal of Neurophysiology, 108,* 956–975.

Steriade, M. (2001). *Intact and sliced brain.* Cambridge, MA: MIT Press.

Steriade, M. (2003). *Neuronal substrates of sleep and epilepsy.* Cambridge, UK: Cambridge University Press.

Stuart, G., Spruston, N., Sakmann, B., & Häusser, M. (1997). Action potential initiation and backpropagation in neurons of the mammalian CNS. *Trends in Neuroscience, 20,* 125–131.

Sundaram, P., Nummenmaa, A., Wells, W., Orbach, D., Orringer, D., Mulkern, R., & Okada, Y. (2016). Direct neural current imaging in an intact cerebellum with magnetic resonance imaging. *NeuroImage, 132,* 477–490.

Sykova, E., & Nicholson, C. (2008). Diffusion in brain extracellular space. *Physiology Reviews, 88,* 1277–1340.

Telenczuk, B., Baker, S. N., Herz, A. V. M., & Curio, G. (2011). High-frequency EEG covaries with spike burst patterns detected in cortical neurons. *Journal of Neurophysiology, 105,* 2951–2959.

Tesche, C. D., & Karhu, J. (1997). Somatosensory evoked magnetic fields arising from sources in the human cerebellum. *Brain Research, 744,* 23–31.

Traub, R. D., Contreras, D., Cunningham, M. O., Murray, H., LeBeau, F. E. N., Roopun, A., Bibbig, A., Wilent, W. B., Higley, M. J., & Whittington, M. A. (2005). Single-column thalamocortical network model exhibiting gamma oscillations, sleep spindles and epileptogenic bursts. *Journal of Neurophysiology, 93,* 2194–2232.

Traub, R. D., Jefferys, J. G. R., Miles, R., Whittington, M. A., & Toth K. (1994). A branching dendritic model of a rodent CA3 pyramidal neurone. *Journal of Physiology, 481,* 79–95.

Traub, R. D., Middleton S. J., Knopfel T., & Whittington, M. A. (2008). Model of very fast (>75 Hz) network oscillations generated by electrical coupling between the proximal axons of cerebellar Purkinje cells. *European Journal of Neuroscience, 28,* 1603–1616.

Traub, R. D., & Miles, R. (1991). *Neuronal networks of the hippocampus.* New York, NY: Cambridge University Press.

Traub, R. D., Wong, R. K. S., Miles, R., & Michelson, H. (1991). A model of a CA3 hippocampal pyramidal neuron incorporating voltage-clamp data on intrinsic conductances. *Journal of Neurophysiology, 66,* 635–650.

Wu, J., & Okada, Y. C. (1998). Physiological bases of the synchronized population spikes and slow wave of the magnetic field generated by a guinea pig longitudinal CA3 slice preparation. *Electroencephalography and Clinical Neurophysiology, 107,* 361–373.

Wu, J., & Okada, Y. C. (1999). Roles of a potassium afterhyperpolarization current in generating neuromagnetic fields and field potentials in longitudinal CA3 slices of the guinea-pig. *Clinical Neurophysiology, 110,* 1858–1867.

Wu, J., & Okada, Y. C. (2000). Ca2+- and voltage-activated potassium conductances determine the waveform of neuromagnetic signals from hippocampal CA3 longitudinal slice of guinea-pig. *Clinical Neurophysiology, 111,* 150–160.

5

WHICH PART OF THE NEURONAL CURRENT CAN BE DETERMINED BY ELECTROENCEPHALOGRAPHY?

A. S. Fokas, Parham Hashemzadeh, and Richard M. Leahy

5.1. INTRODUCTION

Neuronal activity in the brain generates an intracranial current that gives rise to an electric potential on the scalp measured by electroencephalography (EEG) and a magnetic flux outside the head measured by magnetoencephalography (MEG). Motivated by this physiological situation, the following basic mathematical questions are answered in this work: Assuming that the electric potential is known everywhere on the scalp, which components of the current that gave rise to this potential can be determined? Similarly, assuming that the magnetic flux is known everywhere outside the head, which part of the current that gave rise to this magnetic flux can be determined? In order to answer these questions, we make the following assumptions:

(i) We assume that the brain can be approximated by four different compartments that are distinguished by different values of their electrical conductivities: namely, the domain Ω_c, which represents the space occupied by the cerebral cortex, and three shells surrounding Ω_c, which are respectively denoted by Ω_f, Ω_b, and Ω_s. These spaces denote the cerebrospinal fluid Ω_f, the skull Ω_b, and the scalp Ω_s. The domains have conductivities σ_c, σ_f, σ_b, and σ_s, respectively.

(ii) We assume that the primary current is supported either within Ω_c or on the boundary S_c of Ω_c.

(iii) We assume a continuous distribution of the primary current. This is the direct opposite of the assumption that the current consists of a single dipole or a set of discrete dipoles.

A. S. Fokas, Parham Hashemzadeh, and Richard M. Leahy, *Which Part of the Neuronal Current Can Be Determined by Electroencephalography?* In: *Fifty Years of Magnetoencephalography*. Edited by: Andrew C. Papanicolaou, Timothy P. L. Roberts, and James W. Wheless, Oxford University Press (2020). © Oxford University Press. DOI: 10.1093/oso/9780190935689.003.0005.

A crucial tool for our analysis is provided by the existence of the so-called Helmholtz decomposition. Namely, without loss of generality, we can always represent the current $\mathbf{J}^p(\tau)$ in terms of a scalar function $\Psi(\tau)$ and a vectorial function $\mathbf{A}(\tau)$,

$$\mathbf{J}^p(\tau) = \nabla_\tau \Psi(\tau) + \nabla_\tau \times A(\tau), \quad \tau \in \Omega_c, \quad (1)$$

where $\mathbf{A}(\tau)$ satisfies the constraint $\nabla \cdot \mathbf{A} = 0$ [this constraint implies that the current involves three arbitrary scalar functions, namely $\Psi(\tau)$ and the two independent scalar functions characterizing $\mathbf{A}(\tau)$]. Equation (1) allows us to provide complete answers to the previous questions. Indeed, the following surprising result is valid: Both the electric potential on the scalp and the magnetic flux outside the head are affected only by the values of $\Psi(\tau)$, the radial part $\mathbf{A}(\tau)$, and their gradients, on the surface of the cerebral cortex.

5.1.1. Current With a Three-Dimensional Support

If the primary current has three-dimensional support, we will assume the current vanishes on the surface of the cerebral cortex. This assumption is based on the following argument: suppose that $\mathbf{J}^p$ has support in Ω_c, which is considered to be an open set; therefore, there exists an $\varepsilon > 0$ such that the shell $S_{c-\varepsilon}$ of thickness ε in the interior of Ω_c is free from neuronal sources.

It should be noted that the vanishing of the current $\mathbf{J}^p$ on the above surface does *not* imply the vanishing of the functions $\Psi(\tau)$ and $\mathbf{A}(\tau)$ on this surface. For example, even if $\mathbf{J}^p$ is a dipole source, then $\Psi(\tau)$ and $\mathbf{A}(\tau)$ have support everywhere. Indeed, it is shown (Menendez & Andino, 2015) that if $\mathbf{J}^p(\tau) = Q\delta(\tau - r_0)$, where Q is constant, then

$$\Psi(\tau) = \frac{1}{4\pi} Q \cdot \frac{(\tau - r_0)}{|\tau - r_0|^3}, \quad (2)$$

and

$$A(\tau) = \frac{1}{4\pi} Q \times \frac{(\tau - r_0)}{|\tau - r_0|^3}. \quad (3)$$

It is shown in this chapter that assumptions (1) to (3), together with the assumption that $\mathbf{J}^p(\tau)$ vanishes on $\partial\Omega_c$, yield the following fundamental formula:

$$u(r) = \frac{1}{4\pi} \int_{S_c} \hat{n} \cdot [\Psi(\tau)\nabla_\tau v_s(r,\tau) \\ - v_s(r,\tau)\nabla_\tau \Psi(\tau)] dS(\tau), \quad r \in S_s, \quad (4)$$

where $\hat{n}(\tau)$ denotes the unit vector to the surface of the cerebral cortex denoted by S_c, and $v_s(r,\tau)$ is an auxiliary function defined later in the section on Auxiliary Functions, which depends on the conductivities and the topology of the brain, but it is *independent* of the current.

Equation (4) implies that the electric potential on the scalp is affected only by the value of $\Psi(\tau)$ and it's gradient on the surface of the cerebral cortex.

The previous result implies that it is *impossible* to determine the three-dimensional current without some additional assumptions. A popular such assumption is to impose the minimal L_2 constraint. However, there exists the misconception that it is possible to obtain a unique current by imposing such a constraint *without* first identifying the part of the current that is affected by the data. In what follows, we will demonstrate the previous fallacy by discussing the spherical model, in which case the implications of the L_2 minimization can be computed explicitly.

In Fokas, Gelfand, and Kurylev (1996), L_2 minimization is imposed assuming that only MEG data are known. In this case, using the analogue of (4) for MEG, it is shown that the data $r \cdot \mathbf{B}(r)$ can be expanded in terms of spherical harmonics $Y_l^m(\theta, \phi)$, as follows:

$$r \cdot \mathbf{B}(r) = -\sum_{l=0}^{\infty} \sum_{m=-l}^{l} C_l^m r^{-(l+1)} \nabla_r Y_l^m(\hat{r}), \quad (5)$$

where r denotes the position vector of the MEG sensor outside the head, $\mathbf{B}(r)$ denotes the magnetic flux, and the constants C_l^m are known from the measurements. The L_2 minimization implies that the neuronal current is given by

$$\mathbf{J}^p(\tau, \theta, \phi) = -\frac{1}{\tau \sin(\theta)} \frac{\partial F}{\partial \varphi} \hat{\theta} + \frac{1}{\tau} \frac{\partial F}{\partial \theta} \hat{\phi}, \quad (6)$$

where $\hat{\theta}$ and $\hat{\phi}$ are unit vectors associated with the θ and ϕ coordinates, and $F(\tau)$ is given by

$$F(\tau, \theta, \phi) = \sum_{l=0}^{\infty} \sum_{m=-l}^{l} f_l^m Y_l^m(\theta, \phi), \quad (7)$$

where $f_l^m(\tau)$ can be expressed in terms of the known constants C_l^m via the equation

$$f_l^m = \frac{(2l+1)(2l+3)}{l} r^{l+1} C_l^m. \quad (8)$$

In Fokas and Kurylev (2012), L_2 minimization is imposed assuming both EEG and MEG data are known. In this case, it is shown that $\mathbf{J}^p(\tau)$ is given by equation (1), where $\mathbf{A}(\tau)$ can be expressed in terms of its radial component $\tau \cdot \mathbf{A}(\tau)$, and both this radial component and $\Psi(\tau)$ can be expanded in terms of spherical harmonics with coefficients $a_n^m(\tau)$ and $\psi_n^m(\tau)$ explicitly given in terms of the known coefficients of the spherical expansion of EEG and MEG data. It is straightforward to verify that the expressions of current obtained via the previous procedures are very different.

5.1.2. Current Supported on the Surface of the Cerebral Cortex

In many physiological situations, it can be assumed that the current has support on the surface of the cerebral cortex. Let a point $\tau = (\lambda, \mu, v)$, where $\lambda, \mu,$ and v are orthogonal

coordinates and the cortical surface S_c is defined by equation $\lambda = a$. Assume that $\mathbf{J}^p$ is supported on S_c. Then equation $\mathbf{J}^p$ can be expanded in the form

$$\mathbf{J}^p(\tau) = J_1(\mu, v) \tau_1(\mu, v) + J_2(\mu, v) \tau_2(\mu, v)$$
$$+ J_3(\mu, v) \hat{n}(\mu, v), \quad (9)$$

where

$$\tau_1(\mu, v) = \frac{\partial_\tau(a, \mu, v)}{\partial_\mu},$$
$$\tau_2(\mu, v) = \frac{\partial_\tau(a, \mu, v)}{\partial_\mu}, \quad \hat{n} = \frac{\tau_1 \times \tau_2}{|\tau_1 \times \tau_2|}. \quad (10)$$

It will be shown in the Main Results section that in the particular case that the current $\mathbf{J}^p$ is normal to the surface, that is, $J_1 = J_2 = 0$, the electric potential on the scalp is given by

$$u(r) = \frac{1}{4\pi} \int_{S_c} J_3(\mu, v) \frac{\partial v_s}{\partial \lambda} |\tau_1| |\tau_2| d\mu dv. \quad (11)$$

Equation (11) can be solved uniquely for S_c in terms of $u(r)$. Indeed, in this case, one needs to determine $J_3(\tau)$, that is, a single scalar function supported in a two-dimensional domain. The data also consist of a single scalar function $u(r)$ supported on a two-dimensional domain; thus, it is natural to expect that the relevant inverse problem can be solved uniquely.

The situation with MEG is much simpler in the sense that it is *not* necessary to compute any auxiliary functions. It is shown in Fokas (2009) that the analogue of equation (4) is

$$\frac{4\pi}{\mu} r \cdot \mathbf{B}(r) = -\int_{S_c} \left[\frac{1}{|r-\tau|} \nabla_\tau (\tau \cdot A) \right.$$
$$\left. -(\tau \cdot A) \nabla_\tau \frac{1}{|r-\tau|} \right] \cdot \hat{n}(\tau) dS(\tau)$$
$$+ \frac{1}{4\pi} \int_{S_c} \left[(r \cdot \mathbf{H}(r, \tau))(\nabla_\tau \Psi(\tau)) \right.$$
$$\left. -\Psi(\tau) \nabla_\tau (r \cdot \mathbf{H}(r, \tau)) \right] \cdot \hat{n}(\tau) dS(\tau),$$

$$(12)$$

where $\mathbf{H}(r, \tau)$ is a geometry-dependent vectorial function given by

$$\mathbf{H}(r,\tau) = (\sigma_c - \sigma_f)\int_{S_c} v_f(r',\tau)h(r',r)dS(r')$$
$$+ (\sigma_f - \sigma_h)\int_{S_f} v_b(r',\tau)h(r',r)dS(r')$$
$$+ (\sigma_b - \sigma_s)\int_{S_b} v_s(r',\tau)h(r',r)dS(r')$$
$$+ \sigma_s \int_{S_s} v_s(r',\tau)h(r',r)dS(r'), \quad (13)$$

where $h(r', r)$ is defined as

$$h(r',r) = \hat{n}(r') \times \nabla_{r'}\frac{1}{|r-r'|}. \quad (14)$$

However, $\mathbf{H}(r, \tau)$ only involves differences of conductivities, so $\mathbf{H}(r, \tau)$ is small and hence $r \cdot \mathbf{B}(r)$ can be approximated to

$$\frac{4\pi}{\mu}r \cdot \mathbf{B}(r) \approx -\int\int_{S_c}\left[\frac{1}{|r-\tau|}\nabla_\tau(\tau \cdot A(\tau))\right.$$
$$\left. - (\tau \cdot A(\tau))\nabla_\tau\frac{1}{|r-\tau|}\right] \cdot \hat{n}(\tau)dS(\tau).$$
$$(15)$$

In analogy with (4), there also exists an expression relating $r \cdot \mathbf{B}(r)$ with $J_3(\mu, v)$. Thus, the normal component of a current supported on S_c can be uniquely computed via either EEG or MEG.

Regarding the uniqueness result for the MEG, it is noted that the data again consist of a single scalar function, namely the radial component of the magnetic flux. Now, the data are supported on a three-dimensional domain, but because the radial component of the magnetic flux outside the head satisfies the Laplace equation, knowledge of $r \cdot \mathbf{B}(r)$ on a surface is sufficient to determine $r \cdot \mathbf{B}$ in a three-dimensional domain. Hence, in MEG, the data effectively also consist of a scalar function supported in a two-dimensional domain, so again one expects

that the relevant inverse problem can be solved uniquely.

5.2. MAIN RESULTS

Proposition 2.1. *Consider a four-compartments model specified by the domains* $\Omega_c, \Omega_f, \Omega_b,$ *and* Ω_s *modeling the spaces occupied by the cortex, the cerebrospinal fluid, the skull (bone), and the scalp, which have conductivities* $\sigma_c, \sigma_f, \sigma_b,$ *and* $\sigma_s,$ *respectively. Let* $\mathbf{J}^p$ *be continuously distributed inside* $\Omega_c.$ *Express* $\mathbf{J}^p$ *via the Helmholtz decomposition formula given by (1).*

The electric potential $u(r)$ *on the external surface of the scalp, which is denoted by* $S_s,$ *satisfies the equation*

$$u(r) = \frac{1}{4\pi}\int_{S_c}\hat{n}(\tau) \cdot [\Psi(\tau)\nabla_\tau v_s(r,\tau)$$
$$r \in S_s.$$
$$(16)$$
$$- v_s(r,\tau)\nabla_\tau\Psi(\tau) + v_s(r,\tau)\mathbf{J}^p]dS(\tau),$$

If the normal component $\mathbf{J}^p(\tau)$ *vanishes on* $S_c,$ *then* $u(r)$ *is given by equation (4).*

Proof. It was shown in Fokas (2009) that the electric potential on the scalp is given by

$$u(r) = \frac{1}{4\pi}\int_{\Omega_c}\mathbf{J}^p(\tau) \cdot \nabla_\tau v_s(r,\tau)dV(\tau), \quad r \in S_s.$$
$$(17)$$

However, the divergence theorem,

$$\int_\Omega \nabla \cdot F(\tau)dV(\tau) = \int_{\partial\Omega}\hat{n}(\tau) \cdot F(\tau)dS(\tau), \quad (18)$$

where $\partial\Omega$ is the boundary of Ω and $\hat{n}$ is the unit vector in the outward direction of $\partial\Omega,$ implies

$$\int_{\Omega_c}\nabla_\tau \cdot [v_s(r,\tau)\mathbf{J}^p(\tau)]dV(\tau)$$
$$= \int_{S_c}v_s(r,\tau)[\hat{n}(\tau) \cdot \mathbf{J}^p(\tau)]dS(\tau). \quad (19)$$

Hence, equation (19) becomes

$$\int\limits_{\Omega_c} \mathbf{J}^p \cdot \nabla_\tau v_s(r,\tau) dV(\tau)$$

$$+ \int\limits_{\Omega_c} [\nabla_\tau \cdot \mathbf{J}^p(\tau)] v_s(r,\tau) dV(\tau)$$

$$= \int\limits_{S_c} [\hat{n}(\tau) \cdot \mathbf{J}^p(\tau)] v_s(r,\tau) dS(\tau), \quad r \in S_s. \tag{20}$$

Using (20) in (17) we find

$$u(r) = -\frac{1}{4\pi} \int\limits_{\Omega_c} [\nabla_\tau \cdot \mathbf{J}^p(\tau)] v_s(r,\tau) dV(\tau)$$

$$+ \frac{1}{4\pi} \int\limits_{S_c} [\hat{n}(\tau) \cdot \mathbf{J}^p(\tau)] v_s(r,\tau) dS(\tau), \quad r \in S_s. \tag{21}$$

Replacing in the previous equation $\nabla_\tau \cdot \mathbf{J}^p(\tau)$ with $\Delta_\tau \Psi(\tau)$, we find

$$u(r) = -\frac{1}{4\pi} \int\limits_{\Omega_c} \Delta_\tau \Psi(\tau) v_s(r,\tau) dV(\tau)$$

$$+ \frac{1}{4\pi} \int\limits_{S_c} [\hat{n}(\tau) \cdot \mathbf{J}^p(\tau)] v_s(r,\tau) dS(\tau),$$

$$r \in S_s. \tag{22}$$

The equations defining $v_j(r,\tau)$, $j = c, f, b, s$ remain invariant if r and τ are interchanged, thus v_j not only are harmonic in r but also are harmonic in τ. Green's second identity implies that if a function h is harmonic, then the following identity is valid:

$$\int\limits_{\Omega} (\Delta f) h dV(\tau) = \int\limits_{\partial\Omega} \hat{n}(\tau) \cdot [h\nabla f - f\nabla h] dS(\tau), \tag{23}$$

where $\partial\Omega$ denotes the boundary of Ω. Using the above equation with $f = \Psi$, $h = v_s$, $\Omega = \Omega_c$, in (22), we find (16).

Proposition 2.2. *Suppose that the cortical surface S_c is defined by the equation $\lambda = a$, where $\tau =$*

τ (λ, μ, ν) *and λ, μ, ν are orthogonal coordinates. Assume that $\mathbf{J}^p$ is supported on S_c, namely*

$$\mathbf{J}^p(\tau) = J_1(\mu,\nu)\tau_1(\mu,\nu) + J_2(\mu,\nu)\tau_2(\mu,\nu)$$

$$+ J_3(\mu,\nu)\hat{n}(\mu,\nu),$$

where $\tau_1(\mu,\nu)$, $\tau_2(\mu,\nu)$, and $\hat{n}(\mu,\nu)$ are given by equation (10). Then, the electric potential on the scalp is given by

$$u(r) = \frac{1}{4\pi} \int\limits_{S_c} \left\{ -\left[\frac{\partial(|\tau_1||\tau_2|J_1(\tau))}{\partial\mu} \right. \right.$$

$$\left. + \frac{\partial(|\tau_1||\tau_2|J_2(\tau))}{\partial\nu} \right] \frac{h_\lambda(\tau)}{|\tau_1||\tau_2|}$$

$$\left. + J_3 \frac{\partial v_s(r,\tau)}{\partial\lambda} \right\} dS(\tau), \quad r \in S_s, \tag{24}$$

where h_λ is defined by

$$h_\lambda(\lambda,\mu,\nu) = \left| \frac{\partial\tau(\lambda,\mu,\nu)}{\partial\lambda} \right|. \tag{25}$$

Proof. Suppose that $\tilde{\mathbf{J}}^p$ is independent of λ and has support in a small shell Ω of thickness δ in the interior of Ω_c. Then,

$$u(r) = \frac{1}{4\pi} \int\limits_{\Omega} \tilde{\mathbf{J}}^p(\tau) \cdot (\nabla_\tau v_s(r,\tau)) dV(\tau), \quad r \in S_s. \tag{26}$$

Hence,

$$u(r) = -\frac{1}{4\pi} \int\limits_{\Omega} (\nabla_\tau \cdot \tilde{\mathbf{J}}^p(\tau)) v_s(r,\tau) dV(\tau)$$

$$+ \frac{1}{4\pi} \int\limits_{\partial\Omega} (\hat{n}(\tau) \cdot \mathbf{J}^p(\tau)) v_s(r,\tau) dS(\tau), \quad r \in S_s. \tag{27}$$

We will compute the limit of (27) as $\delta \to 0$. In this connection we recall that $dV(\tau) = h_\lambda h_\mu h_\nu d\lambda d\mu d\nu$, where h_λ is given by the equation (24) and h_μ, h_ν are defined by the equations

$$h_\mu(\lambda,\mu,\nu) = \left| \frac{\partial \tau(\lambda,\mu,\nu)}{\partial \mu} \right|,$$

$$h_\nu(\lambda,\mu,\nu) = \left| \frac{\partial \tau(\lambda,\mu,\nu)}{\partial \nu} \right|. \quad (28)$$

Using the mean value theorem, the volume integral in the rhs of (27) yields

$$-\frac{\delta}{4\pi} \int_{S_c} [(\nabla_\tau \cdot \tilde{\mathbf{J}}^p) v_s h_\lambda h_\mu h_\nu]_{\lambda=a} d\mu d\nu$$

$$= -\frac{1}{4\pi} \int_{S_c} (\nabla_\tau \cdot \mathbf{J}^p) v_s h_\lambda(a,\mu,\nu) |\tau_1||\tau_2| d\mu d\nu, \quad (29)$$

where $\mathbf{J}^p = \delta \tilde{\mathbf{J}}^p$. The lateral sides of $\partial\Omega$ yield a zero contribution as $\delta \to 0$. Furthermore, $\hat{n}$ is the same on the top surface where $\lambda = a$, and on the bottom surface where $\lambda = a - \delta$. Thus, recalling that $dS = h_\mu h_\nu d\mu d\nu$, the second term of the rhs of (27) yields

$$\frac{1}{4\pi} \int_{S_c} (\hat{n} \cdot \tilde{\mathbf{J}}^p) \{ [v_s h_\mu h_\nu]_{\lambda=a} - [v_s h_\mu h_\nu]_{\lambda=a-\delta} \} d\mu d\nu \quad (30)$$

$$= \frac{1}{4\pi} \int_{S_c} (\hat{n} \cdot \mathbf{J}^p) \left[\frac{\partial(h_\mu h_\nu)}{\partial \lambda} \right]_{\lambda=a} d\mu d\nu. \quad (31)$$

Using (27) in equations (30) and (31), we find

$$u(r) = -\frac{1}{4\pi} \int_{S_c} (\nabla \cdot \mathbf{J}^p) v_s h_\lambda(\alpha,\mu,\nu) |\tau_1||\tau_2| d\mu d\nu \quad (32)$$

$$+ \frac{1}{4\pi} \int_{S_c} (\hat{n} \cdot \mathbf{J}^p) \left\{ |\tau_1||\tau_2| \left[\frac{\partial v_s}{\partial \lambda} \right]_{\lambda=a} \right.$$

$$\left. + v_s \left[\frac{\partial(h_\mu h_\nu)}{\partial \lambda} \right]_{\lambda=a} \right\} d\mu d\nu, \quad r \in S_c. \quad (33)$$

Employing in the previous equation the identities (Dassios, Fokas, Hashemzadeh, & Leahy, 2017)

$$\hat{n} \cdot \mathbf{J}^p = J_3, \quad \nabla_\tau \cdot \mathbf{J}^p = \frac{1}{H} \frac{\partial(HJ_1)}{\partial \mu} + \frac{1}{H} \frac{\partial(HJ_2)}{\partial \nu} - \zeta J_3,$$

$$H = |\tau_1||\tau_2|,$$

where ζ denotes the mean curvature of S_c, equation (33) becomes

$$u(r) = \frac{1}{4\pi} \int_{S_c} \left\{ \left[-\frac{1}{H} \frac{\partial(HJ_1)}{\partial \mu} - \frac{1}{H} \frac{\partial(HJ_2)}{\partial \nu} \right. \right.$$

$$\left. + \zeta J_3 \right] v_s h_\lambda(\alpha,\mu,\nu) |\tau_1||\tau_2|$$

$$+ J_3 [|\tau_1||\tau_2| \left[\frac{\partial v_s}{\partial \lambda} \right]_{\lambda=a}$$

$$\left. + v_s \left[\frac{\partial(h_\mu h_\nu)}{\partial \lambda} \right]^{\lambda=a} \right\} d\mu d\nu, \quad r \in S_s. \quad (34)$$

Using in the above equation the identity

$$\zeta = -\left[\frac{1}{h_\lambda h_\mu h_\nu} \frac{\partial(h_\mu h_\nu)}{\partial \lambda} \right]_{\lambda=a}, \quad (35)$$

and recalling that $dS = |\tau_1||\tau_2| d\mu d\nu$, equation (34) simplifies to (24).

5.3. AUXILIARY FUNCTIONS $V_j(R, \tau)$

For a given geometry, the functions $v_j(r, \tau)$, $j = c, f, b, s$ are defined via the following boundary value problem:

$$\nabla^2 v_c(r, \tau) = 0, \quad r \in \Omega_c, \ \tau \in \Omega_c$$

$$\frac{\partial}{\partial n} \left[\frac{1}{|r - \tau|} + v_c(r, \tau) \right] = \sigma_f \frac{\partial v_f(r, \tau)}{\partial n}, \quad r \in S_c; \quad (36)$$

$$\nabla^2 v_f(r, \tau) = 0, \quad r \in \Omega_f, \ \tau \in \Omega_c,$$

$$v_f(r, \tau) = \frac{1}{\sigma_c} \left[\frac{1}{|r - \tau|} + v_c(r, \tau) \right], \quad r \in S_c,$$

$$\sigma_f \frac{\partial v_f(r, \tau)}{\partial n} = \sigma_b \frac{\partial v_b(r, \tau)}{\partial n}, \quad r \in S_f, \tau \in \Omega_c; \quad (37)$$

$$\nabla^2 v_b(r,\tau)=0, \quad r\in\Omega_b, \quad \tau\in\Omega_c,$$
$$v_b(r,\tau)=v_f(r,\tau), \quad r\in S_f,$$
$$\sigma_b\frac{\partial v_b(r,\tau)}{\partial n}=\sigma_s\frac{\partial v_s(r,\tau)}{\partial n}, \quad r\in S_b, \quad \tau\in\Omega_c; \tag{38}$$

$$\nabla^2 v_s(r,\tau)=0, \quad r\in\Omega_s, \quad \tau\in\Omega_c,$$
$$v_s(r,\tau)=v_b(r,\tau), \quad r\in S_b, \tag{39}$$
$$\frac{\partial v_s(r,\tau)}{\partial n}=0, \quad r\in S_s.$$

Equations (37) to (40) are *independent* of the current $\mathbf{J}^p(\tau)$ and depend only on the geometry and on the conductivities σ_c, σ_b, σ_f, and σ_s.

It is shown in Fokas (2009) that the functions $v_j(r,\tau)$ can be related to the functions $u_j(r,\tau)$,

$$u_j(r,\tau), r\in\Omega_j, \tau\in\Omega_c, j\in\{c,f,b,s\}, \tag{40}$$

which are defined in terms of a single dipole via the following equations:

$$\sigma_c\nabla^2 u_c(r)=\nabla\cdot Q\,\delta(r-\tau), \quad r\in\Omega_c,$$
$$\sigma_c\frac{\partial u_c}{\partial n}=\sigma_f\frac{\partial u_f(r)}{\partial n}, \quad r\in S_c; \tag{41}$$

$$\nabla^2 u_f(r)=0, \quad r\in\Omega_f,$$
$$u_f(r)=u_c(r), \quad r\in S_c, \tag{42}$$
$$\sigma_f\frac{\partial u_f(r)}{\partial n}=\sigma_b\frac{\partial u_b}{\partial n}, \quad r\in S_f;$$

$$\nabla^2 u_b(r)=0, r\in\Omega_b,$$
$$u_b(r)=u_f(r), r\in S_f, \tag{43}$$
$$\sigma_b\frac{\partial u_b(r)}{\partial n}=\sigma_s\frac{\partial u_b(r)}{\partial n}, \quad r\in S_b;$$

$$\nabla^2 u_s(r)=0, \quad r\in\Omega_s,$$
$$u_s(r)=u_b(r), \quad r\in S_b, \tag{44}$$
$$\frac{\partial u_s(r)}{\partial n}=0, \quad r\in S_s.$$

The functions u_j and v_j are related by the equation

$$u_j(r,\tau)=\frac{1}{4\pi}Q(\tau)\cdot\nabla_\tau v_j(r,\tau),$$
$$j\in\{f,b,s\}, r\in\Omega_j, \tau\in\Omega_c. \tag{45}$$

5.4. NUMERICAL IMPLEMENTATIONS

We will present numerical results for the case of the ellipsoidal head model shown in Figure 5.1. Several authors have focused on the dipole source problem for the ellipsoidal head model (Giapalaki & Kariotou, 2006; Gutíerrez & Nehorai, 2006, 2008). In contrast to these works, we concentrate on a distributed source problem setting. Ellipsoidal harmonics are the optimal choice of basis functions for analyzing ellipsoidal geometries (Bardhan & Knepley, 2012; Giapalaki & Kariotou, 2006; Gutíerrez & Nehorai, 2006, 2008). However, for the distributed inverse source problem of EEG and MEG, it is shown in Hashemzadeh and Fokas (2018) that the relevant inversion matrices are highly ill-conditioned and unsuitable for inversion.

The conductivities, physical dimensions, and mesh parameters of the compartments of Figure 5.1 are given in Table 5.1.

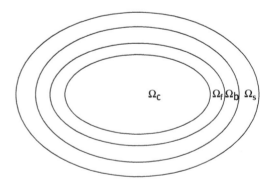

FIGURE 5.1 The different compartments of the head model. Ω_c denotes the cerebrum, which is surrounded by three shells, Ω_f, Ω_b, and Ω_s, denoting the cerebrospinal fluid, the skull, and the scalp. Their conductivities are respectively denoted by σ_c, σ_f, σ_b, and σ_s. The spaces Ω_c, Ω_f, Ω_b, and Ω_s are bounded by the surfaces S_c, (S_c, S_f), (S_f, S_b), and (S_b, S_s).

Table 5.1 Ellipsoidal Head Model and Triangular Surface Mesh Parameters Used in the OpenMEEG Computations

DOMAIN	CONDUCTIVITY (S/M)	A(METERS)	B(METERS)	C(METERS)	NODES	TRIANGLES
Cerebrum	0.3	0.0702	0.0614	0.0527	3,124	6,244
Skull	0.0042	0.0780	0.0683	0.0585	3,124	6,244
Scalp	0.33	0.0867	0.0758	0.0650	3,126	6,248

5.4.1. Electroencephalographic Reconstructions of $J_3(\tau)$

Here, we construct the inversion matrix by using piecewise constant basis functions for the expansion of the normal component $J_3(\tau)$. In order to implement (11), we employ normally oriented discrete dipoles at the nodes of the source mesh in the openMEEG (Gramfort et al., 2010) so that we can compute the integrand term $\dfrac{\partial v_s(r,\tau)}{\partial \lambda}$ in equation (11). The unknown function $\mathbf{J}^p(\tau)$ can be expanded as

$$\mathbf{J}^p(\tau) = \sum_{i=1}^{N} J_3^i \Phi_i(\tau) \hat{n}(\tau), \quad i=1,...,N, \quad (46)$$

where $\{\Phi_i(\tau)\}$ denote the basis function. By substituting equation (46) and $\dfrac{\partial v_s(r,\tau)}{\partial n}$ into equation (11) and employing a suitable surface integration scheme, we arrive at the least squares problem

$$u = E\mathbf{J}_3, \quad (47)$$

where E denotes the gain matrix or the inversion matrix. Recently, a versatile numerical quadrature technique involving local radial basis functions was proposed by Reeger, Fornberg, and Watts (2016). It outlines a numerical scheme for the integration of functions on any smooth, closed, triangulated surface and only requires function values of the integrand at the nodes. The algorithm computes a set of quadrature weights. The surface integral is simply approximated as

$$\int_{S_c} f(\tau) dS(\tau) \approx \sum_{i=1}^{N} w_i f(\tau_i), \quad (48)$$

where $f(\tau_i)$ is the function value of the integrand at the node position vector τ_i.

For a current $\mathbf{J}^p(\tau)$, which is supported only the surface of the cerebral cortex and which is normal to it, there is a one-to-one correspondence between $J_3(\tau)$ and $u(r)$. Thus, in this case, an alternative approach for computing the gain matrix is the following: use OpenMEEG to expand $\mathbf{J}^p(\tau)$ in terms of piecewise constant basis functions and for a given sensor array construct an inversion matrix.

In order to avoid the inverse crime, we generate the data using a different model than the one employed for reconstructions. We assume that the source mesh has N nodes and T triangles. The reconstruction steps are as follows:

(i) Use N normally oriented discrete dipoles and employ OpenMEEG to compute

$$\frac{\partial v_s(r,\tau)}{\partial n}.$$

(ii) Substitute the expansion of (46) with

$$\Phi_i(\tau) = \delta(\tau - \tau_i) \text{ and } \frac{\partial v_s(r,\tau)}{\partial n} \text{ in (11). Employ}$$

the numerical quadrature of Reeger et al. (2016) to compute the relevant inversion matrix. This matrix is denoted here by E_1.

(iii) Compute a second gains matrix using the distributed source option in OpenMEEG, that is, "-SSH", as described in the paragraph that follows (48). This matrix is denoted here by E_2.

(iv) Consider a test function for $J_3(\tau)$ and compute the function values $\{J_3(\tau_i): i = 1, ..., N\}$ at the nodes of the mesh. Denote this vector by $\mathbf{J}_3 \in \mathbb{R}^N$. The synthetic data are generated via equation (47), that is, $u_1(r) = \mathbf{E}_1\mathbf{J}_3$.

(v) For the inversion step, the gain matrix $\mathbf{E}_2$ is employed. The truncated singular value decomposition (TSVD) is used for computing the estimate $\mathbf{J}_3 = \mathbf{E}_2^\dagger \mathbf{u}$.

We choose the following test function:

$$J_3(\tau) = e^{-1500\|\tau - \tau_1\|} + e^{-1500\|\tau - \tau_2\|}, \quad (49)$$

where τ_1, τ_2 denote the position vectors of two sources. A simple approach for comparing inversion matrices $\mathbf{E}_1$ and $\mathbf{E}_2$ is to generate two data sets, using the test function given by equation (49). For, a given $\mathbf{J}_3$, the data sets are generated as given here:

$$\mathbf{u}_1 = \mathbf{E}_1\mathbf{J}_3, \quad \mathbf{u}_2 = \mathbf{E}_2\mathbf{J}_3,$$

where $\mathbf{J}_3 = \{J_3(\tau_i): i = 1, ..., N\}$ denotes the function values of $J_3(\tau)$ at the nodes of the mesh. The results of this comparison are shown in Figure 5.2. It can be observed that $\mathbf{u}_1 \approx \mathbf{u}_2$, which in turn implies that $\mathbf{E}_1 \approx \mathbf{E}_2$.

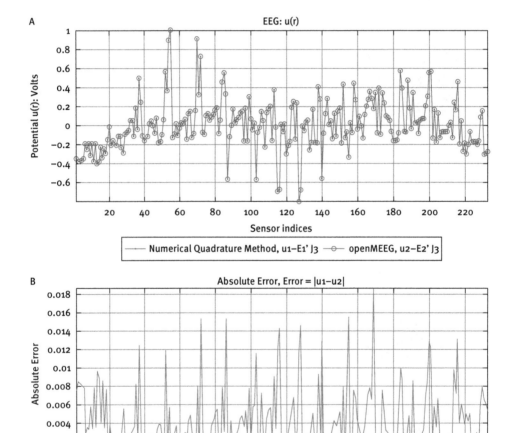

FIGURE 5.2 The potential $u(r)$ (volts) at every sensor index. The test function is given by equation (49). In subplot (a), the *solid blue line with dots* depicts equation $\mathbf{u}_1 = \mathbf{E}_1\mathbf{J}_3$. The *solid red line with circles* depicts equation $\mathbf{u}_2 = \mathbf{E}_2\mathbf{J}_3$. In subplot (b), the absolute error $|u_1(r_j) - u_2(r_j)|$ is shown as a function of indices. EEG = electroencephalography; openMEEG = _____.

For the purpose of visualization, the reconstructions are depicted on an ellipsoidal head model in Figure 5.3.

In order to better quantify the error associated with reconstructions, it is plotted in Figure 5.4 as a two-dimensional plot. Subplot (a) depicts $J_3(\tau_i)$ and $\hat{J}_3(\tau_i)$ at every node index. Subplot (b) depicts the absolute error, that is, $|J_3(\tau_i) - \hat{J}_3(\tau_i)|$, at every node index.

5.4.2. Reconstructions of $\Psi(\tau)$

A rigorous analysis of the Helmholtz decomposition and reconstruction of the relevant components of the current on the ellipsoidal head model is presented in Hashemzadeh and Fokas (2018). Here, we provide an overview of the key steps associated with imaging $\Psi(\tau)$ both for the case of the ellipsoidal head model and for a realistic head model. Furthermore, we present reconstructions for the case of the

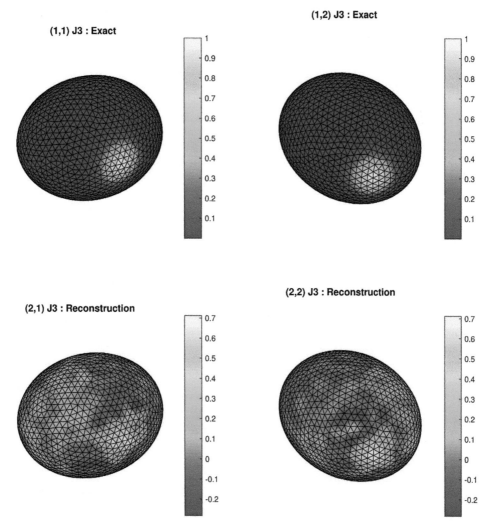

FIGURE 5.3   A reconstruction test case on an ellipsoidal head model for magnetoencephalography. Subplot $(1,1)$ and subplot $(1,2)$ depict the normalized function $J_3(\tau) = e^{-1500\|\tau-\tau_1\|} + e^{-1500\|\tau-\tau_2\|}$. Subplot $(2,1)$ and subplot $(2,2)$ depict the corresponding reconstructions, respectively.

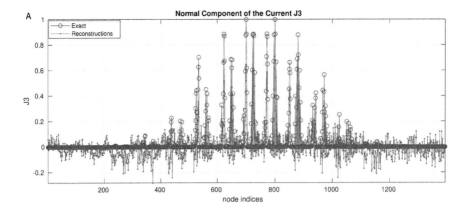

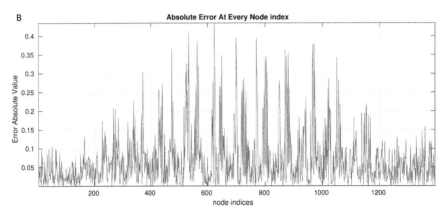

FIGURE 5.4 A reconstruction test case on an ellipsoidal head model for electroencephalography. Subplot (a) depicts the comparison of $J_3(\tau)$ and its corresponding reconstruction $\hat{J}_3(\tau)$. The *blue solid line with circles* depicts $J_3(\tau)$ as given by equation (49), and the *red solid line with dots* depicts $\hat{J}_3(\tau)$. Subplot (b) depicts the absolute error $|J_3(\tau) - \hat{J}_3(\tau)|$ for every node index.

ellipsoidal head model with parameters shown in Table 5.2.

The surfaces S_c, S_b, and S_s shown in Figure 5.1 are now co-focal surfaces with the following characteristics:

S_c: $0 < c_3 < b_3 < a_3$, S_b: $0 < c_2 < b_2 < a_2$, S_s: $0 < c_1 < b_1 < a_1$.

The surface of the cerebrum S_c is defined by the equation

$$\frac{x^2}{a_3^2} + \frac{y^2}{b_3^2} + \frac{z^2}{c_3^2} = 1. \tag{50}$$

In this setting, the inversion equation for EEG is given by equation (4). The challenge

Table 5.2 Ellipsoidal Head Model and Triangular Surface Mesh Parameters Used in the OpenMEEG Computations

DOMAIN	CONDUCTIVITY (S/M)	A(METERS)	B(METERS)	C(METERS)	NODES	TRIANGLES
Cerebrum	0.3	0.0702	0.0614	0.0527	3,124	6,244
Skull	0.0042	0.0780	0.0683	0.0585	3,124	6,244
Scalp	0.33	0.0867	0.0758	0.0650	3,126	6,248

here is to compute both $v_s(r, \tau)$ and $\dfrac{\partial v_s(r, \tau)}{\partial_n}$.

OpenMEEG can solve the boundary value problem described by equations (42) to (45). More precisely, one can directly solve $\dfrac{\partial v_s(r, \tau)}{\partial_{\hat{n}}}$ by employing OpenMEEG. However, presently, there does not exist a direct solver for the boundary value problem described by equations (37) to (40); this means that $v_s(r, \tau)$ needs to be estimated. For the case of the ellipsoidal head model, it is shown in Hashemzadeh and Fokas (2018) that a numerically stable representation for the auxiliary function $v_s(r, \tau)$ is given by

$$v_s(r, \tau) = 4\pi \sum_{n=1}^{\infty} \sum_{p=1}^{2l+1} \frac{C_n^p}{\gamma_n^p} E_n^p(\tau) E_n^p(r), \quad (51)$$

where C_n^p are geometry-dependent coefficients that can be estimated by the output of the OpenMEEG solver, γ_n^p is a normalization, and $\mathbb{E}p_n(\tau)$ denote the ellipsoidal harmonic degree n, order p (see Bardhan & Knepley, 2012; Hashemzadeh & Fokas, 2018). For reasons related to the sign ambiguity issue (Bardhan & Knepley, 2012), we employ the following parametrization:

$$\Psi(\tau) = \sum_{n=1}^{\infty} \sum_{p=1}^{2n+1} \psi_n^p(\lambda) E_n^p(\tau), \quad (52)$$

where we make the assumption that the functions $\psi_n^p(\lambda)$ take the form $\psi_n^p(\lambda) = \lambda a_n^p$. On the surface S_c, $\lambda = a_3$ and $\{a_n^p\}$ are the unknown coefficients linearly related to data. Substituting equations (51) and (52) into equation (4), we arrive at the following least squares problem:

$$\mathbf{u} = \mathrm{E}\alpha, \quad (53)$$

where $\mathbf{u}$ is the data (from EEG electrodes) and $\mathrm{E} \in \mathbb{R}^{Ns \times Np}$ is the ellipsoidal inversion matrix. A detailed analysis of the inversion

matrix E is provided in Hashemzadeh & Fokas (2018). It is shown that E is highly ill-conditioned and unsuitable for reconstruction. However, for a given a, equation (53) can be used to generate synthetic data. For the purposes of inversion, an alternative inversion matrix is constructed using equation (4) and a surface integration technique outlined by Reeger et al. (2016). In this setting, we choose to parametrize $\Psi(\tau)$ using multiquadratic radial basis functions:

$$\Psi(\tau) = \sum_{n=1}^{N} \beta_j \sqrt{\left\| \tau - \tau_j \right\|^2 + c^2}, \quad (54)$$

where $\{\beta_j\}$ are the radial basis coefficients and c is the shape parameter. The shape parameter should be estimated from the data. However, to avoid high computational costs, we have arbitrarily set this parameter to be $c = 10^{-2}$. The construction of the inversion matrix involves employing equation (54) in (4). This leads to the system of linear equations

$$\mathbf{u} = \mathrm{L}\beta, \quad (55)$$

where $\mathrm{L} \in \mathbb{R}^{Ns \times N}$. Here $N_s = 312$ is the number of electrodes and $N = 3124$ and is the number of nodes in the surface mesh of the cerebrum (see Table 5.2 for details of the surface meshes of the head ellipsoidal head model). To avoid the inverse crime (Kaipio & Somersalo, 2004), data are generated using the ellipsoidal harmonic inversion equation (53).

In Hashemzadeh & Fokas (2018), it is shown that $\log[E_{ij}]$ decays quite rapidly with increasing degree n and order p. Furthermore, it is shown that only 25 coefficients can be recovered at most. So, in this simple test case, we consider that data are generated from only the coefficient a_4^5, which corresponds to column entry 22 that multiplies the matrix entries $E_{k,25}$, for all sensor indices k. All other coefficients are set to zero, that is, $\{a_n^p = 0 : n \neq 4, p \neq 5\}$. Moreover, we consider the case that data are contaminated with additive white Gaussian noise (WGN) with a signal-to-noise ratio (SNR) of 20 dB.

The reconstruction steps are outlined here:

(i) Set $\{a_n^p\}=0$, except for $n = 4$, $p = 8$, which is set to $a_4^8=1$, $\lambda = a_3$ on surface S_c and $\psi_n^p(a_3)=a_3a_n^p$ in equation (52), that is, $\psi_4^8(a_3)=a_3$. Compute $\{\Psi(\tau_j): j = 1, ..., N\}$ at the nodes of the surface mesh.

(ii) Generate the synthetic data via equation (53), $u = Ea$, and add noise. The SNR is set at 20 dB, that is, SNR = 20 dB.

(iii) Reconstruct using equation (55), that is, $u = L\beta$. Here, we employ the TSVD to invert the matrix L with 40 of the largest singular values.

(iv) Substitute the estimated $\hat{\beta}$ into equation (54) to obtain the estimated $\hat{\Psi}(\tau)$.

(v) The reconstructions on an ellipsoidal head model are shown in Figure 5.5. The same

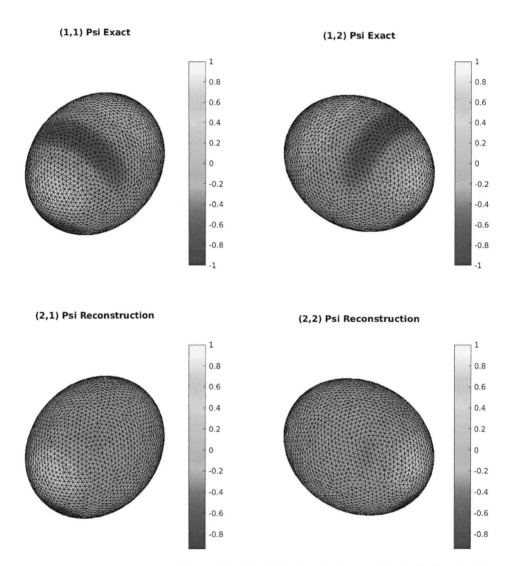

FIGURE 5.5   A reconstruction on an ellipsoidal head model outlined in the text. Subplot $(1,1)$ and subplot $(1,2)$ depict the normalized function $\Psi(\tau)$ corresponding to $\{a_n^p=0,a_4^5=1\}$ from different viewing angles. Subplot $(2,1)$ and subplot $(2,2)$ depict the corresponding reconstructions. The signal-to-noise ratio (SNR) = 20 dB.

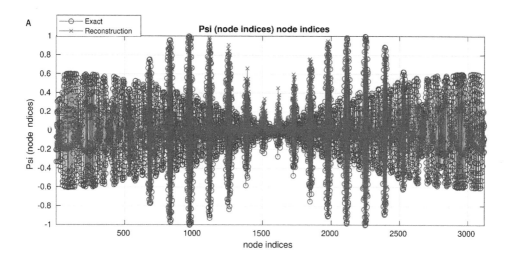

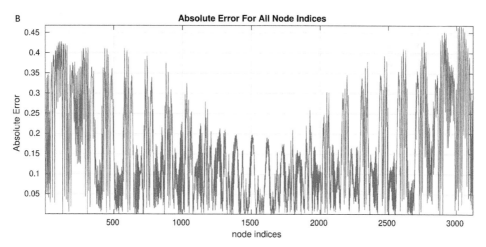

FIGURE 5.6   A reconstruction on an ellipsoidal head model outlined in the text. The signal-to-noise ratio (SNR) = 20 dB. Subplot (a) depicts the comparison of the function $\Psi(\tau)$ and its corresponding reconstruction $\hat{\Psi}(\tau)$. The *blue solid line with circles* depicts $\Psi(\tau)$, and the *red solid line with crosses* depicts $\hat{\Psi}(\tau)$. Subplot (b) depicts the absolute error $E(j):=\left|\Psi(\tau_j)-\hat{\Psi}(\tau_j)\right|$ for every node index.

reconstructions and the error $=\left|\Psi(\tau)-\hat{\Psi}(\tau)\right|$ are shown in Figure 5.6.

ACKNOWLEDGMENT

A. S. Fokas and P. Hashemzadeh are grateful to the Engineering and Physical Sciences Research Council and the Centre for Mathematical Imaging in Healthcare (for partial support. The grant number for this project is EP/N014588/1.

REFERENCES

Bardhan, J. P., & Knepley, M. G. (2012). Computational science and re-discovery: Open-source implementation of ellipsoidal harmonics for problems in potential theory. *Computational Science & Discovery, 5*(1).

Dassios, G., Fokas, A. S., Hashemzadeh, P., & Leahy, R. H. (2017). EEG for current with two dimensional support. *IEEE Transactions on Biomedical Engineering, 65*(9), 2101–2108.

Fokas, A. S. (2009). Electro-magneto-encephalography for a three-shell model: Distributed current in arbitrary, spherical and ellipsoidal geometries. *Journal of the Royal Society Interface, 6*, 479–488.

Fokas, A. S., Gelfand, I. M., & Kurylev, Y. (1996). Inversion method for magnetoencephalography. *Inverse Problems, 12* (3), 651–663.

Fokas, A. S., & Kurylev, Y. Electro-magneto-encephalography for the three-shell model: Minimal L2-norm in spherical geometry. *Inverse Problems, 28*(3).

Giapalaki, S. N., & Kariotou, F. (2006). The complete ellipsoidal shell-model in EEG imaging. *Abstract and Applied Analysis, 2006*.

Gramfort, A., Papadopoulo, T., Olivi, E., & Clerc, M. OpenMEEG opensource software for quasistatic bioelectromagnetics. *BioMedical Engineering OnLine, 9*(45).

Grave de Peralta Menendez, R., & Gonzalez Andino, S. (2015). Electrical neuroimaging with irrotational sources. *Computational and Mathematical Methods in Medicine, 2015*.

Gutiérrez, D., & Nehorai, A. (2006). Array response kernel for EEG in four-shell ellipsoidal geometry. *Fortieth Asilomar Conference on Signals, Systems and Computers*.

Gutiérrez, D., & Nehorai, A. (2008). Array response kernels for EEG and MEG in multilayer ellipsoidal geometry. *IEEE Transactions on Biomedical Engineering, 55*(3), 1103–1111.

Hashemzadeh, P., & Fokas, A. S. (2018). Helmholtz decomposition of the neuronal current for the ellipsoidal head model. *Inverse Problems, 35*(2).

Kaipio, J., & Somersalo, E. (2004). *Statistical and computational inverse problems*. New York, NY: Springer-Verlag.

Reeger, J. A., Fornberg, B., & Watts, M. L. (2016). Numerical quadrature over smooth, closed surfaces. *Proceedings of the Royal Society A: Mathematical, Physical and Engineering Sciences, 472*(2194), 20160401.

6

MAGNETOENCEPHALOGRAPHY SOURCE ESTIMATION

TRANSFORMING THE SENSOR-LEVEL SIGNALS TO ESTIMATES OF BRAIN ACTIVITY

Matti S. Hämäläinen

6.1. INTRODUCTION

In the study of both normal and pathological brain function, the methods of magnetoencephalography (MEG) and electroencephalography (EEG) hold the unique position of being the only noninvasive techniques capable of directly measuring neuronal activity with a millisecond time resolution. These two methods are thus extremely well suited for discovering the spatiotemporal sequences of brain activity while also capturing fundamental brain rhythms and frequency-dependent interactions of brain activity between different regions.

Whereas the first EEG studies were conducted in the 1920s and 1930s, MEG studies were initiated only about 40 years later, using signal averaging with an EEG reference (Cohen, 1968). Real-time MEG measurements were enabled in the beginning

of 1970s with the invention and development of the ultrasensitive superconducting quantum-interference device (SQUID) sensors. The first recordings made by David Cohen at the Massachusetts Institute of Technology (MIT) showed that high-quality recording of the magnetic counterpart of the visual alpha rhythm was possible (Cohen, 1972). During the first decade of MEG, pioneering groups recorded many sensory signals and tediously mapped their spatial distributions with single-site devices (Williamson & Kaufman, 1981). At the same time, the theoretical foundations of MEG were established, and at the end of the decade the first equivalent current dipole (ECD) fitting software was created and marked the start of inverse modeling of MEG signals (Tuomisto et al., 1983). By the beginning of the 1980s, it had become clear that for practical neuroscience and clinical studies, multichannel MEG

Matti S. Hämäläinen, *Magnetoencephalography Source Estimation: Transforming the Sensor-Level Signals to Estimates of Brain Activity* In: *Fifty Years of Magnetoencephalography*. Edited by: Andrew C. Papanicolaou, Timothy P. L. Roberts, and James W. Wheless, Oxford University Press (2020). © Oxford University Press. DOI: 10.1093/oso/9780190935689.003.0006.

systems ultimately covering the entire scalp would be a necessity. The first whole-head MEG system with more than 100 channels was introduced in 1991 (Knuutila et al., 1991). By the end of the century, more than 200 such instruments had been delivered to researchers and clinicians worldwide.

6.2. KEY CHARACTERISTICS OF MAGNETOENCEPHALOGRAPHY

Both MEG and EEG are measures of ongoing neuronal activity and are ultimately generated by the same sources: postsynaptic currents in groups of neurons that have a geometrical arrangement favoring currents with a uniform direction across nearby neurons. The most significant such assembly is that of pyramidal cells in the cerebral cortex. The macroscopic source current generated by these assemblies, often called the *primary current* (Hämäläinen, Hari, Ilmoniemi, Knuutila, & Lounasmaa, 1993; Hari & Ilmoniemi, 1986), creates an electric potential distribution, which can be sampled on the scalp using EEG.

This potential distribution is associated with passive *volume currents* in the conducting medium (Hari & Ilmoniemi, 1986). In general, the primary and volume currents together generate the magnetic field, measured with MEG. Rather surprisingly, however, the effect of the volume currents can be often quite easily taken into account. The integral effect of all the currents to the magnetic field can be computed accurately with a relatively undetailed model of electrical conductivity distribution (Hämäläinen & Sarvas, 1989; Okada, Lahteenmaki, & Xu, 1999), whereas EEG is significantly affected by the conductivity details between the sources and the electrodes. Furthermore, the effect of the real or virtual reference electrode employed has to be correctly taken into account. Since MEG and EEG capture electrical activity patterns of neural populations directly, they allow for functional brain activity to be delineated at a very fine temporal scale and possibly decomposed into its dominating oscillatory frequency components.

The ability to compute the MEG/EEG patterns generated by known sources, commonly called the solution of the *forward problem*, opens up the possibility of finding an estimate of the primary currents given the MEG measurement. However, this *inverse problem* is ill-posed: many different current distributions are capable of explaining the data (non-uniqueness), and the solutions are sensitive to noise in the data (ill-conditioned). Another way to express the non-uniqueness is to state that there are source distributions which are invisible to MEG, EEG, or both. When one wants to go from the MEG recordings at the sensor level to a plausible estimate of its underlying source, one must accept that one has to *always* employ simplifying assumptions and approximations. If one understands the qualities of this simplified equivalent source description, it is possible to gain useful insights to brain function from it, even though the actual complex spatial details cannot be reliably recovered because the measurements are necessarily made far away from the sources. Figure 6.1 illustrates the non-uniqueness of the inverse problem. In this simulation, the data were calculated from a single current dipole in the right auditory cortex. When the current dipole model is applied, the correct solution is, naturally, obtained. However, when these same data are analyzed with the minimum-norm estimate (MNE), the result is a smooth, widespread current distribution because that gives rise to exactly the same field distribution as the current dipole. Vice versa, when a widespread current distribution is analyzed, the result of dipole modeling is, erroneously, a very local source, whereas the MNE approach gives the correct answer. It is thus evident that the result of the analysis depends crucially on the underlying assumptions of the source modeling method.

Recent advances in MEG sensor technology may help partly overcome this problem and give access to finer spatial detail by bringing the sensors closer to the sources. Demonstrations

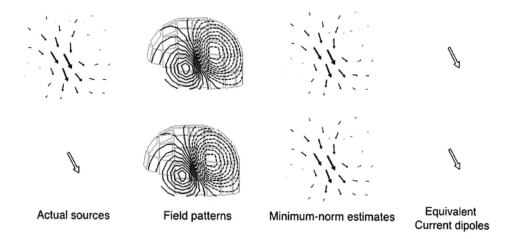

Actual sources   Field patterns   Minimum-norm estimates   Equivalent Current dipoles

FIGURE 6.1   A comparison of minimum-norm estimates and a single current dipole used to represent a distributed source (*top left*) and a current dipole (*top right*). Note that the resulting field patterns are identical, as are the minimum-norm and current dipole solutions.

of the utility of new MEG sensors include measurements with both high-T_c SQUIDs (Andersen et al., 2017; Faley, Poppe, Borkowski, Schiek, & Boers, 2012; Xie et al., 2017) and optically pumped magnetometers (OPMs), which can even be operated when the subject is moving freely (Borna et al., 2017; Boto et al., 2017). Incidentally, other noninvasive brain imaging methods have their challenges as well, but the MEG (and EEG) communities have historically been very vocal about expressing their limitations in the literature.

One can mitigate the non-uniqueness of the inverse problem by imposing anatomically and physiologically meaningful constraints. The noise sensitivity can be reduced by regularization: Exact match between the measured data and those predicted by the model is partly sacrificed to make the estimates more robust (Baillet, Mosher, & Leahy, 2001; Hämäläinen et al., 1993). Interestingly, MEG analysis has from the beginning emphasized the need to work in terms of the source estimates, in the *source space*, rather than with the sensor space signals. In contrast, even today, the vast majority of EEG studies rely on traditional sensor space analyses. The source space approach is, in fact, more straightforward with MEG than

with EEG because of the availability of a reasonably accurate forward model and because, as will be discussed later, MEG sees a specific subset of the sources in the brain. The source estimation approach has gradually made its way to EEG analyses as well, emphasizing the benefits of understanding the data in terms of brain sources rather than their manifestations on the scalp or outside. We will discuss the development of source modeling techniques in the following section.

In limited instances, the phenomena observed noninvasively in MEG or EEG can also be accessed with invasive recordings in *humans*. In particular, diagnosis of abnormal epileptic signals often requires the use of invasive electrodes either on the surface of the cortex (electrocorticogram, ECoG) or in the brain with isolated depth electrodes or arrays thereof.

An important concept related to noninvasive and invasive measurements is the *detectability* or signal strength, particularly as a function of the distance between the sensors and the active sources. This depends on three factors: (i) the spatial characteristics of the source; (ii) temporal synchrony within the source area; and (iii) the spatial selectivity of the sensors. It is well known that, at the level of even single neurons or small assemblies of neurons, the currents may exhibit a "closed" or "open" configuration (Lopes da Silva & Van Rotterdam, 1992). In addition, the contribution of action potentials as opposed to postsynaptic currents is minor at a distance because of the two opposing current dipoles needed to represent the primary currents corresponding to action potentials (Hämäläinen & Hari, 2002). At a macroscopic level, there may be further cancellation effects caused by the macroscopic curvature of the cortex in which the primary currents are normal to the cortical mantle (Ahlfors et al., 2010). In addition to these spatial effects, the strength of the measured signals depends on the length scale on which the activity is synchronous across cells. If this scale is small, measurements made at a distance, effectively averaging the source currents over a larger area or volume, may have a smaller amplitude than the distance dependence determined by the Maxwell's equations governing the physics would alone predict. This characteristic may explain why high-frequency oscillations (e.g., in the gamma band) are often more easily seen in intracranial measures than in extracranial MEG/EEG (Dalal et al., 2009). Finally, the sensor configuration also needs to be taken into account. This is often described as the lead field, which is the sensitivity pattern of the sensor (Tripp, 1983). It is worth pointing out that invasive recordings with macroscopic electrodes are in many ways similar to the surface EEG measurements, except that some of the electrodes are *potentially* located much closer to the sources than any electrode on the scalp. In principle, source estimation methods similar to those used in MEG/EEG (Baillet et al., 2001) can be used to estimate the sources of the invasive recordings pending an accurate forward model (Kakisaka et al., 2012; Murakami et al., 2016). In some cases, simultaneous MEG and invasive recordings are also possible, and a combined source estimation approach would allow better resolution of the brain activity than possible on the basis of the surface measures alone.

Because of the ambiguity of the electromagnetic inverse problem, it is very difficult to determine the actual extent of the activated areas. In this regard, assuming that the sources of MEG will be confined to the cortical mantle can be useful. For example, it might not be possible to explain the observed signals well with a focal source instead of an extended one because the focal source (current dipole) best explaining the data would not be located in the allowed cortical source space. Conversely, if a cortical constraint is not employed a best-fitting dipole source located in the gray matter, this very likely indicates that the true activity has a limited spatial extent. Some investigators (Murakami & Okada, 2015) have also argued that the current density supported by brain tissue is remarkably constant across species and brain structures: There appears to be a maximum value across the brain structures and species ($q_0 = 1$–2 nAm/mm^2). The empirical values presented by Murakami and Okada (2015) closely matched the theoretical values obtained with an independently validated neural network model, indicating that the invariance is not coincidental. This maximum value leads to a lower limit for the source extent. Since the current dipole density q, (average) dipole amplitude Q, and activated area A are related by $q = Q/A$, and $q < q_0$, we have $A > Q/q_0$. For an estimated current dipole amplitude $Q = 20$ nAm, the corresponding active cortical area should be $A \geq 10$ mm^2. Similar conclusions can be drawn from the EEG source estimates. However, the dependence of EEG on the tissue conductivities, which are not precisely known, makes it difficult to arrive at reliable quantitative estimates of the source strengths on the basis of EEG alone.

6.3. MAGNETOENCEPHALO-GRAPHY SOURCE ESTIMATION

As discussed earlier, the ill-posed nature of the inverse problem makes it difficult to prescribe a universally applicable approach to MEG analysis. However, the existence of many different approaches may also be considered an important benefit. After the experiment has been established with a tentative hypothesis, one can outline the optimal analysis pipeline. It is also conceivable that the experimental design can be informed by the available analysis approaches. Such iterative interaction, illustrated in Figure 6.2, clearly requires the existence of interdisciplinary research teams, which has been one of the common characteristics of many leading MEG centers to date.

Despite the wide variety of source estimation approaches, to be discussed in section 3.2, they all share some important common characteristics. First, the elementary *source model* in all approaches is a current dipole, which corresponds to a current sink-source pair with a small separation. Second, the measured data are modeled as a sum of a signal and noise:

$$y(t)=s(t)+n(t),$$

where $y(t)=(y_1(t)\dots y_M(t))^T$ is a column vector of the measured data, while $s(t)=(s_1(t)\dots s_M(t))^T$ and $n(t)=(n_1(t)\dots n_M(t))^T$ are the signal and noise vectors, respectively.

Third, because of the linearity of the Maxwell's equations, the signal amplitudes are linearly related to those of the sources $x(t)=(x_1(t)\dots x_N(t))^T$ by a gain matrix:

$s(t)=Ax(t)$. This relationship is not a "model" in the sense that the matrix A incorporates the *biophysics* of the MEG signal generation and is crucial for understanding the spatial characteristics of MEG. The most basic one is that A is dense; that is, every sensor sees every source with different weights, or, equivalently, each sensor sees a combination of all source activities. Since A is an expression of fundamental laws of physics, it is independent of the neuroscience per se or clinical question being addressed. For example, one can study the relative sensitivities of MEG/EEG to sources at different cortical sites and gain understanding to the relative merits of the two types of measurements with help of just the solution of the forward problem and without a need to specify or apply a source estimation procedure first (Goldenholz et al., 2009). The characteristics of A are further discussed in the next section. In practice, the time is discretely sampled, and the relationship between the data, source amplitudes, and noise can be compactly expressed as $Y = AX + N$, where the columns of the matrices Y, X, and N are the samples of the data, source amplitudes at times t_k, $k=1\dots K$.

Finally, it is usually assumed that the noise is uncorrelated across time points and that at each time point, the noises in different channels are jointly Gaussian with time-independent covariance matrix C_n, which is

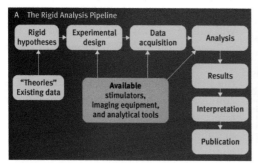
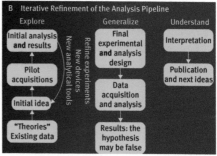

FIGURE 6.2 (A) The rigid analysis pipeline, in which the experiment and analysis workflow uses already available methods without interactions. (B) Iterative refinement of the analysis pipeline to optimize the experimental and analytical process as a whole.

estimated either from data acquired in the absense of a subject ("empty-room data") or from periods of the recording when signals of interest are not present. The former approach is used when sources of spontaneous activity, including epileptic spikes, are to be estimated, while the latter approach applies to evoked-response measurements. After C_n has been estimated, the data y and the gain matrix A are usually whitened to allow for uniform treatment in all source estimation approaches. After whitening, $\tilde{n}_k \sim N(0,1)$ and the whitened noise covariance $\tilde{C}_n = I$, which simplifies the subsequent analysis.

With this background, the task of MEG source estimation is to find best estimates $\hat{x}(t)$ given the measured data $y(t)$, the gain matrix A, and characteristics of noise $n(t)$. We will next discuss the particular approaches used to compute A, that is, the forward models, followed by an overview of different source estimation techniques.

6.3.1. Forward Models

For the MEG source estimation (inverse modeling) task to succeed, we need to possess an accurate-enough forward model, which consists of a description of the distribution electrical conductivity of the head and an analytical or numerical method to compute MEG (and EEG) given the conductivity assumptions and the elementary sources, the *source model*. Notably, the magnetic permeability of the head is close enough to that of the vacuum, and the time derivatives can be ignored from the Maxwell's equations for the computation of MEG. Therefore, the quasistatic approximation (Hämäläinen et al., 1993; Plonsey, 1969) is sufficient. This is means that the effects of the changes in source amplitudes x on the measured data y are instantaneous: There are no propagation delays or capacitive effects. Thus, if there is a change in the measured signal pattern as a function of time, the source constellation and/or the noise pattern has changed. For the

following discussion, it must be noted that the electrical conductivity is not only a location-dependent scalar quantity but also may possess anisotropy: The conductivity differs dependent on the direction it is measured. This anisotropy can be measured not only with direct electrical means but also with help of diffusion-weighted magnetic resonance imaging (MRI) (Tuch et al., 2001).

The simplest, and a surprisingly good, approximation for the head's conductivity distribution for MEG relies on spherical symmetry: The head is assumed to be composed of spherical shells with different electrical conductivities. In this case, a closed-form analytical expression exists for the magnetic field (MEG) outside the sphere (Cuffin & Cohen, 1977; Ilmoniemi, Hämäläinen, & Knuutila, 1985; Sarvas, 1987). This sphere model yields MEG characteristics of remarkable simplicity. First, unlike in EEG, only currents tangential to the surface contribute to the magnetic field. Since the principal direction of the primary currents in the cortex is perpendicular to the cortex, there are important differences between MEG and EEG. Specifically, EEG receives overwhelming contributions from the activity in the gyri, close to the electrodes. This sensitivity to nearby sources may often overshadow the signals from the more distant sulci, which MEG is primarily sensitive to. Furthermore, if the synchronous activity is extended over a large area of cortex covering both walls of a sulcus and the adjacent gyri, the MEG signals from the sulcal walls cancel out, while the gyral activity with currents pointing radially in the same direction will still be seen on EEG (Ahlfors et al., 2010).

Second, the radial component of the magnetic field can be computed directly from the primary current, and even the tangential components can be computed without explicit reference to the volume currents. Third, unlike for EEG, the result is independent of the conductivity profile along the model's radius. While these assertions are not strictly correct under more realistic conductivity assumptions, they serve as a good baseline with respect to which differences can often be considered as small perturbations. Furthermore, while the analytical approach is by far the most efficient and accurate one for the sphere model, the numerical methods described later can be applied in the spherically symmetric case as well, emphasizing the dichotomy between the model assumptions and the actual solution method used. It should also be noted that other simple conductor shapes, including the ellipsoid, can be handled analytically (Cuffin & Cohen, 1977).

If the spherical symmetry is abandoned and the head is assumed to consist of homogeneous compartments of realistic shape, the solution can be obtained with the boundary-element method (BEM) (Hämäläinen & Sarvas, 1989; Mosher, Leahy, & Lewis, 1999). This numerical approach has been finessed and can now even take into account thin layers of cerebrospinal fluid (CSF) (Stenroos & Nummenmaa, 2016). In addition, it has been shown that BEM can incorporate compartment topologies earlier believed to be accessible with the finite-element method (FEM) and finite-difference method (FDM) only (Stenroos, 2016). Specifically, the limitation to nested (layered) and island-in-the-sea geometries can be relaxed. The latter development is particularly important for the infant head: The infant skull consists of separate pieces that are connected by soft tissue (fontanels). In this geometry, each piece of skull shares its single closed boundary surface with the scalp, fontanel, and brain, resulting in piecewise-constant conductivity contrast across this boundary. Previous attempts to model this geometry using BEM have employed an approximation in which the fontanel is taken into account with a thinner region in the skull (Roche-Labarbe et al., 2008). For the purposes of MEG modeling in adults, it is, however, often sufficient to consider the skull to be a perfect insulator (Hämäläinen & Sarvas, 1987, 1989). However, it was later established that a three-compartment model consisting of the intracranial space, skull, and the scalp is preferable even for MEG (Stenroos, Hunold,

& Haueisen, 2014) and certainly if combined analysis of MEG and EEG is contemplated. Routine use of multicompartment models is, however, dependent on using accurate and reliable MRI-based means to estimate the shape of the skull compartment. Furthermore, the determination of the electrical conductivity of each compartment remains a challenge.

The prevailing approach in computing the MEG/EEG forward solutions in complex conductor geometries is the FEM, which has been developed to a great sophistication (Drechsler, Wolters, Dierkes, Si, & Grasedyck, 2009; Lanfer, Wolters, Demokritov, & Pantev, 2007; Lew et al., 2013; Lew, Wolters, Dierkes, Röer, & MacLeod, 2009; Wolters, Anwander, Berti, & Hartmann, 2007a; Wolters, Köstler, Möller, Härdtlein, & Anwander, 2007b; Wolters et al., 2007c). The FEM can incorporate an arbitrary conductivity distribution, including anisotropies. However, especially given the uncertainties in the conductor geometry and the actual electrical conductivities, and possibly the need to resort to atlas-based approximate models, the modern BEM approaches offer several benefits: (i) Since the potential is computed on the boundary surfaces only, the intricate methods to accommodate the source singularities in the volume-based FEM are not needed. (ii) Thin layers of CSF or touching surfaces can be accommodated by locally increasing the density of the surface tessellations rather than having to create a large number of voxel elements. (iii) The computational burden is small enough to allow a detailed study of the effects of the conductivity geometry, conductivities, and surface tessellation density on the accuracy of the solution. On the other hand, the FEM offers the capability to model anisotropic conductivity, possibly important in the white matter (Gullmar, Haueisen, & Reichenbach, 2010) and the skull (Dannhauer, Lanfer, Wolters, & Knosche, 2011).

The refinement of the forward model increases the precision of the source locations estimated (reduces bias). However, in general, an improved forward model does not increase the spatial resolution, if understood as the ability to resolve two close-by, simultaneously active sources. In some cases, the source estimates may actually be relatively insensitive to the accuracy of the forward model (Stenroos & Hauk, 2013).

6.3.2. Source Estimation Approaches

The aim of the solution of the inverse problem is to produce source estimates, which correctly describe the locations and extents of the sources underlying the measured MEG data, and yield the unmixed waveforms of the underlying sources. The MEG/EEG source estimation methods can be divided into three categories: (i) parametric source models, (ii) distributed current estimates, and (iii) scanning approaches.

In the parametric approach, one commonly assumes that the cortical activity underlying the measurements is sparse (i.e., salient activity occurs only in a small number of cortical sites) and that each active area has a small-enough spatial extent to be equivalently accounted for by a point source, a current dipole. This multidipole model has been very successful in the analysis of evoked potentials and fields. Even though the multidipole model is often used to explain measurements of primary and secondary sensory responses, it has also been employed in modeling of more complex cognitive functions (see, e.g., Nishitani, Avikainen, & Hari, 2004; Salmelin, Hari, Lounasmaa, & Sams, 1994) and cortical rhythms (Salmelin & Hari, 1994). The current dipole model is the de facto standard in the analysis of MEG data for the two established clinical applications of MEG: localization of epileptic spikes and mapping of eloquent cortex before surgery. In addition to considering the estimated dipole amplitudes and the locations when evaluating the validity of the dipole model, rigorous statistical criteria have been applied as well. After the model parameters have been estimated, the significance of the model can be evaluated

by using a χ^2 statistic. If one cannot reject the dipole model, the confidence region can be computed to verify that the model parameters are significant, that is, that the model is identifiable. These basic, straightforward statistical criteria are still rather rarely systematically applied, even though they were introduced to MEG analytical tools more than 25 years ago (Sarvas, 1987).

The distributed modeling approaches assume a distribution of sources on the cortex and other structures and apply an additional criterion to select a particular distribution to explain the data and to produce an image of the most likely current distribution. Most, if not all, of these methods can be expressed either by using the Bayesian statistical framework or by expressing the best estimate, $\check{x}$, as a solution of a optimization problem

$$\hat{x} = \underset{x}{argmin}\left\{ y - Ax_2^2 + f(x) \right\}$$

where the first data term promotes agreement of the actual data and those predicted by the model according to the ℓ_2-norm criterion and $f(x)$ is the additional criterion (in Bayesian terms prior) for the source amplitudes x.

To date, the most successful approach of this kind is the cortically constrained MNE (Dale et al., 2000; Dale & Sereno, 1993; Hämäläinen & Ilmoniemi, 1984), which constrains the currents to the cortical mantle and selects a solution, which has the minimum overall power, that is, $f(x) = \lambda^2 x^T x$, where λ^2 is a positive regularization constant. The MNE is a diffuse estimate, usually overestimating the extent of the source, and therefore, the extent of the MNE should not be interpreted literally. In addition to the ℓ_2-norm constraint employed in MNE, it is possible to use a criterion promoting sparsity, for example, the ℓ_1-norm to produce minimum-current estimates (MCEs), which resemble multiple dipole models, with the difference that the constellation of sources is different at each time point (Uutela,

Hämäläinen, & Somersalo, 1999). Subsequent developments of ℓ_1-norm solutions (mixed-norm estimates) have included constraints on the source waveforms and requirement that the set of sources remains unchanged throughout the analysis period (Gramfort, Kowalski, & Hämäläinen, 2012; Gramfort, Strohmeier, Haueisen, Hämäläinen, & Kowalski, 2013; Ou, Hämäläinen, & Golland, 2009).

One way to characterize the different distributed estimation approaches is to employ time-space plots shown in Figure 6.3. As shown, every source location in the standard MNE (ℓ_2) has a nonzero time course (see Figure 6.3A). This means that if the signal-to-noise ratio (SNR) could be increased indefinitely, every location would become significantly active, albeit with different amplitudes. Since this estimate is linear in the data, the time courses of the sources are linear combinations of the sensor time courses and thus have the same general time–frequency structure.

In the MCE (ℓ_1) case, the solution is nonlinear in the data, and each time point is considered separately. Therefore, the constellation of sources changes as a function of time, and the time course at a given source location has a nonphysiological telegraphic characteristic (see Figure 6.3B). When applied MCE to actual source analysis, several nearby source sites are usually averaged together to yield more believable source waveforms. To avoid this heuristic procedure in favor of a more principled approach, we introduced the mixed

ℓ_{21}-norm estimate (Gramfort et al., 2012; Gramfort et al., 2013; Ou et al., 2009). In this method, the source waveforms are assumed to be weighted sums of (orthonormal) temporal functions. The selection of the temporal waveform series coefficients, different for each source location, is based on the ℓ_2 norm, while the ℓ_1 norm is employed over space (see Figure 6.3C). This method results in a sparse constellation of sources, which is constant over time. We employed the singular value of the decomposition (SVD) of the data matrix $Y = U \Lambda V^T$ to yield the series of temporal component waveforms as a subset of columns of V. This particular ℓ_{21}-norm estimate (MxNE) thus has the temporal characteristics of the original data, similar to the ℓ_2-norm MNE. As a result, each of the sources will be active throughout the analysis period.

To comply with a scenario where the source constellation may change over the analysis period, we introduced the Time–Frequency Mixed-Norm Estimate (TF-MxNE, see Figure 6.3D). This method uses a combination of ℓ_{21} and ℓ_1 norms over the time–frequency coefficients of the data. Without going into details, the method promotes source waveforms, which are locally smooth but globally sparse. In other words, the sources may turn on and off, and the source constellation is thus allowed to change over time.

Until now, only the ℓ_2-norm MNE had found its way to the repertoire of widely accepted

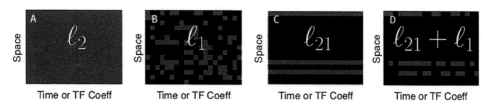

FIGURE 6.3 Sparsity patterns promoted by the different distributed source estimates: (A) ℓ_2 all nonzero, (B) ℓ_1 scattered and unstructured nonzero, (C) ℓ_{21} block row structure, and (D) $\ell_{21} + \ell_1$ block row structure with intrarow sparsity. *Gray* color indicates nonzero coefficients. TF Coeff = time–frequency coefficients. (Figure modified from Gramfort, A., Strohmeier, D., Haueisen, J., Hämäläinen, M. S., & Kowalski, M. [2013]. Time-frequency mixed-norm estimates: Sparse M/EEG imaging with non-stationary source activations *NeuroImage*, *70*, 410–422.)

distributed source estimation approaches. The utility of the sparsity-promoting estimates discussed previously, especially in the analysis of clinical data, is yet to be determined.

In the third approach to source estimation, a suitable scanning function, derived from the input data, is evaluated at each candidate source location. A high value indicates a likely location of a source. Examples of this method are the linearly constrained minimum variance beamformer (Sekihara & Nagarajan, 2008; Van Veen & Buckley, 1988) and MUSIC (Mosher & Leahy, 1998; Mosher, Lewis, & Leahy, 1992) approaches. The beamformer method has gained a lot of popularity among MEG researchers, while its use in EEG has been limited. This is probably because for the beamformer method to work, the forward model needs to be sufficiently accurate (Steinstrater, Sillekens, Junghoefer, Burger, & Wolters, 2010). Finally, the scanning approaches differ from the parametric dipole model and the source imaging approaches in the sense that the "pseudo-images" they produce do not constitute a current distribution that is capable of directly explaining the measured data.

All three types of methods have been widely used for the analysis of cortical activity and have also been validated to varying degrees in patients with invasive recordings (see, e.g., Tanaka et al., 2010). However, subcortical structures and the cerebellum also play important roles in brain function. For example, brainstem and thalamic relay nuclei have a central role in sensory processing (Jones, 1998, 2001). Thalamocortical and hippocampal oscillations govern states of sleep, arousal, and anesthesia (Steriade, McCormick, & Sejnowski, 1993). Striatal regions are crucial for movement planning, while limbic structures like the hippocampus and amygdala drive memory, emotion, and learning (Alexander, DeLong, & Strick, 1986; Graybiel, 2000; Phelps & LeDoux, 2005). Unfortunately, the anatomy of the brain poses two particular challenges for deep source estimation with MEG. First, deep brain structures are farther away from the sensors than the cerebral cortex and thus produce much lower amplitude MEG signals than the cortex. A second, perhaps more fundamental problem stems from the fact that the subcortical structures are surrounded by the cortical mantle. As a result, measurements arising from the activity of deep structures can, in principle, be explained by a surrogate distribution of currents on the cortical surface. This ambiguity also means that it is even harder to estimate subcortical activity when cortical activity is occurring simultaneously.

However, in our recent paper (Krishnaswamy et al., 2017), we reason that these limitations could be mitigated if only a finite number of cortical sites are active together with the subcortical structures. In many neuroscience studies, salient cortical activity at any moment in time tends to be restricted to a small set of well-circumscribed areas. It follows that if we can identify this sparse subset of active cortical sources and eliminate the remaining irrelevant cortical sources (Babadi et al., 2014), we have a chance at recovering the locations and time courses of both cortical and subcortical sources. In our paper (Krishnaswamy et al., 2017), we demonstrate the feasibility of this approach by introducing a new source estimation method capitalizing on this insight. Its general applicability will depend on the degree of overlap amongst the MEG field patterns of these candidate sources and the SNR of the measurements.

6.4. SUMMARY

In the previous sections, we discussed the general characteristics of MEG to give background to the problem of solving the inverse problem of MEG. Emphasizing the fact that that this transformation from the sensor signals to the source space in the brain is done in the presence of noise, we interchangeably refer to this problem as *source estimation*. MEG can be used not only to infer the sites of brain activity but also to estimate the time courses of the cortical activity, to evaluate their time frequency contents, and to compute measures of association between activities at different sites. Therefore, a universally optimal method for sensor-to-source space transformation to cover this wide spectrum of different questions does not exist. Furthermore, depending on the situation, the activity at each of the distributed sites may be focal or extended.

Our discussion of the source estimation methods gives an overview of parametric and distributed source estimation approaches and briefly covers the scanning methods as well. Finally, we consider the feasibility of detecting sources outside the cortex. In this quest, the likely sparsity of salient cortical activity may be a helpful constraint. However, reliably estimating activity in deeper brain structures and in the cerebellum is highly case dependent and requires not only novel analytical tools but also precisely circumscribed hypotheses and clever experimental designs.

In parallel with the advances in source estimation techniques, methodological advances are made in the detection of MEG signals using new sensor technologies. It is becoming possible to routinely measure MEG in close proximity to the scalp with a wide coverage. We expect that this on-scalp MEG technology will further increase the usefulness of MEG to advance our understanding of the functional organization of the brain.

REFERENCES

Ahlfors, S. P., Han, J., Lin, F. H., Witzel, T., Belliveau, J. W., Hämäläinen, M. S., & Halgren, E. (2010). Cancellation of EEG and MEG signals generated by extended and distributed sources. *Human Brain Mapping, 31,* 140–149.

Alexander, G. E., DeLong, M. R., & Strick, P. L. (1986). Parallel organization of functionally segregated circuits linking basal ganglia and cortex. *Annual Review of Neuroscience, 9,* 357–381.

Andersen, L. M., Oostenveld, R., Pfeiffer, C., Ruffieux, S., Jousmäki, V., Hämäläinen, M., . . . Lundqvist, D. (2017). Similarities and differences between on-scalp and conventional in-helmet magnetoencephalography recordings. *PLoS One, 12,* e0178602.

Babadi, B., Obregon-Henao, G., Lamus, C., Hämäläinen, M. S., Brown, E. N., & Purdon, P. L. (2014). A subspace pursuit-based iterative greedy hierarchical solution to the neuromagnetic inverse problem. *NeuroImage, 87,* 427–443.

Baillet, S., Mosher, J. C., & Leahy, R. M. (2001). Electromagnetic brain mapping *IEEE Signal Processing Magazine, 18,* 14–30.

Borna, A., Carter, T. R., Goldberg, J. D., Colombo, A. P., Jau, Y-Y., Berry, C., . . . Schwindt, P. D. D. (2017). A 20-channel magnetoencephalography system based on optically pumped magnetometers. *Physics in Medicine and Biology, 62,* 8909–8923.

Boto, E., Meyer, S. S., Shah, V., Alem, O., Knappe, S., Kruger, P., . . . Brookes, M. J. (2017). A new generation of magnetoencephalography: Room temperature measurements using optically-pumped magnetometers. *NeuroImage, 149,* 404–414.

Cohen, D. (1968). Magnetoencephalography: Evidence of magnetic fields produced by alpha-rhythm currents. *Science, 161,* 784–786.

Cohen, D. (1972). Magnetoencephalography: Detection of the brain's electrical activity with a superconducting magnetometer. *Science, 175,* 664–666.

Cuffin, B. N., & Cohen, D. (1977). Magnetic fields of a dipole in special volume conductor shapes. *IEEE Transactions on Biomedical Engineering, 24,* 372–381.

Dalal, S. S., Baillet, S., Adam, C., Ducorps, A., Schwartz, C., Jerbi, K., . . . Lachaux, J. P. (2009). Simultaneous MEG and intracranial EEG recordings during attentive reading. *NeuroImage, 45,* 1289–1304.

Dale, A. M., Liu, A. K., Fischl, B. R., Buckner, R. L., Belliveau, J. W., Lewine, J. D., & Halgren, E. (2000). Dynamic statistical parametric mapping: Combining fMRI and MEG for high-resolution imaging of cortical activity. *Neuron, 26,* 55–67.

Dale, A. M., & Sereno, M. I. (1993). Improved localization of cortical activity by combining EEG and MEG with MRI cortical surface reconstruction: A linear approach. *Journal of Cognitive Neuroscience, 5,* 162–176.

Dannhauer, M., Lanfer, B., Wolters, C. H., & Knosche, T. R. (2011). Modeling of the human skull in EEG source analysis. *Human Brain Mapping, 32,* 1383–1399.

Drechsler, F., Wolters, C. H., Dierkes, T., Si, H., & Grasedyck, L. (2009). A full subtraction approach for finite element method based source analysis using constrained Delaunay tetrahedralization. *NeuroImage, 46,* 1055–1065.

Faley, M. I., Poppe, U., Borkowski, R. E., Schiek, M., & Boers, F. (2012). Magnetoencephalography using a multilayer hightc DC SQUID magnetometer. *Physics Procedia, 36,* 66–71.

Goldenholz, D. M., Ahlfors, S. P., Hämäläinen, M. S., Sharon, D., Ishitobi, M., Vaina, L. M., & Stufflebeam, S. M. (2009). Mapping the signal-to-noise-ratios of cortical sources in magnetoencephalography and electroencephalography. *Human Brain Mapping, 30*, 1077–1086.

Gramfort, A., Kowalski, M., & Hämäläinen, M. (2012). Mixed-norm estimates for the M/EEG inverse problem using accelerated gradient methods. *Physics in Medicine and Biology, 57*, 1937–1961.

Gramfort, A., Strohmeier, D., Haueisen, J., Hämäläinen, M. S., & Kowalski, M. (2013). Time-frequency mixed-norm estimates: Sparse M/EEG imaging with non-stationary source activations. *NeuroImage, 70*, 410–422.

Graybiel, A. M. (2000). The basal ganglia. *Current Biology, 10*, R509–511.

Gullmar, D., Haueisen, J., & Reichenbach, J. R. (2010). Influence of anisotropic electrical conductivity in white matter tissue on the EEG/MEG forward and inverse solution: A high-resolution whole head simulation study. *NeuroImage, 51*, 145–163.

Hämäläinen, M., & Hari, R. (2002). Magnetoencephalographic characterization of dynamic brain activation: Basic principles and methods of data collection and source analysis. In A. W. Toga & J. C. Mazziotta (Eds.), *Brain mapping: The methods* (pp. 227–253). San Diego: Academic Press.

Hämäläinen, M., Hari, R., Ilmoniemi, R., Knuutila, J., & Lounasmaa, O. V. (1993). Magnetoencephalography: Theory, instrumentation, and applications to noninvasive studies of the working human brain. *Reviews of Modern Physics, 65*, 413–497.

Hämäläinen, M., & Ilmoniemi, R. (1984). *Interpreting magnetic fields of the brain: minimum norm estimates.* Espoo, Finland: Helsinki University of Technology.

Hämäläinen, M. S., & Sarvas, J. (1987). Feasibility of the homogeneous head model in the interpretation of neuromagnetic fields. *Physics in Medicine and Biology, 32*, 91–97.

Hämäläinen, M. S., & Sarvas, J. (1989). Realistic conductivity geometry model of the human head for interpretation of neuromagnetic data. *IEEE Transactions on Biomedical Engineering, 36*, 165–171.

Hari, R., & Ilmoniemi, R. J. (1986). Cerebral magnetic fields. *Critical Reviews in Biomedical Engineering, 14*, 93–126.

Ilmoniemi, R. J., Hämäläinen, M. S., & Knuutila, J. (1985). The forward and inverse problems in the spherical model. In H. Weinberg, G. Stroink, & T. Katila (Eds.), *Biomagnetism: Applications and theory* (pp. 278–282). New York, NY: Pergamon Press.

Jones, E. G. (1998). Viewpoint: The core and matrix of thalamic organization. *Neuroscience, 85*, 331–345.

Jones, E. G. (2001). The thalamic matrix and thalamocortical synchrony. *Trends in Neuroscience, 24*, 595–601.

Kakisaka, Y., Kubota, Y., Wang, Z. I., Piao, Z., Mosher, J. C., Gonzalez-Martinez, J., . . . Burgess, R. C. (2012). Use of simultaneous depth and MEG recording may provide complementary information regarding the epileptogenic region. *Epileptic Disorders, 14*, 298–303.

Knuutila, J., Ahonen, A., Hämäläinen, M., Kajola, M., Lounasmaa, O. V., Simola, J., . . . Vilkman, V. (1991). Design of a 122-channel neuromagnetometer covering the whole head. In M. Hoke (Ed.), *Abstract book of the 8th International Conference on Biomagnetism* (pp. 109–110). University of Münster, Germany.

Krishnaswamy, P., Obregon-Henao, G., Ahveninen, J., Kahn, S., Babadi, B., Iglesias, J. E., . . . Purdon, P. L. (2017). Sparsity enables estimation of both subcortical and cortical activity from MEG and EEG. *Proceedings of the National Academy of Sciences of the United States of America, 114*, E10465–E10474.

Lanfer, B., Wolters, C. H., Demokritov, S. O., & Pantev, C. (2007). Validating finite element method based EEG and MEG forward computations. Paper presented at the 41 Jahrestagung der Deutschen Gesellschaft für Biomedizinische, Technik Aachen, Germany.

Lew, S., Sliva, D. D., Choe, M. S., Grant, P. E., Okada, Y., Wolters, C. H., & Hämäläinen, M. S. (2013). Effects of sutures and fontanels on MEG and EEG source analysis in a realistic infant head model. *NeuroImage, 76C*, 282–293.

Lew, S., Wolters, C. H., Dierkes, T., Röer, C., & MacLeod, R. S. (2009). Accuracy and run-time comparison for different potential approaches and iterative solvers in finite element method based EEG source analysis. *Applied Numerical Mathematics, 59*, 1970–1988.

Lopes da Silva, F., & Van Rotterdam, A. (1992). Biophysical aspects of EEG and MEG generation. In E. Niedermeyer & F. Lopes da Silva (Eds.), Electroencephalography: Basic principles, clinical applications and related fields (2nd ed., pp. 29–41). Baltimore, MD: Urban & Schwarzenberg.

Mosher, J. C., & Leahy, R. M. (1998). Recursive MUSIC: A framework for EEG and MEG source localization. *IEEE Transactions on Biomedical Engineering, 45*, 1342–1354.

Mosher, J. C., Leahy, R. M., & Lewis, P. S. (1999). EEG and MEG: Forward solutions for inverse methods. *IEEE Transactions on Biomedical Engineering, 46*, 245–259.

Mosher, J. C., Lewis, P. S., & Leahy, R. M. (1992). Multiple dipole modeling and localization from spatio-temporal MEG data. *IEEE Transactions on Biomedical Engineering, 39,* 541–557.

Murakami, H., Wang, Z. I., Marashly, A., Krishnan, B., Prayson, R. A., Kakisaka, Y., . . . Alexopoulos, A. V. (2016). Correlating magnetoencephalography to stereo-electroencephalography in patients undergoing epilepsy surgery. *Brain, 139,* 2935–2947.

Murakami, S., & Okada, Y. (2015). Invariance in current dipole moment density across brain structures and species: Physiological constraint for neuroimaging. *NeuroImage, 111,* 49–58.

Nishitani, N., Avikainen, S., & Hari, R. (2004). Abnormal imitation-related cortical activation sequences in Asperger's syndrome. *Annals of Neurology, 55,* 558–562.

Okada, Y., Lahteenmaki, A., & Xu, C. (1999). Comparison of MEG and EEG on the basis of somatic evoked responses elicited by stimulation of the snout in the juvenile swine. *Clinical Neurophysiology, 110,* 214–229.

Ou, W., Hämäläinen, M. S., & Golland, P. (2009). A distributed spatio-temporal EEG/MEG inverse solver. *NeuroImage, 44,* 932–946.

Phelps, E. A., & LeDoux, J. E. (2005). Contributions of the amygdala to emotion processing: From animal models to human behavior. *Neuron, 48,* 175–187.

Plonsey, R. (1969). *Bioelectric phenomena.* New York: McGraw-Hill.

Roche-Labarbe, N., Aarabi, A., Kongolo, G., Gondry-Jouet, C., Dumpelmann, M., Grebe, R., & Wallois, F. (2008). High-resolution electroencephalography and source localization in neonates. *Human Brain Mapping, 29,* 167–176.

Salmelin, R., & Hari, R. (1994). Spatiotemporal characteristics of sensorimotor neuromagnetic rhythms related to thumb movement. *Neuroscience, 60,* 537–550.

Salmelin, R., Hari, R., Lounasmaa, O. V., & Sams, M. (1994). Dynamics of brain activation during picture naming. *Nature, 368,* 463–465.

Sarvas, J. (1987). Basic mathematical and electromagnetic concepts of the biomagnetic inverse problem. *Physics in Medicine and Biology, 32,* 11–22.

Sekihara, K., & Nagarajan, S. S. (2008). *Adaptive spatial filters for electromagnetic brain imaging.* Berlin, Germany: Springer.

Steinstrater, O., Sillekens, S., Junghoefer, M., Burger, M., & Wolters, C. H. (2010). Sensitivity of beamformer source analysis to deficiencies in forward modeling. *Human Brain Mapping, 31,* 1907–1927.

Stenroos, M. (2016). Integral equations and boundary-element solution for static potential in a general piece-wise homogeneous volume conductor. *Physics in Medicine and Biology, 61,* N606–N617.

Stenroos, M., & Hauk, O. (2013). Minimum-norm cortical source estimation in layered head models is robust against skull conductivity error. *NeuroImage, 81,* 265–272.

Stenroos, M., Hunold, A., & Haueisen, J. (2014). Comparison of three-shell and simplified volume conductor models in magnetoencephalography. *NeuroImage, 94,* 337–348.

Stenroos, M., & Nummenmaa, A. (2016). Incorporating and compensating cerebrospinal fluid in surface-based forward models of magneto- and electroencephalography. *PLoS One, 11,* e0159595.

Steriade, M., McCormick, D. A., & Sejnowski, T. J. (1993). Thalamocortical oscillations in the sleeping and aroused brain. *Science, 262,* 679–685.

Tanaka, N., Hämäläinen, M. S., Ahlfors, S. P., Liu, H., Madsen, J. R., Bourgeois, B. F., . . . Stufflebeam, S. M. (2010). Propagation of epileptic spikes reconstructed from spatiotemporal magnetoencephalographic and electroencephalographic source analysis. *NeuroImage, 50,* 217–222.

Tripp, J. H. (1983). Physical concepts and mathematical models. In S. J. Williamson, G. L. Romani, I. Kaufman, & I. Modena (Eds.), *Biomagnetism: An interdisciplinary approach* (pp. 101–139). New York, NY: Plenum Press.

Tuch, D. S., Wedeen, V. J., Dale, A. M., George, J. S., & Belliveau, J. W. (2001). Conductivity tensor mapping of the human brain using diffusion tensor MRI. *Proceedings of the National Academy of Sciences of the United States of America, 98,* 11697–11701.

Tuomisto, T., Hari, R., Katila, T., Poutanen, T., & Varpula, T. (1983). Studies of auditory evoked magnetic and electric responses: Modality specificity and modelling. *Il Nuovo Cimento D, 2:*471–494.

Uutela, K., Hämäläinen, M., & Somersalo, E. (1999). Visualization of magnetoencephalographic data using minimum current estimates. *NeuroImage, 10,* 173–180.

Van Veen, B., & Buckley, K. (1988). Beamforming: A versatile approach to spatial filtering. *IEEE ASSP Magazine, 5,* 4–24.

Williamson, S. J., & Kaufman, L. (1981). Biomagnetism. *Journal of Magnetism and Magnetic Materials, 22,* 129–202.

Wolters, C. H., Anwander, A., Berti, G., & Hartmann, U. (2007a). Geometry-adapted hexahedral meshes improve accuracy of finite-element-method-based EEG source analysis. *IEEE Transactions on Biomedical Engineering, 54,* 1446–1453.

Wolters, C. H., Köstler, H., Möller, C., Härdtlein, J., & Anwander, A. (2007b). Numerical approaches for dipole modeling in finite element method based source analysis. *Elsevier International Congress Series, 1300,* 189–192.

Wolters, C. H., Köstler, H., Möller, C., Härtlein, J., Grasedyck, L., & Hackbusch, W. (2007c). Numerical mathematics of the subtraction method for the modeling of a current dipole in EEG source reconstruction using finite element head models. *SIAM Journal on Scientific Computing, 30,* 24–45.

Xie, M., Schneiderman, J. F., Chukharkin, M. L., Kalabukhov, A., Riaz, B., Lundqvist, D., ... Winkler, D. (2017). Benchmarking for on-scalp MEG sensors. *IEEE Transactions on Biomedical Engineering, 64,* 1270–1276.

7

THE NEED FOR AND ROAD TO HYBRID MAGNETOENCEPHALOGRAPHY– MAGNETIC RESONANCE IMAGING

Risto J. Ilmoniemi

7.1. INTRODUCTION

After 50 years of magnetoencephalography (MEG), multiple novel technical approaches and new methodologies are now being developed. Optically pumped magnetometers (OPMs), high-transition-temperature (high-T_c) superconducting quantum-interference devices (SQUIDs), nitrogen-vacancy, and other new types of sensors may replace traditional low-temperature SQUIDs, at least in specialized applications. Sophisticated signal-separation and noise-canceling methods, as well as source-determination algorithms, are better than ever. Machine learning and other advanced data analysis tools are applied, and methods to better solve the inverse problem by using a priori information about the neuronal sources are being developed. However, many of these wonderful techniques are not reliable or accurate so long as geometrical information about the head and the brain with respect to the sensor array is not sufficiently precise.

This chapter will describe, after some historical background, new efforts to help solve this problem. If the head geometry (its location with respect to the sensor array, detailed shape of the scalp, skull, cerebrospinal fluid, cortex, and their conductivities) were precisely known, we would be able to take full advantage of the fine mathematical tools that have already been developed. This presentation tries to avoid unnecessary technical detail, with the emphasis being on issues regarding MEG instrumentation that may be of interest to the neuroscientist or clinician.

As explained elsewhere in this section, it took about 10 years from the first high-quality neuromagnetic measurements (Cohen, 1972) until MEG was used for other purposes than for demonstrating its technical ability to

Risto J. Ilmoniemi, *The Need for and Road to Hybrid Magnetoencephalography–Magnetic Resonance Imaging* In: *Fifty Years of Magnetoencephalography*. Edited by: Andrew C. Papanicolaou, Timothy P. L. Roberts, and James W. Wheless, Oxford University Press (2020). © Oxford University Press. DOI: 10.1093/oso/9780190935689.003.0007.

measure various spontaneous and evoked signals in healthy volunteers. Barth, Sutherling, Engel, & Beatty (1982) showed the potential of MEG in epilepsy studies, and Romani, Williamson, & Kaufman (1982) reported that the location of source activity explaining measured auditory evoked magnetic fields appears to depend on sound frequency. At the same time, efforts to develop multichannel MEG instruments had begun, with the hope that in this way neuroscientific and clinical applications would start to thrive. In the Low Temperature Laboratory of Helsinki University of Technology (HUT), we built a seven-channel magnetometer (Ehnholm, Ilmoniemi, & Wiik, 1981), which did not prove to be practical but gave a lot of useful technical experience, followed by a quite successful four-channel device (Ilmoniemi, Hari, & Reinikainen, 1984). Soon thereafter, the San Diego company SHE (later, Biomagnetic Technologies Inc., or BTi; still later, 4-D Neuroimaging), in collaboration with the Neuromagnetism Laboratory of New York University, introduced a five-channel MEG device (Williamson et al., 1985) and a two-dewar system with a seven-channel magnetometer in each (Williamson & Kaufman, 1989). New multichannel devices were subsequently built by several groups and companies. Here I focus on developments in Finland, where MEG technology was commercialized by Neuromag Ltd.

(later, part of 4-D Neuroimaging; still later, part of Elekta Ltd.; now MEGIN Ltd.), and where we are now developing a hybrid MEG–MRI system.

After the installation of the four-channel MEG device, our work at HUT continued with a reliable and low-noise seven-channel instrument (Knuutila et al., 1987), a 24-channel MEG device (Ahlfors et al., 1990; Kajola et al., 1989), and, finally, the first full-head system with 122 channels (Ahonen et al., 1993) (Figure 7.1). The full-head systems, introduced also by BTi and by CTF (Vancouver, Canada) in the 1990s, were a game changer. It was now possible to obtain a comprehensive view of brain activity at once, without moving the sensor array over different parts of the brain. In Helsinki, the device was installed at the Low Temperature Laboratory of HUT and also at the new BioMag Laboratory at the Helsinki University Hospital (Ilmoniemi et al., 2000). The BioMag Laboratory was organized by Professor Toivo Katila of HUT together with the technical director of the Hospital, Dr. Pekka Karp; the director of the Hospital, Arvo Relander; and the rector of the University of Helsinki, Professor Risto Ihamuotila, as a joint research center of the two universities and the hospital. This was another game changer because it brought the instrument close to neurological patients and was easily accessible to clinicians eager to perform neuromagnetic studies, first with healthy

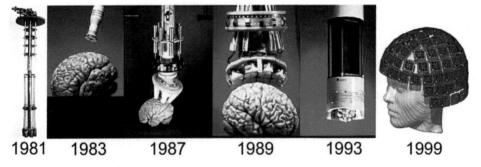

FIGURE 7.1 Development of multichannel magnetoencephalography (MEG) systems at the Helsinki University of Technology and the Neuromag company (Ahonen et al., 1993; Ehnholm et al., 1981; Ilmoniemi et al., 1984; Kajola et al., 1989; Knuutila et al., 1987). (Images by R. Ilmoniemi [1981, 1983], J. Knuutila [1987, 1989], Elekta Ltd. [1993], and M. Seppä [1999]).

volunteers and somewhat later with patients. Some of the first research patients with the new whole-head MEG systems at HUT and BioMag were those with Alzheimer disease (Pekkonen et al., 1996), schizophrenia (Tiihonen et al., 1998), and stroke (Wikström et al., 1999). However, the foremost clinical application of MEG proved to be epilepsy (Hari et al., 1993; Paetau, Kajola, & Hari, 1990; Simos, Rezaie, & Papanicolaou, 2019).

7.2. THE NEED FOR HYBRID MAGNETOENCEPHALOGRAPHY AND MAGNETIC RESONANCE IMAGING SYSTEMS

The importance of combining MEG with MRI was realized early (Ilmoniemi, 1985). The most important benefit of MEG over the widely available electroencephalography (EEG) is its ability to locate brain activity. To relate the location coordinates to individual anatomy, structural MRI is needed. In addition, structural MRI can help constrain the estimated source currents to the cortex (Ilmoniemi, 1985), making the three-dimensional source volume a two-dimensional layer. Later, after the invention of functional MRI (fMRI; Belliveau et al., 1991), it was realized that the new kind of data could be used as additional information to help solve the MEG inverse problem. Namely, one could assume that locations where hemodynamic changes are found would be the most probable sites also for electrophysiological signal sources. We performed the first pioneering MEG–fMRI studies together with Jack Belliveau and his colleagues in 1995 at the BioMag Laboratory (where MEG was done) and at Massachusetts General Hospital (where fMRI was done) (see Ahlfors et al., 1999; Korvenoja et al., 1999).

Thus, structural MRI benefits MEG data interpretation in three main ways: first, MEG localization results can be displayed on top of anatomical images; second, one obtains geometrical information (conductivity structure and cortical shape) for the analysis of the inverse problem, for example, in beamforming; third, a priori information regarding source locations will be more accurate. Because MEG and MRI are normally done separately, the two data sets have to be combined. This requires co-registration of the MEG and MRI coordinate systems. A common way to do this is to find the same landmark points in MEG and MRI studies, for example, preauricular points and the nasion. Several mechanisms tend to make this procedure inaccurate: (a) distortion of the overall head shape in high-field MRI, in particular by differences in susceptibility between tissues and the air; (b) inaccuracy of determining landmarks in the MRI; (c) inaccuracy of determining landmarks in MEG; (d) movement of the brain within the head between MRI and MEG sessions, in particular if MEG is performed in sitting position and MRI in supine position; and (e) movement of the head in the course of the MEG study. The typical overall error of co-registration may be in the range of 5 to 10 mm, depending on how carefully the registration is performed, although with special techniques, head movement can be minimized and repeatability of registration can be improved (Meyer et al., 2017).

However, even in favorable cases, the brain may move relative to the skull and scalp between MRI and MEG sessions, and some of the geometrical distortions in high-field MRI are unavoidable. Some improvement for solving the inverse problem can be gained by using simultaneous EEG with MEG (Virtanen, Rinne, Ilmoniemi, & Näätänen, 1996; Virtanen, Parkkonen, Ilmoniemi, Pekkonen, & Näätänen, 1997), but since the electromagnetic inverse problem has no unique solution, supplementary or a priori information about the neuronal sources in addition to MEG or EEG data is needed.

7.3. ULTRA-LOW-FIELD MAGNETIC RESONANCE IMAGING

It was demonstrated by John Clarke's group at the University of California, Berkeley

(McDermott et al., 2004) that one can obtain high-quality magnetic resonance images at ultra-low magnetic fields, that is, at fields of the order of 100 mT (0.0001 T). This is surprising because we have learned that the signal level in nuclear magnetic resonance (NMR, the basic phenomenon in MRI) is proportional to the square of the magnetic field strength B. This is because both determinants of the MRI signal strength (the polarization of spins and their precession frequency) are proportional to B. At 0.0001 T, the signal amplitude would thus be only about one-billionth (1/1,000,000,000) of that at 3 T. So how is ultra-low-field (ULF) MRI possible?

McDermott et al. (2004) combined two well-known techniques: (a) To measure the MRI magnetic field, they used a SQUID magnetometer, which has a frequency-independent sensitivity and is thus suitable for measurements at low Larmor frequencies. (b) They used prepolarization, meaning that before the manipulation of the spins with gradient fields for MRI, the sample was polarized at a relatively high magnetic field (130 mT). Subsequently, the group at Los Alamos developed the technique for human studies (Zotev et al., 2007); this group also performed the first combined MEG and ULF-MRI recordings (Zotev et al., 2008). After learning from John Clarke at a meeting in Dubrovnik in 2006 about the prospects of ULF MRI, we started the development of the technique at HUT, and in 2008, in an EU-funded international effort (MEGMRI, 2008–2012), we began to develop whole-head MEG–MRI technology, with Professor Clarke as an advisor.

7.4. MOTIVATION FOR ULTRA-LOW-FIELD MAGNETIC RESONANCE IMAGING AND ITS COMBINATION WITH MAGNETOENCEPHALO-GRAPHY

Several benefits can be expected if MEG and MRI can be combined into a hybrid device. First, the co-registration error can be essentially eliminated if the system is properly calibrated (Mäkinen, Zevenhoven, & Ilmoniemi, 2019). Second, at low fields, we will avoid susceptibility artefacts, which cause geometrical distortions in MRI. Third, workflow in MEG studies will become easier and faster because both MEG and MRI can be measured in the same session. Fourth, ULF MRI provides unique information; for example, T1 contrast is dramatically better below 1 mT than at high magnetic fields (Clarke, Hatridge, & Mössle, 2007). This improved contrast may turn out to be useful in characterizing pathological tissue in cases in which high-field MRI is not sufficiently sensitive (Busch et al., 2012). Fifth, there is a possibility that tissue conductivities of different head compartments can be obtained more accurately with ULF MRI–based current imaging than with other methods (Nieminen, Zevenhoven, Vesanen, Hsu, & Ilmoniemi, 2014; Vesanen, Nieminen, Zevenhoven, Hsu, & Ilmoniemi, 2014); this would improve the accuracy and reliability of inverse-problem solutions for both MEG and EEG and make even the targeting of transcranial magnetic stimulation (TMS) or transcranial direct current stimulation (tDCS) more accurate than before. Additional benefits include quiet operation and avoiding the need to put the patient in the narrow MRI tube, making the device more suitable for small children and for people with claustrophobia or excess weight.

As mentioned earlier, the MEG inverse problem (even when combined with high-resolution EEG) is non-unique, meaning that infinitely many different source-current distributions could produce the measured field values. Therefore, additional information or knowledge (a priori or supplementary knowledge) about the source currents usually has to be available to obtain any meaningful estimate of the source currents. In some cases, for example, if one knows a priori (or correctly guesses) that a single source would dominate the creation of the recorded MEG signals, or if one can assume independent time courses for a small number of distinct sources, the underlying neuronal activity can be quite reliably located using, for example, single-dipole fitting, the MUSIC algorithm, or beamforming (see Ilmoniemi & Sarvas, 2019). However, very often the case is not that simple; and if the forward problem solution is not sufficiently accurate (because of inaccurate co-registration of MEG and MRI coordinate systems or inaccurately known conductivity structure), even the sophisticated techniques mentioned previously cannot be relied on.

A considerable improvement in the reliability of source estimation is obtained if one can assume that the neuronal sources generating MEG or EEG signals are located in the gray matter. This highly plausible assumption can be used to constrain the inverse-problem solution to the cortex. However, if the co-registration error is more than about 2 mm, such a constraint could force the sources to reside in the white matter, in the cerebrospinal fluid, or even within the skull. One might at first think that a co-registration error of, say, 6 mm would produce an error in source localization of just 6 mm. But this is unfortunately not the case in general; since a source displaced by 6 mm from its real location cannot produce the same magnetic field pattern as the real one, the solution for a localized source must be formed by a distribution of sources, possibly and probably quite far from the original real source. Such false sources in the inverse solution, called *ghost sources,* can lead to misinterpretation of the results. Chella et al. (2019) have in simulation studies investigated this problem by evaluating errors in source localization and connectivity measures due to co-registration errors. Their study shows that one should aim at co-registration accuracy of 2 mm or better. In reality, as pointed out earlier, further errors arise from inaccurate head models; it seems clear that we will need improved knowledge of conductivity values as well to benefit from state-of-the art electromagnetic modeling of the head structure (Matti Stenroos, private communication).

Simultaneous ULF MRI will reduce the geometrical uncertainties in MEG studies: Sensor locations with respect to the head will be known with submillimeter accuracy; the shapes of the cerebrospinal fluid compartments, the cortex, and the white matter will be known more accurately. This will enable one, for the first time, to take advantage of the full potential of sophisticated data analysis tools, many of which have already been developed. We "only" need to get the technology ready.

7.5. TECHNOLOGY FOR MAGNETOENCEPHALOGRAPHY–MAGNETIC RESONANCE IMAGING

The first helmet-shaped sensor array for MEG–MRI was built at Aalto University (Vesanen et al., 2013). Figure 7.2 shows the present, more advanced, MEG–MRI prototype at Aalto University (group led by Koos Zevenhoven), built in the European BREAKBEN project (Ilmoniemi et al., 2016) in close collaboration with VTT Technical Research Center of Finland (SQUID development, led by Mikko Kiviranta) and MEGIN Ltd. (in particular dewar and data acquisition; group led by Jukka Nenonen). The helmet-shaped dewar houses 120 SQUID magnetometers for measuring both MEG and MRI signals as well as the superconducting coil for producing the prepolarization magnetic field in the head. The other magnetic fields for MRI are produced by coils on the sides of the dewar. Note that access to the MEG device is not hindered by the MRI coils.

Although the typical sensitivity of SQUID magnetometers, on the order of several $fT/Hz^{1/2}$ (1 $fT/Hz^{1/2}$ means that the root-mean-square noise in 1-Hz bandwidth is 1 fT) is excellent for most MEG studies, it is not quite sufficient for ULF MRI.

Four key factors determine the ultimate image quality in ULF MRI: (a) SQUID noise level, (b) prepolarization field, (c) bandwidth of the Larmor frequencies when gradients are used, and (d) number of independent

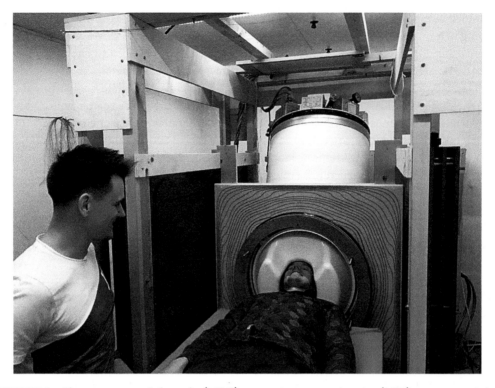

FIGURE 7.2 The magnetoencephalography (MRG)–magnetic resonance imaging (MRI) prototype at Aalto University that features white-noise levels below 1 fT/Hz$^{1/2}$. The liquid helium container contains the helmet-shaped SQUID-sensor array that measures the neuromagnetic and MRI fields surrounding the head as well as a superconducting magnet that produces the prepolarization field for MRI. The strength of the prepolarization field is about 100 mT, that is, 14 orders of magnitude (100,000,000,000,000) higher than the smallest fields that can be measured after the prepolarization field has been turned off. Two of the key developers of the system are in the picture: Marko Havu (standing) and Antti Mäkinen (supine).

measurement channels (sensors). One can think about the requirements in terms of information obtained from the brain to obtain the images. The images consist of pixels (or voxels in three dimensions), and the required amount of information in bits is equal the number of pixels (or voxels) times the average number of informative bits per pixel. For example, if we aim at about 2-mm resolution, we would have approximately 300,000 voxels in the head image. With 4 bits per voxel, we would need 1.2 million bits of information to form the image. With 120 independent SQUID sensors, this would make 10,000 bits per sensor. If the relevant bandwidth were on the order of 200 Hz, the measurement time 10% of the total time, and signal-to-noise ratio (SNR) of order

one, this would result in a data rate of about 20 bits per second per channel. Then, one could in principle obtain the desired image in about 500 seconds. Please note that this is only an idealized order-of-magnitude computation, but from it one can get an idea of what is of importance. In particular, the SNR is a crucial limiting factor of ULF MRI.

7.6. NEW SENSOR TECHNOLOGIES

In addition to MEG–MRI, several other new technologies for MEG are being developed. Two of them, high-T_c SQUIDs and OPMs, have the benefit that cooling to liquid-helium temperatures is no more needed. Hybrid quantum interference devices (hyQUIDs) need cooling, but their developer, York Instruments Ltd., has a cooling method without liquid helium. Other interesting sensor types have been developed, for example, those based on giant magnetoresistance (Caruso et al., 2017; Pannetier et al., 2004; Sergeeva-Chollet et al., 2011) and nitrogen vacancies in diamonds (Karadas et al., 2018).

High-T_c SQUIDs can be cooled with inexpensive liquid nitrogen instead of helium. The use of liquid nitrogen enables one to build thin-wall dewars with sensors very close (~1 mm) to the scalp. Although this will enhance the magnetic-field signals from the brain, the noise level in high-T_c SQUID magnetometers is still too high for high-quality MRI.

Also, OPMs can be placed close to the scalp, but not quite as close as high-T_c SQUIDs because they require a certain volume of alkali-metal gas (heated to at least 120° C); the center of mass of the gas contained will need to be perhaps a distance of 3 to 4 mm from the scalp in practical devices. Currently, OPMs are not sufficiently sensitive for high-quality MRI, and their limited bandwidth may also limit ULF MRI use.

It is conceivable that the benefits of different magnetometer types will someday be combined by using multiple sensor technologies in the same MEG system.

7.7. CONCLUSION

Multichannel sensor arrays developed in the 1980s and later have made MEG measurements faster, more reliable, and more accurate. However, because the inverse problem is non-unique, data interpretation always requires either explicit a priori information or assumptions about the nature of the neuronal currents in the brain. Sophisticated powerful methods such as MUSIC and beamforming have been developed for MEG source determination, but even when their assumptions of a small number of localized sources is correct, they suffer from inaccurate volume conductor models or inaccurate co-registration of MEG and MRI data sets.

Hybrid MEG–MRI systems, when perfected, will eliminate the co-registration inaccuracy and promises to inform us also about the individual conductivity structure if conductivity imaging with ultra-low-field MRI will succeed.

ACKNOWLEDGMENT

This project has received funding from the European Union Horizon 2020 research and innovation programme under grant agreement No. 686865. I gratefully acknowledge the collaboration and valuable contributions to this work by Dr. Rainer Körber of Physikalisch Technische Bundesanstalt Berlin, Professor Gian Luca Romani of the University of Chieti–Pescara, Professor Jens Haueisen of the Technical University of Ilmenau, Dr. Jyrki Mäkelä of the BioMag Laboratory at Helsinki University Hospital, and their team members as well as the teams at Aalto University, VTT, and MEGIN who have worked toward hybrid MEG–MRI.

REFERENCES

Ahlfors, S., Ahonen, A., Ehnholm, G., Hämäläinen, M., Ilmoniemi, R., Kajola, M., . . . Vilkman, V. (1990). A 24-SQUID gradiometer for magnetoencephalography. *Physica B: Condensed Matter, 165–166*, 97–98.

Ahlfors, S. P., Simpson, G. V., Dale, A. M., Belliveau, J. W., Liu, A. K., Korvenoja, A., . . . Ilmoniemi, R. J. (1999). Spatiotemporal activity of a cortical network for processing visual motion revealed by MEG and fMRI. *Journal of Neurophysiology, 82*, 2545–2555.

Ahonen, A. I., Hämäläinen, M. S., Kajola, M. J., Knuutila, J. E. T., Laine, P. P., Lounasmaa, O. V., . . . Tesche, C. D. (1993). 122-channel SQUID instrument for investigating the magnetic signals from the human brain. *Physica Scripta, T49A*, 198–205.

Barth, D. S., Sutherling, W., Engel, J., & Beatty, J. (1982). Neuromagnetic localization of epileptiform spike activity in the human brain. *Science, 218*, 891–894.

Belliveau, J. W., Kennedy, D. N., McKinstry, R. C., Buchbinder, B. R., Weisskoff, R., Cohen, M. S., . . . Rosen, B. R. (1991). Functional mapping of the human visual cortex by magnetic resonance imaging. *Science, 254*, 716–719.

Busch, S., Hatridge, M., Mößle, M., Myers, W., Wong, T., Mück, M., . . . Clarke, J. (2012). Measurements of T1-relaxation in *ex vivo* prostate tissue at 132 μT. *Magnetic Resonance in Medicine, 67*, 1138–1145.

Caruso, L., Wunderle, T., Lewis, C. M., Valadeiro, J., Trauchessec, V., Rosillo, J. T., . . . Pannetier-Lecoeur, M. (2017). *In vivo* magnetic recording of neuronal activity. *Neuron, 95*, 1283–1291.

Chella, F., Marzetti, L., Stenroos, M., Parkkonen, L., Ilmoniemi, R. J., Romani, G. L., & Pizzella, V. (2019). The impact of improved MEG–MRI co-registration on MEG connectivity analysis. *NeuroImage, 197*, 354–367.

Clarke, J., Hatridge, M., & Mössle, M. (2007). SQUID-detected magnetic resonance imaging in microtesla fields. *Annual Review of Biomedical Engineering, 9*, 389–413.

Cohen, D. (1972). Magnetoencephalography: Detection of the brain's electrical activity with a superconducting magnetometer. *Science, 175*, 664–666.

Ehnholm, G. J., Ilmoniemi, R. J., & Wiik, T. O. (1981). A seven channel SQUID magnetometer for brain research. *Physica B + C, 107*, 29–30.

Hari, R., Ahonen, A., Forss, N., Granström, M. L., Hämäläinen, M., Kajola, M., . . . Paetau, R. (1993). Parietal epileptic mirror focus detected with a whole-head neuromagnetometer. *Neuroreport, 5*, 45–48.

Ilmoniemi, R. (1985). Neuromagnetism: Theory, techniques, and measurements. PhD Thesis, Helsinki University of Technology, Helsinki, Finland.

Ilmoniemi, R., Hari, R., & Reinikainen, K. (1984). A four-channel SQUID magnetometer for brain research. *Electroencephalography and Clinical Neurophysiology, 58*, 467–473.

Ilmoniemi, R. J., Ahonen, A., Alho, K., Aronen, H. J., Huttunen, J., Karhu, J., . . . Pekkonen, E. (2000). MEG and MCG in a clinical environment: In C. J. Aine, G. Stroink, C. C. Wood, Y. Okada, & S. J. Swithenby (Eds.), *Biomag 96*. New York, NY: Springer.

Ilmoniemi, R. J., Haueisen, J., Kiviranta, M., Körber, R., Mäkelä, J. P., Nenonen, J., . . . Zevenhoven, K. (2016). Breaking the nonuniqueness barrier in electromagnetic neuroimaging: the BREAKBEN project. In *Biomag 2016: The 20th International Conference on Biomagnetism,* Seoul, South Korea.

Ilmoniemi, R. J., & Sarvas, J. (2019). *Brain signals: Physics and mathematics of MEG and EEG.* Cambridge, MA: MIT Press.

Kajola, M., Ahlfors, S., Ehnholm, G. J., Hällström, J., Hämäläinen, M. S., Ilmoniemi, . . . Vilkman, V. (1989). A 24-channel magnetometer for brain research. In S. J. Williamson, M. Hoke, G. Stroink, & M. Kotani (Eds.), *Advances in biomagnetism* (pp. 673–676). New York, NY: Springer.

Karadas, M., Wojciechowski, A. M., Huck, A., Dalby, N. O., Andersen, U. L., & Thielscher, A. (2018). Feasibility and resolution limits of opto-magnetic imaging of neural network activity in brain slices using color centers in diamond. *Scientific Reports, 8*, 4503.

Knuutila, J., Ahlfors, S., Ahonen, A., Hällström, J., Kajola, M., Lounasmaa, O. V., . . . Tesche, C. (1987). Large-area low-noise seven-channel dc SQUID magnetometer for brain research. *Review of Scientific Instruments, 58*, 2145–2156.

Korvenoja, A., Huttunen, J., Salli, E., Pohjonen, H., Martinkauppi, S., Palva, J. M., . . . Aronen, H. J. (1999). Activation of multiple cortical areas in response to somatosensory stimulation: Combined magnetoencephalographic and functional magnetic resonance imaging. *Human Brain Mapping, 8*, 13–27.

Mäkinen A. J., Zevenhoven K. C. J., & Ilmoniemi R J. (2019). Automatic spatial calibration of ultra-low-field MRI for high-accuracy hybrid MEG–MRI. *IEEE Transactions in Medical Imaging, 38*, 1317–1327.

McDermott, R., Lee, S., Ten Haken, B., Trabesinger, A. H., Pines, A., & Clarke, J. (2004). Microtesla MRI with a superconducting quantum interference device. *Proceedings of the National Academy of Sciences of the United States of America, 101*, 7857–7861.

Meyer, S. S., Bonaiuto, J., Lim, M., Rossiter, H., Waters, S., Bradbury, D., . . . Barnes, G. R. (2017). Flexible head-casts for high spatial precision MEG. *Journal of Neuroscience Methods, 276*, 38–45.

Nieminen, J. O., Zevenhoven, K. C. J., Vesanen, P. T., Hsu, Y.-C., & Ilmoniemi, R. J. (2014). Current-density imaging using ultra-low-field MRI with adiabatic pulses. *Magnetic Resonance Imaging, 32*, 54–59.

Paetau, R., Kajola, M., & Hari, R. (1990). Magnetoencephalography in the study of epilepsy. *Neurophysiologie Clinique/Clinical Neurophysiology, 20*, 169–187.

Pannetier, M., Fermon, C., Le Goff, G., Simola, J., & Kerr, E. (2004). Femtotesla magnetic field measurement with magnetoresistive sensors. *Science, 304*, 1648–1650.

Pekkonen, E., Huotilainen, M., Virtanen, J., Näätänen, R., Ilmoniemi, R. J., & Erkinjuntti, T. (1996). Alzheimer's disease affects parallel processing between the auditory cortices, *NeuroReport, 7*, 1365–1368.

Romani, G. L., Williamson, S. J., & Kaufman, L. (1982). Tonotopic organization of the human auditory cortex. *Science, 216*, 1339–1340.

Sergeeva-Chollet, N., Dyvorne, H., Dabek, J., Herreros, Q., Polovy, H., Goff, G. L., . . . Fermon, C. (2011). Low field MRI with magnetoresistive mixed sensors. *Journal of Physics: Conference Series, 303*, 012055.

Simos, P. G., Rezaie, R., & Papanicolaou, A. C. (2019). Applications of magnetoencephalography in epilepsy and tumor surgery. In K. Fountas & E. Z. Kapsalaki (Eds.), *Epilepsy surgery and intrinsic brain tumor surgery* (pp. 51–65). New York, NY: Springer.

Tiihonen, J., Katila, H., Pekkonen, E., Jääskeläinen, I. P., Huotilainen, M., Aronen, H. J., . . . Karhu, J. (1998). Reversal of cerebral asymmetry in schizophrenia measured with magnetoencephalography. *Schizophrenia Research, 30*, 209–219.

Vesanen, P. T., Nieminen, J. O., Zevenhoven, K. C. J., Dabek, J., Parkkonen, L. T., Zhdanov, A. V., . . . Ilmoniemi, R. J. (2013). Hybrid ultra-low-field MRI and magnetoencephalography system based on a commercial whole-head neuromagnetometer. *Magnetic Resonance in Medicine, 69*, 1795–1804.

Vesanen, P. T., Nieminen, J. O., Zevenhoven, K. C., Hsu, Y. C., & Ilmoniemi, R. J. (2014). Current-density imaging using ultra-low-field MRI with zero-field encoding. *Magnetic Resonance Imaging, 32*, 766–770.

Virtanen, J., Rinne, T., Ilmoniemi, R. J., & Näätänen, R. (1996). MEG-compatible multichannel EEG electrode array. *Electroencephalography and Clinical Neurophysiology, 99*, 568–570.

Virtanen, J., Parkkonen, L., Ilmoniemi, R. J., Pekkonen, E., & Näätänen, R. (1997). Biopotential amplifier for simultaneous operation with biomagnetic instruments. *Medical and Biological Engineering and Computing, 35*, 402–408.

Wikström, H., Roine, R. O., Salonen, O., Buch Lund, K., Salli, E., Ilmoniemi, R. J., . . . Huttunen, J. (1999). Somatosensory evoked magnetic fields from the primary somatosensory cortex (SI) in acute stroke. *Clinical Neurophysiology, 110*, 916–923.

Williamson, S. J., Pelizzone, M., Okada, Y., Kaufman, L., Crum, D. B., & Marsden, J. R. (1985). Magnetoencephalography with an array of SQUID sensors. In H. Collan, P. Berglund, & M. Krusius (Eds.), *Proceedings of the 10th Internation Cryogenic Engineering Conference* (pp. 339–348). Guildford, UK: Butterworths.

Williamson, S. J., & Kaufman, L. (1989). Advances in neuromagnetic instrumentation and studies of spontaneous brain activity. *Brain Topography, 2*, 129–139.

Zotev, V. S., Matlashov, A. N., Volegov, P. L., Savukov, I. M., Espy, M. A., Mosher, J. C., . . . Kraus Jr., R. H. (2008). Microtesla MRI of the human brain combined with MEG. *Journal of Magnetic Resonance, 194*, 115–120.

Zotev, V. S., Matlashov, A. N., Volegov, P. L., Urbaitis, A. V., Espy, M. A., & Kraus Jr., R. H. (2007). SQUID-based instrumentation for ultralow-field MRI. *Superconductor Science and Technology, 20*, S367–S373.

8

MAGNETOENCEPHALOGRAPHY USING OPTICALLY PUMPED MAGNETOMETERS

Elena Boto, Niall Holmes, Tim M. Tierney, James Leggett,
Ryan Hill, Stephanie Mellor, Gillian Roberts, Gareth R. Barnes,
Richard Bowtell, and Matthew J. Brookes

8.1. INTRODUCTION

For more than 40 years, magnetoencephalography (MEG) (Cohen, 1972) systems have been based on magnetic field measurements made using superconducting quantum interference devices (SQUIDs) (Hämäläinen, Hari, Ilmoniemi, Knuutila, & Lounasma, 1993; Jaklevic, Lambe, Silver, A. H., Mercereau, 1964). These remarkable devices exploit superconductivity, and the well-known Josephson effect (Josephson, 1962, 1974), to enable measurement of extremely small changes in magnetic field. At the time of writing, the vast majority of the installed base of MEG systems worldwide are based on SQUIDs because this has traditionally been the only practical solution to detecting the very-low-amplitude magnetic fields generated by the human brain. The SQUID has a number of properties that make it ideal for MEG recording: The noise floor is less than 10 fT/sqrt(Hz) (and

in the vast majority of cases more like 2–5 fT/sqrt [Hz]), giving SQUIDs high sensitivity. The bandwidth is about 0 to 12,000 Hz, enabling coverage of the signals of interest generated by the brain. Dynamic range is high (can be fT to μT), meaning that MEG measurements can be made even in the presence of relatively high static field (e.g., generated by a metal implant in the patient). These properties have enabled the development of whole-head SQUID-based sensor arrays, with several hundred sensors enabling coverage of the entire scalp. Problems such as crosstalk between sensors, and sensor tuning, have been all but eliminated, allowing SQUID-based MEG to become "plug and play," providing an extremely powerful platform for state-of-the-art neuroscientific experimentation.

However, despite the utility and high levels of success of SQUID-based MEG, there are significant limitations related to the current

Elena Boto, Niall Holmes, Tim M. Tierney, James Leggett, Ryan Hill, Stephanie Mellor, Gillian Roberts, Gareth R. Barnes, Richard Bowtell, and Matthew J. Brookes, *Magnetoencephalography Using Optically Pumped Magnetometers* In: *Fifty Years of Magnetoencephalography*. Edited by: Andrew C. Papanicolaou, Timothy P. L. Roberts, and James W. Wheless, Oxford University Press (2020). © Oxford University Press. DOI: 10.1093/oso/9780190935689.003.0008.

generation of MEG systems. The requirement for superconductivity means that sensors must be sited inside a cryogenic dewar, immersed in liquid helium. Consequently, sensors are fixed in position inside a one-size-fits-all helmet (into which the subject's head is placed). This is problematic because MEG systems cannot adapt to different head shapes or sizes, meaning that in people with small heads (e.g., infants), the brain is further from the sensors. Given the inverse square relation between signal magnitude and brain to sensor distance, this results in a dramatically lower signal (and hence signal-to-noise [SNR] ratio). Bespoke SQUID systems can be built to accommodate smaller heads (Okada et al., 2006), but this requires fabrication of a separate helmet that is then inappropriate for adult measurements. In addition, since sensors are fixed in position, any movement of the head relative to the array can degrade data quality (Gross et al., 2013). In recent years, algorithms have been introduced to help compensate for such motion (Nenonen et al., 2012; Taulu & Simola, 2006). However, despite successful utilization in a range of studies, such algorithms cannot cope with large movements (e.g., on a scale of several centimeters), where a subject's head moves sufficiently far to alter SNR ratio. This significant problem limits the participant cohorts who can be scanned using MEG (since it is challenging to keep some participants still) and the type of neuroscientific question that can be addressed. The requirement for cooling (to ~4 K) also means that a vacuum must be maintained between the sensors and the outer shell of the helmet. Consequently, even in a subject whose head fits the helmet perfectly, the closest one can place a field detector is about 15 to 20 mm from the scalp, again limiting the available signal. Finally, the complexity of SQUID circuitry and associated cryogenics, coupled with the necessary magnetic shielding to attenuate background magnetic interference, makes MEG systems expensive to buy and run. It follows that the introduction of new magnetic field detectors that could lift these limitations might offer a step change in the utility of MEG as a neuroimaging tool.

Recent years have seen the introduction of a number of promising alternatives to SQUIDs as the fundamental building block of MEG systems. For example, **high-T_c SQUIDs** use a superconducting material with a higher transition temperature, T_c, allowing a standard SQUID to be fabricated that can operate at liquid nitrogen (77 K), rather than liquid helium (4 K), temperatures. Insulation requirements are thus reduced, which means that sensor-to-scalp distance could be reduced from a few centimeters to less than 1 mm (Andersen et al., 2017), thus promising higher signal strength. Further, high-T_c SQUIDs have the potential to be more flexible (Riaz, Pfeiffer, & Schneiderman, 2017), potentially enabling better adaptation to different head shapes and sizes. A new variant of the SQUID, known as the **hyQUID,** has also recently been developed (Shelly, Matrozova, & Petrashov, 2016). Similar to a SQUID, the hyQUID consists of a superconducting loop, with the difference being that that the weak link is made of a conductor (rather than an oxide layer). Field detection is based on a process called *Andreev reflection*. At the time of writing, a commercial hyQUID-based MEG device is in development, and despite the fact that hyQUIDs require extremely low temperature (lower than liquid helium) to operate, this system is cryogen-free, with a superconducting state maintained by pulse tube refrigeration.

Nitrogen vacancy (NV) sensors exploit the isolated electronic spin system of the NV center in diamond to offer a sensitive measure of weak magnetic fields (Rondin et al., 2014). They operate at room temperature and have recently been miniaturized, potentially offering a route to mounting MEG sensors on the scalp, offering higher signal

(Dale & Morely, 2017). Currently, the sensitivity of these sensors remains somewhat lower than that of a SQUID; however, this limitation could be lifted in the near future. Finally, **optically pumped magnetometers** (OPMs) exploit the spin properties of alkali atoms, and a technique known as optical pumping, to prepare a gas of atoms such that its opacity to laser light becomes a sensitive marker of local magnetic field. The theoretical sensitivity of the OPM surpasses even that of the SQUID (Dang, Maloof, & Romalis, 2010), and OPMs operate without cryogenic cooling. They have recently been miniaturized (Sander et al., 2012) and commercialized (Shah & Wakai, 2013) and can be placed directly on the scalp. When operated in the spin exchange relaxation-free (SERF) regime, their bandwidth is suited to MEG acquisition (~0–150 Hz), and their dynamic range (~±1.5 nT; see also later), although limited, is acceptable.

Any of the nascent technologies mentioned previously has the potential to replace SQUID as the primary building block of a MEG system (and indeed for all biomagnetic measurements). Each has significant advantages over the SQUID (and each other), and it is currently unclear which might emerge as the technique of choice. However, of all the emerging technologies, arguably the one with the greatest extant potential to fundamentally revolutionize MEG as a functional neuroimaging tool is the OPM. OPMs are small and lightweight, offering the potential for development of a flexible MEG system, which could be adapted to any head shape, and in principle could become wearable (similar to an electroencephalography [EEG] cap) such that subjects could move freely during data acquisition. Because the external surface of an OPM is at approximately body temperature, the sensing volume can be placed close to the head, increasing the signal strength. And, of course, there is no need for cryogenics. In the section that follows, we describe the fundamental operating principles of the OPM and the technical requirements that are necessary to produce an environment in which OPMs work. We also review the extant literature on the application of OPMs in MEG measurement.

8.2. THE PHYSICS OF AN OPTICALLY PUMPED MAGNETOMETER

8.2.1. Basic Principle

There are a number of different types of OPM design in the literature; however, most rely on a measurement of the evolution of an atomic spin ensemble in an external magnetic field (nominally the neuromagnetic field). Consequently, the fundamental working principle can be outlined with a single description, summarized in three steps:

1. Atoms are prepared in a well-defined "spin state" (i.e., the orientations of the atomic magnetic moments, with respect to the environment, are aligned). The atomic ensemble therefore becomes spin-polarized (a bit like an array of tiny bar magnets (or compass needles) would align to point north in the earth's magnetic field) (Figure 8.1B).

2. The aligned atomic spins interact with a magnetic field in their environment (e.g., the magnetic field from the brain), causing a precession at the Larmor frequency, given by

$$\omega_L = \gamma \left| B_0 \right| \qquad [1]$$

That is, the atomic magnetic moments ("bar magnets") rotate away from alignment at a rate proportional to the magnitude of the environmental field, B_0 (γ is the atomic gyromagnetic ratio) (see Figure 8.1C).

3. The altered state of the atoms can be measured through assessment of the change in magnetization, and the external magnetic field

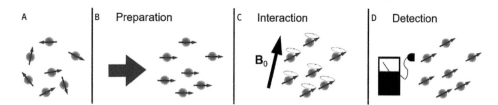

FIGURE 8.1   Principle of operation of an optically pumped magnetometer. (A) An ensemble of atomic spins is initially randomly oriented. (B) Atomic spins are spin-polarized, aligning the atomic magnetic moments. (C) Interaction with an external magnetic field, $\mathbf{B_0}$, causes precession of spins about the field at a rate proportional to the magnitude of the magnetic field. (D) Detection of the evolution of spins provides an indirect but quantitative measurement of the magnetic field. (Adapted from Boto, E. [2019]. *Wearable magnetoencephalography*. PhD thesis submitted to the University of Nottingham, UK.)

generating that change is characterized with high precision (see Figure 8.1D).

These three steps are depicted in Figure 8.1, where the *arrows* correspond to the alignment of the atomic magnetic moments.

The most common technique used to spin-polarize the atoms is optical pumping (Happer, 1972), hence the name *OPM*. Through this mechanism, the angular momentum of atoms (which dictates the orientation of their magnetic moment) can be altered by illuminating them with circularly polarized light, the frequency of which is resonant with a transition between atomic energy levels. This process produces a coherent alignment of the spins in the ensemble. The light used to polarize the atoms can also be used to read out the spin state of the atoms, and along with it, the effect of the external magnetic field on the spins (thus forming a magnetometer). Figure 8.2 shows a schematic diagram of a simple, miniaturized OPM (Shah & Wakai, 2013). Panel A shows the path of laser light through the sensor head, through a vapor cell filled with a gas of alkali atoms that sits within the sensor (approximately 6 mm from the outer casing). The internal optical components are labeled in panel B. For rubidium-87 (^{87}Rb; the alkali metal that is most commonly used in such devices; see later), a laser diode emitting 795-nm light is used for optical pumping. The laser light

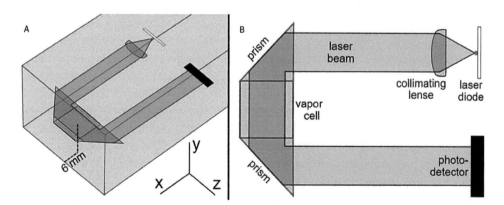

FIGURE 8.2   Schematic diagram of an optically pumped magnetometer. (A) Three-dimensional schematic showing the path of a laser beam through a sensor head. The cell containing the atomic vapor is placed about 6 mm from the end of the sensor. (B) Two-dimensional schematics with labels showing the relevant optics. (Adapted from Boto [2019]. *Wearable magnetoencephalography*. PhD thesis submitted to the University of Nottingham, UK.)

is collimated by a plano-convex lens and reflected through 90 degrees using a prism before passing through the cell. The light transmitted is then reflected again and directed toward a photodetector, which monitors its intensity. This scheme allows simultaneous optical pumping and monitoring of transmitted light. We now turn to a more detailed description of the physics of this system.

8.2.2. Quantum Mechanics and Optical Pumping

Atomic electrons orbit the nucleus in different shells, which are denoted by the principle quantum number, n. In simple terms, the higher the value of n, the further from the nucleus the electron orbits (and consequently the higher its energy). Alkali metals, like ^{87}Rb, are useful in many applications because their outer shell (highest n) contains just a single electron, which can be manipulated experimentally, allowing precise control of a spin ensemble. In addition, rubidium has a low melting temperature, and its atomic energy levels are easily accessible using infrared laser diodes, making it an attractive choice for OPM design. OPMs exploit the energy structure of the ground and excited states to polarize the ^{87}Rb atoms (Figure 8.1B). To understand this phenomenon, it proves useful to review briefly some basic atomic physics.

In addition to the principle quantum number, the outer (valence) electron also possesses orbital angular momentum, L (in a classical model, this is due to its motion around the nucleus) and spin angular momentum, S (because, again classically, it is thought of as spinning on its own axis). Quantum mechanics tells us that these properties are also quantized (i.e., can only take discrete values); for example, L can only take integer values between 0 and $n - 1$, and importantly, the shape of the atomic orbital changes for different values of L, with higher values being associated with higher energy. In ^{87}Rb, the ground state of the valence electron has orbital angular momentum, $L = 0$,

and the first excited state has $L = 1$. To move the electron between these states, it needs to absorb an amount of energy equal to the energy difference between the two states. This can be achieved by using resonant light, whose frequency is set such that photon energies are tuned to the appropriate energy difference.

To complicate matters, the separate energy levels ($L = 0$ and $L = 1$) are also affected by interactions within the atom. For example, loosely we think of an electron as orbiting the nucleus, and so equivalently, from the frame of reference of the electron, the positively charged nucleus appears to rotate around the electron. This means that the relative motion of the positively charged nucleus acts like a current loop, generating a magnetic field that passes through the electron. Since the electron itself possesses both charge and spin, it has its own magnetic field. Thus, there will be interaction between these two fields, which in part gives rise to the *fine structure* of atomic spectra. A full treatment of this interaction is provided by Tierney et al. (2019), and the result is that an excited valence electron (in the $L = 1$ state) can take one of two possible values of energy, depending on the interaction. This means that in order to induce a transition between energy levels using incident laser light, one can tune the light to one of two frequencies; these are known as the D1 and D2 transitions. For ^{87}Rb, the D1 transition corresponds to a wavelength of 795 nm, and it is this transition that is mostly used in OPMs.

In addition to interaction between orbital and spin angular momentum, there is a smaller but nevertheless important interaction between the magnetic field generated by the electron spin and the atomic nucleus (which also has spin). This interaction, known as the *hyperfine interaction*, results in a further splitting of the energy levels. Here, both the ground state ($L = 0$) and the first excited state ($L = 1$) can now take two different values of energy, known as the $F = 1$ and $F = 2$ states, where F refers to the total atomic angular momentum (i.e., the combination of the orbital angular momentum of the electron, electron spin, and nuclear spin).

This is known as *hyperfine splitting*; it is a small effect compared to the fine structure (in fact, for all practical purposes, the bandwidth of a laser is such that specific transitions between separate hyperfine states cannot be selectively targeted).

Finally, interaction with an external magnetic field further modifies the hyperfine structure. Not only is the total atomic angular momentum quantized, but also its orientation is quantized, and this is denoted by a quantum number, m_F, which can take integer values between $-F$ and F. In the absence of a magnetic field, these different states are degenerate (i.e., they all have the same energy). However, in the presence of a magnetic field, the orientation of the atomic angular momentum (relative to the field) becomes important, and different values of m_F result in different atomic energy levels (a process known as *Zeeman splitting*). The overall result of the fine, hyperfine, and Zeeman terms is that an electron can take a number of different discrete energy levels (each corresponding to a different quantum state) where the energy itself depends not only on fundamental physical interactions within the atom but also on the external magnetic field. For the ground and first excited states, these energies are shown by the *black lines* in Figure 8.3.

Optical pumping allows us to drive transitions between states, and so the valence electron will change energy level (i.e., undergo a D1 transition) between the ground and first excited state, when the atomic sample is irradiated using 795-nm laser light. Ordinarily, such irradiation would induce transitions, and the electron could exist at any one of the Zeeman sublevels shown in Figure 8.3. However, to better control precisely which sublevel it occupies, circularly polarized light is used. In left circularly polarized light, photons have angular momentum of +1, which (if that photon is absorbed) will add to the angular momentum of the atom. Therefore, only transitions causing a change of $\Delta m_F = +1$ are allowed to occur. At the same time, atoms

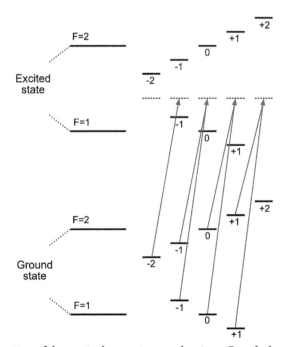

FIGURE 8.3 Schematics of the optical pumping mechanism. Circularly polarized light only causes atomic transitions with $\Delta m_F = +1$. (Adapted from Boto [2019]. *Wearable magnetoencephalography*. PhD thesis submitted to the University of Nottingham, UK.)

may spontaneously emit light, decaying back to the ground state. They do so by emitting a randomly polarized resonant photon that can depolarize another atom if reabsorbed. These two effects (D1 transition and spontaneous emission) will eventually force the atoms into the level with the lowest orbital angular momentum ($L = 0$), that is, the ground state, and highest atomic angular momentum ($F = 2$, $m_F = +2$). An example of this process is depicted by the *red lines* in Figure 8.3. When an atom is in this state, which is known as the "dark" state, it is unaffected by the laser light, because of the unavailability of an atomic energy level with $m_F > +2$ in the excited state. The atomic ensemble thus becomes transparent to the laser light, which passes through the vapor cell unaffected.

As the laser optically pumps the atoms into this transparent steady state, the atomic angular momenta align (recall that m_F relates to the orientation of angular momentum, and consequently orientation of the atomic magnetic moment). This means that a strong net magnetization, aligned along the laser axis, is produced in the gas. The gas is said to be spin-polarized and becomes magnetically sensitive. This is the fundamental basis of how a gas of atoms can be forced into a state in which it is highly sensitive to magnetic fields, through the optical pumping process. When in this state, influence of an external magnetic field causes a precessional motion of the atomic magnetic moments about the applied magnetic field.

8.2.3. Zero-Field and Spin Exchange Suppression

Unfortunately, the polarization that is induced by optical pumping can be eliminated by collisions between polarized and unpolarized atomic species because the atoms can exchange their spin through collisions (either with each other or with the walls of the cell). This process is known as spin exchange (SE) relaxation and counters the effect of the laser optical

pumping, returning the gas to its initial state of poor magnetic sensitivity. However, it is possible to minimize the SE effect by working in a very low magnetic field and at high atomic density.

At high atomic densities, spin-exchange collisions will occur frequently. In such a collision between two atoms, the electron spin orientation in both atoms can be reversed, causing a redistribution among the Zeeman sublevels, leading to a loss of polarization. The sensitivity of a magnetometer generally improves as the number of atoms increases, but this improvement is negated by the SE collisions, which limit the polarization lifetime. However, Happer and Tang (1973) discovered that at extremely high atomic densities, and near zero fields, the SE rate will be larger than the frequency of precession, and an individual atom will precess by only a small angle between SE collisions. Each atom samples the different sublevels in a short period of time, and the entire atomic ensemble precesses coherently. This is referred to as the SERF regime (Allred, Lyman, Kornack, & Romalis, 2002), and OPMs are often described as zero-field or SERF magnetometers. This is shown in Figure 8.4, with the SE rate increasing by a factor of 10 between each plot (top to bottom, left to right). If the SE rate is small compared with the Larmor frequency, then an individual atom spends a longer period of time in one hyperfine level. The coherence time of the entire ensemble is limited. As the SE rate increases, atoms spend shorter times in a particular state between collisions, and a single precession frequency is observed. To optimize [87]Rb density in the vapor cell and hence maintain a SERF environment, heaters can be placed around the cell and used to heat the gas to about 150° C. This increases the density such that the SE rate exceeds the Larmor precession frequency. This has the undesirable effect that the center of an OPM must be heated. However, insulation and effective heat exchange can maintain a reasonable surface temperature.

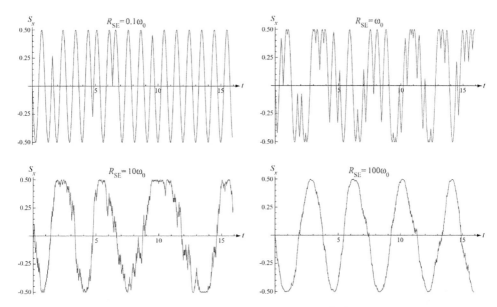

FIGURE 8.4   Spin exchange relaxation-free regime. The spin exchange (SE) rate is increasing by a factor of 10 between plots. ω_0 represents the Larmor frequency. When SE is sufficiently fast, the atomic ensemble precesses coherently at a net frequency slower than ω_0.

8.3. MEASURING THE MAGNETIC FIELD

To now understand how this quantum system interacts with an external magnetic field, we turn to a description of the bulk magnetization of the spin ensemble. After optical pumping and SE suppression using SERF, a large steady-state polarization exists within the vapor cell, along the direction of the laser, which we assume to be the z-direction. Assuming that the magnetic field is zero, after all of the atoms are pumped into the dark state (their magnetic moments aligned), the cell then becomes completely transparent to the light (since the atoms cannot absorb any more photons). The signal at the photodetector in the OPM, which is sensitive to the amount of laser light passing through the cell, is a maximum. This situation is shown schematically in Figure 8.5. However,

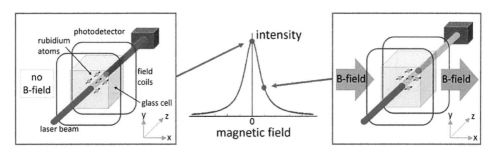

FIGURE 8.5   Optically pumped magnetometer response to magnetic field. In zero-field condition (*left*), laser light passes through the cell. An external field applied in the x-direction (*right*) causes rotation of the polarization vector away from z and consequently a drop in laser intensity at the photodetector. Mathematically, polarization along the axis of the laser (hence the signal at the photodetector) is a Lorentzian function of applied field (*middle*). (Adapted from Boto, E., Holmes, N., Leggett, J., Roberts, G., Shah, V., Meyer, S. S., . . . Brookes, M. J. [2018]. Moving magnetoencephalography towards real-world applications with a wearable system. *Nature, 555*, 657.)

the bulk polarization vector in the gas (i.e., sum of all of the atomic magnetic moments) can be influenced by an external magnetic field (e.g., generated by the brain); this interaction can be modeled mathematically by the Bloch equations (Bloch, 1946). Assuming an external field along the x-direction, this interaction causes a rotation of the polarization away from the z-axis. This causes a redistribution of the atoms across the hyperfine states, and so the atoms can begin to absorb light again. When this happens, we see a measurable drop in laser light passing through the cell and thus the reduced signal at the photodetector. This is shown in the right panel of Figure 8.5. The result of this change in polarization is that the photodetector signal is a Lorentzian function of field, peaking at zero. This is referred to as the *zero-field* or *Hanle resonance* (Hanle, 1925).

Measurement of signals in this way provides a marker of magnetic field; however, there are a number of difficulties with this approach. First, the Lorentzian is symmetric about zero, meaning that the photodetector signal will give the same output regardless of the direction of the magnetic field through the cell. Second, the top of the Lorentzian is relatively flat, meaning relatively low sensitivity for very small (e.g.,

femtotesla) changes from zero field. Third, the system is highly sensitive to noise (Kastler, 1973). However, these limitations are overcome by using an electromagnetic coil, placed at either side of the cell (i.e., a Helmholtz coil), to generate an oscillating magnetic field inside the cell. This effectively modifies the Bloch equation by the addition of an extra sinusoidal term, and the solution, which was expounded by Tannoudji, Dupont-Roc, Haroche, & LaLoe (1970) shows that the polarization in the z-direction becomes:

$$P_z \infty \frac{\gamma \tau B_x}{1 + \left(\gamma \tau B_x^2\right)^2} P_0' \sin(\omega t) \qquad [2]$$

This is a sinusoidal function at the modulation frequency, ω (P_0, γ, and τ are constants). This solution has desirable properties: first, lock-in detection can be used to demodulate the signal (remove the influence of the sinusoid) and the fact that we seek a signal at a known and well-defined frequency reduces noise. Second, polarization plotted against field takes the form of a dispersion curve (Figure 8.6); positive and negative changes in magnetic field can be discriminated, and the steepest slope is around zero field, providing greatest sensitivity to very

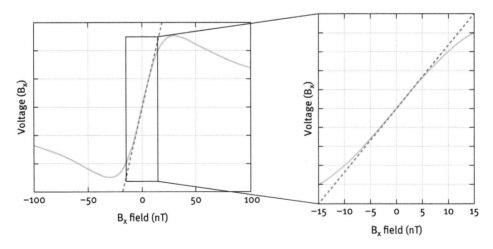

FIGURE 8.6 Magnetometer response. The voltage output of an optically pumped magnetometer is a function of the magnetic field along the sensor's sensitive axis (x) and has a dispersion shape, with maximum slope at zero field. The response is also close to linear near zero field (Adapted from Boto [2019]. *Wearable magnetoencephalography*. PhD thesis submitted to the University of Nottingham, UK.)

small field changes from zero. Additionally, the response of the sensor is approximately linear around zero field, as shown in the *inset* of Figure 8.6. However, a deviation from linear is seen with increasing field.

It should be noted that the deviation from linear as magnetic fields increase effectively manifests as an apparent change in the gain of the sensor. In fact, it has been shown (Boto et al., 2018) that an offset field of approximately 1.5 nT causes approximately a 5% change in the gain. This (somewhat arbitrary) value has been used here as an effective measure of the operational dynamic range of an OPM, meaning that the absolute field in which an OPM sensor must operate is within the ±1.5 nT range because outside that range, the error in gain will begin to degrade the sensor performance. This has implications for the environment in which an OPM can operate, which is discussed further later. However, given the magnitude of the typical neuromagnetic field is about 1 pT (when measured at the scalp surface) assuming that other (larger) fields can be nulled then the sensor exhibits an approximately linear output with respect to magnetic field inside the cell, making it an ideal magnetometer for MEG measurements.

An interesting point here relates to the basis of operation of the sensor. When run in the configuration described previously, the sensor would be operating in so-called open-loop mode, meaning that the sensor output is simply the voltage at the photodetector. While this is a sensitive measure of field with linear gain close to zero field, it has the significant problem of the gain errors mentioned previously and very limited dynamic range, which could be problematic for some applications. However, in principle, a closed-loop (or feedback) mode could be introduced whereby any change in voltage measured by the photodetector would, in real time, be fed back to a set of on-board sensor coils. These coils would then compensate by applying an equal and opposite field back through the cell. This closed-loop (or feedback) mode would, ostensibly,

have the advantage of higher dynamic range and guaranteed linearity of response. However, application of currents through on-board sensor coils also generates stray fields outside the OPM, and if sensors are operated in close proximity, this could mean increased cross-talk between sensors. Therefore, while this is a potentially desirable development, technical problems would need to be resolved before operation of a viable sensor array. At present, we are not aware of any closed-loop sensors operating in the field.

8.3.1. Miniaturizing Optically Pumped Magnetometer Sensors and Initial Magnetoencephalography Measurements

OPMs designed based on the working principles described previously (or variants of those principles) have been proved to reach sensitivities comparable (Allred et al., 2002) or in some cases better than SQUIDs (Dang et al., 2010; Kominis, Kornack, Allred, & Romalis, 2003). The experimental setup required for achieving such sensitivity was initially very bulky and laboratory-based. Nevertheless, the first MEG recording using a laboratory OPM setup was reported in 2006 (Xia, Baranga, Hoffman, & Romalis, 2006) inside a human-sized shield during auditory stimulation. Results showed clearly that the auditory evoked response was measurable with a high SNR. However, the physical size of these initial OPMs would have negated the possibility of mounting them comfortably on the head, or indeed of having a large number of measurement sites across the scalp.

The past two decades have seen rapid advances in the miniaturization of OPMs. Methods originally developed for chip-scale atomic clocks were used to build the first microfabricated OPMs (Schwindt, Knappe, Shah, Hollberg, & Kitching, 2004; Schwindt et al., 2007). This initial work, while still far from reaching the sensitivity of a SQUID (sensitivities were of the order of a few picotesla), showed the potential of the technology to be scaled down in size and weight and consequently leave the laboratory bench and become the building block of a viable MEG device. A few years later, a "tabletop" setup showed sensitivities of a few 10s of femtotesla (Shah, Knappe, Schwindt, & Kitching, 2007) and even reached below 10 fT (Griffith, Knappe, & Kitching, 2010; Shah & Romalis, 2009); this had been the generic target for early SQUIDs used for MEG measurements. The introduction of techniques used in manufacturing microelectromechanical systems added to the excitement of having compact magnetometers for biomedical applications and led to the first "packaged" microfabricated OPMs. Some examples of compact packaged OPMs are shown in Figure 8.7. The sensors in panels A, B, and F were developed at the National Institute of Standard and Technology (NIST); the sensor in panel C at Sandia National Laboratories; the sensor in panel D at Kyoto University; and the sensor in panel E at QuSpin Inc. (Louisville, CO).

A number of groups worldwide have now shown that small and lightweight OPM devices are able to successfully measure the MEG signal. For example, Johnson, Schwindt, & Weisend (2010) used a single SERF magnetometer (which operated using two laser beams, with Faraday rotation of the polarization of the second (probe) beam providing optical interrogation of the atoms) to measure evoked responses from both median nerve and auditory stimulation. The same group then demonstrated the first MEG measurements using a multisensor OPM array, again detecting the auditory evoked field (Johnson, Schwindt, & Weisend, 2013). Sander et al. (2012) used a chip-scale OPM (similar to the size of an EEG electrode) to measure not only the somatosensory evoked field but also occipital alpha oscillations. Kamada et al. (2015) fabricated an OPM, to again measure occipital alpha and its modulation by opening and closing the eyes. These latter demonstrations were of significant importance given the recent increase in interest in neural oscillations. Potential clinical applicability was also demonstrated by Alem, Benison, Barth, Kitching, and Knappe (2014), who showed that epileptiform activity, in rodents, was measurable using microfabricated OPM sensors. A significant step forward in viability came with the introduction of the first commercial OPM sensor, made by QuSpin Inc. This commercialization opened a path for laboratories whose expertise was centered on imaging physics (rather than atomic physics) to obtain OPMs and build viable systems capable

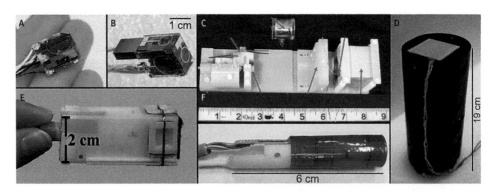

FIGURE 8.7 Examples of the first compact optically pumped magnetometers. (A from Sander, T. H., Preusser, J., Mhaskar, R., Kitching, J., Trahms, L., & Knappe, S. [2012]. Magnetoencephalography with a chip-scale atomic magnetometer. *Biomedical Optics Express, 3,* 981–990.; B from Mhaskar, R., Knappe, S., & Kitching, J. [2012]. A low-power, high-sensitivity micromachined optical magnetometer. *Applied Physics Letters, 101,* 241105 (C from Johnson et al., 2013; D from Kamada et al., 2015; E from Shah & Wakai, 2013; F from Sheng et al., 2017.)

of biomagnetic measurement. This enabled the extremely important translation of the technology from those who develop it to those who wish to exploit it. For example, Boto et al. (2017) showed that QuSpin sensors were able to detect the somatosensory evoked field and modulation of beta oscillations in response to a median nerve stimulus. Taken together, the falling noise floor, miniaturization, and commercialization of OPMs paved the way for their use in MEG experimentation.

8.4. BENEFITS OF ON-SCALP MAGNETOENCEPHALOGRAPHY

Perhaps the most obvious benefit of OPMs for MEG measurement comes from their flexibility. OPMs operate with their external surface at approximately body temperature (the cell containing the atomic vapor is heated in order to place atoms in the SERF regime, but insulation and effective heat dissipation mean that the sensing volume can be placed within a few millimeters of the scalp). This, in turn,

means that OPMs can be placed flexibly on the scalp surface, and the brain-to-sensor distance is less for OPMs than for cryogenically-cooled SQUIDs. This improved proximity has two effects:

1. Since signal falls as the square of distance between the source and sensor, decreasing the brain-to-sensor distance increases the signal magnitude and potentially (assuming equal noise floors) the SNR.

2. Because the spatial topography of the magnetic field pattern is being measured closer to the head, the spatial frequencies measurable on the scalp surface are higher. Consequently, the forward field becomes better resolved spatially (i.e., less spatially diffuse). However, this also means that sensor spacings need to be lower, necessitating the use of a high sensor count.

These two separate effects are shown in Figure 8.8. In Figure 8.8A, an example forward field is shown for a single dipole in the brain; note the

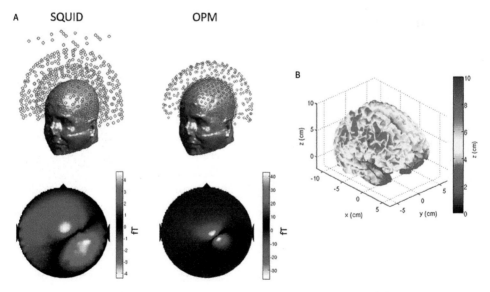

FIGURE 8.8   Simulations showing benefits of on-scalp magnetoencephalography. (A) Example field topographies and magnitudes, for the same dipole location, measured by optically pumped magnetometer (OPM) magnetoencephalography (MEG) and SQUID-based MEG. (B) Improvement in sensitivity afforded by bringing sensors closer to the head. (Adapted from Boto, E., Bowtell, R. W., Krüger, P., Fromhold, M., Morris, P. G., Meyer, S., . . . Brookes, M. J. [2016]. The benefits of atomic magnetometers for MEG: A simulation study. *PLoS One, 11*, e0157655.)

improved signal magnitude and the less diffuse field pattern for OPM MEG. In Figure 8.8B, the ratio of the forward field norm (OPM/ SQUID) is plotted as a function of position in the cortex; as shown, OPMs offer approximately a five-fold higher signal across most of the cortex. This improved signal in OPMs potentially offers greater SNR and therefore improved ability to detect electrophysiological effects of interest. At the time of writing, the noise level of a SQUID remains lower than that of an OPM; however, significant improvements in SNR of OPMs compared with SQUIDs have been realized in practical settings. As time progresses, the noise floor of OPMs will likely drop, enabling even higher fidelity of measurement. The higher spatial frequencies, coupled with increased SNR, also offer improved spatial resolution for source localization; indeed, simulations using a theoretical beamformer formulation suggest that the spatial resolution of an on-scalp MEG system with about 300 channels could be as high as 1 mm (Boto et al., 2016). While there has been no direct experimental validation of this, initial results (Boto et al., 2018) did show that 13 OPMs (over motor cortex) offered better spatial specificity than a 275-channel whole-head SQUID array.

The improved proximity to the brain, shown above in Figure 8.8, is the case for an adult. Difficulties with low SNR in SQUID-based MEG are amplified in cases in which the participant has a small head, for example, in babies and children. The fact that OPMs can be placed flexibly on the scalp surface of any subject means that they can adapt to any head shape. This, in turn, means that one could expect (in principle) equivalent SNR from a baby and an adult. This is not the case in standard SQUID-based MEG scanners, which are configured to be one-size-fits-all, with relatively poor SNR in children. It follows that, while OPM MEG (or indeed any on-scalp measurement) offers exciting potential in adult MEG, that potential is amplified in measurement of pediatric populations.

8.4.1. The "Zero-Field" Problem

One of the significant problems with OPMs is the zero-field resonance condition. As shown in Figure 8.6, the output of an OPM is critically dependent on operation within the linear range of the response curve. This, in turn, means that the device must be operated at close to zero field. As with most MEG installations, OPMs have typically been operated inside a shielded enclosure, which acts to reduce the background field. However, in most practical shields, the static offset field (i.e., the remnant earth's field inside the room) is about 20 to 30 nT—too large for an OPM to operate. OPMs, therefore, are usually fabricated such that the cell containing the atomic vapor is surrounded by a set of electromagnetic (Helmholtz) coils capable of producing a vector field through the cell along any orientation (one of the three pairs of coils are also used to provide the modulation field). The cell itself can be operated (with a broader resonance) to measure the background static magnetic field up to about 200 nT. The current required for the on-board sensor coils to produce an equal and opposite field can then be calculated and applied, creating a zero-field environment within the cell. This simple system enables OPMs to operate within most reasonable shielded environments (e.g., standard magnetically shielded rooms typically used in MEG laboratories). The experimental procedure is such that offset fields are measured and canceled within each OPM at the start of an experiment. For example, in a MEG recording, the OPMs are placed on the head, then current values in the on-board sensor coils are set to zero the field. Subsequently, the MEG measurement can begin, exploiting the high sensitivity of measurement around zero field (see again Figure 8.6).

Although the on-board sensor coils enable effective OPM operation in a nonzero background field, a significant problem arises if the background magnetic field changes appreciably during the experiment. This could be caused by drift in field due to environmental factors such as nearby infrastructure (e.g., an elevator or tramline). However, if sensors are mounted on the head, it is more likely to be caused by movement of the head and attached sensors relative to the background field. For example, in a background field of 30 nT, just a 4-degree rotation of an OPM would generate a field shift large enough to take the sensor outside its dynamic range. To avoid the problem of sensor movement, it is of course possible to mount the sensors in a fixed helmet and have the subject sit with their head stationary inside the helmet (similar to cryogenic MEG). However, this method fails to exploit the lightweight nature of the OPMs, limiting the potential for novel neuroscientific experiments in which subjects are free to move. For this reason, a different approach has been adopted in which large electromagnetic coils, placed around the subject, cancel the background magnetic field in a volume spanning the whole head.

Figure 8.9 shows two examples of coil systems that can be used to cancel the remnant earth's field in a magnetically shielded room. A popular choice for these systems is a Helmholtz cage. A single Helmholtz coil produces uniform fields by applying equal currents to two spatially separated circular loops of wire; the fields from each loop add together, producing a region of uniform field at their center. Applying equal and opposite currents to these loops produces a linear gradient. By constructing these loops on the faces of a cube, complete control over the vector field and the longitudinal (dB_x/dx, dB_y/dy, and dB_z/dz) gradients can be obtained. The transverse (dB_x/dy, dB_x/dz, and dB_y/dz) gradient coils are produced with four loops of wire spatially separated in two dimensions and with current directions carefully chosen to produce the correct field. Figure 8.9A shows a Helmholtz coil arrangement recently described by Iivanainen, Zetter, Groen, Hakkarainen, and Parkkonen (2019). This system used background field measurements to calculate and apply currents to the system, which allowed cancellation of magnetic fields, and all field gradients yielding a close-to-zero-field

environment with reduced (linear) variation in space. Specifically, the static field components over the helmet containing the OPMs were measured and nulled from between −70 and 50 nT to below 1 nT, representing a 40-dB shielding factor. The system was also operated in a feedback loop, meaning that in addition to the temporally static field, it was also able to null dynamic changes in the background field. The feedback loop uses data from OPMs mounted in fixed positions on the head, which are low-pass filtered below 4 Hz to avoid compensating neuromagnetic signals of interest (which were assumed to be >4 Hz). The maximum peak-to-peak drift of a sensor during a 15-minute recording was reduced from 1.3 nT without dynamic correction to 400 pT with dynamic correction (removing the filter, this becomes 30 pT). This system was designed to operate efficiently, generating an environment in which a static OPM array could successfully measure MEG signals, even in a relatively noisy magnetic environment (a two-layer magnetically shielded room). Figure 8.9C shows average evoked responses to median-nerve stimulation collected from six OPMs operated inside this Helmholtz coil arrangement. Recordings were averaged over 143 trials, and data were collected with the field compensation system engaged.

Although a Helmholtz cage provides good cancellation of magnetic field, the enclosure housing the coils limits access to the subject and the range of motions that would be available, constraining the coils to two planes at either side of the subject provides a more open environment. Using techniques adapted from magnetic resonance imaging (MRI) gradient coil design, biplanar coils that produce uniform field and field gradients over a central region can be constructed. Figure 8.9B shows a biplanar coil arrangement, the "fingerprint" coils are mounted on two planes, each with an area of 1.6×1.6 m^2 and separated by 1.5 m. Each plane consists of layers of independent coils, with each coil generating a different field or field gradient (e.g., B_x, B_y, B_z, dB_x/dx, dB_x/dy).

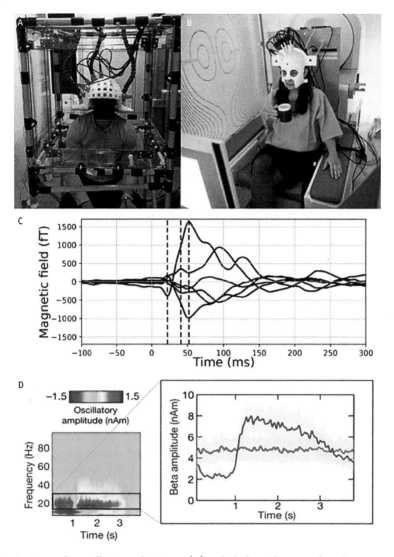

FIGURE 8.9   Background cancellation coil systems. (A) Helmholtz coil surrounding the space occupied by the subject's head. (B) Biplanar coil built on two planes at either side of the subject. (C) Evoked response data measured using the system photographed in part A. (D) Time–frequency data and associated beta-band modulation measured using the system photographed in part B. (C adapted from Iivanainen, J., Zetter, R., Groen, M., Hakkarainen, K., & Parkkonen, L. [2019]. On-scalp MEG system utilizing an actively shielded array of optically-pumped magnetometers. *Neuroimage, 194,* 244–258; D adapted from Boto, E., Holmes, N., Leggett, J., Roberts, G., Shah, V., Meyer, S. S., . . . Brookes, M. J. [2018]. Moving magnetoencephalography towards real-world applications with a wearable system. *Nature, 555,* 657.)

In this way, a set of nine layered coils will yield a similar performance to the Helmholtz cage, without enclosing the subject. As a result of constraining the coils to two planes, the complexity of the wire paths and the scale of the system are significantly increased, leading to a more challenging fabrication. However, easier access and less constraint to the subject yield greater practicality for movement-based studies. In the system shown in Figure 8.9B (which operated inside a three-layer magnetically shielded room), the coils were able to provide an environment in which the magnitude of the offset field was reduced from 28 nT to

740 pT (a shielding factor of 32 dB), and the dominant field gradient was nulled by 22 dB. Again, this shielding level was sufficient to enable an environment in which OPMs could operate effectively. Indeed, Figure 8.9D shows the induced response to a visuomotor task. In this task, a single subject was asked to perform a single finger abduction when visually cued; from an average of 50 trials, a movement-related beta desynchronization, followed by postmovement beta rebound, can be clearly observed.

8.5. WEARABLE MAGNETOENCEPHALOGRAPHY

A close-to-zero background field, generated by coil systems of the type described previously, can allow OPMs to move freely with relatively little measurable change in magnetic field. This being the case, OPMs can be mounted on the surface of the subject's head, with the head allowed to move during MEG data collection. An example is shown in Figure 8.10. Here, a subject executed a "head nod," which was

tracked by a three-dimensional (3D) motion camera. The experiment was performed twice, with and without field nulling, and motion data (Figure 8.10B) showed that the size of the head movement was approximately equivalent in both experiments (a marker on the forehead was shown to move up and down by about 7 cm in both cases). The MEG data (Figure 8.10A) clearly showed that with no nulling (*blue traces*), OPMs measure large background field shifts, which take them outside their dynamic range and render them inoperable. However, with the field nulling on, the OPMs remain operable throughout the movement. A later study using the same field-nulling method demonstrated that OPMs continued to function during controlled translations of up to ±10 cm and rotations of up to ±34 degrees. Residual motion artifacts can be further reduced by regressing motion parameters on to the measured MEG data.

This development offers a new opportunity to measure MEG data continuously, in the presence of subject movement on a scale that has not previously been conceived. For

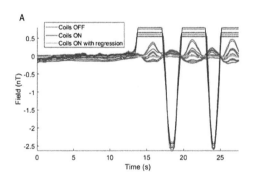 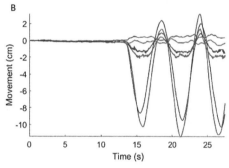

FIGURE 8.10 The effect of field nulling on magnetoencephalography signals recorded during head movement. (A) Magnetic fields measured with an array of optically pumped magnetometers (OPMs) in the head, with (*red*) and without (*blue*) field nulling. Note that without field nulling, head movement induces large shifts in the measured magnetic field, rendering the sensors inoperable (they move outside of their dynamic range, which is defined as the range in which the response is linear to within 5%). However, with field nulling on, the OPMs continue to work. The *green trace* shows the same data following regression of movement parameters that, in this case, were measured using a three-dimensional (3D) tracking camera. Note that the effect of motion can be largely removed. (B) The corresponding movement; subject executed a "head nod," and traces show the 3D motion, in a cartesian coordinate system, of a marker placed on the forehead. Note the large (~7 cm) movement in the foot-to-head direction. (Adapted from Boto, E., Holmes, N., Leggett, J., Roberts, G., Shah, V., Meyer, S. S., . . . Brookes, M. J. [2018]. Moving magnetoencephalography towards real-world applications with a wearable system. *Nature*, 555, 657.)

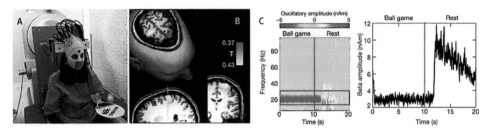

FIGURE 8.11   Magnetoencephalography in motion. (A) Subject is wearing an optically pumped magnetometer helmet while playing a simple ball game (bouncing a ball off a bat). (B) Beamformer images show localization of beta responses to motor and premotor cortex. (C) Time–frequency spectrogram (*left*) and line plot (right) showing the modulation of beta-band oscillations throughout the ball game paradigm. (From Boto, E., Holmes, N., Leggett, J., Roberts, G., Shah, V., Meyer, S. S., . . . Brookes, M. J. [2018]. Moving magnetoencephalography towards real-world applications with a wearable system. *Nature, 555,* 657.)

example, Boto et al. (2018) showed that when a subject undertook a finger movement task, the execution of natural head movements (e.g., stretching or drinking during MEG data acquisition, with head movements of magnitude ~10–15 cm during the task) had little impact on the quality of MEG responses; indeed, both beta-band modulation and evoked responses elicited by the finger movement were measurable, and the SNR of the responses did not differ significantly when the subject was static or moving. Furthermore, the authors were able to show that modulation of beta-band oscillations could be measured, when elicited by the subject playing a ball game (the participant bounced a table tennis ball off a bat for 10 s, followed by 10-s rest, repeated 29 times). These data, which are reproduced in Figure 8.11, show that despite relatively large and unpredictable head, shoulder, and arm/hand movements, MEG data were measurable in response to the ball game paradigm.

This same system has since been used in several other investigations. For example, exploiting the ability to make natural head movements during data acquisition, Holmes et al. (2018) showed that the topological organization of the human visual cortex could be imaged when a subject rotated their head in order to place a visual stimulus into different parts of their visual field. Tierney et al. (2018) showed that OPMs could be used, in

an unconstrained subject, to measure MEG data during a verb generation task (a subject viewed a word on a screen and had to think of a verb relating to that word). The result showed that even a simple OPM MEG system (with 26 channels) was able to lateralize the language network to either left or right hemisphere. The system has also been used to measure MEG data from challenging regions such as the hippocampus (Barry et al., 2019) and cerebellum (Lin et al., 2019). These recent papers suggest not only that OPMs are a viable tool for collection of MEG data but also that subjects who are freely moving can be scanned, and the flexibility of OPM placement allows for traditionally challenging brain areas to be accessed.

8.6. OUTLOOK AND FUTURE PERSPECTIVES

As explained in our introduction, one of the significant problems with the current generation of cryogenic MEG systems is that instrumentation relies on static superconducting sensors. This means that MEG helmets are one-size-fits-all, the requirement for cooling to extremely low temperatures means the pick-up coils are located far from the scalp, and any head movement relative to the helmet causes degradation of data quality. OPMs offer a solution to these problems. First, their lightweight nature, coupled with body-temperature operation, means that they can be mounted in a helmet configuration on the scalp surface, enabling adaptation to any head shape or size. Second, if the system is operated in the presence of field-nulling coils, subjects can move during data acquisition. Finally, by getting closer to the brain, OPM MEG has higher signal and higher SNR than conventional MEG. This, for the first time, offers the promise of a neuroimaging system with the technical advantages of MEG (e.g., high spatial resolution (Baillet, 2017), lower sensitivity to muscle artefacts (Claus, Velis, Lopes da Silva, Viergever, & Kalitzin, 2012, Muthukumaraswamy, 2013), and the practicality of EEG (Boto et al., 2019).

This next-generation MEG system will offer myriad opportunities for neuroscientists to conceive novel experimental paradigms in which naturalistic movement is allowed. For example, paradigms such as that shown in Figure 8.11 potentially offer a new means to study cross-cortical interactions and their role in hand–eye coordination. A more natural environment will better enable experiments probing how humans learn and develop; for example, one could probe brain function while learning to play a musical instrument without the confines of a static head position. Natural interactions between people inside a shielded room, or even scanning two people in the same room at the same time, will be possible, facilitating a new way to study the neural substrates underpinning social interaction. Enabling head movement might also allow the use of new equipment, which can allow a more naturalistic form of stimulation. For example, virtual reality (VR) headsets offer a means to place participants in an immersive virtual environment. The marriage of this technology with neuroimaging techniques has been challenging because the feeling of "presence" in VR is only enabled when subjects' view of their virtual world changes when they move. This critically requires natural head movement on a scale that is not possible in conventional MEG (or functional MRI). However, scalp-mounted MEG, coupled with VR (or indeed any immersive

platform, e.g., a driving simulator), potentially opens up new possibilities for experimentation; for example, understanding how our brains support spatial navigation or how we make decisions when placed in stressful environments. The promise of such stimulation is supported by recent data (Roberts et al., 2019) showing that VR MEG is, in principle, possible, although interference caused by head-mounted displays remains problematic.

Enabling head movement, coupled with the flexibility to adapt to any head shape or size, will allow exciting opportunities for the study of subject cohorts who find conventional scanners difficult to tolerate. The most obvious example is data acquisition in babies and children. Studies of developmental trajectories of neural networks have been challenging in the past because of dramatic changes in head size and increased movement in younger subjects. Conventional MEG systems, built for adults, are limited in studies of children because the sensors are simply too far away from the scalp. Some specialized scanning systems for babies have been developed, using SQUIDs housed within a smaller cryogenic helmet. However, such systems can only be used for infants, precluding scanning of brain development as subjects age. The flexibility of OPMs offers a means to adapt to head size and thus will enable compliance throughout the life span. Further, the extant evidence suggests that children will be able to move, without significant degradation of the data. Perhaps most excitingly, it is possible that future development of electromagnetic coil technology could offer a means to expand the available range of motion. Currently, this is limited to head movement only; however, it is possible to conceive MEG systems in which subjects can stand, or even walk, offering an opportunity for new neuroscientific study, for example, in measuring the maturational trajectory of the motor system as infants learn to walk.

Clinically speaking, OPM MEG also offers the potential to surpass what is possible using current systems. The largest clinical use of

MEG is in epilepsy, where it is used to localize the origins of interictal spikes. It is also used to localize eloquent cortex in regions around the site of a planned resection. The increased SNR that results from bringing sensors closer to the head will likely enable greater sensitivity to abhorrent electrophysiological activity. Further, for reasons outlined previously, OPMs potentially offer greater spatial accuracy for localization. This potentially means an improved system for patient evaluation. The introduction of a MEG system that can cope with patient movement also offers advantages; for example, again it will be easier to scan children, meaning MEG technology can be better deployed in the cohort that stands to gain most from it. In addition, as well as interictal spikes, it might also be easier to measure MEG data during the ictal phase of epilepsy, potentially leading not only to improved localization of the epileptic network but also to a better understanding of the underlying neuropathological mechanisms. Outside epilepsy, the motion robustness of MEG might also allow for other patient populations who find a conventional scanner environment challenging to tolerate, including patients with movement disorders such as those with Parkinson disease who find it challenging to keep still. In addition, an OPM system will likely offer improved measurements and better patient compliance across the gamut of MEG clinical applications, from mental health to brain injury to neurodegeneration. Finally, the use of custom-made (e.g., 3D-printed) helmets alongside motion robustness might enable longer patient recordings, and unlike with EEG, a patient could take a MEG helmet off for a short time for a break and put it back on again without having to reseat sensors.

In summary, OPMs represent a potentially transformative step forward for MEG as an imaging technology. However, at the time of writing, OPM MEG is a nascent technology. The noise floor of OPMs remains somewhat higher than a SQUID, so the complete advantages of smaller brain-sensor distance have not yet been realized. The largest arrays currently in operation contain approximately 30 OPMs, and neither full head coverage nor the applications that go with it (e.g., whole-brain network connectivity measurements) have been achieved. The high spatial resolution that is theoretically achievable using an OPM array has yet to be demonstrated experimentally (although initial evidence suggests spatial resolution is improved compared with conventional MEG). Technical problems like crosstalk between sensors when OPMs are operated in close proximity have yet to be solved. These are just some examples of the hurdles that are yet to be overcome in the development of a viable OPM-based MEG scanning platform. None are insurmountable, and all result from the fact that OPM MEG technology is still in its early phase of development. Therefore, in conclusion, OPM MEG offers a genuine opportunity for a step change in MEG technology. However, it is still in the early phase of development, and time and resources are critical if it is to achieve its true potential.

REFERENCES

Alem, O., Benison, A. M., Barth, D. S., Kitching, J., & Knappe, S. (2014). Magnetoencephalography of epilepsy with a microfabricated atomic magnetrode. *Journal of Neuroscience, 34*, 14324–14327.

Allred, J., Lyman, R., Kornack, T., & Romalis, M. V. (2002). High-sensitivity atomic magnetometer unaffected by spin-exchange relaxation. *Physical Review Letters, 89*, 130801.

Andersen, L. M., Oostenveld, R., Pfeiffer, C., Ruffieux, S., Jousmaki, V., Hämäläinen, M., . . . Lundqvist, D. (2017). Similarities and differences between on-scalp and conventional in-helmet magnetoencephalography recordings. *PLoS One, 12*, e0178602.

Baillet, S. (2017). Magnetoencephalography for brain electrophysiology and imaging. *Nature Neuroscience, 20*, 327–339.

Barry, D. M., Tierney, T. M., Holmes, N., Boto, E., Roberts, G., Leggett, J., . . . Maguire, E. A. (2019). Imaging the human hippocampus with optically-pumped magnetometers. *NeuroImage, 203*, 116192.

Bloch, F. (1946). Nuclear induction. *Physical Review Letters, 70*, 4604–4673.

Boto, E., Bowtell, R. W., Krüger, P., Fromhold, M., Morris, P. G., Meyer, S., . . . Brookes, M. J. (2016).

The benefits of atomic magnetometers for MEG: A simulation study. *PLoS One, 11*, e0157655.

Boto, E., Holmes, N., Leggett, J., Roberts, G., Shah, V., Meyer, S. S., . . . Brookes, M. J. (2018). Moving magnetoencephalography towards real-world applications with a wearable system. *Nature, 555*, 657.

Boto, E., Meyer, S. S., Shah, V., Alem, O., Knappe, S., Kruger, P., . . . Brookes, M. J. (2017). A new generation of magnetoencephalography: Room temperature measurements using optically-pumped magnetometers. *NeuroImage, 149*, 404–414.

Boto, E., Seedat, Z., Holmes, N., Leggett, J., Hill, R. M., Roberts, G., . . . Brookes, M. J. (2019). Wearable neuroimaging: Combining and contrasting magnetoencephalography and electroencephalography. *NeuroImage, 201*, 116099.

Claus, S. C., Velis, D., Lopes da Silva, F. H., Viergever, M. A., & Kalitzin, S. (2012). High frequency spectral components after Secobarbital: The contribution of muscular origin. A study with MEG/EEG. *Epilepsy Research, 100*, 132–141.

Cohen, D. (1972). Magnetoencephalography: Detection of the brains electrical activity with a superconducting magnetometer. *Science, 5*, 664–666.

Dale, M. W., & Morely, G. (2017). Medical applications of diamond magnetometry: Commercial viability. *arXiv*, 170501994.

Dang, H., Maloof, A., & Romalis, M. (2010). Ultrahigh sensitivity magnetic field and magnetization measurements with an atomic magnetometer. *Applied Physics Letters, 97*, 151110.

Griffith, W. C., Knappe, S., & Kitching, J. (2010). Femtotesla atomic magnetometry in a microfabricated vapor cell. *Optics Express, 18*, 27167–27172.

Gross, J., Baillet, S., Barnes, G. R., Henson, R. N., Hillebrand, A., Jensen, O., . . . Schoffelen, J-M. (2013). Good practice for conducting and reporting MEG research. *NeuroImage, 65*, 349–363.

Hämäläinen, M. S., Hari, R., Ilmoniemi, R. J., Knuutila, J., & Lounasma, O. V. (1993). Magnetoencephalography: Theory, instrumentation, and applications to non-invasive studies of the working human brain. *Reviews of Modern Physics, 65*, 413–497.

Hanle, W. (1925). "*Die magnetische Beeinflussung der Resonanzfluoreszenz*". *Ergebnisse der Exakten Naturwissenschaften* (in German). Berlin, Heidelberg: Springer Berlin Heidelberg, 214–232.

Happer, W. (1972). Optical pumping. *Reviews of Modern Physics, 44*, 169.

Happer, W., & Tang, H. (1973). Spin-exchange shift and narrowing of magnetic resonance lines in optically pumped alkali vapors. *Physical Reviews Letters, 31*, 273.

Holmes, M., Leggett, J., Boto, E., Roberts, G., Hill, R. M., Tierney, T. M., . . . Bowtell, R. (2018). A biplanar coil system for nulling background magnetic fields in scalp mounted magnetoencephalography. *NeuroImage, 181*, 760–774.

Iivanainen, J., Zetter, R., Groen, M., Hakkarainen, K., & Parkkonen, L. (2019). On-scalp MEG system utilizing an actively shielded array of optically-pumped magnetometers. *NeuroImage, 194*, 244–258.

Jaklevic, R. C., Lambe, J., Silver, A. H., & Mercereau, J. E. (1964). Quantum interference effects in Josephson tunneling. *Physical Review Letters, 12*, 159–160.

Johnson, C., Schwindt, P. D. D., & Weisend, M. (2010). Magnetoencephalography with a two-color pump-probe, fiber-coupled atomic magnetometer. *Applied Physics Letters, 97*, 243703.

Johnson, C. N., Schwindt, P. D., & Weisend, M. (2013). Multi-sensor magnetoencephalography with atomic magnetometers. *Physics in Medicine & Biology, 58*, 6065–6077.

Josephson, B. D. (1962). Possible new effects in superconductive tunnelling. *Physics Letters, 1*, 251–253.

Josephson, B. D. (1974). The discovery of tunnelling supercurrents. *Reviews of Modern Physics, 46*, 251–254.

Kamada, K., Sato, D., Ito, Y., Natsukawa, H., Okano, K., Mizutani, N., & Kobayashi, T. (2015). Human magnetoencephalogram measurements using newly developed compact module of high-sensitivity atomic magnetometer. *Japanese Journal of Applied Physics, 54*, 026601.

Kastler, A. (1973). The Hanle effect and its use for the measurements of very small magnetic fields. *Nuclear Instruments and Methods, 110*, 259–265.

Kominis, I. K., Kornack, T. W., Allred, J. C., & Romalis, M. V. (2003). A subfemtotesla multichannel atomic magnetometer. *Nature, 422*, 596–599.

Lin, C-H., Tierney, T. M., Holmes, N., Boto, E., Leggett, J., Bestmann, S., . . . Barnes, G. R. (2019). Using optically-pumped magnetometers to measure magnetoencephalographic signals in the human cerebellum. *Journal of Physiology, 597*, 4309–4324.

Muthukumaraswamy, S. D. (2013). High-frequency brain activity and muscle artifacts in MEG/EEG: A review and recommendations. *Frontiers in Human Neuroscience, 7*, 138.

Nenonen, J., Nurminen, J., Kičić, D., Bikmullina, R., Lioumis, P., Jousmäki, V., . . . Kähkönen, S. (2012). Validation of head movement correction and spatiotemporal signal space separation in magnetoencephalography. *Clinical Neurophysiology, 123*, 2180–2191.

Okada, Y., Pratt, K., Atwood, C., Mascarenas, A., Reineman, R., Nurminen, J., & Paulson, D. (2006). BabySQUID: A mobile, high-resolution multichannel magnetoencephalography system for neonatal brain assessment. *Review of Scientific Instruments, 77*, 024301.

Riaz, B., Pfeiffer, C., & Schneiderman, J. F. (2017). Evaluation of realistic layouts for next generation on-scalp MEG: Spatial information density maps. *Scientific Reports, 7*, 6974.

Roberts, G., Holmes, N., Boto, E., Leggett, J., Hill, R. M., Shah, V., . . . Brookes, M. J. (2019). Towards magnetoencephalography in a virtual reality environment. *NeuroImage, 199*, 408–417.

Rondin, L., Tetienne, J-P., Hingant, T., Roch, J-F., Maletinsky, P., & Jacques, V. (2014). Magnetometry with nitrogen-vacancy defects in diamond. *Reports on Progress in Physics, 77*, 056503.

Sander, T. H., Preusser, J., Mhaskar, R., Kitching, J., Trahms, L., & Knappe, S. (2012). Magnetoencephalography with a chip-scale atomic magnetometer. *Biomedical Optics Express, 3*, 981–990.

Schwindt, P. D. D., Knappe, S., Shah, V., Hollberg, L., & Kitching, J. (2004). Chip-scale atomic magnetometer. *Applied Physics Letters, 85*, 26.

Schwindt, P. D. D., Lindseth, B., Knappe, S., Shah, V., Kitching, J., & Liew, L. (2007). Chip-scale atomic magnetometer with improved sensitivity by use of the Mx technique. *Applied Physics Letters, 90*, 081102–081103.

Shah, V., Knappe, S., Schwindt, P. D., & Kitching, J. (2007). Subpicotesla atomic magnetometry with a microfabricated vapour cell. *Nature Photonics, 1*, 649–652.

Shah V, & Romalis, M. V. (2009). Spin-exchange-relaxation-free magnetometrty using elliptically polarised light. *Physical Review A, 80*, 013416.

Shah, V. K., & Wakai, R. T. (2013). A compact, high performance atomic magnetometer for biomedical applications. *Physics in Medicine and Biology, 58*, 8153–8161.

Shelly, C. D., Matrozova, E. A., & Petrashov, V. T. (2016). Resolving thermoelectric "paradox" in superconductors. *Science Advances, 2*, e1501250.

Sletzer, S. (2008). Developments in alkali medal atomic magnetometry. PhD Thesis submitted to Princeton University, Princeton, NJ.

Tannoudji, C., Dupont-Roc, J., Haroche, S., & LaLoe, F. (1970). Diverses résonances de croisement de niveaux sur des atomes pompés optiquement en champ nul i. théorie. *Revue de Physique Appliquee, 5*, 95.

Taulu, S., & Simola, J. (2006). Spatiotemporal signal space separation method for rejecting nearby interference in MEG measurements. *Physics in Medicine & Biology, 51*, 1759.

Tierney, T. M., Holmes, N., Mellor, S., López, J. D., Roberts, G., Hill, R. M., . . . Barnes, G. R. (2019). Optically pumped magnetometers: From quantum origins to multi-channel magnetoencephalography. *NeuroImage, 199*, 598–608.

Tierney, T. M., Holmes, N., Meyer, S. S., Boto, E., Roberts, G., Leggett, J., . . . Barnes, G. R. (2018). Cognitive neuroscience using wearable magnetometer arrays: Non-invasive assessment of language function. *NeuroImage, 181*, 513–520.

Xia, H., Baranga, A. B. A., Hoffman, D., & Romalis, M. V. (2006). Magnetoencephalography with an atomic magnetometer. *Applied Physics Letters, 89*, 211104.

SECTION III

APPLICATIONS TO EPILEPSY

9

GUIDELINES AND PRACTICAL CONSIDERATIONS FOR MAPPING EPILEPTIFORM ACTIVITY AND NETWORK CONNECTIVITY WITH MAGNETOENCEPHALOGRAPHY

Roozbeh Rezaie, James W. Wheless, and Abbas Babajani-Feremi

9.1. VISUAL INSPECTION AND QUALITY ASSESSMENT OF MAGNETOENCEPHALOGRAPHY RECORDINGS

The procedure for identifying epileptiform activity on spontaneous (resting) magnetoencephalography (MEG) recordings is consistent, in many ways, with the approach taken to interpreting conventional scalp electroencephalography (EEG). As endorsed by most clinical MEG users (Bagic et al., 2011; Ebersole & Wagner, 2018; Hari et al., 2018; Hunold, Funke, Eichardt, Stenroos, & Haueisen, 2016; Martinez Castillo et al., 2009), the practice of simultaneously recording scalp EEG with MEG often facilitates the interpretive process, helping dissociate various normal and abnormal neurophysiological phenomena from electrographic signatures of epilepsy and their magnetic counterparts. Moreover,

understanding the appearance of common physiological artifacts, as well as artifacts unique to MEG instrumentation, can further assist the individual interpreting the data to assess the quality of the recordings and influence subsequent signal processing steps, which can affect identification of epileptiform transients and their subsequent localization.

9.1.1. Physiological Artifacts

Physiological artifacts that originate from outside the head but can exceed by orders of magnitude the strength of neuromagnetic signals of interest are typically recognizable on both EEG and MEG recordings. The most salient and well-defined of these artifacts is the cardiac signal, characterized on MEG by the prominent appearance of the R-wave of the QRS complex, often recorded simultaneously in an

Roozbeh Rezaie, James W. Wheless, and Abbas Babajani-Feremi, *Guidelines and Practical Considerations for Mapping Epileptiform Activity and Network Connectivity With Magnetoencephalography* In: *Fifty Years of Magnetoencephalography*. Edited by: Andrew C. Papanicolaou, Timothy P. L. Roberts, and James W. Wheless, Oxford University Press (2020). © Oxford University Press. DOI: 10.1093/oso/9780190935689.003.0009.

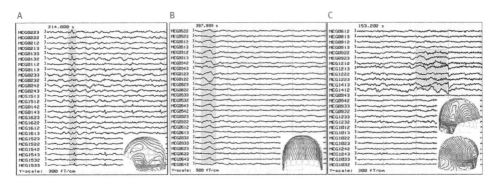

FIGURE 9.1 Morphological and topographic distribution of common physiological artifacts in clinical magnetoencephalography (MEG) recordings. (A) Appearance of the cardiac signal in MEG channels is typically characterized by the R-wave generating a gradient prominent over the left temporal region. (B) Ocular activity seen most prominently in anterior MEG sensors produces a strong bipolar magnetic field in the frontal regions. (C) High-frequency rhythmic activity resulting from contraction of the frontalis and temporalis muscles, characterized by a gradient in frontal and temporal MEG channels.

electrocardiogram channel (Figure 9.1A). The strength of the cardiac signal in MEG channels can vary according to individuals, with infants and children exhibiting a larger signal compared with adults, owing to the proximity of the heart to the MEG sensors. The peak of the cardiac signal typically generates a large gradient over left temporal MEG channels, although some topographical variability across individuals can be appreciated.

In addition to the cardiac signal, ocular activity as the result of blinks or saccadic eye movements, generated by the corneoretinal potential, represent another common source of physiological artifact in MEG recordings. Topographically, blinks and saccades generate prominent magnetic deflections in a broad and bipolar manner across anterior MEG sensors (see Figure 9.1B). Generally, ocular activity can be mitigated by asking patients to keep their eyes closed during testing and is generally less of a problem during interictal recordings, where the patient is void of external visual stimulation. Alternatively, the vertical and horizontal electro-oculograms can also be collected for verification of their counterparts on MEG and removal from the data using advanced off-line statistical processing.

Muscle artifact, associated with contraction of the frontalis and temporalis muscles, is also a common occurrence in MEG recordings and can be expected given the length of recording time and the position that the patient must maintain. Typically, clenching of the jaws generates high-frequency, low-voltage bursts of activity, which could variably result in moderate-to-large gradients visible in the temporal and frontal MEG channels (see Figure 9.1C).

In contrast to the cardiac signal, ocular activity, and muscle artifact, the respiratory signal is a characteristically low-frequency response that can typically be eliminated using a high-pass filter, although this may adversely affect MEG signal quality by amplifying the effects of ferromagnetic objects that are not removed from an individual.

9.1.2. Nonphysiological Artifacts

While environmental (e.g., traffic, elevators, moving magnetic resonance imaging [MRI] field) and instrumentation (e.g., thermal noise, flux traps, superconducting quantum-interference device [SQUID] jumps) artifacts are inherent to MEG, appropriate advances in hardware design and noise cancellation techniques can, in theory, optimize recording environments to mitigate their effects. However, nonphysiological artifacts specifically affecting MEG and not EEG typically originate from within patients in the form of dental implants and orthodontic devices, ventriculoperitoneal (VP) shunts, vagus nerve stimulators (VNS), and gastrostomy tubes (G-tubes) (many of which are not uncommon in pediatric epilepsy settings). Similarly, in cases of patients undergoing sedation, which includes a large number of pediatric patients referred for MEG testing, the introduction of artifacts from infusion pumps and auxiliary monitoring devices may further obscure epileptiform transients that, like physiological artifacts, are orders of magnitude smaller than magnetic fields generated by the aforementioned sources. While contemporary signal processing techniques have evolved to minimize their unwanted contributions to MEG signals (Taulu, Kajola, Simola, et al., 2004; Taulu, Simola, Nenonen, & Parkkonen, 2014), the moderate likelihood that they will be encountered in a clinical setting encourages familiarization of their appearance to individuals tasked with interpreting the data (Figure 9.2).

9.2. IDENTIFICATION AND LOCALIZATION OF EPILEPTIFORM TRANSIENTS IN MAGNETOENCEPHALOGRAPHY

The definition of epileptiform transients on MEG, in the case of both lesional and nonlesional epilepsies, generally adheres to that of paroxysmal events identified electrographically using scalp EEG. Using simultaneous EEG as a guide, MEG recordings have been shown to reliably identify sources of interictal epileptiform discharges (e.g., sharp waves, spikes, polyspikes, or spike–wave complexes) in a variety of epilepsies and epilepsy syndromes (Knowlton et al., 2006, 2009; Otsubo et al., 2001; Papanicolaou et al., 2005; Stefan et al., 2017; Sutherling et al., 2008). While empirical studies have addressed the variability in the attributes of epileptiform spikes identified electrographically (intracranially and extracranially) to their magnetic

counterparts (Fernandes et al., 2005; Merlet et al., 1997; Nowak, Santiuste, & Russi, 2009), it remains common practice to use the scalp EEG as a guide for identifying these transients. An important consideration when addressing the utility of MEG in the evaluation of patients with epilepsy is the fact that MEG primarily characterizes the irritative zone, mainly capturing interictal activity, rather than the ictal onset zone. In practice, given the variables associated with testing patients (e.g., levels of antiepileptic medication, state of arousal, level of sedation, absence of seizure triggers, limited recording time), predicting and capturing ictal onset is a rare occurrence during MEG recordings. Furthermore, with the exception of absence seizures, motor symptoms associated with ictal events confound the quality of the recorded MEG signal because of high-frequency myogenic artifacts and significant head motion, the latter of which can affect the accuracy of localizing the underlying source generators of activity.

9.2.1. Source Localization Approach

While slight differences exist in approaches taken to collecting clinical MEG data across users, the cardinal steps in patient preparation and data acquisition parameters should be observed by all practitioners to ensure optimal yield from a recording. Following general review of the recordings for quality as well as application of appropriate measures to minimize the contributions of physiological, environmental, and instrumentation artifacts, a bandpass filter with low cutoff frequency of 1 to 3 Hz and high cutoff frequency of 50 to 70 Hz (50/60-Hz notch filter) is typically deemed adequate for identifying epileptiform discharges, without distortion, on simultaneous EEG/MEG traces. In selecting filter settings, it bears mentioning that nonepileptiform abnormal patterns of electrographic activity, as well as their MEG counterparts, can also be present in patients with epilepsy. Specifically, the presence of focal slow waves (~1–4 Hz) may be

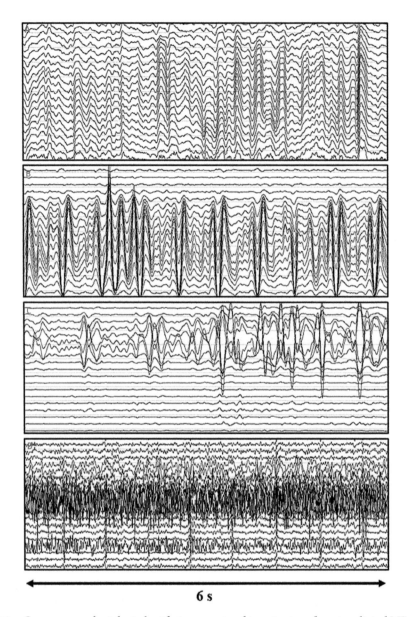

6 s

FIGURE 9.2 Common nonphysiological artifacts encountered in patients undergoing clinical MEG recordings. Low-frequency signals associated with (A) vagus nerve stimulator and (B) dental implants are generally amplified by respiration. Moderate- to high-frequency electromagnetic artifact can also saturate magnetoencephalography sensors from sources such as (C) ventriculoperitoneal shunt or (D) auxiliary monitoring devices attached to the patient inside the shielded room during recordings performed under anesthesia.

consistent with local structural lesions (e.g., vascular malformations, tumors, and stroke) or an epileptic focus, and as such their localization may add context and value to the overall interpretation of clinical MEG recordings (Ishibashi et al., 2002).

Although not without theoretical limitations, the single equivalent current dipole (ECD) model remains the most commonly adopted and clinically valid approach to reconstructing MEG sources of epileptiform activity (Alkawadri, Burgess, Kakisaka, Mosher,

& Alexopoulos, 2018; Ochi et al., 2001; Paetau et al., 1994; Wheless et al., 1999, 2004). In the present context, the ECD model assumes that epileptiform discharges detected by MEG can be modeled as discrete generators made up of a current source and sink, separated by an insulator. For a given point along the temporal evolution of an epileptiform transient (e.g., spike peak), an iterative algorithm is applied to determine the location, orientation, and strength of the ECD that best describe the surface-recorded magnetic field at the corresponding time sample. While some variability in ECD acceptance criteria exists, because of either signal quality or physiological factors, the parameters of interest that are recommended for consideration when accepting or rejecting source solutions include the (a) correlation between the forward-calculated magnetic field and the measured magnetic field; (b) strength of the dipolar source to ensure physiological plausibility; (c) root-mean-square amplitude of the field integrated across channels selected for dipole fitting to ensure sufficient signal-to-noise ratio (SNR); and (d) confidence volume corresponding to the region that was most likely to contain the source of the observed magnetic field distribution.

On selection of ECDs meeting acceptable statistical criteria, the anatomical distribution of the activity sources (and their orientations) can subsequently be visualized by projecting each dipole onto an individual's high-resolution MRI. In practice, this is achieved by precise co-registration of the MEG coordinate system onto the MRI through alignment of the MEG fiducial points (nasion, and left and right auricular points) to analogous points typically identified by high-contrast markers on the MRI.

9.2.2. Spikes, Spike–Wave Complexes, and Polyspikes

Consistent with the electrographic definition, a MEG spike is characterized by a sharply contoured paroxysmal deviation from the background rhythm, with a duration of about 20 to 70 ms, followed by a slow wave before a return to baseline. As expected, spikes can appear focal, multifocal, or generalized, with their rhythmic recurrence being manifest as either spike–wave complexes or polyspikes, which may be focal or generalized in nature.

While time-intensive, the most fundamental aspect of localizing epileptiform discharges on MEG recordings is the process of visual inspection. Following appropriate signal preprocessing steps and review of data for quality, emphasis should be placed on using the scalp EEG to identify a sufficient number of temporally independent epileptiform discharges of similar morphology, to create an event category. The rate of occurrence, as well as the morphology and topographical distribution, of spikes during a typical MEG recording session may be challenging to predict and could depend on a number of situational variables. However, localizing events that are classified, with confidence, as spikes should begin by topographically assessing the spatial distribution of time samples encompassing the event of interest. In the context of the single ECD model, the temporal evolution of the epileptiform spike should be associated with the gradual formation of a dipolar isofield pattern, increasing in strength and focality, approaching the peak amplitude of the event.

Although convention suggests spatiotemporal modeling of a spike at the peak of the event, where SNR is highest, thus yielding statistically optimal source (ECD) estimates, this practice may oversimplify characterization of the irritative zone (for further theoretical discussion, see Chapter 10). Specifically, the onset and propagation phases of a spike may be accounted for by activity sources unique in location and orientation from each other as well as from the source underlying the peak latency (Figure 9.3). This approach merits some consideration, particularly in view of the evidence of an asynchrony between interictal epileptiform spike onset on EEG and MEG, with the latter having been shown to precede

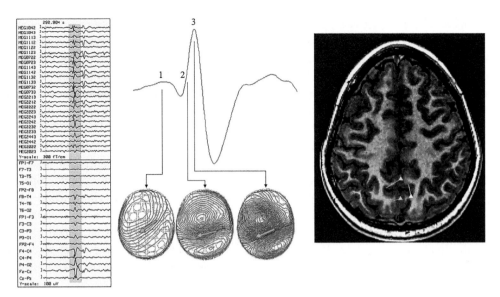

FIGURE 9.3   Spatiotemporal profile of an epileptiform spike in simultaneous magnetoencephalography (MEG) (400 fT/cm) and scalp electroencephalography (EEG) (100 μV) recordings from a 9-year-old boy with cryptogenic focal-onset seizures of right hemisphere origin (1–50 Hz band-pass filter). The concurrent appearance of spike activity on the EEG (maximal at Fz-Cz) and MEG sensors is highlighted in *red*. The *middle* portion of the figure exhibits the spike–wave time course from a MEG sensor exhibiting maximum amplitude, and isofield maps detail the dipolar patterns emerging from the (1) period immediately preceding the (2) rising phase, followed by the (3) peak of the spike. On the *right* side of the figure, ECD modeling demonstrates the spatial variability in MEG spike localization, as characterized by an anterior-to-posterior shift in the activity sources accounting for the early phase (*yellow triangle*), rising period (*white triangle*), and peak (*magenta triangle*) of the event.

the former, suggestive of temporal and spatial variability in defining the irritative zone (Kakisaka et al., 2012; Martinez Castillo et al., 2009; Merlet et al., 1997). Furthermore, given that the various phases composing the spatiotemporal profile of a spike may be generated by different neuronal assemblies, the orientation of the corresponding ECDs may also be an indicator of the underlying pathology. It has been advanced by some that dipole orientation is an important parameter when using MEG to predict seizure foci, particularly in temporal lobe epilepsy (Ebersole, 1997, 1999; Ebersole, Squires, Eliashiv, & Smith, 1995; Ebersole, Squires, Gamelin, Lewine, & Scherg, 1993; Fuchs, Kastner, Tech, Wagner, & Gasca, 2017; Martinez Castillo et al., 2009). Quantitively, however, the decision to characterize the spatial profile of interictal MEG on the basis of localizing activity leading up to the peak of the

spike may require acceptance of less rigid ECD criteria, owing to lower SNR. Ultimately, the time points selected for localization should be considered in the interpretation of the results, along with other clinical evidence that may help elucidate the significance of MEG findings as they relate to the patient's diagnosis.

Although traditionally emphasis has been placed on using scalp EEG as a confirmatory marker of epileptiform discharges on MEG recordings, the advantage of the latter is further highlighted in scenarios in which these events may not be clearly distinguishable on the simultaneously recorded EEG waveforms (Figure 9.4). Qualitatively, differences in the morphology of spikes, such as shape, sharpness, and duration, can be attributed to the fact that magnetic fields are not susceptible to conductivity distortions inherent from scalp EEG (Iwasaki et al., 2005; Kakisaka et al., 2012; Kirsch, Mantle,

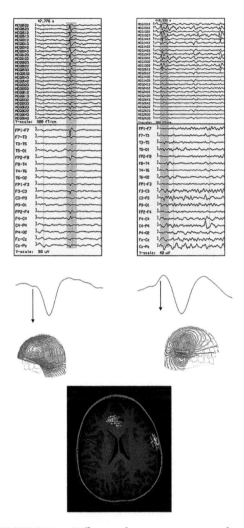

FIGURE 9.4 Differences between magnetic and electrographic epileptiform spike manifestation in a 10-year-old girl with benign childhood focal epilepsy, exhibiting temporally independent multifocal epileptiform discharges (1- to 50-Hz band-pass filter). The first category of events (*left panel*) have a clear appearance on the magnetoencephalography (MEG) (300 fT/cm) and electroencephalography (EEG) (90 µV) studies, maximal at Fp1-F7, with robust isofield contours resulting in a tight equivalent current dipole (ECD) cluster in the left anterior cingulate region. In contrast, independent discharges over the right frontotemporal region clearly present on the MEG waveforms (300 fT/cm), but not scalp EEG (40 µV), generated a strong dipolar pattern, the sources of which form a tight ECD cluster in the inferior precentral region (*right panel*).

& Nagarajan, 2007; Lin et al., 2003; Ossenblok, de Munck, Colon, Drolsbach, & Boon, 2007). Moreover, the evidence and rationale for the existence of epileptiform spikes "unique" to MEG have led to the suggestion that this phenomenon may be governed by the extent and cortical complexity of the irritative zone as well as the orientation and strength of sources generating interictal discharges. Nevertheless, to increase confidence, it is recommended that interictal MEG mapping be performed with simultaneous scalp EEG, given the standard of the latter as a diagnostic tool in epilepsy.

As stated earlier, the frequency with which spikes are detected during a given recording session may vary owing to a number of factors. The ideal scenario in a clinical MEG recording session would consist of localizing a sufficient number of ECD sources that would yield a reliable and reproducible spatiotemporal map of the irritative zone. However, this may, albeit rarely, represent a trade-off in cases in which mapping of eloquent cortex is warranted. Generally, occurrence of high-amplitude spikes during functional mapping is infrequent enough to not interfere with signals averaged in response to external stimuli (auditory, visual, mechanical, or electrical). While band-pass filtering appropriate for evoked magnetic fields may not be sufficient to eliminate spike activity, they can, because of their infrequent occurrence, either be decomposed from the raw signal using advanced signal processing techniques (but with the limitation that other signals of interest may also be removed), suppressed through signal averaging, or removed by omitting epochs contaminated with epileptiform events before averaging. However, in rare cases in which interictal discharges (focal or generalized) occur at or exceed the rate of stimulus presentation, saturation of the evoked fields may in effect result in a spatial representation of "averaged" epileptiform spikes, which could prove problematic if their modeled underlying sources overlap with the eloquent cortex being mapped (Figure 9.5).

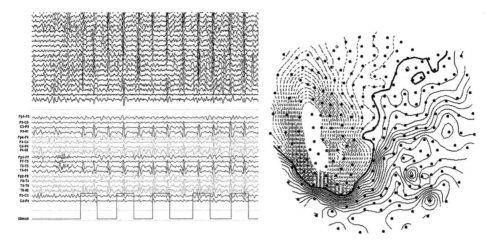

FIGURE 9.5   Frequent spike–wave discharges in a 10-year-old boy with symptomatic focal seizures of bilateral posterior onset, during a magnetoencephalography (MEG) language mapping task (20=Hz low-pass filter). The *red* vertical columns at the *bottom* of the trace indicate the onset of auditory (spoken word) stimuli at a rate of 1 to 2 s. Saturation of the MEG recordings (1 pT) by frequent 2.5-Hz spike-and-slow wave discharges, confirmed on simultaneous scalp electroencephalogram (80 μV) and maximal at P3-O1/T5-O1, are visible throughout the trace, resulting in a posterior dominant magnetic gradient on the isofield contour map.

Unlike spikes without temporal overlap, localizing onset in complex and temporally overlapping events such as typical or atypical generalized spike and slow wave discharges, and polyspikes, can be a challenge for MEG. Characteristic of primary generalized epilepsies, the complex isofield contours generated by these epileptiform discharges typically do not conform to a focal and stable dipolar pattern (Figure 9.6), often yielding solutions with excessive source strength, poor correlation measures, and implausible anatomical distribution. In some cases, however, MEG may lend itself well to confirming or disambiguating the onset of spike and slow wave discharges with diffuse or bisynchronous EEG appearance, such as those exhibiting an amplitude asymmetry (Figure 9.7). Moreover, onset of electrographic seizures in juvenile and childhood absence epilepsy may also be localized on MEG recordings, particularly in cases in which patients exhibit focal interictal spikes in between, or before, ictal onset (Figure 9.8).

9.2.3. Sharp Waves

Different in their morphological characteristics compared with spikes, sharp waves are also of clinical significance in patients with epilepsy, and their appearance on MEG recordings is consistent with that of scalp EEG, defined by a steep rising paroxysmal potential with a duration of about 70 to 200 ms. Although lacking the focality of spikes, MEG nevertheless is useful in localizing the sources of sharp waves, which often have a broad anatomical distribution, perhaps indicative of a wider underlying epileptogenic network (Figure 9.9).

9.3. MAPPING EPILEPTOGENIC NETWORKS USING MAGNETOENCEPHALOGRAPHY: METHODOLOGICAL CONSIDERATIONS

We briefly introduce the technical aspects of brain connectivity analysis using MEG in this section. An example of the application of MEG connectivity analysis in patients

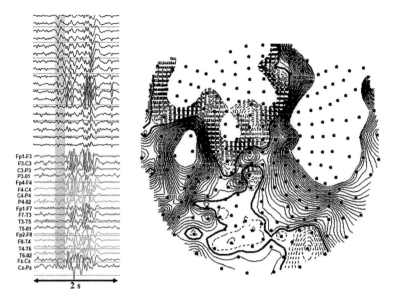

FIGURE 9.6   Simultaneous magnetoencephalogram (5 pT) and scalp electroencephalogram (100 μV) high-amplitude, diffuse irregular spike- and polyspike and slow wave discharges in a 2-year-old girl with a history of intractable symptomatic focal epilepsy secondary to right temporal cyst (3- to 70-Hz band-pass filter). As evident from the leading waveform of the event, isofield contour maps are not suggestive of a focality, as demonstrated by the absence of a single, stable dipolar pattern.

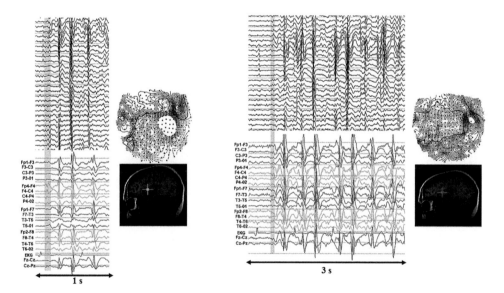

FIGURE 9.7   Magnetoencephalography (MEG) and scalp electroencephalography (EEG) localization of onset in a 16-year-old girl with intractable childhood absence epilepsy (3- to 70-Hz band-pass filter). The *left panel* shows that initial occurrence of 3-Hz spike and slow wave activity was preceded by a clear phase reversal that was maximal at Fp2-F4/F4-C4 on the EEG (100 μV) and was associated with a right anterior dipolar pattern on the MEG (5 pT), which localized to the right insular cortex. As presented in the *right panel,* inspection of subsequent high-amplitude 3- to 4-Hz spike and slow wave discharges showed a focality on the waveforms preceding diffuse onset, which localized to the location of the previous interictal discharge.

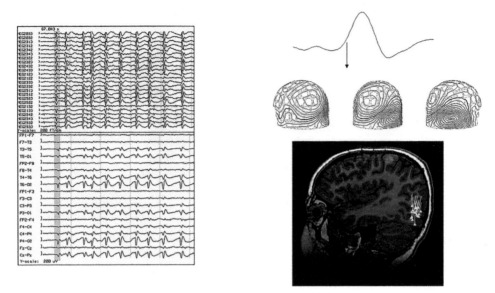

FIGURE 9.8   Localization of lateralized onset in a 7-year-old boy with idiopathic focal epilepsy, with high-voltage bisynchronous occipital spike waves showing amplitude asymmetry (*left panel*). As seen in the *right panel*, the amplitude asymmetry on scalp EEG (200 μV) was verified by a focal dipolar pattern detected by MEG (200 fT/cm), which resulted in a dense ECD cluster in the lateral-mesial occipital region (1- to 50-Hz band-pass filter).

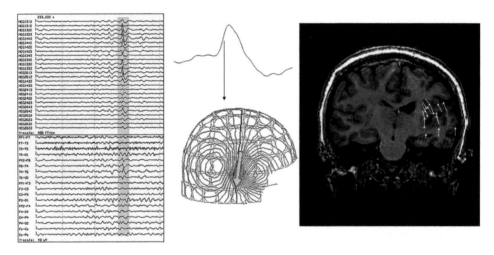

FIGURE 9.9   Appearance and localization of sharp wave activity on simultaneous magnetoencephalography (MEG) (400 fT/cm) and scalp electroencephalography (EEG) (40 μV) in an 18-year-old woman with focal epilepsy secondary to right perisylvian polymicrogyria and gray matter heterotopia (1- to 50-Hz band-pass). As evident from the *left panel,* focal sharp wave activity is visible on both the EEG (maximal at T4–T6) and MEG waveforms, with a clearer morphology on the latter time series. In the *right panel,* inspection of the MEG time course of sharp wave activity is characterized by a robust dipolar pattern and ECD distribution in the vicinity of the lesion. Note that the spatial distribution of activity sources underlying sharp waves has a broader distribution than that seen with spikes.

with epilepsy is presented to highlight the technique's application.

9.3.1. Functional Versus Effective Connectivity

The brain connectivity analysis can be subdivided into *structural, functional,* and *effective* connectivity (Friston, 1994). *Structural connectivity* can be derived through various invasive and noninvasive tract-tracking methods that identify the fiber pathways between different brain regions. MRI diffusion tensor imaging (DTI) is the most commonly used noninvasive method for measuring structural connectivity. *Functional connectivity* is defined as the "temporal correlations between remote neurophysiological events" (Friston, 1994), representing the deviation from statistical independence across these events (Fingelkurts, Fingelkurts, & Kahkonen, 2005). *Effective connectivity* is defined as the direct or indirect influence that a brain area exerts on others (Fingelkurts et al., 2005). Unlike functional connectivity, which can only provide information about temporal correlation, effective connectivity explains the direction of interactions and the casual flow of information between brain regions. The high temporal resolution (<1 ms) of MEG makes it an excellent choice for exploring functional and effective connectivity. Functional and effective connectivity analysis based on MEG have been used in the diagnosis and prognosis of various neurological and psychiatric diseases (Stam, 2010; Tsiaras et al., 2011). For example, resting-state MEG connectivity analysis has been used in several epilepsy studies to investigate the alteration of the brain network from interictal to preictal (Hamandi, Routley, Koelewijn, & Singh, 2016), lateralize and localize the seizure onset zone (Nissen et al., 2017), and relate the alteration of the brain network to the duration and the severity of epilepsy (Englot et al., 2015). (See Chapter 11 of this volume for more details about the applications of the MEG connectivity analysis.)

9.3.2. Sensor Space Versus Source Space

MEG connectivity analysis can be performed in either sensor space or source space. In sensor space connectivity analysis, the functional or effective interactions between signals of MEG sensors are calculated, and a subsequent adjacency matrix (with size of n-by-n, where n is the number of sensors) is created using the values of the connectivity between each pair of sensors. In source space analysis, the MEG sensor signals are first mapped to source space using an inverse solution method, for example, the minimum-norm estimation (MNE). Then the source signals are used in connectivity analysis to calculate an adjacency matrix with size of m-by-m, where m is the number of sources. The number of sources in a typical inverse solution method (e.g. MNE or beamformer) is large ($m \sim 10,000$), and the resulting adjacency matrix is called a *dense-connectome*. This dense connectome is computationally intensive, difficult to visualize, and challenging to interpret. In addition, MEG data rarely contain more than 100 independent sources because of the limited number of MEG sensors ($n \sim 200 – 300$), and thus a dense-connectome is not an appropriate representation for a MEG connectivity analysis. A common solution for this issue is to parcellate the cortex to a limited number of regions (~100 parcels), using, for example, the automated anatomical labeling (AAL) atlas (Tzourio-Mazoyer et al., 2002), and to calculate the connectivity measure based on representative time series of the parcellated regions.

Both source space and sensor space connectivity analyses have some limitations. Although sensor space connectivity is more straightforward to perform than source space connectivity because it does not involve the inverse problem, it is hindered by the "field spread" effect. The field spread effect is a phenomenon that occurs when multiple MEG sensors pick up signals from a single source, resulting in an "artifactual" and erroneous inflation of the MEG connectivity between brain sources (Srinivasan, Winter, Ding, &

Nunez, 2007; Winter, Nunez, Ding, & Srinivasan, 2007). On the other hand, source space connectivity analysis provides more reliable information about the communication between brain areas. However, source space connectivity analysis is limited by the ill-posedness of the inverse problem (Helmholtz, 1853). A unique map of brain activity from measured signals in MEG sensors cannot be generated without imposing major restrictions on the inverse solution. Several methods have been proposed for solving the inverse problem (Baillet, Mosher, & Leahy, 2001), including MNE (Sarvas, 1987) and linearly constrained minimum variance (LCMV) beamformer (Van Veen, van Drongelen, Yuchtman, & Suzuki, 1997). The sensitivity and specificity of each method depend on the assumptions regarding the properties of the neural sources and on the incorporation of a priori information. Similar to the artificial inflation of sensor space connectivity due to the field spread effect, the MEG source space connectivity can also be greatly affected by the "source leakage" effect (Brookes et al., 2012). Source leakage is the spread of reconstructed sources over a relatively large brain volume. A number of connectivity measures have been introduced (e.g. imaginary coherence) to correct the field spread and source leakage effects (Table 9.1).

9.3.3. Preprocessing and Artifact Removal

Before calculating connectivity measures, one important preprocessing step is to identify and potentially remove artifacts from the data. Physiological and nonphysiological artifacts in MEG data were introduced in sections 1.1 and 1.2. Although the effects of artifacts can be reduced by the preprocessing of data, it is recommended to minimize artifacts during MEG data acquisition by following several practical guidelines (Puce & Hamalainen, 2017). A combination of visual inspection and (semi-)automatic detection is often used to remove artifacts or select artifact-free segments of data. Independent component analysis (ICA)

(Bell & Sejnowski, 1995), signal-space projection (SSP) (Uusitalo & Ilmoniemi, 1997), and signal-space separation (SSS) (Taulu, Kajola, & Simola, 2004; Taulu & Simola, 2006) are popular methods for removing artifacts from MEG signals. (See (Puce & Hämäläinen, 2017; Gross et al., 2013) for more details about identification and removal of artifacts in MEG data.)

9.3.4. Connectivity Measures

Various connectivity measures have been proposed for electrophysiological data (Greenblatt et al., 2012), and several studies have evaluated their strengths and weaknesses (Colclough et al., 2016; Garces, Martin-Buro, & Maestu, 2016; Gross et al., 2013; Pereda, Quiroga, & Bhattacharya, 2005; van Diessen et al., 2015; H. E. Wang et al., 2014). Some popular connectivity measures are listed in Table 9.1. Choosing the most appropriate connectivity measure from such a wealth of options may be difficult, and the following issues and criteria should be considered in selecting the optimal measure for a given data and research question: (a) linear or nonlinear relationship between the time courses of signals; (b) time or frequency domain analysis; (c) assessing relations between the phase or the amplitude of signals; (d) investigating directed (effective connectivity) or undirected (functional connectivity) information flow between the sources; (e) evaluating interdependency by considering direct or indirect (i.e., bivariate or multivariate) connectivity; and (f) the effects of field spread (for MEG), volume conduction (for EEG), and source leakage (for MEG and EEG).

Correlation and coherence are linear methods that are relatively straightforward in terms of interpretation and computation and have been used to investigate the connectivity between brain regions for decades (Adey et al., 1967; Shaw, 1984). However, these linear methods are unable to incorporate the intrinsic nonlinearity of the neural activities, and thus several nonlinear connectivity measures have been proposed (Pereda et al., 2005; van Mierlo et al., 2014; Vindiola,

Table 9.1 Overview of Some Conventional Magnetoencephalography and Electroencephalography Connectivity Measures

CONNECTIVITY MEASURE	TYPE	ASSUME LINEARITY?	FIELD SPREAD OR SOURCE LEAKAGE CONTROL?	DIRECTED? (EFFECTIVE CONNECTIVITY?)	INDIRECT CONNECTIVITY (MULTIVARIATE)?	CONCEPT OF MEASURE	COMMENTS "+" ADVANTAGE(S); "−" DISADVANTAGE(S)
Correlation (Brazier & Barlow, 1956)	Amplitude coupling	Yes	No	No	No	The time domain linear relation between the amplitude of two signals	+ Commonly used and straightforward method
Coherence (Adey, Elul, Walter, & Crandall, 1967)	Spectral coherence	Yes	No	No	No	The frequency domain linear relation between the amplitude of two signals	+ Commonly used and straightforward method
Granger Causality (Bressler & Seth, 2011; Granger, 1969; Hesse, Moller, Arnold, & Schack, 2003)	Autoregressive modeling	Yes	Disputed	Yes	Yes	If the future values of signal X is predicted by past and present values of signal Y, then signal Y is said to be a Granger cause of signal X.	+ Well-established and widely used in many fields of research − Methodological choices (e.g., choice of reference in EEG), as well as other confounders (e.g., volume conduction) could interfere with the actual causality
Directed Coherence (G. Wang & Takigawa, 1992)	Autoregressive modeling	Yes	No	Yes	No	The directed linear relation between two signals based on the Granger causality in the frequency domain	− Difficult to estimate an optimal order for the multivariate model

(continued)

Table 9.1 Continue

CONNECTIVITY MEASURE	TYPE	ASSUME LINEARITY?	FIELD SPREAD OR SOURCE LEAKAGE CONTROL?	DIRECTED? (EFFECTIVE CONNECTIVITY?)	INDIRECT CONNECTIVITY (MULTIVARIATE)?	CONCEPT OF MEASURE	COMMENTS "+" ADVANTAGE(S); "−" DISADVANTAGE(S)
Directed Transfer Function (Kaminski & Blinowska, 1991)	Autoregressive modeling	Yes	Yes	Yes	No	The Granger causal relation between the outflow of node X toward node Y (normalized by all inflows towards node Y) in the frequency domain	+ Distinction between common source and interconnectedness − Noisy channels affect the directionality − Difficult to estimate an optimal order for the multivariate model
Partial Directed Coherence (Baccala & Sameshima, 2001)	Autoregressive modeling	Yes	Disputed	Yes	Yes	The Granger causal relation between the outflow of node X toward node Y (normalized by all outflows from node X) in the frequency domain	− No conclusion about the strength of coupling, owing to normalization − Difficult to estimate an optimal order for the multivariate model
Imaginary Part of Coherency (Nolte et al., 2004)	Spectral coherence	Yes	Yes	No	No	By including only the imaginary part of the coherency, the influence of volume conduction is excluded	− Imaginary part is mostly small, thereby causing risk of missing meaningful interactions

Mutual Information (Fraser & Swinney, 1986)	Amplitude or phase coupling	No	No	No	Provides the amount of information in signal X that can be explained by signal Y and vice versa, based on P(X), P(Y), and P(X,Y) where P(.) is the probability distribution function	+ Mutual information is sensitive in narrow-frequency band analysis −Weak coupling could be missed −Complicated computational measure to obtain from experimental time series
Synchronization Likelihood (Stam & van Dijk, 2002)	Generalized synchronization	No	No	No	Provides the normalized strength of the mutual information between two signals X and Y in state space	+ Adequately deals with complexity caused by interacting systems
Phase Locking Value (Lachaux, Rodriguez, Martinerie, & Varela, 1999)	Phase coupling	No	No	No	A measure of the phase synchrony based on the modules of the averaged instantaneous phase differences between two signals	−The size of the instantaneous phase difference is included, but there is no evidence that the size of the phase difference is important for the coupling strength
Phase Slope Index (Nolte et al, 2008)	Phase coupling	Yes	Yes	Yes	Provides an estimate for the direction of information flow, based on the slope of the phase difference of the cross-spectral density between two signals	+ Weighs the contribution of different time series + Not affected by mixture of independent sources (e.g, background activity) −Complicated computational method

(continued)

Table 9.1 Continue

CONNECTIVITY MEASURE	TYPE	ASSUME LINEARITY?	FIELD SPREAD OR SOURCE LEAKAGE CONTROL?	DIRECTED? (EFFECTIVE CONNECTIVITY?)	INDIRECT CONNECTIVITY (MULTIVARIATE)?	CONCEPT OF MEASURE	COMMENTS "+" ADVANTAGE(S); "−" DISADVANTAGE(S)
Phase Lag Index (PLI) (Stam, Nolte, & Daffertshofer, 2007)	Phase coupling	No	Yes	No	No	Provides the asymmetry of the distribution of phase differences between signals X and Y	– Risk for missing linear but functionally meaningful interactions The instantaneous phase differences are binarized, therefore, small phase differences may also be missed under noisy conditions
Weighted PLI (Vinck, Oostenveld, van Wingerden, Battaglia, & Pennartz, 2011)	Phase coupling	Yes	Yes	No	No	Contribution of the observed phase leads and lags is weighted by the magnitude of the imaginary component of the coherency	+ Reduced sensitivity to noise (compared with PLI) + Improved detection of phase synchronization changes (compared with PLI) – The size of the instantaneous phase difference is included, but there is no evidence that the size of the phase difference is important for the coupling strength – Relative insensitive to phase differences around 0 and 180 degrees – Not possible to make a distinction between direct and indirect relations

Method	Type of coupling					Description	
Directed Phase Lag Index (Stam & van Straaten, 2012)	Phase coupling	No	Yes	Yes	No	Direction of information flow between signals X and Y is determined based on the probability that the instantaneous phase of X was smaller than the phase of Y (module π) over time	− Directionality can be ambiguous because leading with a small difference is similar to lagging with a large phase difference
Amplitude Envelope Correlation (AEC) (Liu, Fukunaga, de Zwart, & Duyn, 2010)	Amplitude coupling	Yes	No	No	No	The envelope of the band-limited power (BLP) of signal is calculated, and then the temporal correlation between the BLP signals is calculated	+ Straightforward method
Leakage Controlled AEC (Brookes, Woolrich, & Barnes, 2012; Colclough, Brookes, Smith, & Woolrich, 2015; Hipp, Hawellek, Corbetta, Siegel, & Engel, 2012)	Amplitude coupling	Yes	Yes	No	No	Provides the nonzero lag interactions between the power envelopes of signals based on a multivariate statistical framework	− The orthogonalization may result in so-called secondary leakage or ghost connections, where a genuine connection between two nodes spreads in space because of leakage from these nodes to other proximal regions

(continued)

Table 9.1 Continue

CONNECTIVITY MEASURE	TYPE	ASSUME LINEARITY?	FIELD SPREAD OR SOURCE LEAKAGE CONTROL?	DIRECTED? (EFFECTIVE CONNECTIVITY?)	INDIRECT CONNECTIVITY (MULTIVARIATE)?	CONCEPT OF MEASURE	COMMENTS "+" ADVANTAGE(S); "−" DISADVANTAGE(S)
Phase Difference Derivative (Breakspear, 2004)	Phase coupling	Yes	No	No	No	Provides a direct observation of the temporal behavior of the phase difference derivative to overcome the problem of differentiating between moderate phase-locking and alternations between phase-locking and desynchronization.	+ Provides an instantaneous measure of connectivity
Transfer Entropy (Schreiber, 2000)	Amplitude or phase coupling	No	Yes	Yes	No	An information theoretic implementation of Wiener-type causality to investigate causal interactions, without a need for a prespecified interaction model	+ It is "model agnostic" since it depends only on estimation of multivariate entropies directly from probability distributions

| Phase Difference Derivative (Breakspear, 2004) | Phase coupling | Yes | No | No | No | Provides a direct observation of the temporal behavior of the phase difference derivative to overcome the problem of differentiating between moderate phase-locking and alternations between phase-locking and desynchronization | + Provides an instantaneous measure of connectivity |

See Greenblatt, Pflieger, & Ossadtchi (2012), O'Neill et al. (2018), and van Diessen et al. (2015) for more details.
EEG = electroencephalography.

Vettel, Gordon, Franaszczuk, & McDowell, 2014; Wendling, Ansari-Asl, Bartolomei, & Senhadji, 2009). An important category of the nonlinear methods is phase-based connectivity measures, such as phase locking value (PLV) (Lachaux et al., 1999). Besides linearity, another important aspect of connectivity measures is the ability to identify causal interactions (effective connectivity). Causal interactions can be calculated using bivariate or multivariate connectivity measures. Bivariate measures, such as the phase slope index (PSI) (Nolte et al., 2008), compute the interaction between two signals of interest and ignore the influence of all other signals. On the other hand, the multivariate measures, such as partial directed coherence (PDC) (Baccala & Sameshima, 2001), incorporate the influence of other signals on causal interactions between two signals of interest and attempt to separate direct and indirect interrelations.

Multiple connectivity measures, such as imaginary part of coherency (Nolte et al., 2004) and phase lag index (PLI) (Stam et al., 2007),

have been introduced to address the problems of field spread (MEG), volume conduction (EEG) effects, and leakage of reconstructed sources (MEG/EEG). The source leakage and field spread generate zero-lagged signals that can be misidentified as connections between sources. Therefore, a zero-lagged connectivity between two signals (generated by the source leakage or field spread effect) should be removed from the data, but this is at the expense of removing real zero-lagged connectivity in data.

The majority of MEG/EEG connectivity measures are in frequency domain, including all phase-based measures. The results of MEG/EEG connectivity analysis can be widely affected by the selection of the frequency of interest. A typical approach is to calculate the connectivity measures in classical frequency bands, namely delta (0.5–4) Hz, theta (4–8) Hz, alpha (8–13) Hz, beta (13–30) Hz, low gamma (30–50) Hz, and high gamma (30–150) Hz. Figure 9.10 shows the adjacency matrixes of three connectivity measures

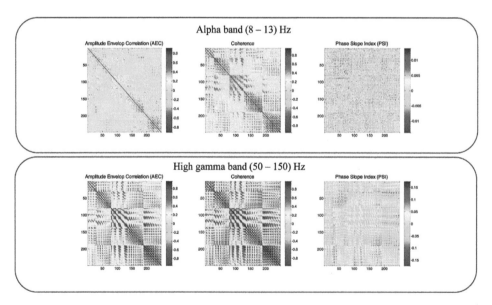

FIGURE 9.10   Results of resting-state magnetoencephalography (rs-MEG) connectivity analysis in sensor space. The adjacency matrixes of three connectivity measures (amplitude envelop correlation [AEC], coherence, and phase slope index [PSI]) in alpha (8–13) Hz and low gamma (30–50) Hz frequency bands are shown. Ten minutes of rs-MEG data were collected in a healthy control subject (a 28-year-old woman) using a whole-head MAGNES 3600 (4D Neuroimaging, San Diego, CA) MEG magnetometer system. Methods similar to those detailed by Babajani-Feremi, Noorizadeh, Mudigoudar, and Wheless (2018) were used for preprocessing, removing artifacts, and calculating the connectivity measures.

(amplitude envelop correlation [AEC], coherence, and PSI) in two frequency bands (alpha and high gamma). These connectivity measures were calculated in sensor space using a resting-state eyes-open MEG dataset in a healthy control subject (a 28-year-old woman). As shown in this figure, values of the connectivity measures are frequency dependent, and their values in the high gamma band are smaller than in the alpha band. In addition, a difference between the PSI and other two measures (AEC and coherence) are illustrated in this figure. The PSI removes the MEG field spread effect, but AEC and coherence cannot remove this effect. A zero-lagged connection between two signals is removed with PSI, and thus the values of connectivity based on this measure are not artificially inflated by the field spread effect.

9.3.5. Network Topology: Graph Metrics

A network can be constructed after calculating the connectivity measure in either sensor or source space. In graph theory, a network is defined as a set of nodes (or vertices) and edges (or lines between the nodes). In MEG applications, nodes are sensors or brain regions, and edges represent the value of connectivity between a pair of nodes. After calculating the values of connectivity between all pairs of nodes in a network, an adjacency matrix is constructed (see Figure 9.10 for a sample adjacency matrix). The adjacency matrix corresponding to an undirected (functional) connectivity measure is symmetric, and it is asymmetric for a directed (effective) connectivity measure. A network can be weighted or binary (unweighted). In weighted network, the strength of connections between all nodes are considered. However, in binary network, nodes are either connected or disconnected. Binary networks are generated by applying a threshold to a weighted network and removing small, spurious connections that are potentially produced by noise. While mitigating the effects of noise through the use of binary

networks may improve the results of network analysis, selecting a value for the threshold is challenging and somehow arbitrary. Although the optimal value of the threshold may vary between subjects and groups (van Wijk, Stam, & Daffertshofer, 2010), some methods have been proposed to address this challenge (Bassett et al., 2009).

After constructing a network and calculating the corresponding adjacency matrix, parameters of the brain network topology can be calculated using various global and local graph metrics. A global graph metric summarizes a specific characteristic (e.g., modularity) of a network, while a local graph metric represents a specific characteristic (e.g., betweenness centrality) of a network at a node level. Various global (e.g., average degree, average strength, average eccentricity, radius, diameter, characteristic path length, clustering coefficient, transitivity, global efficiency, local efficiency, modularity, assortativity coefficient, and small-worldness) and local (e.g., degree, strength, eccentricity, path length, triangles, clustering coefficient, closeness centrality, betweenness centrality, local efficiency, within-module z-score, and participation coefficient) graph metrics have been proposed for neuroimaging applications (Rubinov & Sporns, 2010).

In previous epilepsy studies, the most commonly used graph metrics are based on path length (PL; metrics of integration of the network) and clustering coefficient (CC, metrics of segregation of the network) (Adebimpe, Aarabi, Bourel-Ponchel, Mahmoudzadeh, & Wallois, 2016; Horstmann et al., 2010; Quraan, McCormick, Cohn, Valiante, & McAndrews, 2013; B. Wang & Meng, 2016; C. Wu et al., 2017). The functional brain networks have a "small-world" organization that is characterized by a short average PL and a high average CC (Sporns & Honey, 2006). Compared with random networks, small-world networks are significantly more clustered and also have approximately the same average path length (Watts & Strogatz, 1998). It has been reported that the brain networks of healthy controls and patients with epilepsy have a small-world property (J. Wang et al., 2014). A MEG study in patients with absence epilepsy reported increases in CC and decreases in PL preceding the onset of slow wave discharges (SWDs) (Gupta, Ossenblok, & van Luijtelaar, 2011). This indicates a tendency toward small-worldness before and at the onset of SWD in these patients.

9.3.6. An Application of Magnetoencephalography Network Topology: Predicting Seizure Outcome of Vagus Nerve Stimulation

In this section, we present the results of our recent study as a practical application of MEG for investigating the brain network topology in patients with epilepsy (Babajani-Feremi et al., 2018). We investigated the possibility of predicting seizure outcome of vagus nerve stimulation (VNS) based on the resting-state MEG (rs-MEG) network topology before VNS implantation. VNS is a low-risk surgical option for patients with drug-resistant epilepsy (DRE), but it is only effective in reducing the seizure frequency in about 50% of patients (responders) (Englot, Chang, & Auguste, 2011). Despite decades of application of VNS

for patients with DRE, it is still not possible to predict which patients will respond to VNS treatment. The aim of our study was to evaluate the heritability and reliability of MEG-based graph metrics as potential biomarkers and to predict VNS seizure outcome using these metrics that were calculated based on rs-MEG data before VNS implantation.

Twenty-three patients with epilepsy (14 responders and nine nonresponders) and 89 healthy control subjects were included in this study (Figure 9.11). The rs-MEG recordings were conducted using a whole-head MAGNES 3600 (4D Neuroimaging, San Diego, CA) MEG system. After the preprocessing of rs-MEG data, we performed connectivity analysis in sensor space and calculated the PLV in theta, alpha, and beta frequency bands. Then we computed three global graph metrics: modularity, transitivity, and characteristic path length (CPL). These three graph metrics have been widely used in several studies to characterize the brain network topology of healthy controls and patients with psychiatric or neurological diseases (Khazaee, Ebrahimzadeh, & Babajani-Feremi, 2015; C. Y. Wu et al., 2017).

The modularity, transitivity, and CPL in the three groups (nonresponders, responders, and controls) are shown in Figure 9.12. Our results

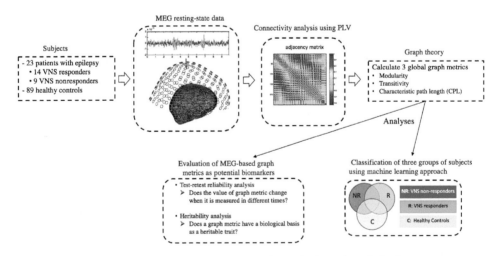

FIGURE 9.11   Overall procedures of our magnetoencephalography (MEG) study (Babajani-Feremi et al., 2018) investigating the application of the brain network topology in vagus nerve stimulation (VNS) responsiveness.

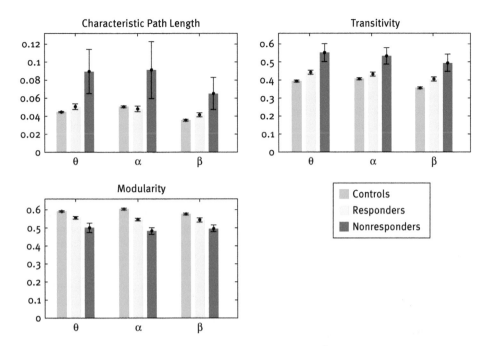

FIGURE 9.12 Comparison of the values of three global graph metrics (characteristic path length [CPL], transitivity, and modularity) in three frequency bands in three groups of subjects: healthy controls, nonresponders to vagus nerve stimulation (VNS); and responders to VNS. See Babajani-Feremi et al. (2018) for more details.

revealed that (a) the modularity and transitivity in three frequency bands were significantly different in responders versus nonresponders ($p < 0.05$, false discovery rate [FDR]-adjusted); (b) there was no significant difference in CPL in any of the three frequency bands in responders versus nonresponders ($p > 0.11$, FDR-adjusted); (c) the modularity and transitivity in all three frequency bands were significantly different in controls versus responders and controls versus nonresponders ($p < 0.006$, FDR-adjusted).

We also evaluated the heritability and reliability of the graph metrics. We found that transitivity, modularity, and CPL were significantly heritable (heritability value [h^2] > 0.51, $p < 0.005$). These results are in agreement with previous studies demonstrating that the network topology is heritable (Sinclair et al., 2015) ($h^2 = 0.42 – 0.60$). We also found an overall good test–retest reliability for the rs-MEG graph measures (intraclass correlation coefficient [ICC] > 0.6), which also concur with previous

MEG studies (Deuker et al., 2009; Jin, Seol, Kim, & Chung, 2011). Overall, our results demonstrate the heritability and reliability of these three global graph metrics, and, thus, they may have a biological basis and be used as potential biomarkers. We employed a machine learning approach using the modularity and transitivity as input features of a naïve Bayes classifier and achieved an accuracy of 87% in classifying nonresponders, responders, and controls.

REFERENCES

Adebimpe, A., Aarabi, A., Bourel-Ponchel, E., Mahmoudzadeh, M., & Wallois, F. (2016). EEG resting state functional connectivity analysis in children with benign epilepsy with centrotemporal spikes. *Frontiers in Neuroscience, 10,* 143.

Adey, W. R., Elul, R., Walter, R. D., & Crandall, P. H. (1967). The cooperative behavior of neuronal populations during sleep and mental tasks. *Electroencephalography and Clinical Neurophysiology, 23*(1), 88.

Alkawadri, R., Burgess, R. C., Kakisaka, Y., Mosher, J. C., & Alexopoulos, A. V. (2018). Assessment of the utility of ictal magnetoencephalography in the localization of the epileptic seizure onset zone. *JAMA Neurology*, 75(10), 1264–1272.

Babajani-Feremi, A., Noorizadeh, N., Mudigoudar, B., & Wheless, J. W. (2018). Predicting seizure outcome of vagus nerve stimulation using MEG-based network topology. *Neuroimage: Clinical*, 19, 990–999.

Baccala, L. A., & Sameshima, K. (2001). Partial directed coherence: A new concept in neural structure determination. *Biological Cybernetics*, 84(6), 463–474.

Bagic, A. I., Knowlton, R. C., Rose, D. F., Ebersole, J. S., Stefan, H., & Trinka, E. (2011). American Clinical Magnetoencephalography Society Clinical Practice Guideline 1: Recording and analysis of spontaneous cerebral activity. *J Clin Neurophysiol*, 28(4), 348–354.

Baillet, S., Mosher, J. C., & Leahy, R. M. (2001). Electromagnetic brain mapping. *Ieee Signal Processing Magazine*, 18(6), 14–30.

Bassett, D. S., Bullmore, E. T., Meyer-Lindenberg, A., Apud, J. A., Weinberger, D. R., & Coppola, R. (2009). Cognitive fitness of cost-efficient brain functional networks. *Proceedings of the National Academy of Sciences of the United States of America*, 106(28), 11747–11752.

Bell, A. J., & Sejnowski, T. J. (1995). An information-maximization approach to blind separation and blind deconvolution. *Neural Computation*, 7(6), 1129–1159.

Brazier, M. A., & Barlow, J. (1956). Some applications of correlation analysis to clinical problems in electroencephalography. *Electroencephalography and Clinical Neurophysiology*, 8(2), 325–331.

Breakspear, M. (2004). "Dynamic" connectivity in neural systems: Theoretical and empirical considerations. *Neuroinformatics*, 2(2), 205–225.

Bressler, S. L., & Seth, A. K. (2011). Wiener-Granger causality: A well established methodology. *Neuroimage*, 58(2), 323–329.

Brookes, M. J., Woolrich, M. W., & Barnes, G. R. (2012). Measuring functional connectivity in MEG: A multivariate approach insensitive to linear source leakage. *Neuroimage*, 63(2), 910–920.

Colclough, G. L., Brookes, M. J., Smith, S. M., & Woolrich, M. W. (2015). A symmetric multivariate leakage correction for MEG connectomes. *Neuroimage*, 117, 439–448.

Colclough, G. L., Woolrich, M. W., Tewarie, P. K., Brookes, M. J., Quinn, A. J., & Smith, S. M. (2016). How reliable are MEG resting-state connectivity metrics? *Neuroimage*, 138, 284–293.

Deuker, L., Bullmore, E. T., Smith, M., Christensen, S., Nathan, P. J., Rockstroh, B., & Bassett, D. S. (2009). Reproducibility of graph metrics of human brain functional networks. *Neuroimage*, 47(4), 1460–1468.

Ebersole, J. S. (1997). Magnetoencephalography/magnetic source imaging in the assessment of patients with epilepsy. *Epilepsia*, 38(Suppl. 4), S1–S5.

Ebersole, J. S. (1999). Classification of MEG spikes in temporal lobe epilepsy. In T. Yoshimoto, M. Kotani, S. Kuriki, H. Karibe, & N. Nakasoto (Eds.), *Recent advances in biomagnetism* (pp. 758–761). Sendai, Japan: Tohoku University Press.

Ebersole, J. S., Squires, K. C., Eliashiv, S. D., & Smith, J. R. (1995). Applications of magnetic source imaging in evaluation of candidates for epilepsy surgery. *Neuroimaging Clinics of North American*, 5(2), 267–288.

Ebersole, J. S., Squires, K. C., Gamelin, J., Lewine, J., & Scherg, M. (1993). *Simultaneous MEG and EEG provide complementary dipole models of temporal lobe spikes*. Paper presented at the AES Proceedings.

Ebersole, J. S., & Wagner, M. (2018). Relative yield of MEG and EEG spikes in simultaneous recordings. *Journal of Clinical Neurophysiology*, 35(6), 443–453.

Englot, D. J., Chang, E. F., & Auguste, K. I. (2011). Vagus nerve stimulation for epilepsy: A meta-analysis of efficacy and predictors of response. *Journal of Neurosurgery*, 115(6), 1248–1255.

Englot, D. J., Hinkley, L. B., Kort, N. S., Imber, B. S., Mizuiri, D., Honma, S. M., . . . Nagarajan, S. S. (2015). Global and regional functional connectivity maps of neural oscillations in focal epilepsy. *Brain*, 138(Pt. 8), 2249–2262.

Fernandes, J. M., da Silva, A. M., Huiskamp, G., Velis, D. N., Manshanden, I., de Munck, J. C., . . . Cunha, J. P. (2005). What does an epileptiform spike look like in MEG? Comparison between coincident EEG and MEG spikes. *Journal of Clinical Neurophysiology*, 22(1), 68–73.

Fingelkurts, A. A., Fingelkurts, A. A., & Kahkonen, S. (2005). Functional connectivity in the brain: Is it an elusive concept? *Neuroscience and Biobehavioral Reviews*, 28(8), 827–836.

Fraser, A. M., & Swinney, H. L. (1986). Independent coordinates for strange attractors from mutual information. *Physical Review A: General Physics*, 33(2), 1134–1140.

Friston, K. J. (1994). Functional and effective connectivity in neuroimaging: A synthesis. *Human Brain Mapping*, 2(1–2), 56–78.

Fuchs, M., Kastner, J., Tech, R., Wagner, M., & Gasca, F. (2017). MEG and EEG dipole clusters from extended cortical sources. *Biomedical Engineering Letters*, 7(3), 185–191.

Garces, P., Martin-Buro, M. C., & Maestu, F. (2016). Quantifying the test-retest reliability of magnetoencephalography resting-state functional connectivity. *Brain Connectivity*, 6(6), 448–460.

Granger, C. W. (1969). Investigating causal relations by econometric models and cross-spectral methods. *Econometrica: Journal of the Econometric Society*, 37, 424–438.

Greenblatt, R. E., Pflieger, M. E., & Ossadtchi, A. E. (2012). Connectivity measures applied to human brain electrophysiological data. *Journal of Neuroscience Methods*, 207(1), 1–16.

Gross, J., Baillet, S., Barnes, G. R., Henson, R. N., Hillebrand, A., Jensen, O., . . . Schoffelen, J. M. (2013). Good practice for conducting and reporting MEG research. *Neuroimage*, 65, 349–363.

Gupta, D., Ossenblok, P., & van Luijtelaar, G. (2011). Space-time network connectivity and cortical activations preceding spike wave discharges in human absence epilepsy: A MEG study. *Medical and Biological Engineering and Computing*, 49(5), 555–565.

Hamandi, K., Routley, B. C., Koelewijn, L., & Singh, K. D. (2016). Non-invasive brain mapping in epilepsy: Applications from magnetoencephalography. *Journal of Neuroscience Methods*, 260, 283–291.

Hari, R., Baillet, S., Barnes, G., Burgess, R., Forss, N., Gross, J., . . . Taulu, S. (2018). IFCN-endorsed practical guidelines for clinical magnetoencephalography (MEG). *Clinical Neurophysiology*, 129(8), 1720–1747.

Helmholtz, H. V. (1853). Ueber einige Gesetze der Vertheilung elektrischer Ströme in körperlichen Leitern, mit Anwendung auf die thierisch-elektrischen Versuche (Schluss.). *Annalen der Physik*, 165(7), 353–377.

Hesse, W., Moller, E., Arnold, M., & Schack, B. (2003). The use of time-variant EEG Granger causality for inspecting directed interdependencies of neural assemblies. *Journal of Neuroscience Methods*, 124(1), 27–44.

Hipp, J. F., Hawellek, D. J., Corbetta, M., Siegel, M., & Engel, A. K. (2012). Large-scale cortical correlation structure of spontaneous oscillatory activity. *Nature Neuroscience*, 15(6), 884–U110.

Horstmann, M. T., Bialonski, S., Noennig, N., Mai, H., Prusseit, J., Wellmer, J., . . . Lehnertz, K. (2010). State dependent properties of epileptic brain networks: Comparative graph-theoretical analyses of simultaneously recorded EEG and MEG. *Clinical Neurophysiology*, 121(2), 172–185.

Hunold, A., Funke, M. E., Eichardt, R., Stenroos, M., & Haueisen, J. (2016). EEG and MEG: Sensitivity to epileptic spike activity as function of source orientation and depth. *Physiological Measures*, 37(7), 1146–1162.

Ishibashi, H., Simos, P. G., Castillo, E. M., Maggio, W. W., Wheless, J. W., Kim, H. L., . . . Papanicolaou, A. C. (2002). Detection and significance of focal, interictal, slow-wave activity visualized by magnetoencephalography for localization of a primary epileptogenic region. *Journal of Neurosurgery*, 96(4), 724–730.

Iwasaki, M., Pestana, E., Burgess, R. C., Luders, H. O., Shamoto, H., Nakasato, N., . . . Stufflebeam, S. M. (2005). Detection of epileptiform activity by human interpreters: Blinded comparison between electroencephalography and magnetoencephalography. *Epilepsia*, 46(1), 59–68.

Jin, S. H., Seol, J., Kim, J. S., & Chung, C. K. (2011). How reliable are the functional connectivity networks of MEG in resting states? *Journal of Neurophysiology*, 106(6), 2888–2895.

Kakisaka, Y., Wang, Z. I., Mosher, J. C., Nair, D. R., Alexopoulos, A. V., & Burgess, R. C. (2012). Magnetoencephalography's higher sensitivity to epileptic spikes may elucidate the profile of electroencephalographically negative epileptic seizures. *Epilepsy Behavior*, 23(2), 171–173.

Kaminski, M. J., & Blinowska, K. J. (1991). A new method of the description of the information flow in the brain structures. *Biological Cybernetics*, 65(3), 203–210.

Khazaee, A., Ebrahimzadeh, A., & Babajani-Feremi, A. (2015). Identifying patients with Alzheimer's disease using resting-state fMRI and graph theory. *Clinical Neurophysiological*, 126(11), 2132–2141.

Kirsch, H. E., Mantle, M., & Nagarajan, S. S. (2007). Concordance between routine interictal magnetoencephalography and simultaneous scalp electroencephalography in a sample of patients with epilepsy. *Journal of Clinical Neurophysiology*, 24(3), 215–231.

Knowlton, R. C., Elgavish, R., Howell, J., Blount, J., Burneo, J. G., Faught, E., . . . Burgess, R. C. (2006). Magnetic source imaging versus intracranial electroencephalogram in epilepsy surgery: A prospective study. *Annals of Neurology*, 59(5), 835–842.

Knowlton, R. C., Razdan, S. N., Limdi, N., Elgavish, R. A., Killen, J., Blount, J., . . . Kuzniecky, R. (2009). Effect of epilepsy magnetic source imaging on intracranial electrode placement. *Annals of Neurology*, 65(6), 716–723.

Lachaux, J. P., Rodriguez, E., Martinerie, J., & Varela, F. J. (1999). Measuring phase synchrony in brain signals. *Human Brain Mapping*, 8(4), 194–208.

Lin, Y. Y., Shih, Y. H., Hsieh, J. C., Yu, H. Y., Yiu, C. H., Wong, T. T., . . . Chang, M. S. (2003). Magnetoencephalographic yield of interictal spikes in temporal lobe epilepsy: Comparison with scalp EEG recordings. *Neuroimage*, 19(3), 1115–1126.

Liu, Z. M., Fukunaga, M., de Zwart, J. A., & Duyn, J. H. (2010). Large-scale spontaneous fluctuations and correlations in brain electrical activity observed with magnetoencephalography. *Neuroimage, 51*(1), 102–111.

Martinez Castillo, E., Papanicolaou, A. C., Stefan, H., Wheless, J., Otsubo, H., Santiuste, M., . . . Kaltenhäuser, M. (2009). Spontaneous brain activity. In A. C. Papanicolaou (Ed.), *Clinical magnetoencephalography and magnetic source imaging*. Cambridge, UK: Cambridge University Press.

Merlet, I., Paetau, R., Garcia-Larrea, L., Uutela, K., Granstrom, M. L., & Mauguiere, F. (1997). Apparent asynchrony between interictal electric and magnetic spikes. *Neuroreport, 8*(5), 1071–1076.

Nissen, I. A., Stam, C. J., Reijneveld, J. C., van Straaten, I. E., Hendriks, E. J., Baayen, J. C., . . . Hillebrand, A. (2017). Identifying the epileptogenic zone in interictal resting-state MEG source-space networks. *Epilepsia, 58*(1), 137–148.

Nolte, G., Bai, O., Wheaton, L., Mari, Z., Vorbach, S., & Hallett, M. (2004). Identifying true brain interaction from EEG data using the imaginary part of coherency. *Clinical Neurophysiology, 115*(10), 2292–2307.

Nolte, G., Ziehe, A., Nikulin, V. V., Schlogl, A., Kramer, N., Brismar, T., & Muller, K. R. (2008). Robustly estimating the flow direction of information in complex physical systems. *Physical Review Letters, 100*(23).

Nowak, R., Santiuste, M., & Russi, A. (2009). Toward a definition of MEG spike: Parametric description of spikes recorded simultaneously by MEG and depth electrodes. *Seizure, 18*(9), 652–655.

Ochi, A., Otsubo, H., Chitoku, S., Hunjan, A., Sharma, R., Rutka, J. T., . . . Snead, O. C., 3rd. (2001). Dipole localization for identification of neuronal generators in independent neighboring interictal EEG spike foci. *Epilepsia, 42*(4), 483–490.

O'Neill, G. C., Tewarie, P., Vidaurre, D., Liuzzi, L., Woolrich, M. W., & Brookes, M. J. (2018). Dynamics of large-scale electrophysiological networks: A technical review. *Neuroimage, 180*(Pt. B), 559–576.

Ossenblok, P., de Munck, J. C., Colon, A., Drolsbach, W., & Boon, P. (2007). Magnetoencephalography is more successful for screening and localizing frontal lobe epilepsy than electroencephalography. *Epilepsia, 48*(11), 2139–2149.

Otsubo, H., Ochi, A., Elliott, I., Chuang, S. H., Rutka, J. T., Jay, V., . . . Snead, O. C. (2001). MEG predicts epileptic zone in lesional extrahippocampal epilepsy: 12 Pediatric surgery cases. *Epilepsia, 42*(12), 1523–1530.

Paetau, R., Hamalainen, M., Hari, R., Kajola, M., Karhu, J., Larsen, T. A., . . . Salonen, O. (1994). Magnetoencephalographic evaluation of children and adolescents with intractable epilepsy. *Epilepsia, 35*(2), 275–284.

Papanicolaou, A. C., Pataraia, E., Billingsley-Marshall, R., Castillo, E. M., Wheless, J. W., Swank, P., . . . Simos, P. G. (2005). Toward the substitution of invasive electroencephalography in epilepsy surgery. *Journal of Clinical Neurophysiology, 22*(4), 231–237.

Pereda, E., Quiroga, R. Q., & Bhattacharya, J. (2005). Nonlinear multivariate analysis of neurophysiological signals. *Progress in Neurobiology, 77*(1–2), 1–37.

Puce, A., & Hämäläinen, M. S. (2017). A review of issues related to data acquisition and analysis in EEG/MEG studies. *Brain Science, 7*(6), 58.

Quraan, M. A., McCormick, C., Cohn, M., Valiante, T. A., & McAndrews, M. P. (2013). Altered resting state brain dynamics in temporal lobe epilepsy can be observed in spectral power, functional connectivity and graph theory metrics. *PLoS One, 8*(7), e68609.

Rubinov, M., & Sporns, O. (2010). Complex network measures of brain connectivity: Uses and interpretations. *Neuroimage, 52*(3), 1059–1069.

Sarvas, J. (1987). Basic mathematical and electromagnetic concepts of the biomagnetic inverse problem. *Physics in Medicine and Biology, 32*(1), 11–22.

Schreiber, T. (2000). Measuring information transfer. *Physical Review Letters, 85*(2), 461–464.

Shaw, J. C. (1984). Correlation and coherence analysis of the EEG: A selective tutorial review. *International Journal of Psychophysiology, 1*(3), 255–266.

Sinclair, B., Hansell, N. K., Blokland, G. A., Martin, N. G., Thompson, P. M., Breakspear, M., . . . McMahon, K. L. (2015). Heritability of the network architecture of intrinsic brain functional connectivity. *Neuroimage, 121*, 243–252.

Sporns, O., & Honey, C. J. (2006). Small worlds inside big brains. *Proceedings of the National Academy of Science United States of America, 103*(51), 19219–19220.

Srinivasan, R., Winter, W. R., Ding, J., & Nunez, P. L. (2007). EEG and MEG coherence: Measures of functional connectivity at distinct spatial scales of neocortical dynamics. *Journal of Neuroscientific Methods, 166*(1), 41–52.

Stam, C. J. (2010). Use of magnetoencephalography (MEG) to study functional brain networks in neurodegenerative disorders. *Journal of the Neurological Sciences, 289*(1-2), 128–134.

Stam, C. J., Nolte, G., & Daffertshofer, A. (2007). Phase lag index: Assessment of functional connectivity from multi channel EEG and MEG with diminished bias from common sources. *Human Brain Mapping, 28*(11), 1178–1193.

Stam, C. J., & van Dijk, B. W. (2002). Synchronization likelihood: An unbiased measure of generalized synchronization in multivariate data sets. *Physica D: Nonlinear Phenomena, 163*(3-4), 236–251.

Stam, C. J., & van Straaten, E. C. (2012). Go with the flow: Use of a directed phase lag index (dPLI) to characterize patterns of phase relations in a large-scale model of brain dynamics. *Neuroimage, 62*(3), 1415–1428.

Stefan, H., Trinka, E., Fernandes, J. M., da Silva, A. M., Huiskamp, G., Velis, D. N., . . . Cunha, J. P. (2017). Magnetoencephalography (MEG): Past, current and future perspectives for improved differentiation and treatment of epilepsies. *Seizure, 44*(1), 121–124.

Sutherling, W. W., Mamelak, A. N., Thyerlei, D., Maleeva, T., Minazad, Y., Philpott, L., & Lopez, N. (2008). Influence of magnetic source imaging for planning intracranial EEG in epilepsy. *Neurology, 71*(13), 990–996.

Taulu, S., Kajola, M., & Simola, J. (2004). Suppression of interference and artifacts by the signal space separation method. *Brain Topography, 16*(4), 269–275.

Taulu, S., & Simola, J. (2006). Spatiotemporal signal space separation method for rejecting nearby interference in MEG measurements. *Physics in Medicine and Biology, 51*(7), 1759–1768.

Taulu, S., Simola, J., Nenonen, J., & Parkkonen, L. (2014). Novel noise reduction methods. In S. Supek & C. Aine (Eds.), *Magnetoencephalography from signals to dynamic cortical networks* (pp. 35–71). Berlin (Heidelberg): Springer-Verlag.

Tsiaras, V., Simos, P. G., Rezaie, R., Sheth, B. R., Garyfallidis, E., Castillo, E. M., & Papanicolaou, A. C. (2011). Extracting biomarkers of autism from MEG resting-state functional connectivity networks. *Computational Biology and Medicine, 41*(12), 1166–1177.

Tzourio-Mazoyer, N., Landeau, B., Papathanassiou, D., Crivello, F., Etard, O., Delcroix, N., . . . Joliot, M. (2002). Automated anatomical labeling of activations in SPM using a macroscopic anatomical parcellation of the MNI MRI single-subject brain. *Neuroimage, 15*(1), 273–289.

Uusitalo, M. A., & Ilmoniemi, R. J. (1997). Signal-space projection method for separating MEG or EEG into components. *Medical and Biological Engineering and Computing, 35*(2), 135–140.

van Diessen, E., Numan, T., van Dellen, E., van der Kooi, A. W., Boersma, M., Hofman, D., . . . Stam, C. J. (2015). Opportunities and methodological challenges in EEG and MEG resting state functional brain network research. *Clinical Neurophysiology, 126*(8), 1468–1481.

van Mierlo, P., Papadopoulou, M., Carrette, E., Boon, P., Vandenberghe, S., Vonck, K., & Marinazzo, D. (2014). Functional brain connectivity from EEG in epilepsy: Seizure prediction and epileptogenic focus localization. *Progress in Neurobiology, 121*, 19–35.

Van Veen, B. D., van Drongelen, W., Yuchtman, M., & Suzuki, A. (1997). Localization of brain electrical activity via linearly constrained minimum variance spatial filtering. *IEEE Transactions on Biomedical Engineering, 44*(9), 867–880.

van Wijk, B. C. M., Stam, C. J., & Daffertshofer, A. (2010). Comparing brain networks of different size and connectivity density using graph theory. *PLoS One, 5*(10).

Vinck, M., Oostenveld, R., van Wingerden, M., Battaglia, F., & Pennartz, C. M. A. (2011). An improved index of phase-synchronization for electrophysiological data in the presence of volume-conduction, noise and sample-size bias. *Neuroimage, 55*(4), 1548–1565.

Vindiola, M. M., Vettel, J. M., Gordon, S. M., Franaszczuk, P. J., & McDowell, K. (2014). Applying EEG phase synchronization measures to non-linearly coupled neural mass models. *Journal of Neuroscientific Methods, 226*, 1–14.

Wang, B., & Meng, L. (2016). Functional brain network alterations in epilepsy: A magnetoencephalography study. *Epilepsy Research, 126*, 62–69.

Wang, G., & Takigawa, M. (1992). Directed coherence as a measure of interhemispheric correlation of EEG. *International Journal of Psychophysiology, 13*(2), 119–128.

Wang, H. E., Benar, C. G., Quilichini, P. P., Friston, K. J., Jirsa, V. K., & Bernard, C. (2014). A systematic framework for functional connectivity measures. *Frontiers in Neuroscience, 8*, 405.

Wang, J., Qiu, S., Xu, Y., Liu, Z., Wen, X., Hu, X., . . . Huang, R. (2014). Graph theoretical analysis reveals disrupted topological properties of whole brain functional networks in temporal lobe epilepsy. *Clinical Neurophysiology, 125*(9), 1744–1756.

Watts, D. J., & Strogatz, S. H. (1998). Collective dynamics of "small-world" networks. *Nature, 393*(6684), 440–442.

Wendling, F., Ansari-Asl, K., Bartolomei, F., & Senhadji, L. (2009). From EEG signals to brain connectivity: A model-based evaluation of interdependence measures. *Journal of Neuroscientific Methods, 183*(1), 9–18.1

Wheless, J. W., Castillo, E., Maggio, V., Kim, H. L., Breier, J. I., Simos, P. G., & Papanicolaou, A. C. (2004). Magnetoencephalography (MEG) and magnetic source imaging (MSI). *Neurologist, 10*(3), 138–153.

Wheless, J. W., Willmore, L. J., Breier, J. I., Kataki, M., Smith, J. R., King, D. W., . . . Papanicolaou, A. C. (1999). A comparison of magnetoencephalography, MRI, and V-EEG in patients evaluated for epilepsy surgery. *Epilepsia, 40*(7), 931–941.

Winter, W. R., Nunez, P. L., Ding, J., & Srinivasan, R. (2007). Comparison of the effect of volume conduction on EEG coherence with the effect of field spread on MEG coherence. *Statistics in Medicine, 26*(21), 3946–3957.

Wu, C., Xiang, J., Jiang, W., Huang, S., Gao, Y., Tang, L., . . . Wang, X. (2017). Altered effective connectivity network in childhood absence epilepsy: A multi-frequency MEG study. *Brain Topography, 30*(5), 673–684.

10

BEYOND THE IRRITATIVE ZONE

USE OF MAGNETOENCEPHALOGRAPHY TO CHARACTERIZE ASPECTS OF THE EPILEPTOGENIC ZONE

Eduardo M. Castillo, Tara Kleineschay, Milena Korostenskaja, James Baumgartner, and Ki Hyeong Lee

10.1. INTRODUCTION

In the context of the presurgical evaluation of patients with refractory epilepsy, magnetoencephalography (MEG) has gained recognition as a noninvasive, clinically valid method for the localization of the sources of epileptiform activity (Barth, Sutherling, Engel J., Beatty, 1982; Eisenberg, Papanicolaou, Baumann, Rogers, & Brown, 1991; Modena et al., 1982; Ricci et al., 1987; Rose, Smith, & Sato, 1987; Rose, Sato, et al., 1987; Sutherling & Barth, 1989; Sutherling, Crandall, Cahan, & Barth, 1988; Sutherling et al., 1987). Over the past two decades, it has been demonstrated that MEG provides additional and complementary information to that obtained from electroencephalography (EEG) (Ebersole & Ebersole, 2010); can facilitate decisions regarding the optimal placement of invasive electrodes (Knowlton et al., 2009; Sutherling et al., 2008);

and when combined with magnetic resonance imaging (MRI) and surface EEG, may reduce dependence on invasive electrophysiology for epileptic foci localization (Ebersole, Squires, Eliashiv, & Smith, 1995; Papanicolaou et al., 2005). These contributions helped to generalize the use of MEG as an increasingly important tool to characterize different aspects of the epileptogenic network in a noninvasive fashion, helping to guide clinical decisions, particularly when surgery is a considered as a treatment option.

Interestingly, while the value of MEG as a noninvasive tool for epilepsy localization has been consolidated, little insight has been provided by clinicians and experts regarding the interpretation of MEG results in individual cases in the light of findings from other evaluation methods used at the same time. In this chapter, we will reflect on the uses of MEG

Eduardo M. Castillo, Tara Kleineschay, Milena Korostenskaja, James Baumgartner, and Ki Hyeong Lee, *Beyond the Irritative Zone: Use of Magnetoencephalography to Characterize Aspects of the Epileptogenic Zone* In: *Fifty Years of Magnetoencephalography*. Edited by: Andrew C. Papanicolaou, Timothy P. L. Roberts, and James W. Wheless, Oxford University Press (2020). © Oxford University Press. DOI: 10.1093/oso/9780190935689.003.0010.

to better characterize different cortical zones within the epileptic network in epilepsy surgery candidates before the surgical treatment. First, we will review the role of MEG in the presurgical workout under the classical model of epileptic zones proposed by Rosenow and Lüders (2001). In the context of this framework, MEG has typically been incorporated as a noninvasive tool to record interictal events and localize their sources, helping to identify the irritative zones (IZs). We will review evidence that supports, given certain conditions, the use of MEG to make valid inferences about two other zones: the ictal onset zone (IOZ) and the functional deficit zone (FDZ). One of these indications comes from simultaneous intracranial EEG and MEG recordings, where we had the rare opportunity to test the sensitivity of MEG to interictal events arising from the IOZ and other zones, defined on the basis of the "gold standard," that is, the invasive recordings. Similarly, we will review how in certain subpopulations it has been demonstrated that the patterns of propagation of interictal activity, recorded by MEG, can help to better characterize the extent of the FDZ. As a conclusion, we will propose a workflow that integrates the described findings and modality-specific features and that reflects our experience in evaluating epileptic patients. This workflow describes a dynamic process in which information derived from MEG should be interpreted in the light of other findings, particularly those obtained from noninvasive methods (e.g., MRI, or ictal and interictal EEG) in order to maximize the value of the predictions made using MEG and other noninvasive tools.

10.2. PRESURGICAL ASSESSMENT OF CORTICAL ZONES INVOLVED IN EPILEPSY IN THE CONTEXT OF THE CLASSICAL MODEL

The success of epilepsy surgery in patients with drug-resistant focal epilepsy is contingent on several factors, foremost among which is the accurate identification of the area necessary for generating seizures (i.e., the epileptogenic zone [EZ]). The evaluation of patients leading to the identification of the EZ and to the decision to perform surgery consists of two phases (Figure 10.1).

The diagnostic procedures during the initial noninvasive evaluation (phase I) include clinical, neurological, and neuropsychological examination, MRI exam, and continuous monitoring of scalp EEG in the epilepsy monitoring unit (EMU) in order to obtain video-EEG (vEEG) recordings of interictal and ictal events. vEEG monitoring is continued until a number of seizures are recorded (typically a minimum of three). At the conclusion of the phase I evaluation, a consensus decision is made by the multidisciplinary team based on the collected data, resulting in three alternative recommendations: (a) the patient is not deemed a suitable surgical candidate, usually because he/she does not have epilepsy or the disease is multifocal or diffuse; (b) sufficient information to define the EZ is available, and surgery is recommended; or (c) additional evaluation is recommended (phase II). At this point, when a patient becomes a surgical candidate or a phase II evaluation candidate, he/she undergoes the MEG evaluation.

MEG, being a noninvasive technique, is typically requested after the phase I procedures have established the existence of refractory epilepsy that could potentially benefit from surgery and a more detailed localization of the EZ needs to be achieved. Although incidental ictal MEG recordings occur (in approximately 10% of MEG sessions) and can provide relevant information regarding the IOZ (Alkawadri, Burgess, Kakisaka, Mosher, & Alexopoulos, 2018), in practice, the use of MEG in epilepsy localization is confined to recordings for the characterization and source localization of epileptiform interictal activity (i.e., sharps, spikes). This form of use of MEG has been incorporated into the presurgical evaluation workflows in epileptic patients with functions similar to those of ambulatory EEG,

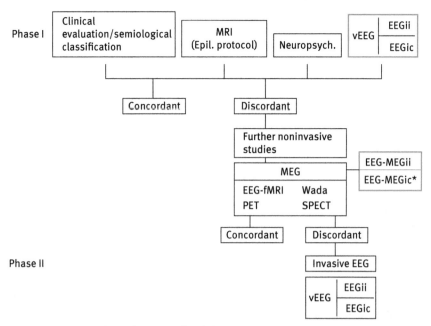

FIGURE 10.1 Diagnostic procedures during presurgical evaluation of patients with refractory epilepsy. When available, samples of interictal and ictal electroencephalography (EEGii, EEGic) are collected during phase I and can be used to support the hypothesis that the ictal onset zone (IOZ) may also generate interictal discharges (when a certain level of spatial overlap between an IOZ and an irritative zone [IZ] is evident). This information should be compared with results obtained during the magnetoencephalography (MEG) session (EEG-MEGii) in order to ascertain that adequate sampling of the interictal activity has been achieved. SPECT = single photon emission computed tomography; vEEG = video electroencephalography.

even though it provides a higher level of spatial accuracy in identifying epileptiform activity sources.

If phase II evaluation is recommended, the patient is readmitted to the hospital, where he/she undergoes surgical implantation of subdural grids, and/or depth electrodes, through which ictal and interictal activity is, again, monitored in the EMU for several days. This invasive monitoring is also supplemented by video monitoring (invasive vEEG). The decision as to what types of invasive procedure need to be used (depth electrodes, strips, or grids) and what brain regions should be monitored depends on all available diagnostic information collected, that is, phase I data, the Wada procedure results, and, when available, the structural and metabolic imaging data and, in some cases, the MEG data. At the conclusion of phase II evaluation, a consensus

decision is formulated defining the EZ, and its surgical resection/disconnection is considered. Converging evidence between clinical, structural, and functional measurements allows clinicians to generate hypotheses regarding the localization and extent of the EZ and the other cortical zones involved in epilepsy for a given patient. Table 10.1 shows the phase I and phase II neurodiagnostic techniques contributing to the characterization of distinct cortical zones within the epileptic network (for a review, see Rosenow & Lüders, 2001).

Under this model (Rosenow & Lüders, 2001), three cortical areas (the IOZ, symptomatogenic zone [SZ], and epileptogenic lesion [EL]) make a significant contribution in defining the EZ, with only limited value of the IZ (Figure 10.2).

In 2001, when this model was first presented (Rosenow & Lüders, 2001), MEG was regarded

Table 10.1 Classical Model of Zones Included in the Epileptic Network and Neurodiagnostic Techniques Used to Characterize Them During Phase I and Phase II Evaluation

ZONE	DEFINITION	TECHNIQUE (PHASE I)	TECHNIQUE (PHASE II)
Functional deficit zone (FDZ)	Areas with functional abnormalities	Neurological and neuropsychological examination, EEG, fMRI, PET, SPECT	Intracranial EEG
Irritative zone (IZ)	Areas that generates interictal spikes	EEG, MEG, EEG-fMRI	Intracranial EEG
Epileptogenic lesion (EL)	Structural abnormality that is the direct cause of seizures	MRI	Tissue pathology
Symptomatogenic zone (SZ)	Areas that produce the initial semiology	Patient report and ictal video-EEG	Intracranial EEG, SPECT/SISCOM
Ictal onset zone (IOZ)	Areas that generate the seizures	Video-EEG	Intracranial EEG
Epileptogenic zone (EZ)	Areas necessary for generating SZ (removal/disconnection abolished SZ)	Hypothesis based on converging evidences	Hypothesis based on converging evidences to be tested after surgical outcome is available

Note that MEG has been considered a tool to characterize the irritative zones.

EEG = electroencephalography; fMRI = functional MRI; MEG = magnetoencephalography; MRI = magnetic resonance imaging; PET = positron emission tomography; SISCOM = subtraction ictal single photon emission computed tomography co-registered to MRI; SPECT = single photon emission computed tomography.

Modified from Rosenow, F., & Lüders, H. (2001). Presurgical evaluation of epilepsy. *Brain, 124*(Pt 9), 1683–1700.

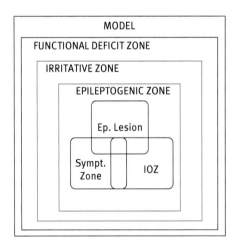

FIGURE 10.2   Classical model (adapted from Rosenov & Luders, 2001) of cortical areas in epilepsy. The epileptogenic lesion (EL), ictal onset zone (IOZ), and symptomatogenic zone (SZ) are the three most relevant cortical areas for the localization of the epileptogenic zone (EZ).

as an experimental technique, and its contribution, limited to the characterization of the IZs, was of limited value for the localization of the EZ. In the past 20 years, this position has been challenged by many studies, especially those documenting surgical outcomes, and MEG has proved to make valid contributions to the prediction of the EZ (Bear & Kirsch, 2016; Englot et al., 2015; Garcia-Tarodo et al., 2018; Papanicolaou et al., 2005; Pataraia et al., 2004; RamachandranNair et al., 2007). Being based on interictal recordings, MEG should not have a significant role in the definition of the EZ for a given patient unless one (or several) of the cortical areas constituting the EZ is an active generator of interictal discharges. Therefore, a part of the analysis and interpretation of MEG findings of our epileptic patients is devoted to finding evidence (from phase I evaluations) supporting

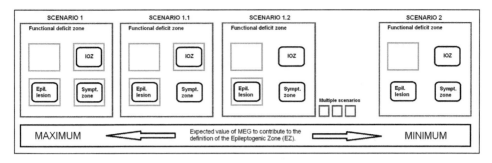

FIGURE 10.3 Some of the possible scenarios regarding the overlap between the irritative zones (*blue squares*) and other cortical zones. The contribution of magnetoencephalography (MEG) to the localization of the epileptogenic zone (EZ) will depend on what cortical areas generate interictal discharges. A documented existence of interictal events arising from the ictal onset zone (IOZ), EZ, or symptomatogenic zone (SZ) (scenarios 1, 1.1, and 1.2) supports the use of MEG to make valid contributions in defining the EZ. Lack of interictal activity, arising from the IOZ, EZ, or SZ (scenario 2) will limit the contribution of MEG.

the hypothesis that the IOZ, SZ, or EL is an active generator of interictal discharges recorded during the MEG session. Following this argument, if the IOZ, SZ, or EL is an active generator of interictal discharges, then MEG data and source modeling used to localize those interictal discharges will contribute to the definition of the EZ. But this is only one of the possible scenarios (see scenario 1 in Figure 10.4, later). Likewise, it is possible that none of the three cortical areas contributing to the definition of the EZ (i.e., IOZ, SZ, EL) are active generators of interictal discharges recorded by MEG (scenario 2 in Figure 10.3), making MEG findings irrelevant for the characterization of the EZ.

Clinicians should consider findings from phase I and contemplate all possible scenarios to correctly integrate the results of MEG evaluations. While all the results from phase I are relevant and can provide evidence that can be used in this process, some of the findings from vEEG and MRI have special importance. A detailed review of these findings and basic understanding regarding the differences in sensitivity and specificity of the modalities used will serve clinicians well in formulating hypotheses regarding the most fitting clinical scenario, thus better predicting the value of MEG for any particular patient. Some of the factors to be considered are described next.

10.3. GENERAL CONSIDERATIONS REGARDING ELECTRO-ENCEPHALOGRAPHY AND MAGNETIC RESONANCE IMAGING FINDINGS AFFECTING MAGNETOENCEPHALOGRAPHY INTERPRETATION

EEG and MEG are modalities with different sensitivity (Funke, Constantino, Van Orman, & Rodin, 2009; Goldenholz et al., 2009; Stefan et al., 2003) that complement each other in characterizing epileptiform activity (Ebersole & Ebersole, 2010). In simultaneous EEG-MEG recordings, it is not rare to find MEG-only spikes (without EEG correlate) and/or EEG-only spikes (without MEG correlate), and source modeling using both modalities is recommended (Ebersole & Wagner, 2018). It is important to acknowledge that the sensitivity of EEG and MEG in detecting epileptiform activity is affected by region-specific differences in signal-to-noise-ratios (SNRs) of the cortical sources (de Jongh, de Munck, Gonçalves, & Ossenblok, 2005; Goldenholz et al., 2009). In a large group with 113 consecutive epilepsy patients, Pataraia et al. (2004) found that MEG was able to localize the EZ (i.e., resected region) in 72% of patients, while prolonged scalp vEEG monitoring did so in only in 40%. In the same study, MEG

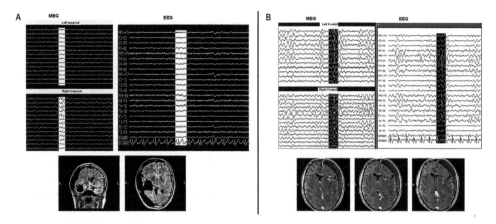

FIGURE 10.4   Magnetoencephalography (MEG) and electroencephalography (EEG) recordings (*top*) and magnetic source imaging (MSI; *bottom*) in two patients with epilepsy diagnosis serve to illustrate the effects of magnetic resonance imaging abnormalities on EEG findings. Large structural abnormalities are present in both patients. (A) A 29-year-old patient with a subdural hygroma (right hemisphere). MEG shows sharp epileptiform events over the right temporal region, notably, without the corresponding EEG events. (B) A 35-year-old patient with cystic hydroma. EEG shows left hemispheric suppression pattern and right hemispheric preponderance for interictal epileptiform activity, while MEG indicates left hemispheric onset of interictal discharges with fast generalization.

contributed to the localization of the EZ in 58% of the patients with nonlocalizing vEEG.

In cases of negative or nonlocalizing MRI, the agreement between MEG localization with subtraction ictal single photon emission computed tomography co-registered to MRI (SISCOM) (Seo et al., 2011) and/or fluorodeoxyglucose positron emission tomography (FDG-PET) (Widjaja et al., 2013) provides good prediction of intracranial EEG results for localization of the EZ. In a recent study, Duez et al. (2016) have demonstrated an additional diagnostic value yielded by MEG in patients with epilepsy, accompanied by 18% of negative EEG findings. These results favor the argument that MEG evaluations should be conducted when the conventional EEG workup was unrevealing. Therefore, MEG should be considered in cases with negative or nonlocalizing EEG findings, particularly when there are significant MRI abnormalities and/or if clinical semiology is congruent with an EZ localized in areas where EEG sensitivity is comparatively limited (i.e., frontal, operculoinsular, cingulate, medial frontoparietal).

In addition to the intrinsic differences in sensitivity between EEG and MEG, it is important to consider the effect that structural abnormalities (e.g., lesions, postsurgical defects) can have on EEG recordings. It is not rare to encounter lack of EEG-MEG concordance when a significant structural brain abnormality is distorting volume conduction (van den Broek, Reinders, Donderwinkel, & Peters, 1998) and affecting the sensitivity of EEG to interictal and/or ictal activity, while this effect on MEG is negligible. Figure 10.4 shows two examples that illustrate the differences in sensitivity between EEG and MEG recordings in patients with significant structural brain abnormalities, interfering with volume conduction and, therefore, reducing EEG sensitivity and/or distorting its topography.

10.4. LOOKING FOR EVIDENCE OF CORTICAL ZONE WITHIN THE EPILEPTOGENIC ZONE GENERATING INTERICTAL DISCHARGES

From intracranial recordings, we know that the IOZ is frequently, but not always, a generator of interictal discharges. Bartolomei et al. (2016)

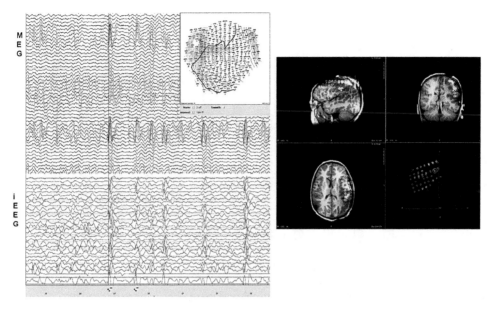

FIGURE 10.5   Simultaneous recordings from grids of subdural electrodes (intracranial electroencephalography [icEEG]) and magnetoencephalography (MEG) of interictal discharges. (*Left*) Note the correspondence between intracranial EEG discharges and MEG discharges. (*Right*) Co-registration of dipoles (*yellow*) corresponding to the onset of individual epileptiform discharges onto the patient's magnetic resonance image and the active iEEG electrodes for the same events (*red*).

found that in patients with focal cortical dysplasia (FCD), the level of concordance between the IZ and the IOZ increases to 75%, while in other groups it stays closer to 33%. Therefore, predictions of the IOZ made using interictal discharges, modeled using MEG, should only be made at the individual level, after taking into account this variability and many other individual factors. Part of the interpretation of MEG results should be devoted to better understanding whether there is evidence, suggesting that the cortical zones within the EZ are active generators of the recorded interictal discharges.

10.4.1. Lessons From Simultaneous Intracranial Electroencephalography and Magnetoencephalography Recordings

From comparisons between scalp EEG, MEG, and subsequent intracranial EEG recordings, conducted in the same patients, we have learned that while MEG may help to uncover additional irritative zones, which are not detected by scalp

EEG, it may miss some of the irritative zones detected by intracranial EEG (Agirre-Arrizubieta, Huiskamp, Ferrier, van Huffelen, & Leijten, 2009; Kim et al., 2016; Minassian et al., 1999, Tanaka et al., 2018). In rare occasions, instead of subsequent testing, simultaneous intracranial EEG and MEG have been conducted to perform a spike-to-spike sensitivity test (Figure 10.5). These studies allow direct comparison of epileptiform events, arising from the IOZ and other IZs, and define sensitivity of these two modalities.

Here, we briefly describe our experience and conclusions following a study of 11 pediatric patients, where simultaneous recordings from the dense grids arrays of subdural electrodes and MEG were conducted (for preliminary results of six cases, see Castillo et al., 2010). The cortical area, corresponding to each interictal intracranial EEG discharge, was calculated, and the presence/absence of an associated MEG discharge was tested. Those interictal intracranial EEG events, sharing topography with the IOZ (previously defined from prolonged intracranial vEEG), were identified.

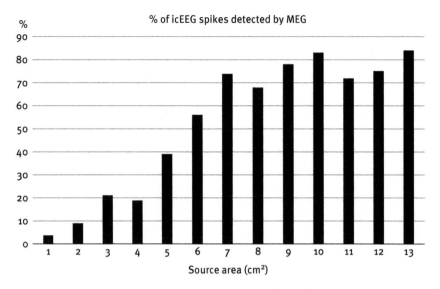

FIGURE 10.6   Percentage of intracranial electroencephalography (icEEG) spikes detected by magnetoencephalography (MEG) as a function of source area.

We found that out of the 1,181 interictal spikes detected by intracranial EEG, approximately 40% did not produce an associated MEG spike. MEG detected less than 25% of the discharges with a source area under 5 cm^2 and close to 75% of the discharges with a source area of 7 cm^2 or higher. A significant percentage (61%) of interictal discharges arising from the IOZ were detected. Importantly, in 10 out of 11 patients, interictal discharges arising from the IOZ were detected by MEG. Source area (estimated from intracranial EEG) had a major impact in MEG spike detectability (Figure 10.6). Similar results have been reported by other groups (e.g., Oishi et al., 2002), who used subdural electrodes. These studies described a relationship between MEG sensitivity and two parameters: the extent of the activated area (or number of contacts) and its voltage.

10.4.2. Level of Agreement Between Interictal and Ictal Electroencephalography Preceding Magnetoencephalography

From vEEG recordings conducted during phase I, a detailed description of the interictal and ictal events (topographic distribution and morphology of events) should be obtained. Interictal epileptiform events, sharing topographic distribution with ictal events, should be noted and labeled (Figure 10.7). Although at the stage of noninvasive recordings these are indirect indications, they can be used to support (or falsify) the hypothesis that, for a given patient, the IOZ is an active generator of interictal discharges. If that is the case, the subset of interictal events (those in topographic agreement with the IOZ defined using EEG) should be given more weight during MEG analysis to generate a valid prediction of the IOZ and, therefore, contribute significantly to defining the EZ. This prediction can be later confirmed or dismissed with the use of invasive EEG recordings.

Figure 10.7 shows recorded focal interictal EEG activity (spike–wave complex) that is in topographic agreement with the area showing an evolving pattern during seizure onset (ictal EEG). Since MEG is typically based on interictal recordings, it is reasonable to assume that the contribution of MEG to the definition of the EZ will be greater if it is based on interictal discharges, showing topographic overlap with the IOZ, rather than with other irritative zones not necessarily associated with the EZ.

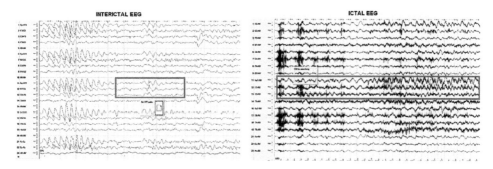

FIGURE 10.7   Phase I electroencephalography (EEG) recordings, showing an example of topographic concordance between one of the areas recording interictal discharges (left temporal) and the evolving pattern present during seizure onset. Under this scenario, with an area of overlapping interictal and ictal EEG activity, magnetoencephalography could be used to generate a hypothesis regarding the localization of the ictal onset zone, based on those specific interictal events.

It is important as well to consider that the lack of topographic concordance between the ictal EEG and interictal EEG does not necessarily imply that the IOZ is not generating interictal activity. Neither this should be used to dismiss the uses of MEG based on the idea that "if the patient does not have interictal activity, then MEG will not help." Given the intrinsic differences of sensitivity between EEG and MEG, it is not rare to find cases in which the level of their agreement is partial or inexistent. Indeed, in many cases we should expect disagreement between MEG and EEG findings, if we consider (a) how volume conduction is affected by the presence of a lesion, significantly distorting EEG signals; and (b) the different region-specific sensitivity of these two modalities (Mohamed et al., 2013; Ossenblok, de Munck, Colon, Drolsbach, & Boon, 2007).

10.4.3. Ictal and Interictal Magnetoencephalography

Occasionally, in about 10% of MEG sessions, both ictal and interictal events are recorded in a given patient, allowing localization of the IZs and the IOZ. This scenario, which can be expected in patients with frequent clinical or subclinical seizures, gives us the rare opportunity to compare the spatial distribution of sources of interictal and ictal activity in MEG

recordings. Figure 10.8 shows ictal MEG-EEG recordings and source localization of both ictal and interictal activity, demonstrating spatial overlap between the IOZ and one of the IZs. Although ictal MEG recordings are incidental, they have proved their value in delineating the IOZ in agreement with intracranial EEG (Alkawadri et al., 2018; Assaf et al., 2003) as well as in engendering a favorable surgical outcome in patients considered otherwise unsuitable for epilepsy surgery (Ramanujam et al., 2017).

10.5. SPIKE PROPAGATION AND FUNCTIONAL DEFICIT ZONE: THE CASE OF BENIGN CHILDHOOD EPILEPSY WITH CENTROTEMPORAL SPIKES

The relationships between the FDZ and MEG-derived localization of epileptiform activity have been studied in atypical benign partial epilepsies (Shiraishi et al., 2014; Wolff et al., 2005). Relevant information regarding the cortical areas, presenting with distorted functionality, can be extracted not only from the localization of the MEG-derived sources calculated at the onset, rising period, or the peak of the discharges but also from the patterns of propagation (e.g., intralobar, extralobar, intrahemispheric, extrahemispheric) of those epileptiform discharges (Castillo,

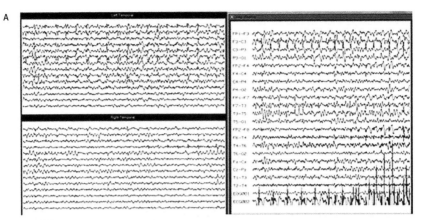

MEG: ictal recordings

EEG: ictal onset left centroparietal

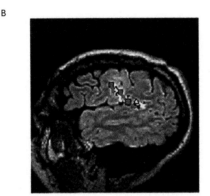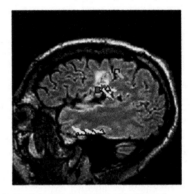

MSI showing two clusters of interictal activity (yellow), and one of ictal activity (blue). Source of somatosensory response indicates postcentral gyrus (green).

FIGURE 10.8 (A) Magnetoencephalography (MEG) and electroencephalography (EEG) recordings, corresponding to ictal event. (B) Sources corresponding to the leading spikes of an ictal event (*blue*), interictal events (*yellow*), and somatosensory responses (*green*). Notice two clusters of interictal events, but only in one of them are the overlapping sources found at the onset of the ictal event (inferior aspects of perirolandic region and a perirolandic epileptogenic lesion). MSI = magnetic source imaging.

Kleineschay, & Baumgartner, 2015). In the case of benign childhood epilepsy with centrotemporal spikes (BECTS), these abnormalities have been repeatedly characterized by EEG and MEG studies (Gregory & Wong, 1984; Loiseau et al., 1973; Minami et al., 1996). Some of the studies (Otsubo et al., 2001; Perkins et al., 2008) indicate that a subgroup of patients presents with an atypical evolution, developing cognitive and developmental deficits, while maintaining the same electrographic signature as others without cognitive decline. To characterize the patterns of spike propagation in these two groups of patients and its relationship with the clinical evolution, we reviewed the interictal MEG recordings from 14 patients after their clinical evolution was established as typical (six cases) and atypical (eight cases) forms of BECTS on the basis of neuropsychological and clinical features (Castillo et al., 2015).

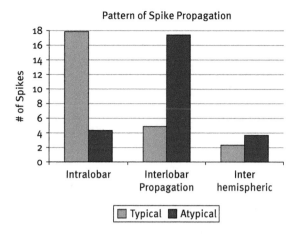

FIGURE 10.9   Histograms showing the topographic patterns of spike propagation in two groups (typical and atypical benign childhood epilepsy with centrotemporal spikes [BECTS]). An average of 24 and 23.4 spikes, respectively, were analyzed for each patient in each group. Notice the trend of interlobar propagation in the group with atypical variants of BECTS.

Briefly, from MEG-EEG recordings, a minimum of 20 individual spikes, simultaneously present in EEG and MEG, were selected and reviewed for each case. Intracranial sources were calculated at three stages of each spike (i.e., onset, peak, propagation), and the resulting patterns of activation were labeled as intralobar, interlobar, and interhemispheric (Figure 10.9).

The results (Castillo et al., 2015) indicated that in the benign/typical group, intralobar propagation was the dominant pattern (six out of six cases), while interlobar and interhemispheric propagation was present in all atypical cases (eight out of eight cases). In summary, propagation of abnormal activity to distant cortical areas and an extended FDZ was clearly associated with the presence of cognitive and developmental disturbances in children with BECTS.

10.6. CONCLUSION: PROPOSED WORKFLOW FOR THE CLINICAL INTERPRETATION OF MAGNETOENCEPHALOGRAPHY ESTIMATES IN EPILEPSY

The analysis of MEG recordings is typically conducted by clinicians and specialists with ample experience in the analysis of electromagnetic signals. After analysis is done and a report is completed, it is important to reflect on the actual use of these findings in the context of a comprehensive evaluation that incorporates results from multiple clinical evaluations, including additional structural and functional modalities. As clinicians with different backgrounds and specialties (neurologists, neurophysiologists, neurosurgeons, neuropsychologists) are being involved in the decision-making process, it is important to conceive the integration of MEG results as a dynamic process. During this process, MEG findings should be integrated with findings from the phase I evaluation first, and then with the phase II results if conducted, for validation of results (Figure 10.10).

After phase I, and for the correct interpretation of MEG results, the following hypothesis should be tested: is the IOZ, SZ, or EL an active generator of interictal discharges? We can search for indirect evidence supporting or dismissing this hypothesis using phase I findings. For example, if there is a topographic agreement between ictal and interictal EEG events, recorded during phase I, it will suggest that the IOZ is an active generator of interictal discharges. The presence of a lesion together with congruent ictal and interictal EEG and

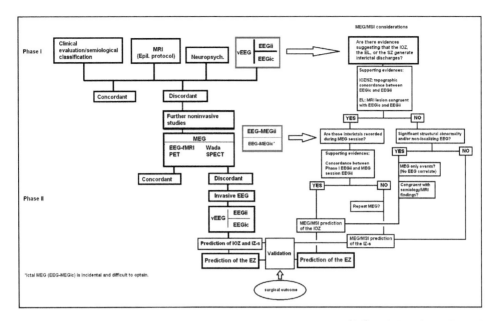

FIGURE 10.10 Workflow describing the presurgical evaluation in epilepsy (*left*) and the effects of that the flow of information, derived during this evaluation, on the magnetoencephalography interpretation (*right*) and its estimated predictive value.

EEG findings could reinforce this hypothesis. In principle, under this scenario, MEG could be used to formulate predictions of the IOZ (therefore, at least a part of the EZ) as long as during the MEG session an adequate sampling of the patient's interictal activity is collected. Logistically, this implies trying to reproduce, during the MEG recording, conditions similar to those most successful for the EEG recording (e.g., sleep deprivation, drug dosages). In the search for correspondences between ictal and interictal EEG, it is important to acknowledge the differences in sensitivity of these two modalities. Presence of structural abnormalities, distorting EEG findings, and differences in regional sensitivity between EEG and MEG should also be considered in this process.

For clinicians interpreting MEG results, it is important to acknowledge that a diversity of scenarios and factors modulate the predictive value of MEG localization in epilepsy. An active search for evidence to support or dismiss the idea that cortical areas within the EZ are also contributing to the interictal activity,

recorded during the MEG session, is a critical process during the interpretation of MEG results.

REFERENCES

Agirre-Arrizubieta, Z., Huiskamp, G. J., Ferrier, C. H., van Huffelen, A. C., & Leijten, F. S. (2009). Interictal magnetoencephalography and the irritative zone in the electrocorticogram. *Brain, 132*(Pt. 11), 3060–3071.

Alkawadri, R., Burgess, R. C., Kakisaka, Y., Mosher, J. C., & Alexopoulos, A. V. (2018). Assessment of the utility of ictal magnetoencephalography in the localization of the epileptic seizure onset zone. *JAMA Neurology, 75*(10), 1264–1272.

Assaf, B. A., Karkar, K. M., Laxer, K. D., Garcia, P. A., Austin, E. J., Barbaro, N. M., & Aminoff, M. J. (2003). Ictal magnetoencephalography in temporal and extratemporal lobe epilepsy. *Epilepsia, 44*(10), 1320–1327.

Barth, D. S., Sutherling, W., Engel J., Jr., Beatty, J. (1982). Neuromagnetic localization of epileptiform spike activity in the human brain. *Science, 218*(4575), 891–894.

Bartolomei, F., Trébuchon, A., Bonini, F., Lambert, I., Gavaret, M., Woodman, M., Giusiano, B., Wendling, F., & Bénar, C. (2016). What is the concordance between the seizure onset zone and the irritative zone? A SEEG quantified study. *Clinical Neurophysiology, 127*(2), 1157–1162.

Bear, J., & Kirsch, H. (2016). Concordance between interictal MEG and stereo-EEG predicts seizure freedom after epilepsy surgery. *Brain, 139*(11), 2821–2823.

Castillo, E., Li, Z., von Allmen, G., Baumgartner, J., Slater, J., & Papanicolaou, A. (2010). Sensitivity of MEG to interictal events arising from the irritative and ictal onset zones: Findings from simultaneous MEG-iEEG recordings. American Epilepsy Society 64th Annual Meeting, San Antonio, Texas. *Epilepsy Currents, 11*(Suppl. 1).

Castillo, E. M., Kleineschay, T., & Baumgartner, J. (2015). Contributions of magnetoencephalography to characterizing brain function in pediatric epilepsy: evidences of validity and added value. *Journal of Pediatric Epilepsy, 4*(4), 207–215.

de Jongh, A., de Munck, J. C., Gonçalves, S. I., & Ossenblok, P. (2005). Differences in MEG/EEG epileptic spike yields explained by regional differences in signal-to-noise ratios. *Journal of Clinical Neurophysiology, 22*(2), 153–158.

Duez, L., Beniczky, S., Tankisi, H., Hansen, P. O., Sidenius, P., Sabers, A., & Fuglsang-Frederiksen, A. (2016). Added diagnostic value of magnetoencephalography (MEG) in patients suspected for epilepsy, where previous, extensive EEG workup was unrevealing. *Clinical Neurophysiology, 127*(10), 3301–3305.

Ebersole, J. S., & Ebersole, S. M. (2010). Combining MEG and EEG source modeling in epilepsy evaluations. *Journal of Clinical Neurophysiology, 27*(6), 360–371.

Ebersole, J. S., Squires, K. C., Eliashiv, S. D., & Smith, J. R. (1995). Applications of magnetic source imaging in evaluation of candidates for epilepsy surgery. *Neuroimaging Clinics of North America, 5*(2), 267–288.

Ebersole, J. S., & Wagner, M. (2018). Relative yield of MEG and EEG spikes in simultaneous recordings. *Journal of Clinical Neurophysiology, 35*(6), 443–453.

Eisenberg, H. M., Papanicolaou, A. C., Baumann, S. B., Rogers, R. L., & Brown, L. M. (1991). Magnetoencephalographic localization of interictal spike sources: Case report. *Journal of Neurosurgery, 74*(4), 660–664.

Englot, D. J., Nagarajan, S. S., Imber, B. S., Raygor, K. P., Honma, S. M., Mizuiri, D., . . . Chang, E. F. (2015). Epileptogenic zone localization using magnetoencephalography predicts seizure freedom in epilepsy surgery. *Epilepsia, 56*(6), 949–958.

Funke, M., Constantino, T., Van Orman, C., & Rodin, E. (2009). Magnetoencephalography and magnetic source imaging in epilepsy. *Clinical EEG and Neuroscience, 40*(4), 271–280.

Garcia-Tarodo, S., Funke, M., Caballero, L., Zhu, L., Shah, M. N., & Von Allmen, G. K. (2018). Magnetoencephalographic recordings in infants: A retrospective analysis of seizure-focus yield and postsurgical outcomes. *Journal of Clinical Neurophysiology, 35*(6), 454–462.

Goldenholz, D. M., Ahlfors, S. P., Hämäläinen, M. S., Sharon, D., Ishitobi, M., Vaina, L. M., & Stufflebeam, S. M. (2009). Mapping the signal-to-noise-ratios of cortical sources in magnetoencephalography and electroencephalography. *Human Brain Mapping, 30*(4), 1077–1086.

Gregory, D. L., & Wong, P. K. (1984). Topographical analysis of the centrotemporal discharges in benign rolandic epilepsy of childhood. *Epilepsia, 25*(6), 705–711.

Kim, D., Joo, E. Y., Seo, D. W., Kim, M. Y., Lee, Y. H., Kwon, H. C., . . . Hong SB. (2016). Accuracy of MEG in localizing irritative zone and seizure onset zone: Quantitative comparison between MEG and intracranial EEG. *Epilepsy Res, 127*, 291–301.

Knowlton, R. C., Razdan, S. N., Limdi, N., Elgavish, R. A., Killen, J., Blount, J., . . . Kuzniecky, R. (2009). Effect of epilepsy magnetic source imaging on intracranial electrode placement. *Annals of Neurology, 65*(6), 716–723.

Loiseau, P., & Beaussart, M. (1973). The seizures of benign childhood epilepsy with Rolandic paroxysmal discharges. *Epilepsia, 14*(4), 381–389.

Minami, T., Gondo, K., Yamamoto, T., Yanai, S., Tasaki, K., & Ueda, K. (1996). Magnetoencephalographic analysis of Rolandic discharges in benign childhood epilepsy. *Annals of Neurology, 39*(3), 326–334.

Minassian, B. A., Otsubo, H., Weiss, S., Elliott, I., Rutka, J. T., & Snead, O. C., 3rd. (1999). Magnetoencephalographic localization in pediatric epilepsy surgery: Comparison with invasive intracranial electroencephalography. *Annals of Neurology, 46*(4), 627–633.

Modena, I., Ricci, G. B., Barbanera, S., Leoni, R., Romani, G. L., & Carelli, P. (1982). Biomagnetic measurements of spontaneous brain activity in epileptic patients. *Electroencephalography and Clinical Neurophysiology, 54*(6), 622–628.

Mohamed, I. S., Gibbs, S. A., Robert, M., Bouthillier, A., Leroux, J. M., & Khoa Nguyen, D. (2013). The utility of magnetoencephalography in the presurgical evaluation of refractory insular epilepsy. *Epilepsia, 54*(11), 1950–1959.

Oishi, M., Otsubo, H., Kameyama, S., Morota, N., Masuda, H., Kitayama, M., & Tanaka, R. (2002). Epileptic spikes: Magnetoencephalography versus simultaneous electrocorticography. *Epilepsia, 43*(11), 1390–1395.

Ossenblok, P., de Munck, J. C., Colon, A., Drolsbach, W., & Boon, P. (2007). Magnetoencephalography is more successful for screening and localizing frontal lobe epilepsy than electroencephalography. *Epilepsia, 48*(11), 2139–2149.

Otsubo, H., Chitoku, S., Ochi, A., Jay, V., Rutka, J. T., Smith, M. L., . . . Snead, O. C., 3rd. Malignant Rolandic-sylvian epilepsy in children: diagnosis, treatment, and outcomes. *Neurology, 57*(4):590–596.

Papanicolaou, A. C., Pataraia, E., Billingsley-Marshall, R., Castillo, E. M., Wheless, J. W., . . . Simos, P. G. (2005). Toward the substitution of invasive electroencephalography in epilepsy surgery. *Journal of Clinical Neurophysiology, 22*(4), 231–237.

Pataraia, E., Simos, P. G., Castillo, E. M., Billingsley, R. L., Sarkari, S., Wheless, J. W., . . . Papanicolaou, A. C. (2004). Does magnetoencephalography add to scalp video-EEG as a diagnostic tool in epilepsy surgery? *Neurology, 62*(6), 943–948.

Perkins, F. F., Jr., Breier, J., McManis, M. H., Castillo, E., Wheless, J., McGregor, A. L., . . . Clarke, D. F. (2008). Benign rolandic epilepsy—perhaps not so benign: Use of magnetic source imaging as a predictor of outcome. *Journal of Child Neurology, 23*(4), 389–393.

RamachandranNair, R., Otsubo, H., Shroff, M. M., Ochi, A., Weiss, S. K., Rutka, J. T., & Snead, O. C., 3rd. (2007). MEG predicts outcome following surgery for intractable epilepsy in children with normal or nonfocal MRI findings. *Epilepsia, 48*(1), 149–157.

Ramanujam, B., Bharti, K., Viswanathan, V., Garg, A., Tripathi, M., Bal, C., . . . Tripathi, M. (2016). Can ictal-MEG obviate the need for phase II monitoring in people with drug-refractory epilepsy? A prospective observational study. *Seizure, 45*, 17–23.

Ricci, G. B., Romani, G. L., Salustri, C., Pizzella, V., Torrioli, G., Buonomo, S., . . . Modena, I. (1987). Study of focal epilepsy by multichannel neuromagnetic measurements. *Electroencephalography and Clinical Neurophysiology, 66*(4), 358–368.

Rose, D. F., Sato, S., Smith, P. D., Porter, R. J., Theodore, W. H., Friauf, W., . . . Jabbari, B. (1987). Localization of magnetic interictal discharges in temporal lobe epilepsy. *Annals of Neurology, 22*(3), 348–354.

Rose, D. F., Smith, P. D., & Sato, S. (1987). Magnetoencephalography and epilepsy research. *Science, 238*(4825), 329–335.

Rosenow, F., & Lüders, H. (2001). Presurgical evaluation of epilepsy. *Brain, 124*(Pt 9), 1683–1700.

Seo, J. H., Holland, K., Rose, D., Rozhkov, L., Fujiwara, H., Byars, A., . . . Lee, K. H. (2011). Multimodality imaging in the surgical treatment of children with nonlesional epilepsy. *Neurology, 76*(1), 41–48.

Shiraishi, H., Haginoya, K., Nakagawa, E., Saitoh, S., Kaneko, Y., Nakasato, N., . . . Otsubo, H. (2014). Magnetoencephalography localizing spike sources of atypical benign partial epilepsy. *Brain Development, 36*(1):21–27.

Stefan, H., Hummel, C., Scheler, G., Genow, A., Druschky, K., Tilz, C., . . . Romstöck, J. (2003). Magnetic brain source imaging of focal epileptic activity: A synopsis of 455 cases. *Brain, 126*(Pt. 11), 2396–2405.

Sutherling, W. W., & Barth, D. S. (1989). Neocortical propagation in temporal lobe spike foci on magnetoencephalography and electroencephalography. *Annals of Neurology, 25*(4), 373–381.

Sutherling, W. W., Crandall, P. H., Cahan, L. D., & Barth, D. S. (1988). The magnetic field of epileptic spikes agrees with intracranial localizations in complex partial epilepsy. *Neurology, 38*(5), 778–786.

Sutherling, W. W., Crandall, P. H., Engel, J., Jr., Darcey, T. M., Cahan, L. D., & Barth, D. S. (1987). The magnetic field of complex partial seizures agrees with intracranial localizations. *Annals of Neurology, 21*(6), 548–558.

Sutherling, W. W., Mamelak, A. N., Thyerlei, D., Maleeva, T., Minazad, Y., . . . Lopez, N. (2008). Influence of magnetic source imaging for planning intracranial EEG in epilepsy. *Neurology, 71*(13), 990–996.

Tanaka, N., Papadelis, C., Tamilia, E., Madsen, J. R., Pearl, P. L., & Stufflebeam, S. M. (2018). Magnetoencephalographic mapping of epileptic spike population using distributed source analysis: Comparison with intracranial electroencephalographic spikes. *Journal of Clinical Neurophysiology, 35*(4), 339–345.

van den Broek, S. P., Reinders, F., Donderwinkel, M., & Peters, M. J. (1998). Volume conduction effects in EEG and MEG. *Electroencephalography and Clinical Neurophysiology, 106*(6):522–534.

Widjaja, E., Shammas, A., Vali, R., Otsubo, H., Ochi, A., Snead, O. C., . . . Charron, M. (2013). FDG-PET and magnetoencephalography in presurgical workup of children with localization-related nonlesional epilepsy. *Epilepsia, 54*(4), 691–699.

Wolff, M., Weiskopf, N., Serra, E., Preissl, H., Birbaumer, N., & Kraegeloh-Mann, I. (2005). Benign partial epilepsy in childhood: selective cognitive deficits are related to the location of focal spikes determined by combined EEG/MEG. *Epilepsia, 46*(10), 1661–1667.

11

USE OF MULTIPLE FREQUENCY BANDS IN MAGNETOENCEPHALOGRAPHY FOR CHARACTERIZATION OF EPILEPSY

Woorim Jeong and Chun Kee Chung

11.1. LOCALIZATION OF PATHOLOGICAL OSCILLATIONS

The recent advancement of analytical methodology for magnetoencephalography (MEG) signals enables us to detect and localize pathological oscillations in multiple frequency ranges besides detecting interictal spikes in MEG traces and localizing their courses using the equivalent current dipole (ECD) model. These methodologies include, among others, various types of time–frequency analysis for visualization and detection of pathological oscillations and minimum-norm estimation (MNE), standardized low-resolution electromagnetic tomography (sLORETA), multiple signal classification (MUSIC), and MEG beamformers for source localization (Tamilia, Madsen, Grant, Pearl, & Papadelis, 2017). To improve noninvasive localization of epileptic activity, these techniques have been applied to the detection and localization of MEG ictal and interictal activity in multiple frequency bands, including conventional frequency bands (1–70 Hz) and faster frequency bands.

Of various frequency bands, there has been special interest in fast oscillations exhibited by the epileptic brain for more than a decade. The fast oscillations in this chapter denote gamma (30–80 Hz), ripple (80–250 Hz), and fast ripple (250–500 Hz) bands, and the high-frequency oscillation (HFO) indicates fast oscillations of origin in both ripple and fast ripple frequency bands. Previous studies have suggested that ictal and interictal fast oscillations are a good indicator of the seizure onset zone (SOZ) and that removal of the areas generating pathological fast oscillations are related to a good surgical outcome (Bragin, Engel, & Staba, 2010; Worrell & Gotman, 2011; Jacobs et al., 2012; Zijlmans et al., 2012). Although pathological fast oscillations are mostly reported in invasive studies, recent studies suggested that these oscillations can

Woorim Jeong and Chun Kee Chung, *Use of Multiple Frequency Bands in Magnetoencephalography for Characterization of Epilepsy* In: *Fifty Years of Magnetoencephalography.* Edited by: Andrew C. Papanicolaou, Timothy P. L. Roberts, and James W. Wheless, Oxford University Press (2020). © Oxford University Press. DOI: 10.1093/oso/9780190935689.003.0011.

also be reliably measured by using noninvasive recordings of MEG (Frauscher et al., 2017; Hamandi, Routley, Koelewijn, & Singh, 2016; Papadelis, Poghosyan, Fenwick, & Ioannides, 2009; Tamilia et al., 2017). From a clinical perspective, MEG is advantageous to invasive electroencephalography (EEG) for initial localization of the epileptogenic zone owing to freedom from selection bias because they cover the whole brain. In addition, in a study of fast oscillations, MEG is advantageous to another noninvasive method, scalp EEG, because MEG is less susceptible to contamination from muscle activity than scalp EEG (Muthukumaraswamy, 2013; Zimmermann & Scharein, 2004).

11.1.1. Ictal Oscillations in Multiple Frequency Bands

Although rare, several previous studies reported successful recordings of ictal activities through high-resolution whole-head MEG systems (Ray & Bowyer, 2010). For source localization of ictal MEG signals, previous studies used both low- and high-frequency activities near ictal onset. This is reasonable because increased preictal activities in multiple frequency bands beginning several seconds before the ictal onset were reported in several invasive and noninvasive studies (Ochi et al., 2007; Perucca, Dubeau, & Gotman, 2013; Worrell et al., 2004). In early ictal MEG studies, ictal onset zone (IOZ) was evaluated from source localization of ictal spikes by using single ECD method, and results were found consistent with invasive EEG (Alkawadri, Burgess, Kakisaka, Mosher, & Alexopoulos, 2018; Assaf et al., 2003; Eliashiv, Elsas, Squires, Fried, & Engel, 2002; Medvedovsky et al., 2012; Shiraishi et al., 2001). However, failures of IOZ localization were also reported, which may accrue to a movement artifact from a seizure event and the low signal-to-noise ratio (SNR) of early spikes in ictal MEG. In addition, the assumption of an ECD model that spatially restricted generators may not be suitable for localizing

ictal activities. Moreover, in general, fast oscillation decreases according to the power law; thus, fast activity may undergo subtle change. In this sense, the standard ECD model might not be suitable for the localization of fast frequency components of ictal activities (Sakuma, Sekihara, & Hashimoto, 1999). To improve the accuracy of IOZ localization, several previous studies have adopted newer distributed source localization techniques, such as dynamic statistical parametric maps (Tanaka et al., 2009), wavelet-based maximum entropy on the mean (wMEM) (Pellegrino et al., 2016), and MNE (Alkawadri et al., 2018). Those studies reported successful and more accurate IOZ localization in comparison to the standard ECD technique.

Several other studies used time–frequency analysis for identification and localization of MEG ictal onset and IOZ (Fujiwara et al., 2012; Sueda et al., 2013; Yagyu et al., 2010). By reviewing the power spectrum, prominent activities in alpha to beta bands were observed at ictal MEG onset (Sueda et al., 2013; Yagyu et al., 2010). Another study reported that ictal onset patterns varied considerably from patient to patient but included low-amplitude faster frequency rhythmic discharges (Fujiwara et al., 2012). Although exact frequency bandwidth was not explicitly provided, prominent activities in the gamma band (>35 Hz) were shown in the power spectrum of two patients. In summary, previous studies demonstrated that prominent activities in multiple frequency bands at ictal onset can be detected in MEG recordings.

Source localization of selected frequency band signals over time at ictal onset, rather than localization of ictal spike at a single time point (e.g., spike peak), has been performed in several MEG studies with focal epilepsy patients (Fujiwara et al., 2012; Jeong, Kim, & Chung, 2016; Velmurugan et al., 2018). The particular freqency bandwidth that showed earliest spectral power change in ictal MEG, which belongs to gamma frequency band in some patients, was chosen for source analysis in one previous study with eight pediatric epilepsy patients (Fujiwara et al., 2012). They reported that ictal MEG proved better than interictal MEG in terms of concordance with SOZ in intracranial EEG. In another ictal MEG study with 13 adult epilepsy patients, objective approaches of predefined time windows and frequency bands were used for ictal source localization in contrast to other previous studies that used manually selected specific frequency bands and time windows by reviewing the power spectrum, which is subjective and possibly biased (Jeong et al., 2016). Several seconds (15, 10, 5, and 2 s) of preictal data were localized in the theta (3–7 Hz), alpha (8–12 Hz), beta (13–29 Hz), and gamma (30–70 Hz) frequency bands by using wavelet transformation and the sLORETA algorithm. They found that source localization in the gamma band for a 10-second window before ictal onset showed best concordance to the resection cavity, which is better than all other predefined as well as subjectively selected windows and frequency bands. They also found that all seizure-free patients with focal cortical dysplasia (FCD) showed sublobar concordance in their ictal source localization. These results provide evidence that source localization of ictal MEG fast oscillation at gamma frequency band could be a useful tool for presurgical evaluation in patients with medically intractable epilepsy.

The usefulness of ictal MEG at a faster frequency (>80 Hz) was also investigated (Xiang et al., 2010; Velmurugan et al., 2018). In an ictal MEG study with 20 medically intractable focal epilepsy patients, transient bursts of high-frequency oscillatory cycles (80–200 Hz) in the preictal and ictal epoch continuum (peri-ictal) was observed (Velmurugan et al., 2018). Its source localization using sLORETA and beamformers showed consistent results that ictal HFO sources were concordant with presumed epileptogenic zone evaluated by magnetic resonance imaging (MRI), ictal and interictal scalp EEG, and positron emission tomography (PET)-computed tomography (CT). They also found that in patients who underwent surgery, ictal MEG HFO was concordant with the surgical resection site, and all were seizure-free during follow-up. By using the wavelet-based beamformer algorithm, another study also demonstrated successful source localization of ictal HFO (110–910 Hz) to the epileptogenic zone determined by intracranial EEG in four pediatric patients with epilepsy (Xiang et al., 2010). These studies demonstrate that ictal HFO (>80 Hz) could be detected in MEG and its sources accurately localized to the epileptogenic zone.

In addition to focal epilepsy, MEG ictal HFO was also successfully detected and localized in generalized epilepsy (Miao et al., 2014; Tenney et al., 2014). Ictal HFOs ranging from 80 to 500 Hz were used to localize SOZ in 10 children with absence epilepsy (Miao et al., 2014). HFO spectral power in real-time spectrograms was assessed using Morlet continuous wavelet transform, and magnetic sources were localized through dynamic magnetic source imaging. They found that HFOs were identified in all patients, and the rate of fast ripples (250–500 Hz) was associated with seizure frequency. Compared with spikes, HFOs were localized more focally to medial prefrontal cortex during the absence seizure. In another study with 12 children with absence epilepsy, significant power in the time–frequency analysis was observed within 1- to 20-Hz, 20- to 70-Hz, and 70- to 150-Hz bandwidths at ictal onset (Tenney et al., 2014). Source localization using the sLORETA algorithm revealed that sources within HFO bandwidth (70–150 Hz) localized primarily to the frontal regions. Although the clinical and pathophysiological implications of HFOs in absence seizure should be further investigated, these two previous studies suggested that HFOs can be used for the explanation of epileptic activity generation in childhood absence epilepsy.

In summary, recent MEG studies used multiple frequency band signals over time instead of only using a single time point of an ictal spike in localization of IOZ, which often showed better concordance to SOZ of invasive EEG. Previous studies also consistently reported that pathological fast oscillations (>30 Hz) could successfully be detected in ictal MEG, and its magnetic sources were accurately localized to SOZ. These results provide the possibility that MEG ictal activities in multiple frequency bands, especially fast oscillations, can be used for the clinical purpose of noninvasive delineation of SOZ in the future.

11.1.2. Interictal Fast Oscillations

As for the interictal activities in multiple frequency bands, interictal fast oscillations as a biomarker for epileptogenicity are well-documented in invasive EEG studies (Frauscher et al., 2017; Jacobs et al., 2012; Ren et al., 2015). Fast oscillations in the time domain are generally defined as short spontaneous MEG patterns consisting of at least four oscillations above baseline in the filtered signal (e.g., >30 Hz for gamma, >80 Hz for ripple, >250 Hz for fast ripple). It has been shown that interictal fast oscillations are often superimposed on interictal spikes but can occur independently with interictal spikes. Although clinical significance of the distinction between fast oscillations with and without spikes is not known yet, previous studies have suggested that interictal fast oscillations are more specific and accurate than spikes in delineation of the epileptogenic zone.

Compared with ictal, MEG interictal fast oscillations were more often reported previously (Guggisberg, Kirsch, Mantle, Barbaro, & Nagarajan, 2008; Jeong, Kim, & Chung, 2013; Rampp et al., 2010; Papadelis et al., 2016; van Klink, Hillebrand, & Zijlmans, 2016; van Klink et al., 2017; von Ellenrieder et al., 2016; Xiang et al., 2009). Earlier studies showed that high-frequency components of MEG interictal spikes are reliably localized to the epileptogenic zone (Guggisberg et al., 2008; Mohamed, Gaetz, Otsubo, Snead, & Cheyne, 2007). In a study of 27 focal epilepsy patients, beta/gamma (~12–55 Hz) components were investigated at the time of MEG spikes (Guggisberg et al., 2008). The investigators reported that the sources of spike-locked fast oscillations were accurately localized to the surgical resection area by 85% in patients with a favorable surgical outcome, which is better than 69% of ECD model of single spikes.

In another study of three children with refractory epilepsy using an event-related beamformer, sources of beta/gamma oscillations (20–70 Hz) of interictal spikes were concordant with the localization results of the ECD model and the intracranial EEG findings (Mohamed et al., 2007). The study showed that localization of interictal fast oscillations could be a reliable alternative to conventional MEG techniques for localizing interictal epileptic activities.

MEG interictal high-frequency components without the aid of interictal spikes were also successfully detected and localized (Rampp et al., 2010; Xiang et al., 2009). In the first study that investigated the high-frequency content independent of spikes, sums of divided time segment spectrograms of 2-minute MEG recordings were used in 30 children with focal epilepsy (Xiang et al., 2009). They found that interictal high-frequency components (100–1,000 Hz) were detected in 26 (86%) patients, and sources localized by using an accumulated source imaging method were concordant with SOZ identified by intracranial EEG in nine of 11 (82%) patients who underwent epilepsy surgery. In addition, the HFO activity was concordant with MRI lesion in 21 (70%) patients. In another study, fast oscillations detected in simultaneously recorded intracranial EEG were used as a "trigger" event for MEG (Rampp et al., 2010). Detected high gamma oscillations (64–84 Hz) in invasive EEG were superimposed on and independent of interictal spikes. The minimum-norm source analysis of MEG high gamma oscillations showed concordant localization with SOZ in five of six (83%) patients. These results proved that MEG fast oscillations correspond directly to the fast oscillations in invasive EEG and demonstrated that correctly localizing, spike-independent fast oscillations seem to be present in interictal MEG.

Taken together, previous studies showed that MEG can detect high-frequency components related to the epileptogenic zone, and MEG fast oscillations can be measured independently from interictal spikes. More recently, as is typically performed in invasive EEG, studies identified individual events of MEG fast oscillations in the time domain without relying on the timing of interictal spikes or invasive EEG (Jeong et al., 2013; Papadelis et al., 2016; van Klink et al., 2016; von Ellenrieder et al., 2016). Given the lower occurrence rates of pathological fast oscillations and more high-frequency artifacts in the MEG data compared with the invasive EEG (Muthukumaraswamy, 2013) and the workload of visual analysis from the high number of physical MEG channels (>300), semiautomatic approaches with automatic detection followed by a visual review are most popularly used for detection of fast oscillations in MEG. The criteria used for automatic detection vary between studies. However, the criteria of presence of at least four peaks that were standing out from the ongoing background activity (>~3 standard deviations) in the frequency range of interest is commonly used in previous MEG studies (Migliorelli et al., 2017;

Tamilia et al., 2017; van Klink et al., 2017). In the next step, any possible artifacts were visually inspected and excluded. Possible artifacts could include any oscillations with very high amplitude in comparison to the background, showing irregular morphology or large frequency variability, or co-occurring with muscle, movement, and electrode artifacts as identified with electrooculogram (EOG), electrocardiogram (ECG), and electromyogram (EMG) data at the timing of the detected fast oscillations (Jeong et al., 2013; von Ellenrieder et al., 2016).

The clinical value of fast oscillations in MEG as an independent diagnostic measure was evaluated previously by comparing independently identified gamma and interictal spike events (Jeong et al., 2013). Interictal spikes were detected in 24 of 30 patients with FCD. Gamma oscillations were detected in 28 patients in bandpass-filtered data (30–70 Hz) of 10-minutet spontaneous MEG (Figure 11.1). They found

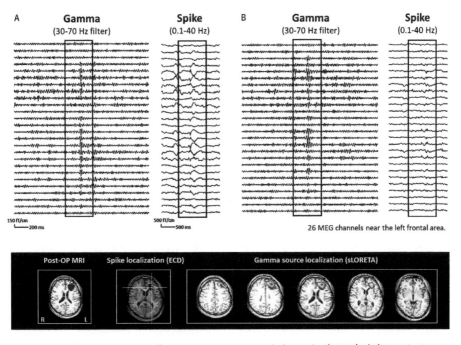

FIGURE 11.1 Pathologic gamma oscillations in magnetoencephalography (MEG). (A) Graph shows 26 MEG channels near the left frontal area. Gamma oscillations co-occurred with interictal spike. (B) Gamma oscillations occurred without interictal spike. (C) Source maps of interictal spike and gamma oscillations from (A) signals. ECD = equivalent current dipole; sLORETA = standardized low-resolution electromagnetic tomography. (Modified from Jeong, W., Kim, J. S., & Chung, C. K. [2013]. Localization of MEG pathologic gamma oscillations in adult epilepsy patients with focal cortical dysplasia. *Neuroimage: Clinical, 3,* 507–514.)

that interictal spikes and gamma oscillations can co-occur (~20%) but more often occurred independently. The ECD and sLORETA algorithms were used for source localization of interictal spikes and gamma oscillations, respectively. Compared with interictal spikes, the source of gamma oscillations showed a better concordance rate to the surgical resection cavity in patients who achieved a seizure-free outcome. In summary, pathological fast oscillations (e.g., gamma) can be detected in the time domain independently from interictal spike and localized to the epileptogenic zone, which suggests that the use of pathological gamma oscillation events as an independent diagnostic measure is feasible.

The interictal HFO events above 80 Hz can also be detected in MEG traces without the aid of MEG interictal spikes or HFOs detected by invasive EEG (Papadelis et al., 2016; van Klink et al., 2016, 2017; von Ellenrieder et al., 2016). Studies reported that the rate of visually detected HFOs (>80 Hz) in MEG is usually low (<0.5/min), and they often, but not exclusively, co-occur with epileptic spikes. In one study, interictal HFO events in the ripple frequency band (80–150 Hz) were detected in MEG traces by using a semiautomatic algorithm, and their sources were compared with the SOZ in two children with surgically treated epilepsy (Papadelis et al., 2016). In this study, HFO events, not accompanied by an isolated high-frequency peak at the power spectrum, were discarded in order to automatically reject possible artifacts. To compare HFOs in MEG and simultaneously recorded scalp EEG, they kept only HFO events that occurred in both the EEG and the MEG signals at the same time. In both patients, HFOs were always overlying interictal spikes. They found that the sources of HFOs that were estimated using wMEM were concordant between MEG and scalp EEG as well as SOZ. In another study, MEG fast oscillations above 80 Hz were also detected and compared with scalp EEG and invasive EEG in 17 patients with focal epilepsy (von Ellenrieder et al., 2016). They showed that fast oscillation events (40–160 Hz) can be identified independently of information

obtained from spikes in MEG. The wMEM was used to localize the sources of detected fast oscillations and found that sources were concordant with the epileptogenic region in most patients. They further demonstrated that, compared with scalp EEG, detection sensitivity was lower but the specificity was higher in MEG. Regarding detection sensitivity of MEG, an increase of sensitivity to fast oscillations by using virtual channels constructed with beamforming techniques has been suggested (van Klink et al., 2016, 2017). They reported that virtual sensors identified epileptic HFOs (80–250 Hz) that are not discernible by the actual MEG sensors and that HFOs were even visible in unfiltered virtual sensor signals.

In summary, reliable measurement of epileptic fast oscillations (>30 Hz) in MEG has been demonstrated during the past decade. Interictal fast oscillations of MEG can be detected independently of interictal spikes, and their sources seem to be more specific and accurate than interictal spikes in delineating the epileptogenic zone. Although use of MEG fast oscillations as an independent diagnostic measure for epilepsy in clinical settings seems to be promising, more intensive investigations are required for validation of the usefulness of MEG fast oscillations in presurgical evaluation. Moreover, methods that could differentiate between pathological and physiological fast oscillations and that detect only fast oscillations of cerebral origin but not of muscular origin should also be validated for future clinical applications.

11.2. CONNECTIVITY AND FUNCTIONAL NETWORKS

The advances in brain connectivity and its network analyses have provided unprecedented opportunities to investigate how brain regions are interconnected and how the complex network is organized (Bullmore & Sporns, 2009; van Diessen et al., 2015). Efforts to investigate large-scale brain networks in epilepsy for understanding underlying brain pathophysiology have increased (Kramer & Cash, 2012; Pittau et al., 2014; Stam, 2014). Generally, connectivity in MEG refers to interactions between time series in terms of amplitude or phase. There are different ways to characterize functional interactions among brain regions. One is functional and effective connectivity (Pittau & Vulliemoz, 2015). Functional connectivity measures the statistical dependency between signals recorded from different brain areas without implying any directionality of influence. Effective connectivity measures directionality or causal interactions between signals. Such connectivity measures across multiple sources are commonly used to construct cross-correlation matrices, which are subsequently used in network analysis (e.g., graph-theory analysis). Detailed methods for connectivity and network measures are described elsewhere (Bullmore & Sporns, 2009; Hart, Ypma, Romero-Garcia, Price, & Suckling, 2016).

Epilepsy is nowadays thought of as a large-scale network disorder rather than a focal disorder (Kramer & Cash, 2012; Pittau et al., 2014; Stam, 2014). Although noninvasive investigation of whole-brain large-scale network in epilepsy has been implemented through the use of functional MRI (fMRI), MEG has the advantage of a high temporal resolution compared with that of fMRI, which can only cover brain oscillations under 0.1 Hz. This high temporal resolution of MEG allows us to investigate brain connectivity and network topology of epilepsy in various frequency bands. From a clinical perspective, the motivation for studying connectivity of networks in epilepsy is to improve on the value of diagnostic and prognostic information, such as the differentiation of an epileptic brain from a healthy brain, characterization of epileptogenic networks, or prediction of postsurgical outcome (Hamandi et al., 2016; Pang & Snead, 2016; Pittau & Vulliemoz, 2015).

Since connectivity and network analysis of MEG were recently adopted in an epilepsy study, a large body of subsequent studies has focused on characterizing specific connectivity or network properties of an epileptic brain that differ from a healthy brain by using resting-state recordings with no interictal epileptiform discharges. These studies have reported abnormally rich connectivity with a clear modular structure in the theta-alpha range (5–14 Hz) in five patients with absence seizure (Chavez, Valencia, Navarro, Latora, & Martinerie, 2010), widespread increases of network connectivity in the alpha-beta bands (8–29 Hz) in 13 patients with idiopathic generalized epilepsy (Elshahabi et al., 2015), increased functional connectivity between the areas of the so-called default mode network in the delta (1–4 Hz) and the theta (4–8 Hz) bands in 16 patients with temporal lobe epilepsy (Hsiao et al., 2015), greater variability in oscillatory amplitude in the beta band (13–30 Hz) in the sensorimotor network of 23 patients with benign epilepsy with centro-temporal spikes (Koelewijn et al., 2015), altered whole-brain cortical network hubs in various frequency bands (theta, alpha, beta, and gamma) in 44 medial temporal lobe epilepsy cases with hippocampal sclerosis (Jin, Jeong, & Chung, 2015b) (Figure 11.2) and 35 epilepsy patients with FCD (Jin, Jeong, & Chung, 2015a), and higher global functional connectivity and network efficiency in the beta (13–30 Hz) and gamma (31–45 Hz) bands in 35 epilepsy patients with FCD (Jeong, Jin, Kim, Kim, & Chung, 2014). A more recent study even reported that not only patients and healthy controls but also left and right medial temporal lobe epilepsy patients can be successfully distinguished by applying a machine learning algorithm of a support vector machine to resting-state functional connectivity data (Jin & Chung, 2017).

The usefulness of MEG connectivity and network analysis in identification of epileptogenic networks has also been assessed in several previous studies and seems to provide promising results. By applying connectivity analysis, the dynamics of epileptic networks were successfully characterized in patients with generalized epilepsy (Dominguez et al., 2005; Foley et al., 2014) and focal epilepsy

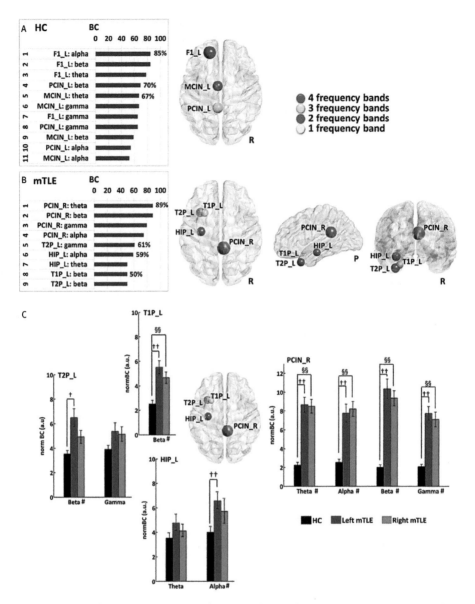

FIGURE 11.2 Altered functional hubs in medial temporal lobe epilepsy patients with hippocampal sclerosis (mTLE). (A and B) Ranked distribution of hubs in healthy controls (HC, A) and mTLE (B). Shown are the hubs selected on the basis of the aggregated ranking percentage across subjects (>50% of ranking percent; *left panels*) and their topologic maps projected onto a cortical surface derived from the betweenness centrality (BC) measure irrespective of frequency band. Network hub color indicates the number of frequency bands identified at the hubs at the same location. Hub size corresponds to the largest aggregated ranking percentage of the hub location. (C) Group differences in BC at patients' hubs. Shown are BC values (mean and standard error, in arbitrary units) at hubs identified in mTLE patients, and their group-wise differences. #$p < 0.05$ (corrected, between HC and mTLE); †$p < 0.05$ (corrected, between HC and left mTLE); ††$p < 0.01$ (corrected, between HC and left mTLE); §§$p < 0.01$ (corrected, between HC and right mTLE). F1 = dorsolateral superior frontal gyrus; HIP = hippocampus; MCIN = middle cingulate gyrus; PCIN = posterior cingulate gyrus; T1P = superior temporal gyrus (temporal pole); T2P = middle temporal gyrus (temporal pole). (Modified from Jin, S. H., Jeong, W., & Chung, C. K. [2015]. Mesial temporal lobe epilepsy with hippocampal sclerosis is a network disorder with altered cortical hubs. *Epilepsia, 56*[5], 772–779.)

(Coito et al., 2015; Dai, Zhang, Dickens, & He, 2012; Jin, Jeong, & Chung, 2013). For example, enhanced local-phase synchrony compared with long-range phase synchrony (3–55 Hz) was observed during generalized seizures (Dominguez et al., 2005). In focal epilepsy, effective connectivity analysis successfully estimated the primary epileptogenic source and epileptic propagation from sources of interictal MEG spikes (Coito et al., 2015; Dai et al., 2012; Jin et al., 2013). As for the network analysis, despite its potential importance for clinical applications, the direct relationship between network topology and the epileptogenic zone has not been well-addressed, with the exception of one recent study, which in fact suggested such a direct relationship (Nissen, van Klink, Zijlmans, Stam & Hillebrand, 2016).

In addition to diagnosis, MEG connectivity and network analysis could help in improving prognostic information for epilepsy. Regarding the prediction of postsurgical seizure outcome, one study reported that patients with enhanced regional connectivity within the resection area were more likely to achieve postoperative seizure freedom than those with neutral or decreased regional connectivity (Englot et al., 2015). Changes of specific network features after epilepsy surgery have also been investigated in tumor-related epilepsy (Douw et al., 2010) and lesional epilepsy (van Dellen et al., 2014). In a study with lesional epilepsy, only in patients who became seizure-free, regions close to the resection area demonstrated postsurgical decreases in one of the network measures (van Dellen et al., 2014). In addition to the seizure outcome, given that MEG network topology is associated with the memory function of epilepsy patients (Ibrahim et al., 2014; Jin & Chung, 2015), functional network analysis could also be used for the prediction of cognitive function after surgery in the future.

In summary, connectivity and network analysis of spontaneous MEG in epilepsy have the potential to become useful in improving diagnostic and prognostic information. Connectivity and network analyses of resting-state MEG recordings without epileptic discharges successfully differentiate an epileptic brain from a healthy one. The dynamics of epileptic networks can be identified by using functional connectivity analysis. Its application has suggested the feasibility of using cortical source connectivity analysis from interictal MEG for potential localization of epileptiform activities. Recent studies also suggested the possibility of using functional connectivity analysis for the prediction of postsurgical seizure and cognitive outcome. Although the data accumulating from MEG functional connectivity studies showed a potential clinical use for epilepsy, the clinical significance needs to be further demonstrated, especially for the network analysis. Moreover, since selected connectivity/network measures and frequency bands vary from study to study, a consensus on reliable functional network biomarkers of epilepsy should be made for future clinical applications of a functional connectivity analysis of MEG data.

11.3. CONCLUSION

To improve clinical use of MEG in epilepsy, various analytical approaches using multiple frequency band signals of spontaneous MEG have begun to be applied in epilepsy studies, which provided promising results. During the past decade, one special frequency of interest among others is fast oscillations (>30 Hz) in both ictal and interictal MEG studies. Several studies demonstrated reliable measurement of epileptic fast oscillations during ictal and interictal periods using noninvasive MEG. Moreover, interictal fast oscillations can be detected independently of interictal spikes in MEG traces. Magnetic sources of ictal and interictal fast oscillations over time accurately localized the epileptogenic areas and often showed better performance than the use of a single time point of ictal or interictal spikes. Apart from the localization of fast oscillations, connectivity and network analysis using multiple frequency band MEG signals potentially can be used to improve diagnostic and prognostic information in epilepsy. For future applications, more intensive studies are needed to increase the reliability of detection and localization of MEG recorded events using multiple frequency bands, especially fast oscillations, and to validate the clinical significance of functional network properties in epilepsy.

ACKNOWLEDGMENT

This research was supported by the Basic Science Research Program through the National Research Foundation of Korea (NRF) funded by the Ministry of Science, ICT and Future Planning (2016M3C7A1904984).

REFERENCES

Alkawadri, R., Burgess, R. C., Kakisaka, Y., Mosher, J. C., & Alexopoulos, A. V. (2018). Assessment of the utility of ictal magnetoencephalography in the localization of the epileptic seizure onset zone. *JAMA Neurology*, 75(10), 1264–1272 .

Assaf, B. A., Karkar, K. M., Laxer, K. D., Garcia, P. A., Austin, E. J., Barbaro, N. M., & Aminoff, M. J. (2003). Ictal magnetoencephalography in temporal and extratemporal lobe epilepsy. *Epilepsia*, 44(10), 1320–1327.

Bragin, A., Engel, J., Jr., & Staba, R. J. (2010). High-frequency oscillations in epileptic brain. *Current Opinion in Neurology*, 23(2), 151–156.

Bullmore, E., & Sporns, O. (2009). Complex brain networks: Graph theoretical analysis of structural and functional systems. *Nature Reviews Neuroscience*, 10, 186.

Chavez, M., Valencia, M., Navarro, V., Latora, V., & Martinerie, J. (2010). Functional modularity of background activities in normal and epileptic brain networks. *Physical Review Letters*, 104(11), 118701.

Coito, A., Plomp, G., Genetti, M., Abela, E., Wiest, R., Seeck, M., & Vulliemoz, S. (2015). Dynamic directed interictal connectivity in left and right temporal lobe epilepsy. *Epilepsia*, 56(2), 207–217.

Dai, Y., Zhang, W., Dickens, D. L., & He, B. (2012). Source connectivity analysis from MEG and its application to epilepsy source localization. *Brain Topography*, 25(2), 157–166.

Dominguez, L. G., Wennberg, R. A., Gaetz, W., Cheyne, D., Snead, O. C., & Velazquez, J. L. P. (2005). Enhanced synchrony in epileptiform activity? Local versus distant phase synchronization in generalized seizures. *Journal of Neuroscience*, 25(35), 8077–8084.

Douw, L., van Dellen, E., de Groot, M., Heimans, J. J., Klein, M., Stam, C. J., & Reijneveld, J. C. (2010). Epilepsy is related to theta band brain connectivity and network topology in brain tumor patients. *BMC Neuroscience*, 11(1), 103.

Eliashiv, D. S., Elsas, S. M., Squires, K., Fried, I., & Engel, J., Jr. (2002). Ictal magnetic source imaging as a localizing tool in partial epilepsy. *Neurology*, 59(10), 1600–1610.

Elshahabi, A., Klamer, S., Sahib, A. K., Lerche, H., Braun, C., & Focke, N. K. (2015). Magnetoencephalography reveals a widespread increase in network connectivity in idiopathic/genetic generalized epilepsy. *PLoS One*, 10(9), e0138119.

Englot, D. J., Hinkley, L. B., Kort, N. S., Imber, B. S., Mizuiri, D., Honma, S. M., . . . Nagarajan, S. S. (2015). Global and regional functional connectivity maps of neural oscillations in focal epilepsy. *Brain*, 138(8), 2249–2262.

Foley, E., Cerquiglini, A., Cavanna, A., Nakubulwa, M. A., Furlong, P. L., Witton, C., & Seri, S. (2014). Magnetoencephalography in the study of epilepsy and consciousness. *Epilepsy and Behavior*, 30, 38–42.

Frauscher, B., Bartolomei, F., Kobayashi, K., Cimbalnik, J., van 't Klooster, M. A., Rampp, S., . . . Gotman, J. (2017). High-frequency oscillations: The state of clinical research. *Epilepsia*, 58(8), 1316–1329.

Fujiwara, H., Greiner, H. M., Hemasilpin, N., Lee, K. H., Holland-Bouley, K., Arthur, T., . . . Rose, D. F. (2012). Ictal MEG onset source localization compared to intracranial EEG and outcome: Improved epilepsy presurgical evaluation in pediatrics. *Epilepsy Research*, 99(3), 214–224.

Guggisberg, A. G., Kirsch, H. E., Mantle, M. M., Barbaro, N. M., & Nagarajan, S. S. (2008). Fast oscillations associated with interictal spikes localize the epileptogenic zone in patients with partial epilepsy. *Neuroimage*, 39(2), 661–668.

Hamandi, K., Routley, B. C., Koelewijn, L., & Singh, K. D. (2016). Non-invasive brain mapping in epilepsy: Applications from magnetoencephalography. *Journal of Neuroscience Methods*, 260, 283–291.

Hart, M. G., Ypma, R. J., Romero-Garcia, R., Price, S. J., & Suckling, J. (2016). Graph theory analysis of complex brain networks: New concepts in brain mapping applied to neurosurgery. *Journal of Neurosurgery*, 124(6), 1665–1678.

Hsiao, F. J., Yu, H. Y., Chen, W. T., Kwan, S. Y., Chen, C., Yen, D. J., . . . Lin, Y. Y. (2015). Increased intrinsic connectivity of the default mode network in temporal lobe epilepsy: Evidence from resting-state MEG recordings. *PLoS One, 10*(6), e0128787.

Ibrahim, G. M., Cassel, D., Morgan, B. R., Smith, M. L., Otsubo, H., Ochi, A., . . . Doesburg, S. (2014). Resilience of developing brain networks to interictal epileptiform discharges is associated with cognitive outcome. *Brain, 137*(Pt, 10), 2690–2702.

Jacobs, J., Staba, R., Asano, E., Otsubo, H., Wu, J. Y., Zijlmans, M., . . . Gotman, J. (2012). High-frequency oscillations (HFOs) in clinical epilepsy. *Progress in Neurobiology, 98*(3), 302–315.

Jeong, W., Jin, S. H., Kim, M., Kim, J. S., & Chung, C. K. (2014). Abnormal functional brain network in epilepsy patients with focal cortical dysplasia. *Epilepsy Research, 108*(9), 1618–1626.

Jeong, W., Kim, J. S., & Chung, C. K. (2013). Localization of MEG pathologic gamma oscillations in adult epilepsy patients with focal cortical dysplasia. *Neuroimage: Clinical, 3*, 507–514.

Jeong, W., Kim, J. S., & Chung, C. K. (2016). Usefulness of multiple frequency band source localizations in ictal MEG. *Clinical Neurophysiology, 127*(2), 1049–1056.

Jin, S. H., & Chung, C. K. (2015). Functional substrate for memory function differences between patients with left and right mesial temporal lobe epilepsy associated with hippocampal sclerosis. *Epilepsy and Behavior, 51*, 251–258.

Jin, S. H., & Chung, C. K. (2017). Electrophysiological resting-state biomarker for diagnosing mesial temporal lobe epilepsy with hippocampal sclerosis. *Epilepsy Research, 129*, 138–145.

Jin, S. H., Jeong, W., & Chung, C. K. (2013). Information source in multiple MEG spike clusters can be identified by effective connectivity in focal cortical dysplasia. *Epilepsy Research, 105*(1–2), 118–124.

Jin, S. H., Jeong, W., & Chung, C. K. (2015a) Focal cortical dysplasia alters electrophysiological cortical hubs in the resting-state. *Clinical Neurophysiology, 126*(8), 1482–1492.

Jin, S. H., Jeong, W., & Chung, C. K. (2015b). Mesial temporal lobe epilepsy with hippocampal sclerosis is a network disorder with altered cortical hubs. *Epilepsia, 56*(5), 772–779.

Koelewijn, L., Hamandi, K., Brindley, L. M., Brookes, M. J., Routley, B. C., Muthukumaraswamy, S. D., . . . Singh, K. D. (2015). Resting-state oscillatory dynamics in sensorimotor cortex in benign epilepsy with centro-temporal spikes and typical brain development. *Human Brain Mapping, 36*(10), 3935–3949.

Kramer, M. A., & Cash, S. S. (2012). Epilepsy as a disorder of cortical network organization. *Neuroscientist, 18*(4), 360–372.

Medvedovsky, M., Taulu, S., Gaily, E., Metsähonkala, E. L., Makela, J. P., Ekstein, D., . . . Paetau, R. (2012). Sensitivity and specificity of seizure-onset zone estimation by ictal magnetoencephalography. *Epilepsia, 53*(9), 1649–1657.

Miao, A., Xiang, J., Tang, L., Ge, H., Liu, H., & Wu, T. (2014). Using ictal high-frequency oscillations (80–500Hz) to localize seizure onset zones in childhood absence epilepsy: A MEG study. *Neuroscience Letters, 566*, 21–26.

Migliorelli, C., Alonso, J. F., Romero, S., Nowak, R., Russi, A., & Mañanas, M. A. (2017). Automated detection of epileptic ripples in MEG using beamformer-based virtual sensors. *Journal of Neural Engineering, 14*(4).

Mohamed, I. S., Gaetz, W., Otsubo, H., Snead, O. C., & Cheyne, D. (2007). Localization of interictal spikes using an event-related beamformer. *International Congress Series, 1300*, 669–672.

Muthukumaraswamy, S. D. (2013). High-frequency brain activity and muscle artifacts in MEG/EEG: A review and recommendations. *Frontiers in Human Neuroscience, 7*, 138.

Nissen, I. A., van Klink, N. E. C., Zijlmans, M., Stam, C. J., & Hillebrand, A. (2016). Brain areas with epileptic high frequency oscillations are functionally isolated in MEG virtual electrode networks. *Clinical Neurophysiology, 127*(7), 2581–2591.

Ochi, A., Otsubo, H., Donner, E. J., Elliott, I., Iwata, R., Funaki, T., . . Snead, O. C. (2007). Dynamic changes of ictal high-frequency oscillations in neocortical epilepsy: Using multiple band frequency analysis. *Epilepsia, 48*(2), 286–296.

Pang, E. W., & Snead, O. C., III. (2016). From structure to circuits: The contribution of MEG connectivity studies to functional neurosurgery. *Frontiers in Neuroanatomy, 10*, 67.

Papadelis, C., Poghosyan, V., Fenwick, P. B. C., & Ioannides, A. A. (2009). MEG's ability to localise accurately weak transient neural sources. *Clinical Neurophysiology, 120*(11), 1958–1970.

Papadelis, C., Tamilia, E., Stufflebeam, S., Grant, P. E., Madsen, J. R., Pearl, P. L., & Tanaka, N. (2016). Interictal high frequency oscillations detected with simultaneous magnetoencephalography and electroencephalography as biomarker of pediatric epilepsy. *Journal of Visualized Experiments, 2016*(118).

Pellegrino, G., Hedrich, T., Chowdhury, R., Hall, J. A., Lina, J. M., Dubeau, F., . . . Grova, C. (2016). Source localization of the seizure onset zone from ictal EEG/MEG data. *Human Brain Mapping, 37*(7), 2528–2546.

Perucca, P., Dubeau, F., & Gotman, J. (2013). Widespread EEG changes precede focal seizures. *PLoS One, 8*(11), e80972.

Pittau, F., Megevand, P., Sheybani, L., Abela, E., Grouiller, F., Spinelli, L., . . . Vulliemoz, S. (2014). Mapping epileptic activity: Sources or networks for the clinicians? *Frontiers in Neurology, 5*, 218.

Pittau, F., & Vulliemoz, S. (2015). Functional brain networks in epilepsy: Recent advances in noninvasive mapping. *Current Opinion in Neurology, 28*(4), 338–343.

Rampp, S., Kaltenhäuser, M., Weigel, D., Buchfelder, M., Blümcke, I., Dörfler, A., & Stefan, H. (2010). MEG correlates of epileptic high gamma oscillations in invasive EEG. *Epilepsia, 51*(8), 1638–1642.

Ray, A., & Bowyer, S. M. (2013). Clinical applications of magnetoencephalography in epilepsy. *Annals of Indian Academy of Neurology, 13*(1), 14–22.

Ren, L., Kucewicz, M. T., Cimbalnik, J., Matsumoto, J. Y., Brinkmann, B. H., Hu, W., . . . Worrell, G. A. (2015). Gamma oscillations precede interictal epileptiform spikes in the seizure onset zone. *Neurology, 84*(6), 602–608.

Sakuma, K., Sekihara, K., & Hashimoto, I. (1999). Neural source estimation from a time–frequency component of somatic evoked high-frequency magnetic oscillations to posterior tibial nerve stimulation. *Clinical Neurophysiology, 110*(9), 1585–1588.

Shiraishi, H., Watanabe, Y., Watanabe, M., Inoue, Y., Fujiwara, T., & Yagi, K. (2001). Interictal and ictal magnetoencephalographic study in patients with medial frontal lobe epilepsy. *Epilepsia, 42*(7), 875–882.

Stam, C. J. (2014). Modern network science of neurological disorders. *Nature Reviews Neuroscience, 15*, 683.

Sueda, K., Takeuchi, F., Shiraishi, H., Nakane, S., Sakurai, K., Yagyu, K., . . . Saitoh, S. (2013). Magnetoencephalographic analysis of paroxysmal fast activity in patients with epileptic spasms. *Epilepsy Research, 104*(1), 68–77.

Tamilia, E., Madsen, J. R., Grant, P. E., Pearl, P. L., & Papadelis, C. (2017). Current and emerging potential of magnetoencephalography in the detection and localization of high-frequency oscillations in epilepsy. *Frontiers in Neurology, 8*, 14.

Tanaka, N., Cole, A. J., von Pechmann, D., Wakeman, D. G., Hämäläinen, M. S., Liu, H., . . . Stufflebeam, S. M. (2009). Dynamic statistical parametric mapping for analyzing ictal magnetoencephalographic spikes in patients with intractable frontal lobe epilepsy. *Epilepsy Research, 85*(2), 279–286.

Tenney, J. R., Fujiwara, H., Horn, P. S., Vannest, J., Xiang, J., Glauser, T. A., & Rose, D. F. (2014). Low- and high-frequency oscillations reveal distinct absence seizure networks. *Annals of Neurology, 76*(4), 558–567.

van Dellen, E., Douw, L., Hillebrand, A., de Witt Hamer, P. C., Baayen, J. C., Heimans, J. J., . . . Stam, C. J. (2014). Epilepsy surgery outcome and functional network alterations in longitudinal MEG: A minimum spanning tree analysis. *Neuroimage, 86*, 354–363.

van Diessen, E., Numan, T., van Dellen, E., van der Kooi, A. W., Boersma, M., Hofman, D., . . . Stam, C. J. (2015). Opportunities and methodological challenges in EEG and MEG resting state functional brain network research. *Clinical Neurophysiology, 126*(8), 1468–1481.

van Klink, N., Hillebrand, A., & Zijlmans, M. (2016). Identification of epileptic high frequency oscillations in the time domain by using MEG beamformer-based virtual sensors. *Clinical Neurophysiology, 127*(1), 197–208.

van Klink, N., van Rosmalen, F., Nenonen, J., Burnos, S., Helle, L., Taulu, S., . . . Hillebrand, A. (2017). Automatic detection and visualisation of MEG ripple oscillations in epilepsy. *Neuroimage: Clinical, 15*, 689–701.

Velmurugan, J., Nagarajan, S. S., Mariyappa, N., Ravi, S. G., Thennarasu, K., Mundlamuri, R. C., . . . Sinha, S. (2018). Magnetoencephalographic imaging of ictal high-frequency oscillations (80–200 Hz) in pharmacologically resistant focal epilepsy. *Epilepsia, 59*(1), 190–202.

von Ellenrieder, N., Pellegrino, G., Hedrich, T., Gotman, J., Lina, J. M., Grova, C., & Kobayashi, E. (2016). Detection and magnetic source imaging of fast oscillations (40–160 Hz) recorded with magnetoencephalography in focal epilepsy patients. *Brain Topography, 29*(2), 218–231.

Worrell, G., & Gotman, J. (2011). High-frequency oscillations and other electrophysiological biomarkers of epilepsy: Clinical studies. *Biomarkers in Medicine, 5*(5), 557–566.

Worrell, G. A., Parish, L., Cranstoun, S. D., Jonas, R., Baltuch, G., & Litt, B. (2004). High-frequency oscillations and seizure generation in neocortical epilepsy. *Brain, 127*(Pt. 7), 1496–1506.

Xiang, J., Liu, Y., Wang, Y., Kirtman, E. G., Kotecha, R., Chen, Y., . . . Rose, D. (2009). Frequency and spatial characteristics of high-frequency neuromagnetic signals in childhood epilepsy. *Epileptic Disorders, 11*(2), 113–125.

Xiang, J., Wang, Y., Chen, Y., Liu, Y., Kotecha, R., Huo, X., . . . deGrauw, T. (2008). Noninvasive localization of epileptogenic zones with ictal high-frequency neuromagnetic signals. *Journal of Neurosurgery Pediatrics, 5*(1), 113–122.

Yagyu, K., Takeuchi, F., Shiraishi, H., Nakane, S., Sueda, K., Asahina, N., . . . Saitoh, S. (2010). The applications of time-frequency analyses to ictal magnetoencephalography in neocortical epilepsy. *Epilepsy Research, 90*(3), 199–206.

Zijlmans, M., Jiruska, P., Zelmann, R., Leijten, F. S., Jefferys, J. G., & Gotman, J. (2012). High-frequency oscillations as a new biomarker in epilepsy. *Annals of Neurology, 71*(2), 169–178.

Zimmermann, R., & Scharein, E. (2004). MEG and EEG show different sensitivity to myogenic artifacts. *Neurology and Clinical Neurophysiology, 2004,* 78.

12

CAN MAGNETOENCEPHALOGRAPHY IDENTIFY THE EPILEPTOGENIC PATHOLOGY IN CHILDREN?

Won Seok Chang and Hiroshi Otsubo

12.1. INTRODUCTION

Epilepsy is one of the most common and serious neurological disorders affecting children that causes functional disabilities. The prevalence of epilepsy is reported to range from 3.2 to 5.5 per 1,000 people in developed countries and from 3.6 to 44 per 1,000 in developing countries (Bearden, Ciccone, & Patel, 2018). Chronic epilepsy in children can result in cognitive decline and psychomotor disabilities; therefore, it is recommended to attempt to control the seizures as early and aggressively (i.e., epilepsy surgery) as possible (Cross et al., 2006). However, despite optimized medical treatment, approximately 30 to 35% of all patients continue to experience seizures; that is, they have medically refractory epilepsy. For some of these patients, epilepsy surgery can be one of the important treatment options because it results in better reduction of seizure

activity compared with best medical treatment (Del Felice et al., 2010; Jobst & Cascino, 2015).

The presentation of intractable localization-related epilepsy is often heterogeneous in childhood. Pediatric patients with hemispheric or unilateral focal etiologies can have generalized seizure semiologies and bilateral electroencephalography (EEG) patterns, rapid evolution of electroclinical features, progressive neurological disorders, and bilateral congenital brain syndromes (Jonas et al., 2005). Therefore, if epilepsy surgery is planned, careful presurgical evaluation, including EEG, structural imaging, metabolic imaging, and neuropsychological evaluation, should be undertaken and carefully analyzed for the exact identification of the epileptogenic region or hemisphere. These diagnostic modalities can offer crucial information about the epileptogenic region; however, they also have their own drawbacks, such as low

Won Seok Chang and Hiroshi Otsubo, *Can Magnetoencephalography Identify the Epileptogenic Pathology in Children?* In: *Fifty Years of Magnetoencephalography*. Edited by: Andrew C. Papanicolaou, Timothy P. L. Roberts, and James W. Wheless, Oxford University Press (2020).

spatial resolution in the case of EEG and low temporal resolution in the case of structural and metabolic imaging. To overcome these limitations, magnetoencephalography (MEG) was introduced, and its role in presurgical evaluation and mapping has been proved in recent years. Nowadays, MEG has become an essential part of the diagnostic workup of pediatric patients undergoing presurgical evaluation in many institutions and also has been applied for eloquent brain mapping in addition to localization of the epileptogenic zone (Ito et al., 2015). In this chapter, specific characteristics of MEG findings for each epileptogenic lesion and their correlation with findings of other modalities will be reviewed, and the surgical strategy for children showing these specific findings in the presurgical evaluation will be suggested.

12.2. FOCAL CORTICAL DYSPLASIA

Focal cortical dysplasia (FCD) is a neuronal migration disorder and represents the most common structural brain lesion in children with drug-resistant focal epilepsies undergoing epilepsy surgery (Palmini & Holthausen, 2013). It is divided into types I, II, and III. Type I FCD refers to isolated lesions, which present either as radial (FCD type Ia) or tangential (FCD type Ib) dyslamination of the neocortex, microscopically identified in one or multiple lobes. FCD type II is an isolated lesion characterized by cortical dyslamination and dysmorphic neurons without (type IIa) or with (type IIb) balloon cells. On the other hand, type III has a combined pathology such as hippocampal sclerosis (type IIIa), tumor (type IIIb), and vascular malformation (type IIIc) (Blümcke et al., 2011).

Epilepsy surgery for FCD has been regarded as one of the standard treatments, and structural and metabolic images play crucial roles for both diagnosis and treatment planning. However, there are still unsolved issues. The exact localization of the epileptogenic zone and eloquent cortical regions is essential for epilepsy surgery planning for FCD; however, predictions of their anatomical locations may not be confirmed with conventional neuroimaging. Structural magnetic resonance image (MRI) that includes T1-weighted, T2-weighted, and fluid-attenuated inversion recovery (FLAIR) sequence is a "gold standard" for detecting FCD. However, approximately 25% of FCD cases do not show abnormalities on a structural MRI. Positron emission tomography (PET) may give additional information for localization and delineation of the FCD, but PET-negative FCD occurs in about 25% of types I and II FCD (Halac et al., 2017).

Combined with neuroimaging tools, interictal EEG is a widely available tool for evaluating the extent and location of the seizure focus (So, 2000). The role of EEG for diagnosis and localization of FCD has been investigated, and some EEG features have been suggested as typical features of FCD. Especially in FCD type II, such a feature is the frequent occurrence of a focal interictal scalp EEG pattern of rhythmic epileptiform discharges that correlate with the location and extent of the lesion, and a striking pattern of continuous or subcontinuous rhythmic spikes or sharp waves—so-called electrocardiography-like rhythm—is described in about 50% of cases (Chassoux et al., 2012; Lerner et al., 2009). Another EEG feature, delta brush, is also seen in FCD and occurs in less than 20% of FCD seizures, although patients with anti–N-methyl-D-aspartate (NMDA) receptor encephalitis and premature infants can also show this pattern on scalp EEG (Perucca, Dubeau, & Gotman, 2014). However, there are limitations in characterizing the pathology only by EEG findings because EEG patterns of many seizures associated with FCD are still nonspecific. Furthermore, small FCDs located in the depth of the sulcus can be associated with a normal scalp EEG (Guerrini et al., 2015). In these cases, another diagnostic tool such as MEG can provide valuable information for localization of the epileptogenic region and for prediction of the underlying pathology.

MEG detects magnetic fields generated by postsynaptic intracellular currents, and its temporal resolution is of as high precision as that of EEG. However, the spatial resolution of MEG is much higher because magnetic fields are not distorted by the various intracranial tissues such as the cerebrospinal fluid, skull, and scalp. With respect to data acquisition, EEG and MEG detect the same signals generated by postsynaptic potentials at the axon of pyramidal cells. Detection of postsynaptic potentials with EEG and MEG requires the synchronized activation of neurons in a certain area. However, the extent of the area needed to be synchronized for signal detection is different between EEG and MEG. It has been reported that cortical areas of at least 6 cm^2 must be involved in synchronous or near synchronous activity before that activity is detected by scalp EEG (Cooper, Winter, Crow, & Walter, 1965). In contrast, synchronized neuronal activities of 3 cm^2 are sufficient to be detected by MEG. With these advantages, MEG has become one of the most important tools for epilepsy evaluation because of its role in predicting surgical outcome (Merlet & Gotman, 1999; Murakami et al., 2016; Okanishi et al., 2016; RamachandranNair et al., 2007).

As mentioned previously, MEG requires a smaller area of synchronized activity for signal detection (Oishi et al., 2002). For this reason, focal discharges from the epileptic cortex are usually detected by MEG when compared with scalp EEG, which needs a larger area of synchronized neurons to produce a recordable signal. In the case of FCDs, the associated epileptiform discharges are produced by a focal area, and MEG spikes usually precede the EEG spikes. This finding may differentiate between focal and bilateral onset of the epilepsy.

For epileptic source localization by MEG, the equivalent current dipole (ECD) model is usually employed for all well-defined interictal epileptiform discharges, and there is a minimum standard recommendation for the routine clinical recording and analysis of spontaneous MEG and EEG (Bagic, Knowlton,

Rose, Ebersole, & Committee, 2011). We analyze spontaneous MEG for pediatric epilepsy patients using that protocol, which reflects the guidelines of the American Clinical Magnetoencephalography Society.

Although MEG can be used to plan intracranial electrode placement, historically there were limitations in detecting epileptic spikes that have a source located distant from the detectors (i.e., mesial frontal or temporal), although even this may be improved with new-generation MEG equipment. This issue may make the use of MEG difficult for assessment of pathology in cases of bottom of sulcus cortical dysplasia (BOSD). According to our experience, the spatial congruence between the MEG results and BOSD was true for only half of the patients, and it was much less accurate than in cases of FCD, in which the lesions are located in superficial regions (accuracy of 89%) (Nakajima et al., 2016). To overcome this kind of limitation of MEG, novel analysis techniques have been developed, such as minimum-norm estimate (MNE), Laplacian weighted minimum norm, local autoregressive average, and EPIFOCUS (Tanaka & Stufflebeam, 2014). Among these analysis techniques, an MNE-based technique called advanced dynamic statistical parametric mapping (AdSPM) was recently introduced to detect the epileptogenic network and localize deeply located epileptogenic sources.

In the early 2000s, dynamic statistical parametric mapping (dSPM) was developed to generate highly precise spatiotemporal estimates of evoked potential sources by combining the anatomical cortical surface derived from MRI with MEG information. And, combined with noise normalization, dSPM could provide spatiotemporal estimates of source distribution with high temporal resolution by calculating source distribution at any time point of the waveform (Dale et al., 2000; Liu, Dale, & Belliveau, 2002). The dSPM technique was also applied to epilepsy, and it also showed some advantages for localizing epileptogenic networks, compared with the single dipole method, in cases with widespread spikes. Moreover, it can also give information about the spike propagation, which is important for understanding the epileptic network (Tanaka et al., 2009, 2014). However, there are operator-dependent biases in the dSPM analysis method, and these can render its result subjectively biased. To address this problem, the AdSPM analysis was developed. For AdSPM analysis, the resulting dSPM estimates at each time point and at each cortical location are summed across all analyzed spikes, and the largest threshold such that only a single contiguous suprathreshold patch remained is considered as the spike source. The AdSPM technique can be usefully applied for the prediction of epileptogenic regions, with deep-seated FCD presenting scattered or mixed dipoles when the ECD method is used.

12.3. OLIGODENDROGLIOSIS

Clusters of oligodendroglia-like cells (OLCs) constitute a benign condition and are frequently observed in patients with epilepsy. Primarily, oligodendrocytes have the same role as the myelinating cells of the central nervous system, which is essential for signal transduction, and they are the end product of a cell lineage that has to undergo a complex and precisely timed program of proliferation, migration, differentiation, and myelination to finally produce the insulating sheath of axons (Bradl & Lassmann, 2010). Considering that epilepsy requires functionally and anatomically abnormal neuronal networks to propagate seizures, it can be assumed that abnormalities in oligodendrocytes can create abnormal epileptic networks. Aberrant oligodendrocytes are frequently found in various focal epilepsies, including oligodendroglial hamartoma, temporal lobe epilepsy, and low-grade glioma with an oligodendroglial component. Imaging findings of oligodendroglial hyperplasia are usually similar to FCD type I, showing decreased gray-white matter signal differentiation and signal alteration within subcortical white matter on a high-resolution MRI (Schurr et al., 2017).

Although OLCs have similar morphology and myelination activity to oligodendrocytes, there are some differences between normal oligodendrocytes and OLCs. The property that distinguishes OLCs from oligodendrocytes best is the immunoreactivity to Olig2. Olig2 is known to play a central role in directing cell fate choices and controlling cell proliferation during embryogenesis, and it directs the formation of oligodendrocyte precursors and mature oligodendrocytes later in development (Gaber & Novitch, 2011). Under pathological conditions, Olig2 overexpression in oligodendroglial lineage promotes oligodendroglial precursor cell migration and differentiation into mature oligodendrocytes, and subsequently leads to precocious central nervous system myelination (Wegener et al., 2014). Considering that proliferation of pathological networks between epileptogenic regions can lead to generalized epilepsy syndromes, it can be assumed that OLCs that overexpress Olig2 may contribute to the creation of interconnections among regions that constitute the epileptogenic zone. However, it remains unclear whether increased OLCs are the cause or the consequence of generalized epileptogenesis.

In pediatric patients requiring epilepsy surgery for intractable seizures, OLCs across cortical and subcortical regions are increased compared with nonepileptic cortex regardless of the cause of the epilepsy (Sakuma, Halliday, Nomura, Ochi, & Otsubo, 2014). Sakuma et al. (2016) investigated surgical specimens from 30 children who underwent epilepsy surgery and assessed the relationship between the presence of OLCs and the semiology of epilepsy (i.e., EEG and MRI findings, extent of surgical resection, and seizure outcome). In this study, the authors found that increased OLC population in the white matter and at the junction of white and gray matter was closely related to epileptic spasm (ES). EEG had the tendency to show nonfocal interictal patterns, and the probability of multilobar resection was increased when OLC population in white matter was increased. These findings suggested that the interrelation between epileptogenic neurons and abnormal myelination of OLCs might play a role in connecting the extensive epileptogenic zone, which can contribute to the development of ES.

Clusters of OLCs have been recently introduced as a disease entity, and MEG findings of this are rarely investigated. However, based on the previous facts, it is suggested that MEG in oligodendrogliosis will show a wider distribution of epileptic dipoles. In cases of epileptic spasms, it has been recognized that there exist unique neurophysiological profiles. Asano et al. (2005) analyzed the cortical involvement pattern of ES-associated spikes using intracranial electrodes and found that the spikes came from the same lobe; however, they varied in their extent of cortical involvement. MEG studies in ES reported similar findings to those from intracranial EEG recordings, such as clustered MEG dipoles with or without scattering in one hemisphere and paroxysmal fast activity generally confined in one hemisphere (Kakisaka et al., 2011; RamachandranNair et al., 2008; Sueda et al., 2013). In our experience, MEG patterns seen in patients with clusters of OLCs showed differential findings, which was similar to the findings of MEG in ES. As in focal epilepsies, MEG usually leads EEG. The MEG dipole in this condition presented in clusters, and epileptiform dipoles could be confined to one hemisphere with or without scattering. Spike and slow waves were not frequently observed in MEG, and trains of spikes were a more common feature.

12.4. FILAMINOPATHY WITH ASTROCYTIC INCLUSIONS

Recently, there has been increasing interest in astrocytic inclusions (AIs) and their relationship with medically refractory epilepsy in childhood. AIs in brain tissues are more commonly observed in inclusion-bearing disorders such as neurodegenerative tauopathies, synucleinopathies, and polyglutamine disease. And, if the inclusions are located exclusively in astrocytes, Rosenthal fibers in Alexander disease and eosinophilic granular bodies in astrocytic neoplasms could be suspected. However, it has been recognized that some brain tissues from epilepsy patients also have AIs, and there has been increasing evidences that AIs contained substances that might affect epileptogenesis or epileptic networks (Horoupian, Hattab, & Heit, 2003; Kato et al., 1992; Minagawa, Shioda, Shimizu, & Isshiki, 1992). There was an investigation about the content of the AIs by Hazrati et al. (2008). They used light and electron microscopic examination of the surgical specimens from five pediatric patients with early-onset intractable seizures and mild to moderate developmental delay who displayed AIs. In this study, they found that these inclusions were almost exclusively juxtanuclear, highly refractile, spared distal subpial, or perivascular astrocytic processes and were strongly and exclusively immunopositive for filamin A, an actin-binding protein involved in neuronal migration. That finding suggested that intractable epilepsy with AIs can be regarded as a spectrum of disease of filamin or filamin-interaction proteins.

Filamin A is a member of a family of genetically highly conserved filamin proteins that are widely expressed during development (Feng & Walsh, 2004). Filamins are large cytoplasmic proteins with an important role in actin cross-linking; they are thought to be essential for mammalian cell locomotion and for serving as interfaces for protein–protein interactions. Indeed, they have been reported to interact with more than 30 functionally diverse proteins, and if the function of filamin is lost, it is impossible to create peripheral actin gel networks by orthogonal cross-linking of actin filaments (Stossel et al., 2001). Null and missense mutations in filamin A and B are known to cause a wide range of developmental malformations of brain, bone, and other organs. And, in cases with filaminopathy having AIs containing filamin A and accompanied by epilepsy, the clinical course was characterized by early onset (before 6 months of age) of refractory epilepsy presenting as clusters of epileptic spasms, global developmental delay, abnormal neuroimaging, and initial focal surgical resection failure (Whitney et al., 2017).

To our knowledge, there are no established diagnostic criteria of filaminopathy with AIs except for pathology examination. However, some findings from clinical semiology, EEG, MRI, and MEG can suggest the diagnosis of filaminopathy with AIs. Alshafai et al. (2014) compared the presurgical evaluations and surgical outcomes between six children with filaminopathy with AIs and 27 children with FCD. According to the results of this study, there were some similarities on the clinical, EEG, and MRI findings between filaminopathy with AIs and FCD. However, epilepsy patients with AIs were more likely to present with early-onset periodic spasms and to have unusual interictal epileptiform discharges, abnormal sulcation, and gyration pattern and gray matter heterotopia. MEG shows diffuse scattered dipoles rather than clusters of dipoles in most of the cases with hemispheric high-amplitude spikes, and the lesion did not express a spike and slow wave pattern on MEG. In this view, filaminopathy with AIs is expected to be associated with diffuse/hemispheric epileptic encephalopathy, although whether filaminopathy is the cause or the consequences of epileptogenicity and formation of diffuse epileptic networks is still unclear. If the patients have a hemispheric epileptogenic zone, surgical intervention can be helpful, although it needs more extensive resection or hemispherectomy.

12.5. STRATEGY OF EPILEPSY SURGERY AND MAGNETOENCEPHALOGRAPHY FOR PEDIATRIC EPILEPSY PATIENTS

The most common pathological finding in pediatric epilepsy surgery is FCD, and resective surgery can give a chance of cure to the patients (Hidalgo & Weiner, 2017). The International League Against Epilepsy recommends multimodal imaging including EEG, MRI, MEG,

and fluorodeoxyglucose (FDG)-PET as valuable tools for improving the rate of seizure freedom or reducing postoperative neurological deficits. A better understanding of MEG use in evaluation of children for epilepsy surgery will be beneficial because the volume of presurgical candidates is growing over time (Cloppenborg et al., 2016; Guerrini et al., 2015). The seizure-free rate after surgical resection for FCD is greater than 60%, and complete resection of epileptogenic area and unilobar localization are regarded as positive prognostic factors after surgical resection, even though various other factors can affect the surgical outcomes. Withdrawal of anticonvulsant medication can be achieved more frequently in patients with FCD type 2 compared with FCD type 1 (Fauser et al., 2015). In this view, comprehensive analysis for the prediction of the epileptogenic region and pathology can play a key role for successful epilepsy surgery.

Many clinical and diagnostic data can offer clues for these predictions. The history of seizures might indicate the network of the epilepsy, and the developmental status or intellectual functioning could indicate the influence of the epileptic brain on the normal/nonepileptic brain. MRI can show anatomic abnormalities; however, a lesion visible on MRI can be either epileptogenic or nonepileptogenic. PET can demonstrate dysfunctional brain areas, which typically are more extensive than the epileptogenic zone. Ictal single photon emission computed tomography (SPECT) can identify the ictal onset zone during seizures, and a repeat ictal SPECT can give critical information even for the most controversial cases (Takayama et al., 2018). MEG is one of the source localization tools for the epileptiform discharges, and the high spatial and temporal resolution of MEG superimposed on MRI improves the accuracy of the localization of the sources of epileptiform discharges. Even in single-lesion epilepsy cases, MEG can demonstrate asymmetric epileptogenic zones around the lesion, which influences the surgical approach (Otsubo et al., 2001) The interictal spike sources on MEG can be located in the epileptogenic, ictal onset, ictal symptomatogenic, or irritative zone (Rosenow & Lüders, 2001). However, considering that the epileptiform discharges are expressions of neuronal activity of the various zones within the epileptic network, epileptic dipoles on MEG can only represent one part of the epileptic network.

The diagnostic findings among imaging methods are not always concordant, and discordant findings can affect the decision-making process in epilepsy management. If there are concordant findings, a short history of seizures, and focal-onset seizures without cognitive delay, it is easy to make treatment plans for epilepsy surgery. On the contrary, if there are discordant findings, such as can be seen in cases with lesions that are separate or not wholly overlapping with the expected epileptic networks, or if the child has multiple types of seizures with cognitive delay, this can render the delineation of the resection margin difficult.

As described earlier, FCD, oligodendrogliosis, and filaminopathy with AIs have different histories, semiologies, EEG patterns, and MEG findings, although the findings are not always concordant. Considering that each epilepsy case entails a different degree of epileptogenicity, relevant epileptogenic networks, and optimal extents of surgical resection, comprehensive examination of the available clinical and diagnostic data is necessary for more accurate prediction of epileptogenic pathology. For example, the extent of epileptogenic area is most limited in FCD type 2, whereas filaminopathy with AIs tends to have wider epileptogenic networks. Therefore, the extent of epilepsy surgery for filaminopathy with AIs should be more extensive than FCD type 2.

12.6. CONCLUSION

Prediction of epileptogenic pathology is still challenging. However, because optimal treatment strategies for each epilepsy type are quite different, we should keep trying to identify the epileptogenic pathology and localize the epileptic networks before surgical resection. Many diagnostic modalities are applied for achieving these aims because it is still difficult to achieve them through the use of a single modality. Comprehensive understanding of MEG, EEG, MRI, PET, and SPECT, along with neuropsychology, clinical history, and seizure history and semiology, can provide clues for predicting not only the epileptogenic zone but also epileptogenic pathology, and among them, MEG can play a major role in the child with epilepsy.

REFERENCES

Alshafai, L., Ochi, A., Go, C., McCoy, B., Hawkins, C., Otsubo, H., . . . Widjaja, E. (2014). Clinical, EEG, MRI, MEG, and surgical outcomes of pediatric epilepsy with astrocytic inclusions versus focal cortical dysplasia. *Epilepsia, 55*(10), 1568–1575.

Asano, E., Juhász, C., Shah, A., Muzik, O., Chugani, D. C., Shah, J., . . . Chugani, H. T. (2005). Origin and propagation of epileptic spasms delineated on electrocorticography. *Epilepsia, 46*(7), 1086–1097.

Bagic, A. I., Knowlton, R. C., Rose, D. F., Ebersole, J. S., & ACMEGS Clinical Practice Guideline Committee. (2011). American Clinical Magnetoencephalography Society clinical practice guideline 1: Recording and analysis of spontaneous cerebral activity. *Journal of Clinical Neurophysiology, 28*(4), 348–354.

Bearden, D. R., Ciccone, O., & Patel AA. (2018). Global health: Pediatric neurology. *Semin Neurol, 38,* 200–207.

Blümcke, I., Thom, M., Aronica, E., Armstrong, D. D., Vinters, H. V., Palmini, A., . . . Battaglia, G. (2011). The clinicopathologic spectrum of focal cortical dysplasias: A consensus classification proposed by an ad hoc task force of the ILAE Diagnostic Methods Commission 1. *Epilepsia, 52*(1), 158–174.

Bradl, M., & Lassmann, H. (2010). Oligodendrocytes: Biology and pathology. *Acta Neuropathologica, 119*(1), 37–53.

Chassoux, F., Landré, E., Mellerio, C., Turak, B., Mann, M. W., Daumas-Duport, C., . . . Devaux, B. (2012). Type II focal cortical dysplasia: Electroclinical phenotype and surgical outcome related to imaging. *Epilepsia, 53*(2), 349–358.

Cloppenborg, T., May, T. W., Blümcke, I., Grewe, P., Hopf, L. J., Kalbhenn, T., . . . Woermann, F. G. (2016). Trends in epilepsy surgery: Stable surgical numbers despite increasing presurgical volumes. *J Neurol Neurosurg Psychiatry, 87*(12), 1322–1329.

Cooper, R., Winter, A., Crow, H., & Walter, W. G. (1965). Comparison of subcortical, cortical and scalp activity using chronically indwelling electrodes in man. *Electroencephalography and Clinical Neurophysiology, 18*(3), 217–228.

Cross, J. H., Jayakar, P., Nordli, D., Delalande, O., Duchowny, M., Wieser, H. G., . . . Mathern, G. W. (2006). Proposed criteria for referral and evaluation of children for epilepsy surgery: Recommendations of the Subcommission for Pediatric Epilepsy Surgery. *Epilepsia, 47*(6), 952–959.

Dale, A. M., Liu, A. K., Fischl, B. R., Buckner, R. L., Belliveau, J. W., Lewine, J. D., & Halgren, E. (2000). Dynamic statistical parametric mapping: combining fMRI and MEG for high-resolution imaging of cortical activity. *Neuron, 26*(1), 55–67.

Del Felice, A., Beghi, E., Boero, G., La Neve, A., Bogliun, G., De Palo, A., & Specchio, L. M. (2010). Early versus late remission in a cohort of patients with newly diagnosed epilepsy. *Epilepsia, 51*(1), 37–42.

Fauser, S., Essang, C., Altenmüller, D. M., Staack, A. M., Steinhoff, B. J., Strobl, K., . . . Wiegand, G. (2015). Long-term seizure outcome in 211 patients with focal cortical dysplasia. *Epilepsia, 56*(1), 66–76.

Feng, Y., & Walsh, C. A. (2004). The many faces of filamin: A versatile molecular scaffold for cell motility and signalling. *Nature Cell Biology, 6*(11), 1034.

Gaber, Z. B., & Novitch, B. G. (2011). All the embryo's a stage, and Olig2 in its time plays many parts. *Neuron, 69*(5), 833–835.

Guerrini, R., Duchowny, M., Jayakar, P., Krsek, P., Kahane, P., Tassi, L., . . . Cepeda, C. (2015). Diagnostic methods and treatment options for focal cortical dysplasia. *Epilepsia, 56*(11), 1669–1686.

Halac, G., Delil, S., Zafer, D., Isler, C., Uzan, M., Comunoglu, N., . . . Halac, M. (2017). Compatibility of MRI and FDG-PET findings with histopathological results in patients with focal cortical dysplasia. *Seizure-European Journal of Epilepsy, 45*, 80–86.

Hazrati, L.-N., Kleinschmidt-DeMasters, B., Handler, M. H., Smith, M. L., Ochi, A., Otsubo, H., . . . Hawkins, C. E. (2008). Astrocytic inclusions in epilepsy: Expanding the spectrum of filaminopathies. *Journal of Neuropathology & Experimental Neurology, 67*(7), 669–676.

Hidalgo, E. T., & Weiner, H. L. (2017). Surgery for epileptogenic cerebral dysplasia in children. *Developmental Medicine & Child Neurology, 59*(3), 270–275.

Horoupian, D. S., Hattab, E. M., & Heit, G. (2003). Astrocytic cytoplasmic inclusions within an epileptic focus in an otherwise neurologically intact patient. *Human Pathology, 34*(7), 714–716.

Ito, T., Otsubo, H., Shiraishi, H., Yagyu, K., Takahashi, Y., Ueda, Y., . . . Kohsaka, S. (2015). Advantageous information provided by magnetoencephalography for patients with neocortical epilepsy. *Brain and Development, 37*(2), 237–242.

Jobst, B. C., & Cascino, G. D. (2015). Resective epilepsy surgery for drug-resistant focal epilepsy: a review. *JAMA, 313*(3), 285–293.

Jonas, R., Asarnow, R., LoPresti, C., Yudovin, S., Koh, S., Wu, J., . . . Mathern, G. (2005). Surgery for symptomatic infant-onset epileptic encephalopathy with and without infantile spasms. *Neurology, 64*(4), 746–750.

Kakisaka, Y., Gupta, A., Wang, Z. I., Dubarry, A.-S., Alexopoulos, A. V., Mosher, J. C., & Burgess, R. C. (2011). Different cortical involvement pattern of generalized and localized spasms: A magnetoencephalography study. *Epilepsy & Behavior, 22*(3), 599–601.

Kato, S., Hirano, A., Umahara, T., Herz, F., Shioda, K., & Minagawa, M. (1992). Immunohistochemical studies on the new type of astrocytic inclusions identified in a patient with brain malformation. *Acta Neuropathologica, 84*(4), 449–452.

Lerner, J. T., Salamon, N., Hauptman, J. S., Velasco, T. R., Hemb, M., Wu, J. Y., . . . Fried, I. (2009). Assessment and surgical outcomes for mild type I and severe type II cortical dysplasia: A critical review and the UCLA experience. *Epilepsia, 50*(6), 1310–1335.

Liu, A. K., Dale, A. M., & Belliveau, J. W. (2002). Monte Carlo simulation studies of EEG and MEG localization accuracy. *Human Brain Mapping, 16*(1), 47–62.

Merlet, I., & Gotman, J. (1999). Reliability of dipole models of epileptic spikes. *Clinical Neurophysiology, 110*(6), 1013–1028.

Minagawa, M., Shioda, K., Shimizu, Y., & Isshiki, T. (1992). Inclusion bodies in cerebral cortical astrocytes: A new change of astrocytes. *Acta Neuropathologica, 84*(1), 113–116.

Murakami, H., Wang, Z. I., Marashly, A., Krishnan, B., Prayson, R. A., Kakisaka, Y., . . . Bingaman, W. E. (2016). Correlating magnetoencephalography to stereo-electroencephalography in patients undergoing epilepsy surgery. *Brain, 139*(11), 2935–2947.

Nakajima, M., Widjaja, E., Baba, S., Sato, Y., Yoshida, R., Tabei, M., . . . Ochi, A. (2016). Remote MEG dipoles in focal cortical dysplasia at bottom of sulcus. *Epilepsia, 57*(7), 1169–1178.

Oishi, M., Otsubo, H., Kameyama, S., Morota, N., Masuda, H., Kitayama, M., & Tanaka, R. (2002). Epileptic spikes: Magnetoencephalography versus simultaneous electrocorticography. *Epilepsia, 43*(11), 1390–1395.

Okanishi, T., Akiyama, T., Mayo, E., Honda, Y., Ueda-Kawada, C., Nakajima, M., . . . Widjaja, E. (2016). Magnetoencephalography spike sources interrelate the extensive epileptogenic zone of tuberous sclerosis complex. *Epilepsy Research, 127,* 302–310.

Otsubo, H., Ochi, A., Elliott, I., Chuang, S. H., Rutka, J. T., Jay, V., . . . Snead, O. C. (2001). MEG predicts epileptic zone in lesional extrahippocampal epilepsy: 12 pediatric surgery cases. *Epilepsia, 42*(12), 1523–1530.

Palmini, A., & Holthausen, H. (2013). Focal malformations of cortical development: A most relevant etiology of epilepsy in children. *Handbook of Clinical Neurology, 111,* 549–565.

Perucca, P., Dubeau, F., & Gotman, J. (2014). Intracranial electroencephalographic seizure-onset patterns: effect of underlying pathology. *Brain, 137*(1), 183–196.

RamachandranNair, R., Ochi, A., Imai, K., Benifla, M., Akiyama, T., Holowka, S., . . . Otsubo, H. (2008). Epileptic spasms in older pediatric patients: MEG and ictal high-frequency oscillations suggest focal-onset seizures in a subset of epileptic spasms. *Epilepsy Research, 78*(2–3), 216–224.

RamachandranNair, R., Otsubo, H., Shroff, M. M., Ochi, A., Weiss, S. K., Rutka, J. T., & Snead, O. C., III. (2007). MEG predicts outcome following surgery for intractable epilepsy in children with normal or nonfocal MRI findings. *Epilepsia, 48*(1), 149–157.

Rosenow, F., & Lüders, H. (2001). Presurgical evaluation of epilepsy. *Brain, 124*(9), 1683–1700.

Sakuma, S., Halliday, W. C., Nomura, R., Baba, S., Sato, Y., Okanari, K., . . . Ochi, A. (2016). Increased subcortical oligodendroglia-like cells in pharmacoresistent focal epilepsy in children correlate with extensive epileptogenic zones. *Epilepsia, 57*(12), 2031–2038.

Sakuma, S., Halliday, W. C., Nomura, R., Ochi, A., & Otsubo, H. (2014). Increased population of oligodendroglia-like cells in pediatric intractable epilepsy. *Neuroscience Letters, 566,* 188–193.

Schurr, J., Coras, R., Rössler, K., Pieper, T., Kudernatsch, M., Holthausen, H., . . . Polster, T.

(2017). Mild malformation of cortical development with oligodendroglial hyperplasia in frontal lobe epilepsy: A new clinico-pathological entity. *Brain Pathology, 27*(1), 26–35.

So, E. L. (2000). Integration of EEG, MRI, and SPECT in localizing the seizure focus for epilepsy surgery. *Epilepsia, 41*(Suppl. 3), S48–S54.

Stossel, T. P., Condeelis, J., Cooley, L., Hartwig, J. H., Noegel, A., Schleicher, M., & Shapiro, S. S. (2001). Filamins as integrators of cell mechanics and signalling. *Nature Reviews Molecular Cell Biology, 2*(2), 138.

Sueda, K., Takeuchi, F., Shiraishi, H., Nakane, S., Sakurai, K., Yagyu, K., . . . Saitoh, S. (2013). Magnetoencephalographic analysis of paroxysmal fast activity in patients with epileptic spasms. *Epilepsy Research, 104*(1–2), 68–77.

Takayama, R., Imai, K., Ikeda, H., Baba, K., Usui, N., Takahashi, Y., & Inoue, Y. (2018). Successful hemispherotomy in two refractory epilepsy patients with cerebral hemiatrophy and contralateral EEG abnormalities. *Brain and Development, 40*(7), 601–606.

Tanaka, N., Cole, A. J., von Pechmann, D., Wakeman, D. G., Hämäläinen, M. S., Liu, H., . . . Stufflebeam, S. M. (2009). Dynamic statistical parametric mapping for analyzing ictal magnetoencephalographic spikes in patients with intractable frontal lobe epilepsy. *Epilepsy Research, 85*(2–3), 279–286.

Tanaka, N., Peters, J. M., Prohl, A. K., Takaya, S., Madsen, J. R., Bourgeois, B. F., . . . Stufflebeam, S. M. (2014). Clinical value of magnetoencephalographic spike propagation represented by spatiotemporal source analysis: correlation with surgical outcome. *Epilepsy Research, 108*(2), 280–288.

Tanaka, N., & Stufflebeam, S. M. (2014). Clinical application of spatiotemporal distributed source analysis in presurgical evaluation of epilepsy. *Frontiers in Human Neuroscience, 8,* 62.

Wegener, A., Deboux, C., Bachelin, C., Frah, M., Kerninon, C., Seilhean, D., . . . Nait-Oumesmar, B. (2014). Gain of Olig2 function in oligodendrocyte progenitors promotes remyelination. *Brain, 138*(1), 120–135.

Whitney, R., AlMehmadi, S., McCoy, B., Yau, I., Ochi, A., Otsubo, H., . . . Snead, O. C. (2017). The fault in their stars: Accumulating astrocytic inclusions associated with clusters of epileptic spasms in children with global developmental delay. *Pediatric Neurology, 73,* 92–97, e93.

13

REVISIONAL ANALYSIS OF ELECTROENCEPHALOGRAPHY AND MAGNETOENCEPHALOGRAPHY BASED ON COMPREHENSIVE EPILEPSY CONFERENCE

Nobukazu Nakasato, Akitake Kanno, Makoto Ishida,
Shin-ichiro Osawa, Masaki Iwasaki, Yosuke Kakisaka, and Kazutaka Jin

13.1. INTRODUCTION

Electroencephalography (EEG) and magnetoencephalography (MEG) are some of the most important modern methods for presurgical evaluation of epilepsy (Almubarak et al., 2014; Grondin et al., 2006; Iwasaki et al., 2002; Nakasato et al., 1994; So & Lee, 2014). However, analysis and interpretation of the EEG/MEG findings are not simple nor easy because the EEG/MEG sensors often fail to detect low-intensity deep brain activity, which is masked by the background brain noise (Iwasaki et al., 2005; Park et al., 2004), and any EEG/MEG source estimation method is affected by the "inverse problem" because no a priori information is available about the properties of the current sources, such as total numbers, amplitude, morphology, and orientation, and because the conductivity properties of the head are generally unknown for individual subjects (Bénar & Gotman, 2002; Haueisen, Böttner, Nowak, Brauer, & Weiller, 1999; von Helmholtz, 1853). Consequently, clinical EEG/MEG analysis cannot be used as the only method of investigation.

Presently, EEG and MEG spike source estimation, anatomical magnetic resonance imaging (MRI), and ^{18}F-fluorodeoxyglucose positron emission tomography (FDG-PET) are the three major imaging methods for presurgical evaluation of epilepsy. The epileptogenic zone may be demonstrated by one or more of these methods. Therefore, combined use of these methods is strongly recommended before clinical decision-making (Brodbeck et al., 2010; Chassoux et al., 2010; Duez et al., 2019). For example, EEG/ MEG spike analysis is often useful to identify subtle MRI lesions even if the initial MRI examination found no abnormalities (Itabashi et al., 2014).

Nobukazu Nakasato, Akitake Kanno, Makoto Ishida, Shin-ichiro Osawa, Masaki Iwasaki, Yosuke Kakisaka, and Kazutaka Jin, *Revisional Analysis of Electroencephalography and Magnetoencephalography Based on Comprehensive Epilepsy Conference* In: *Fifty Years of Magnetoencephalography*. Edited by: Andrew C. Papanicolaou, Timothy P. L. Roberts, and James W. Wheless, Oxford University Press (2020). © Oxford University Press. DOI: 10.1093/oso/9780190935689.003.0013.

Our experience also suggests that seizure semiology, MRI, and/or FDG-PET findings are often important to optimize EEG/MEG source analysis (Figure 13.1). However, most

previous clinical EEG/MEG studies have been designed to evaluate the diagnostic value independently from other imaging methods (Duez et al., 2019; Lau, Yam, & Burneo, 2008). In this chapter, we highlight the importance of the revised analysis of EEG/MEG spike source estimation based on comprehensive case conference discussion.

13.2. CASE 1: A SIMPLE SITUATION

A right-handed 19-year-old man had suffered from hyper-motor seizures during night sleep since age 11 years. His seizures became intractable at age 15 years despite administration of eight different antiepileptic drugs. He underwent in-hospital comprehensive study in our epilepsy center at age 19 years.

Scalp EEG indicated interictal spikes in the frontotemporal area, with the highest negative peak located in the left frontal pole area. However, scalp EEG showed that ictal onset of his habitual seizures was not clearly localized. Equivalent current dipoles of interictal MEG spikes were localized on the bilateral (interhemispheric) anterior cingulate areas with horizontal (left/right to right/left) current orientations (Figure 13.2E). Therefore, the maximum negative peak over the left frontal pole area was interpreted as paradoxical lateralization caused by the right interhemispheric source in the scalp EEG.

Fluid-attenuated inversion recovery (FLAIR) MRI showed blurred margin and abnormal high intensity of white matter in the medial aspect of the right anterior cingulate area (see Figure 13.2A). FDG-PET showed hypometabolism in the interhemispheric side of the right anterior cingulate area (see Figure 13.2B and D). Therefore, all of the EEG, MEG, anatomical MRI, and FDG-PET findings agreed completely, indicating the epileptogenic area was located in the mesial aspect of the right frontal lobe.

The patient underwent chronic implantation of subdural electrodes. Intracranial EEG

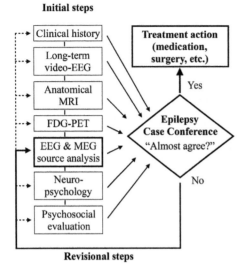

FIGURE 13.1 Clinical decision-making at the Department of Epileptology, Tohoku University Hospital. During 2-week admission, all patients undergo (1) clinical history-taking by physicians, nurses, and psychologists; (2) long-term video-electroencephalography (EEG) monitoring for 4 days; (3) anatomical magnetic resonance imaging (MRI) interpreted by radiologists; (4) ^{18}F-fluorodeoxyglucose positron emission tomography (FDG-PET) interpreted by radiologists; (5) simultaneous recordings of 42-channel scalp EEG and whole-head magnetoencephalography (MEG) using a 160- or 200-channel axial gradiometer system (MEG vision PQ1160C; Yokogawa Electric, Tokyo, Japan) in a magnetically shielded room; (6) neuropsychological evaluation; and (7) psychosocial evaluation. Epilepsy case conference is held every week to review all these reports. The discussion for 30 to 45 minutes per patient involves the neurologists, pediatrician, neurosurgeons, radiologists, psychiatrists, nurses, EEG technicians, pharmacologists, psychologists, and social workers, then the treatment is proposed, such as medication, surgery, psychotherapy, and social care. If some of the initial results do not agree with the others, revisional analysis with or without additional study is recommended. Overall, EEG/MEG spike source analysis is the most difficult method to interpret because this is most often considered to require revisional analysis after the first case conference.

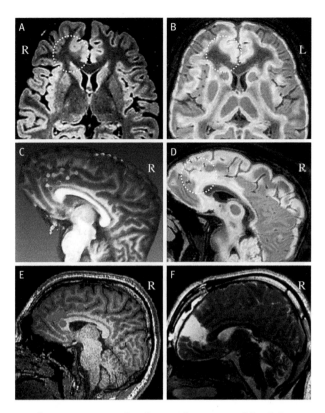

FIGURE 13.2 Summary of neuroimaging study of case 1. This 19-year-old male became seizure-free after surgery. (A) Fluid-attenuated inversion recovery (FLAIR) magnetic resonance imaging (MRI) showing blurred margin and abnormal high intensity of white matter in the medial aspect of the right anterior cingulate area. (B and D) ^{18}F-fluorodeoxyglucose positron emission tomography (FDG-PET) scans showing hypometabolism of the interhemispheric side of the right anterior cingulate area. (C) Intracranial electroencephalography (EEG) studies revealing epileptic spike discharges most frequently in the medial aspect of the right frontal lobe (three red-labeled electrodes). (E) Equivalent current dipoles of interictal magnetoencephalography (MEG) spikes were estimated in the medial aspect of the bilateral (interhemispheric) anterior cingulate areas. (F) MRI after surgery showing the area of cortical resection. A part of the figures were reproduced by permission of the authors from a previous report (Osawa, S. I., Iwasaki, M., Takayama, Y., Jin, K., Nakasato, N., & Tominaga, T. [2018]. Surgical treatment of intractable epilepsy presenting with hyperkinetic seizures originating in the frontal lobe. *Japanese Journal of Neurosurgery [Tokyo]*, 27, 764–772.)

studies revealed that epileptic spike discharges were located most frequently in the medial aspect of the anterior cingulate area (see Figure 13.2C) corresponding to the presurgical interpretation of the anatomical MRI, FDG-PET, and MEG spike dipoles. Consequently, the patient underwent mesial frontal cortical resection (see Figure 13.2F) and achieved complete freedom from seizures.

In this relatively simple case, the EEG and MEG could be conclusively analyzed independently from the other studies.

13.3. CASE 2: A COMPLICATED SITUATION

A right-handed 16-year-old girl suffered from epigastric sensation followed by impaired consciousness and manual and oral automatism. She underwent an in-hospital comprehensive study in our epilepsy center at the age of 16 years.

MRI showed that the right hippocampus was abnormally larger than the left, and FLAIR imaging showed that the right hippocampus

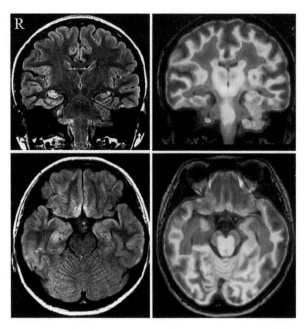

FIGURE 13.3   Magnetic resonance imaging (MRI) and ^{18}F-fluorodeoxyglucose positron emission tomography (FDG-PET) of case 2, a 16-year-old girl. (*Left*) Fluid-attenuated inversion recovery MRI showing enlargement of the right hippocampus. (*Right*) FDG-PET showing hypometabolism of the bilateral hippocampi, especially on the right.

also had increased signal intensity (Figure 13.3). FDG-PET showed hypometabolism of the right hippocampus (see Figure 13.3). All these findings corresponded to mesial temporal lobe epilepsy, as suggested by the seizure semiology.

Scalp EEG (Figure 13.4) indicated the highest negative peak of interictal spikes located in the right frontopolar area. The EEG single current dipole model revealed the radial (anterior-posterior) current source in the right frontal lobe (Figure 13.5 left). MEG spikes occurred as a vertical (inferior-superior) dipole pattern over the right frontotemporal area (see Figure 13.4) with equivalent current dipoles (ECDs) on the right orbitofrontal area (see Figure 13.5).

Long-term video and EEG monitoring recorded no habitual seizures during a 4-day period. Because seizure symptoms, anatomical MRI, and FDG-PET suggested typical mesial temporal lobe epilepsy, the second (revisional) EEG/MEG analysis was requested.

Principal component analysis (PCA) of the averaged spikes of EEG and MEG revealed the first largest (s1; 88.1% in EEG and 67% in MEG) as well as the earlier second largest (s2; 10.9% in EEG and 27.3% in MEG) components (see Figure 13.5, *right*). An ECD model of EEG (see Figure 13.5, *right upper*) and classical low-resolution electromagnetic topography analysis recursively applied (CLARA) of MEG (see Figure 13.5, *right lower*) estimated the s2 sources of EEG and MEG in the right temporal lobe. This patient became seizure-free after administration of perampanel.

Our case conference to discuss the admission study concluded that the patient had right mesial temporal lobe epilepsy with unknown etiology. However, our first EEG/MEG analysis did not correspond to our conclusion. Therefore, a second EEG/MEG study was recommended.

The second study (see Figure 13.5, *right*) using PCA of the averaged spikes identified the first biggest peak (s1; 88.1% in EEG and

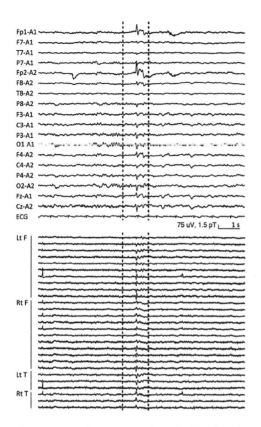

FIGURE 13.4   Electroencephalography (EEG) and magnetoencephalography (MEG) waveforms of case 2. Scalp EEG (*upper*) and MEG (*lower*) showing typical waveforms of an interictal epileptic spike. Note the relatively large peak-to-peak amplitude (>300 μV in scalp EEG and >2 pT in MEG) over the right frontal area.

67% in MEG) and the earlier second biggest peak (s2; 10.9% in EEG and 27.3% in MEG) components. The ECD model of EEG and the CLARA technique estimated the s2 sources in the right temporal lobe. No abnormal antibodies were found in the cerebrospinal fluid. The patient became seizure-free after administration of perampanel.

The EEG and MEG findings in this case were not simple or easy to interpret. The first EEG and MEG analysis did not agree with any of the seizure semiology, anatomical MRI, or FDG-PET results. Prospective studies with an ECD model, for either averaged spikes or nonaveraged single spikes, would indicate incorrect localization of the epileptogenic area in such a case.

13.4. FUTURE PERSPECTIVES FOR ELECTROENCEPHALOGRAPHY AND MAGNETOENCEPHALOGRAPHY ANALYSIS

This chapter discussed two typical cases of localization-related epilepsy: case 1 as a simple situation and case 2 as a complicated situation. No "gold standard" for epileptic spike analysis in EEG or MEG has been established, so several methods must be adopted to achieve the most reasonable interpretation. However, such intense and revisional analyses may be too time-consuming in clinical settings and result in arbitrary conclusions. Therefore, we currently use a simple method first, that is, a single dipole model for the peak or preceding upward slope of unaveraged single spikes. In the following case conference, EEG and MEG data are reviewed with seizure semiology, anatomical MRI, and FDG-PET studies. If all the findings almost agree, the clinical decision can be easily made. If not, revisional analysis of EEG/ MEG is recommended using averaged spikes and PCA models as well as distributed source models such as CLARA. In addition to EEG/ MEG, we often order revisional analysis and additional MRI and FDG-PET studies after the conference. Even history taking will be recommended if necessary.

We have recently introduced our teleconference system for the holding of epilepsy conferences (Figure 13.6). This system offers advantages for the clinical decision-making of each case and allows education of medical staff in our institute as well as other epilepsy centers in Japan, Asia, and even Canada (Kakisaka, Jin, Fujikawa, Kitazawa, & Nakasato, 2018). We appreciate that "no single method" has been established for epilepsy diagnosis. Integration of all available methods would obviously increase the quality of patient care. We also understand that "no perfect method" is available to interpret EEG and MEG findings. Consequently, case-based learning continues to be the best method for education of EEG and MEG

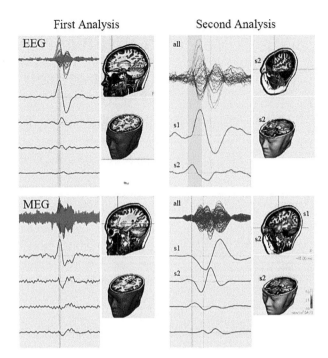

FIGURE 13.5 Comparison of first and second electroencephalography (EEG) and magnetoencephalography (MEG) analyses of case 2. The first EEG/MEG analysis (*left*) estimated the equivalent current dipole (ECD) of a single spike peak in the right frontal lobe with radial (anterior-posterior) orientation in EEG and tangential (inferior-superior) orientation in MEG, suggesting right frontal lobe epilepsy. Note the different source localization between the first and second analyses of EEG and MEG spikes (see text).

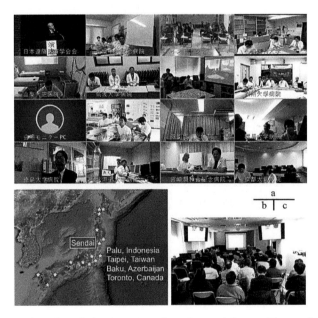

FIGURE 13.6 Snapshots from the Tohoku University tele-epilepsy conference. This conference is held every week using a teleconference system (Polycom HDX 8000; Polycom, Inc., Pleasanton, CA), a real-time multimedia conferencing platform with H.323 high-profile media cards, a high-definition digital camera, and high-quality audio system incorporating technologies for automatic background noise reduction and advanced echo cancellation. A 4 × 4 split screen mode (A) shows multiple connection sites in Japan and other countries (B). During the epilepsy case conference, the teleconference system enables all the participants to ask questions or to give comments freely, including the remote audience, simply by inactivating the "mute" button before speech, and for the in-person audience, simply by talking to the ceiling microphones (C) even without the chairperson's permission.

interpretation until prospective studies can be designed.

ACKNOWLEDGMENTS

This work was supported by Grants-in-Aids for Scientific Research (JP16H05435, 15K15521, and JP15K19143) from the Japan Society for the Promotion of Science and the S-Innovation program, Japan Science and Technology Agency (JST), and Center for Spintronics Research Network, Tohoku University. The authors thank Dr. Curtis Lowery (University of Arkansas) for providing the Polycom teleconference system. The authors also thank Mr. Yuji Ozaki for their support.

REFERENCES

Almubarak, S., Alexopoulos, A., Von-Podewils, F., Wang, Z. I., Kakisaka, Y., Mosher, J. C., . . . Burgess, R. C. (2014). The correlation of magnetoencephalography to intracranial EEG in localizing the epileptogenic zone: A study of the surgical resection outcome. *Epilepsy Research, 108,* 1581–1590.

Bénar, C. G., & Gotman, J. (2002). Modeling of postsurgical brain and skull defects in the EEG inverse problem with the boundary element method. *Clinical Neurophysiology, 113,* 48–56.

Brodbeck, V., Spinelli, L., Lascano, A. M., Pollo, C., Schaller, K., Vargas, M. I., . . . Seeck, M. (2010). Electrical source imaging for presurgical focus localization in epilepsy patients with normal MRI. *Epilepsia, 51,* 583–591.

Chassoux, F., Rodrigo, S., Semah, F., Beuvon, F., Landre, E., Devaux, B., . . . Chiron, C. (2010). FDG-PET improves surgical outcome in negative MRI Taylor-type focal cortical dysplasias. *Neurology, 75,* 2168–2175.

Duez, L., Tankisi, H., Hansen, P. O., Sidenius, P., Sabers, A., Pinborg, L. H., . . . Beniczky, S. (2019). Electromagnetic source imaging in presurgical workup of patients with epilepsy: A prospective study. *Neurology, 92,* e576–e586.

Grondin, R., Chuang, S., Otsubo, H., Holowka, S., Snead, O. C., III, . . . Rutka, J. T. (2006). The role of magnetoencephalography in pediatric epilepsy surgery. *Childs Nervous System, 22,* 779–785.

Haueisen, J., Böttner, A., Nowak, H., Brauer, H., & Weiller, C. (1999). The influence of conductivity changes in boundary element compartments on the forward and inverse problem in electroencephalography and magnetoencephalography. *Biomedical Technology (Berlin), 44,* 150–157.

Itabashi, H., Jin, K., Iwasaki, M., Okumura, E., Kanno, A., Kato, K., . . . Nakasato, N. (2014). Electro- and magneto-encephalographic spike source localization of small focal cortical dysplasia in the dorsal peri-rolandic region. *Clinical Neurophysiology, 125,* 2358–2363.

Iwasaki, M., Nakasato, N., Shamoto, H., Nagamatsu, K., Kanno, A., Hatanaka, K., & Yoshimoto, T. Surgical implications of neuromagnetic spike localization in temporal lobe epilepsy. *Epilepsia, 43,* 415–424.

Iwasaki, M., Pestana, E., Burgess, R. C., Luders, H. O., Shamoto, H., & Nakasato, N. (2005). Detection of epileptiform activity by human interpreters: blinded comparison between electroencephalography and magnetoencephalography. *Epilepsia, 46,* 59–68.

Kakisaka, Y., Jin, K., Fujikawa, M., Kitazawa, Y., & Nakasato, N. Teleconference-based education of epileptic seizure semiology. *Epilepsy Research, 145,* 73–76.

Lau, M., Yam, D., & Burneo, J. G. (2008). A systematic review on MEG and its use in the presurgical evaluation of localization-related epilepsy. *Epilepsy Research, 79,* 97–104.

Nakasato, N., Levesque, M. F., Barth, D. S., Baumgartner, C., Rogers, R. L., & Sutherling, W. W. (1994). Comparison of MEG, EEG, and ECoG source localization in neocortical partial epilepsy in humans. *Electroencephalography and Clinical Neurophysiology, 91,* 171–178.

Osawa, S. I., Iwasaki, M., Takayama, Y., Jin, K., Nakasato, N., & Tominaga, T. (2018). Surgical treatment of intractable epilepsy presenting with hyperkinetic seizures originating in the frontal lobe. *Japanese Journal of Neurosurgery (Tokyo), 27,* 764–772.

Park, H. M., Nakasato, N., Iwasaki, M., Shamoto, H., Tominaga, T., & Yoshimoto, T. (2004). Comparison of magnetoencephalographic spikes with and without concurrent electroencephalographic spikes in extratemporal epilepsy. *Tohoku Journal of Experimental Medicine, 203,* 165–174.

So, E. L., & Lee, R. W. (2014). Epilepsy surgery in MRI-negative epilepsies. *Current Opinions in Neurology, 27,* 206–212.

von Helmholtz, H. Uber einige Gesetze der Vertheilung elektrischer Ströme in körperlichen Leitern mit Anwendung auf die thierischelektrischen Versuche. (1853). *Annalen der Physik, 165*(6), 211–233.

14

EPILEPTIC SLOW WAVE ACTIVITY

Stefan Rampp and Martin Kaltenhäuser

14.1. BACKGROUND

Epilepsy surgery is a viable therapy option in a large percentage of patients suffering from pharmacoresistant epilepsies. Seizure freedom can be achieved in up to 85% depending on etiology (Blumcke et al., 2017; Rosenow & Lüders, 2001), although approximately 40% of patients develop recurrent seizures during the course of 2 to 5 years after surgery (de Tisi et al., 2011). In contrast, chances to become seizure-free if two or three antiepileptic drugs were not effective are below 3% (Mohanraj & Brodie, 2006).

Crucial to the success of epilepsy surgery is the exact localization of the epileptogenic zone, defined as the tissue that needs to be removed to stop the seizures (Rosenow & Lüders, 2001). While the epileptogenic zone is a theoretical concept that can only truly be defined retrospectively based on the postsurgical outcome, it can be approximated by determining the seizure onset zone.

Extensive evidence demonstrates that magnetoencephalography (MEG)-based source imaging (MSI) is able to estimate the epileptogenic zone by localization of interictal epileptic discharges (IEDs), such as epileptic spikes and sharp waves (Englot et al., 2015; Kreidenhuber et al., 2018; Rampp & Stefan, 2007; Stefan et al., 2003). Despite their interictal nature, resection of areas showing frequent IEDs is related to significantly improved postoperative outcome (Stefan et al., 2011). Also, over the course of several years after epilepsy surgery, patients with complete resection of robust MSI results show higher seizure freedom rates compared with patients with incomplete or lack of resection (Mu et al., 2014; Vadera et al., 2013).

With few exceptions, MEG recordings are limited to approximately 1 or 2 hours (De

Stefan Rampp and Martin Kaltenhäuser, *Epileptic Slow Wave Activity* In: *Fifty Years of Magnetoencephalography*. Edited by: Andrew C. Papanicolaou, Timothy P. L. Roberts, and James W. Wheless, Oxford University Press (2020). © Oxford University Press. DOI: 10.1093/oso/9780190935689.003.0014.

Tiège, Lundqvist, Beniczky, Seri, & Paetau, 2017). While longer recordings would be technically feasible, patients become increasingly uncomfortable and are less willing to remain in the scanner. Combined with the general irregularity of IED occurrence, about 20 to 30% of recordings show no or too few IEDs for MSI, and the MEG examination remains negative (Englot et al., 2015; Knake et al., 2006;Stefan et al., 2003).

A number of alternative markers for epileptic focus localization have been described, such as evaluation of fast activity (Rampp et al., 2010; van Klink, Hillebrand, & Zijlmans, 2016; von Ellenrieder et al., 2016; Xiang et al., 2009) or pathological distribution of connectivity (Krishnan et al., 2015). In addition to these comparably recent developments, activity in slow frequency bands in patients with focal epilepsy had been described already in the 1940s (Cobb, 1945) and even earlier in patients with brain tumors (Walter, 1936) and after traumatic brain injury (Jasper, Kershman, & Elvidge, 1940).

14.2. INTERMITTENT RHYTHMIC DELTA ACTIVITY

These early studies indicated that "waves of a period of about one-third of a second did tend to occur in bursts of fair regularity, both of period and of form" (Walter, 1936), which correspond to the family of intermittent rhythmic delta activity (IRDA) patterns on electroencephalography (EEG). Depending on their morphology and topography, subtypes have been recognized with different clinical implications.

IRDA (Cobb, 1945; Di Gennaro et al., 2003; Normand, Wszolek, & Klass, 1995; Reiher, Beaudry, & Leduc, 1989) occurring over the temporal lobes (temporal intermittent rhythmic delta activity, or TIRDA) has a high specificity for epilepsies involving the temporal mesial structures (Gambardella, Gotman, Cendes, & Andermann, 1995; Koutroumanidis et al., 2004) and has been described in up to about half of all patients with temporal lobe

epilepsy (TLE) (Reiher et al., 1989). It frequently displays a unilateral anterior temporal topography, although bilateral TIRDA may occur and is associated with IEDs (Normand et al., 1995; Reiher et al., 1989).

Occipital intermittent rhythmic delta activity (OIRDA) is also observed in patients with epilepsy, but almost exclusively in children (Brigo, 2011; Guilhoto, Manreza, & Yacubian, 2006; Watemberg, Linder, Dabby, Blumkin, & Lerman-Sagie, 2007). Watemberg et al. (2007) describe OIRDA in patients with absence and focal epilepsies and only a single case with encephalopathy. They found slightly faster frequencies (3–4 Hz) in children with absences compared with focal epilepsies (2–3 Hz). Furthermore, OIRDA in patients with absences frequently occurred with intermixed or "occult" IEDs. In contrast, OIRDA in focal epilepsies was not correlated to the timing of either IEDs or seizures. Neuroimaging was unremarkable in all cases with epilepsy and OIRDA.

In contrast, frontal intermittent rhythmic delta activity (FIRDA) does not show a clear association with epilepsy. It occurs in adults and has been described in association with a range of pathologies, such as tumors, edema, degenerative diseases, and metabolic disturbances. FIRDA has not been described in healthy subjects under physiological circumstances; however, hyperventilation may sometimes give rise to such intermittent delta over frontal regions (Accolla, Kaplan, Maeder-Ingvar, Jukopila, & Rossetti, 2011; Brigo, 2011). In patients without a lesion in neuroimaging, FIRDA is frequently associated with an altered state of consciousness (Fariello, Orrison, Blanco, & Reyes, 1982). Furthermore, IRDA and intermittent rhythmic theta activity (IRTA) are increased in patients with attention-deficit hyperactivity disorder (Endres et al., 2017).

Source localization data on IRDA is largely lacking, and evidence on underlying mechanisms is sparse. Similarly, studies using MEG are not available beyond the role of

FIRDA, for example, as nonepileptic variant (Rampp et al., 2018).

14.3. EPILEPSY-RELATED LOW-FREQUENCY MAGNETIC ACTIVITY OR "SLOW WAVE" ACTIVITY

Several studies applied source localization of MEG and EEG data to investigate so-called slow wave or low-frequency magnetic activity (LFMA) patterns. These terms refer to patterns in the delta and theta frequency ranges with some variation in the exact definition of frequency ranges.

Gallen, Tecoma, Iragui, Sobel, Schwartz, and Bloom (1997) reported detection of regional LFMA in 29 of 33 patients undergoing presurgical evaluation for epilepsy surgery. Ten patients had normal magnetic resonance imaging (MRI) results. LFMA had a sensitivity of 75.8% for the consensus of presurgical evaluation. Sensitivity was higher in patients with an abnormal MRI (87%) compared with patients with a normal MRI (50%). Of 20 patients with an Engel class 1 outcome (of 29 operated patients), LFMA localizations were completely concordant with consensus of presurgical evaluation in 11, partially in four, and inconclusive in the remainder. The results were comparable with long-term video-EEG monitoring and were surpassed only by invasive EEG evaluation.

Ishibashi et al. (2002) evaluated visually identified focal trains of low-frequency magnetic activity below 7 Hz (LFMA) in 29 patients with mesial temporal lobe epilepsy. All patients underwent epilepsy surgery. In 17 patients (58.6%), clear LFMA distinguishable from background activity was identified. LFMA showed a predominantly polymorphic appearance with no obvious differences regarding lateralization or localization of activity in the delta (1–3 Hz) and theta (4–7 Hz) frequency bands. Source localization was successful in all and yielded localizations in the lateral temporal lobe on the side of resection. Interestingly, there was no significant difference in comparison with IED localization. Histology confirmed mesial temporal sclerosis in all but three patients, in whom nonspecific gliotic changes were identified. The authors did not evaluate implications of resection of LFMA, respectively IEDs or lack thereof. However, all but five patients were seizure-free after surgery (Engel 1), which would not have enabled such a comparison. Simultaneous EEG was not recorded, preventing a direct comparison of LFMA to IRDA. However, the appearance in MEG, as well as the presence of mesial temporal sclerosis in most of the patients, suggests that the investigated LFMA may have been the magnetic counterpart of TIRDA.

Huppertz et al. (2001) evaluated focal delta activity in association with epileptogenic lesions using EEG source analysis. Both IEDs and delta patterns were identified visually; however, it remains unclear whether the focal delta activity corresponded to classical IRDA. Source analysis of both patterns localized into the lobe containing the lesion. In many cases, a distance of less than 10 mm to the lesion margin could be achieved. Patients with hippocampal atrophy or sclerosis, however, showed however larger distances to areas with focal delta activity, which were found in the adjacent temporal neocortex. Because similar studies are lacking, it remains unclear whether this finding is representative of TIRDA or whether the investigated delta activity constitutes a separate electrophysiological entity.

Overall, localization accuracy of IEDs and focal delta was comparable. Both types of activity revealed the location of the epileptogenic lesion with similar accuracy. Because Huppertz et al. investigated only patients with clear epileptogenic lesions, it is not possible to deduct whether the focal delta activity was caused by epileptic processes and was generated (e.g., in the irritative zone) or whether the slow oscillations must be regarded as a symptom of the lesion.

Vanrumste, Jones, Bones, and Carroll (2005) employed an automated method to detect epochs in EEG that are dominated by a single dipolar source. Their aim was to investigate occurrence and characteristics of activity from areas that also displayed IEDs and seizures. Visual inspection of the detected patterns revealed that while some of the events corresponded to IEDs, in five of eight patients, a notable percentage of patterns consisted of delta and theta waves. Notably, the detected patterns did not clearly correspond to classical IRDA.

Kaltenhäuser, Scheler, Rampp, Paulini, and Stefan (2007) also evaluated slow activity in patients undergoing presurgical evaluation for epilepsy surgery. The automated method provided a statistical overview of the quantity and distribution of activity in the frequency range between 2 and 6 Hz. Detection did not rely on specific morphological characteristics. In fact, the investigators state that some of the detected slow waves were subtle and not immediately apparent to visual inspection. In comparison with a group of healthy subjects, patients with epilepsy presented with significantly higher overall quantities of slow wave activity. The study evaluated patients with different etiologies and included cases with lesion and nonlesional TLE and extratemporal lobe epilepsy (ETLE). Average distance between center of mass of spike localizations and the maximum of the slow wave distribution amounted to 2 cm. Slow wave localizations overlapped with IED localizations and seemed to have a center of gravity in the margin of the IED localization clusters. Slow wave localizations were found in patients both with and without lesions on MRI.

In a follow-up study (Kaltenhäuser, Rampp, Ehrenfried, Heers, & Stefan, 2010), the results could be reproduced. In seven of 10 adult patients, significant increases of slow wave activity were detected, while only six presented with IEDs in MEG. In all seven patients, the slow wave localizations were concordant with findings of conventional presurgical evaluation. Epilepsy surgery resulted in seizure freedom or worthwhile improvement.

Recently, we implemented an automated method for detection and localization of increased focal delta based on frequency domain source imaging (Schönherr et al., 2017). The procedure leverages the significant contrast in slow wave activity between patients with focal epilepsy and healthy controls. We applied the method in patients with previous epilepsy surgery with and without recurrent seizures. Seizure-free patients after surgery still presented with significantly increased levels of focal delta. Because patients with previous brain surgery frequently show slowing over the area of surgery, this was an expected finding. However, patients with recurrent or persisting seizures after surgery exceeded these levels considerably. The overall level of delta could have enabled prediction of recurrent seizures with high specificity and sensitivity (area under the curve of receiver-operator statistics amounted to 0.84).

Furthermore, the study also included two patients who underwent invasive recordings. In both, delta increases were constrained to a few electrodes, which were overlapping with but not identical to areas showing IEDs. In one of the patients, frequent spiking occurred in most of the recorded contacts, while delta increases remained circumscribed. Three patients underwent a second surgery, which included areas of increased focal delta in two. Both were seizure-free after surgery, while the remaining patient did not experience any improvement. Although the sample of invasively recorded and/or operated patients was small, the results suggest a role of delta activity in epileptic processes rather than being only an epiphenomenon of a structural alteration.

Recently, Lin et al. (2018) evaluated the lateralization value of different frequency bands in patients with temporal lobe epilepsy. Etiologies included focal cortical dysplasia, hippocampal sclerosis, and ganglioglioma. Best lateralization values were found in the delta band, with correct results in 10 of 14 patients. Results of spike localizations and video-EEG monitoring were comparable. An additional interesting observation was rhythmic fluctuations of especially delta activity in the vicinity of the epileptogenic region. As in all patients, epileptogenic lesions were identified, but these results cannot resolve whether LFMA is primarily an epileptic or lesional phenomenon.

14.4. SLOW WAVE: EPILEPTIC ACTIVITY OR LESIONAL EPIPHENOMENON?

Slowing in patients with previous brain surgery is a phenomenon well known to clinical epileptologists (Di Gennaro et al., 2003). It is thought to result from disconnection of thalamic inputs to cortical networks, as already suggested by early studies in animal models (Ball, Gloor, & Schaul, 1977). Large lesions could similarly lead to anatomical or functional disconnection, including that due to tumor invasion or perilesional edema. However, this does not imply an interaction with preexisting epilepsy, such as resulting in more seizures or even only interictal activity. It also does not appear obvious how disconnection could lead to generation of epilepsy. Rather, for example, tumoral epileptogenesis is based on glutamatergic and γ-aminobutyric acid (GABA)ergic changes (Pallud, Capelle, & Huberfeld, 2013). Potentially, such alterations could also contribute to the generation of slow activity in EEG and MEG (Kamada et al., 2001).

Slow wave activity, however, has also been detected in patients without lesions (Kaltenhäuser et al., 2007, 2010). While subtle structural alterations may be present in these cases, it seems unlikely that such microscopic lesions are able to lead to disconnection to a degree that would then generate detectable slow activity.

Further evidence that not all of slow activity detected in patients with epilepsy is caused by a lesion or even previous surgery is that after epilepsy surgery, patients with recurrent seizures displayed significantly higher levels of delta than patients in whom the surgical procedure resulted in seizure freedom (Schönherr et al., 2017). According to these results,

postoperative delta may represent a mixture of two subtypes of slow activity: disconnection delta and delta related to epileptic processes.

Consequently, localization of delta in patients without lesions may indeed be an alternative to conventional spike or seizure analysis. In patients with lesional epilepsies, a portion of delta will be a correlate of the structural changes and disconnection, with respective limitations regarding the clinical interpretation. The intensity of focal slow activity may, however, enable distinction of lesional and epileptic slow wave, although corresponding intensity ranges or thresholds have not been elucidated.

14.5. NONEPILEPTIC, PATHOLOGICAL LOW-FREQUENCY MAGNETIC ACTIVITY

Slow activity in the delta and theta range has also been described in the context of other pathologies and is a phenomenon frequently encountered in cortex overlying white matter lesions (Gloor, Ball, & Schaul, 1977). Tumors are sometimes but not always associated with LFMA (Fernández-Bouzas et al., 1999) in the surrounding tissue (Baayen et al., 2003; Kamada et al., 2001; Oshino, Kato, Wakayama, Taniguchi, Hirata, & Yoshimine, 2007) only partially inside the tumor (Baayen et al., 2003). Spectroscopic imaging has demonstrated mild reduction of N-acetyl-aspartate (NAA) and slight accumulation of lactate in these areas, suggesting that LFMA may be an epiphenomenon of locally altered metabolism with lactic acidosis (Kamada et al., 2001) in addition to deafferentation and white matter lesions (Gloor et al., 1977). Edema may also give rise to slow activity, potentially with a peak frequency in the theta band (Fernández-Bouzas et al., 1999). Slow activity has also been reported in patients with traumatic brain injury (Lee & Huang, 2014; Modarres, Kuzma, Kretzmer, Pack, & Lim, 2016) and may be useful to support diagnosis even on a single subject level (Huang et al., 2014).

Independent of any obvious structural alterations, LFMA occurs in patients with dementias (Fernández et al., 2006, 2013), depression (Fernández et al., 2005), and schizophrenia (Fehr et al., 2003). Hypothetically, these observations could be based on pharmacological effects of medication. Fehr et al. (2003) compared LFMA in patients with and without neuroleptic medication and did not find a significant difference in delta or theta frequency bands. In contrast, the relative amount of LFMA correlated with the degree of negative symptoms. In another study, Rockstroh, Wienbruch, Ray, and Elbert (2007) showed that regions with abnormal slow wave activity in patients with schizophrenia correspond to areas that demonstrated gray matter loss, suggesting structural correlates of neuronal network disruption.

Based on currently available evidence, it seems unlikely that the pathological slow activity encountered in different diseases is generated by a single mechanism. Potentially, functional or structural deafferentation and pathological synchronization may represent a common denominator. The wide spectrum of diseases presenting with LFMA limits its specificity and thus its value in localization of focal epilepsies. Focal increases of LFMA should therefore always be interpreted in context with other clinical findings.

14.6. PROCEDURES

In the literature, mainly three procedures are applied to localize slow wave activity for epileptic focus localization. The following section gives an overview of the necessary steps.

14.6.1. Manual Selection and Dipole Localization

This procedure, as used by Ishibashi and Huppertz and their colleagues (Huppertz et al., 2001; Ishibashi et al., 2002), follows the methodology in conventional spike analysis. Patterns in the data are identified visually, usually with the help of frequency filters in the delta, theta, or complete slow wave frequency bands. Individual patterns may then be averaged or analyzed individually. Similar to spike analysis, averaging requires patterns with comparable topography and morphology as well as exact temporal alignment. The choice of the time segment for dipole fitting is of less importance if the identified patterns occur in an oscillatory fashion because the apparent onset of a single cycle depends more on the generator's orientation, phase, and sensor positioning than on propagation or lack thereof. If single delta or theta patterns occur as distinct transients, early time segments should be used because the point of maximal amplitude occurs comparably late in the time course and may thus already be influenced by propagation, similar to what can be expected in other IEDs (Mălîia et al., 2016). The quality of the resulting dipole localizations (regarding, e.g., goodness of fit or residual variance) should similarly be evaluated as in IED analysis (Bagić, Knowlton, Rose, & Ebersole, 2011).

14.6.2. Dipole Density

Kaltenhäuser et al. (2007, 2010) employed an automated method for slow wave detection and localization. The procedure filters the data between 2 and 6 Hz, although using delta- or theta-band filtering may also work. Subsequently, the data are divided into epochs approximately 10 seconds long. A principal component analysis (PCA) of these segments then allows identification of epochs with a single dominant component, suggesting that single dipole modeling may be adequate. Single dipoles are then fitted to each time point within these identified epochs. This results in a large number of dipoles, which are then thresholded according to their fit statistics. Kaltenhäuser et al. (2007) selected dipoles with a minimum correlation of 0.8 between measured and forward modeled field. The density of dipoles, that is, the percentage of dipoles per volume, is then calculated based on a three-dimensional grid with 1-mL voxels covering the intradural volume. The resulting distribution may then be further described by the summed percentage in the most active voxels or the number of voxels above a certain threshold, for example. The location of the maximum then indicates the focus localization. A limitation of the method as implemented by Kaltenhäuser et al. (2007, 2010) is that it was adapted to the sensor layout of a Magnes II system (4D Neuroimaging, San Diego, CA), which consists of two dewars with 37 channels each. This setup allowed only recordings from circumscribed regions of interest. Analytically, the 37 channels constitute a local channel selection, which is suited for dipole localization, if the gradient of a magnetic field is captured. If not, localizations frequently have low-fitting statistics and are rejected by the analysis procedure. In addition, the low number of channels affects the PCA, which more frequently identifies epochs with a dominant component, a side effect of the focused, regional recordings. Adaptation to modern whole-head systems likely would require additional steps or modification of the original method.

14.6.3. Dynamic Imaging of Coherent Sources

Dynamic imaging of coherent sources (DICS) allows imaging of coherent activity in the frequency domain (Gross et al., 2001). DICS can therefore be used to project sensor level slow wave activity into source space (Figure 14.1). Notably, DICS is robust not only for single or few dipolar sources but also for multifocal and distributed activity. The procedure uses several minutes of resting state data (Schönherr et al., 2017), subdivided into consecutive 5-second nonoverlapping epochs. Epochs with movement artifacts or external interference are rejected. The DICS results are then averaged over the frequency bands of interest, for example, 1 to 4 Hz for delta (Schönherr et al., 2017).

In patients with clear focal increases of delta activity, such as patients showing TIRDA already during visual inspection, the results may provide a good estimation of epilepsy-associated slow activity. However, subtle changes may be superimposed by delta oscillations of other pathological or

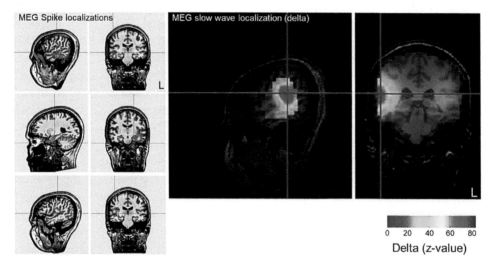

FIGURE 14.1   Example of slow wave localization using the dynamic imaging of coherent sources (DICS) method. The female patient suffered from a pharmacoresistant focal epilepsy since the age of 4 years. Imaging revealed a focal cortical dysplasia type IIb on the left coinciding with the slow wave localization (*right*). Electroencephalography (EEG) and magnetoencephalography (MEG) revealed frequent multifocal spike activity involving both hemispheres (*left*). Note that slow wave localizations show only a single maximum and no significant activation in other spiking areas. The lesion was small and only detected on specialized 3T magnetic resonance imaging including postprocessing.

physiological origins. The setting of resting-state recordings, for example, facilitates reduced vigilance and drowsiness of the patient. Frequently, patients fall asleep, which consequently results in slowing of brain activity, although the stage of slow wave sleep in usually not reached. To compensate such physiological slow wave activity and enhance potentially relevant subtle increases, DICS results can be related to a sample of healthy controls. This can be achieved by recording resting-state data in healthy subjects, using the same protocol, which is used for patients (e.g., 10 minutes, supine positioning, closed eyes, same sample rate and filter settings). All DICS data then need to be normalized to a common coordinate system, such as to an MNI aligned source space. The results of an individual patient can then be compared with healthy controls by z-transforming the data at each source location. Local maxima of the resulting distribution may then suggest the location of an epileptic focus. The total quantity of the DICS projected delta then also correlates with postoperative slowing and recurrent seizures after epilepsy surgery (Schönherr et al., 2017).

14.7. CONCLUSION

Slow wave activity in the delta and theta frequency bands represents an alternative marker of epileptic networks, which may contribute to focus localization in addition to source analysis of spikes and seizure patterns. It may also provide localizing information in cases with negative MEG, that is, without conventional ictal or interictal patterns. However, owing to the limited specificity, interpretation should always take the complete diagnostic context into account.

REFERENCES

Accolla, E. A., Kaplan, P. W., Maeder-Ingvar, M., Jukopila, S., & Rossetti, A. O. (2011). Clinical correlates of frontal intermittent rhythmic delta activity (FIRDA). *Clinical Neurophysiology, 122*, 27–31.

Baayen, J. C., de Jongh, A., Stam, C. J., de Munck, J. C., Jonkman, J. J., Trenité, D-N., . . . Vandertop, W. P. (2003). Localization of slow wave activity in patients with tumor-associated epilepsy. *Brain Topography, 16*, 85–93.

Bagić, A. I., Knowlton, R. C., Rose, D. F., & Ebersole, J. S. (2011). American Clinical Magnetoencephalography Society clinical practice guideline 1: Recording and analysis of spontaneous cerebral activity. *Journal of Clinical Neurophysiology, 28*, 348–354.

Ball, G. J., Gloor, P., & Schaul, N. (1977). The cortical electromicrophysiology of pathological delta waves in the electroencephalogram of cats. *Electroencephalography and Clinical Neurophysiology, 43*, 346–361.

Blumcke, I., Spreafico, R., Haaker, G., Coras, R., Kobow, K., Bien, C. G., . . . EEBB Consortium. (2017). Histopathological findings in brain tissue obtained during epilepsy surgery. *New England Journal of Medicine, 377*, 1648–1656.

Brigo, F. (2011). Intermittent rhythmic delta activity patterns. *Epilepsy Behavior, 20*, 254–256.

Cobb, W. A. (1945). Rhythmic slow discharges in the electro-encephalogram. *Journal of Neurology, Neurosurgery, and Psychiatry, 8*, 65–78.

De Tiège, X., Lundqvist, D., Beniczky, S., Seri, S., & Paetau, R. (2017). Current clinical magnetoencephalography practice across Europe: Are we closer to use MEG as an established clinical tool? *Seizure, 50*, 53–59.

de Tisi, J., Bell, G. S., Peacock, J. L., McEvoy, A. W., Harkness, W. F., Sander, J. W., & Duncan, J. S. (2011). The long-term outcome of adult epilepsy surgery, patterns of seizure remission, and relapse: a cohort study. *Lancet, 378*, 1388–1395.

Di Gennaro, G., Quarato, P. P., Onorati, P., Colazza, G. B., Mari, F., Grammaldo, L. G., . . . Esposito, V. (2003). Localizing significance of temporal intermittent rhythmic delta activity (TIRDA) in drug-resistant focal epilepsy. *Clinical Neurophysiology, 114*, 70–78.

Endres, D., Maier, S., Feige, B., Mokhtar, N. B., Nickel, K., Goll, P., . . . Tebartz van Elst, L. (2017). Increased rates of intermittent rhythmic delta and theta activity in the electroencephalographies of adult patients with attention-deficit hyperactivity disorder. *Epilepsy Behavior, 75*, 60–65.

Englot, D. J., Nagarajan, S. S., Imber, B. S., Raygor, K. P., Honma, S. M., Mizuiri, D., . . . Chang, E. F. (2015). Epileptogenic zone localization using magnetoencephalography predicts seizure freedom in epilepsy surgery. *Epilepsia, 56*, 949–958.

Fariello, R. G., Orrison, W., Blanco, G., & Reyes, P. F. (1982). Neuroradiological correlates of frontally predominant intermittent rhythmic delta activity (FIRDA). *Electroencephalography and Clinical Neurophysiology, 54,*194–202.

Fehr, T., Kissler, J., Wienbruch, C., Moratti, S., Elbert, T., Watzl, H., . . . Gerretsen, P. (2003). Source distribution of neuromagnetic slow-wave activity in schizophrenic patients: Effects of activation. *Schizophrenia Research, 63,* 63–71.

Fernández-Bouzas, A., Harmony, T., Bosch, J., Aubert, E., Fernández, T., Valdés, P., . . . Topjian, A. A. (1999). Sources of abnormal EEG activity in the presence of brain lesions. *Clinical Electroencephalography, 30,* 46–52.

Fernández, A., Rodriguez-Palancas, A., López-Ibor, M., Zuluaga, P., Turrero, A., Maestú, F., . . . Ortiz, T. (2005). Increased occipital delta dipole density in major depressive disorder determined by magnetoencephalography. *Journal of Psychiatry and Neuroscience, 30,* 17–23.

Fernández, A., Turrero, A., Zuluaga, P., Gil-Gregorio, P., del Pozo, F., Maestu, F., & Moratti, S. (2013). MEG delta mapping along the healthy aging–Alzheimer's disease continuum: Diagnostic implications. *Journal of Alzheimer's Disease, 35,* 495–507.

Fernández, A., Turrero, A., Zuluaga, P., Gil, P., Maestú, F., Campo, P., & Ortiz, T. (2006). Magnetoencephalographic parietal δ dipole density in mild cognitive impairment. *Archives of Neurology, 63,* 427.

Gallen, C. C., Tecoma, E., Iragui, V., Sobel, D. F., Schwartz, B. J., & Bloom, F. E. (1997). Magnetic source imaging of abnormal low-frequency magnetic activity in presurgical evaluations of epilepsy. *Epilepsia, 38,* 452–460.

Gambardella, A., Gotman, J., Cendes, F., & Andermann, F. (1995). Focal intermittent delta activity in patients with mesiotemporal atrophy: A reliable marker of the epileptogenic focus. *Epilepsia, 36,* 122–129.

Gloor, P., Ball, G., & Schaul, N. (1977). Brain lesions that produce delta waves in the EEG. *Neurology, 27,* 326–333.

Gross, J., Kujala, J., Hamalainen, M., Timmermann, L., Schnitzler, A., & Salmelin, R. (2001). Dynamic imaging of coherent sources: Studying neural interactions in the human brain. *Proceedings of the National Academy of Science, 98,* 694–699.

Guilhoto, L. M. F. F., Manreza, M. L. G., & Yacubian, E. M. T. (2006). Occipital intermittent rhythmic delta activity in absence epilepsy. *Arquivos de Neuropsiquiatria, 64,* 193–197.

Huang, M-X., Nichols, S., Baker, D. G., Robb, A., Angeles, A., Yurgil, K. A., . . . Lee, R. R. (2014). Single-subject-based whole-brain MEG slow-wave imaging approach for detecting abnormality in patients with mild traumatic brain injury. *NeuroImage: Clinical, 5,* 109–119.

Huppertz, H. J., Hof, E., Klisch, J., Wagner, M., Lücking, C. H., & Kristeva-Feige, R. (2001). Localization of interictal delta and epileptiform EEG activity associated with focal epileptogenic brain lesions. *Neuroimage, 13,* 15–28.

Ishibashi, H., Simos, P. G., Castillo, E. M., Maggio, W. W., Wheless, J. W., Kim, H. L., . . . Papanicolaou, A. C. (2002). Detection and significance of focal, interictal, slow-wave activity visualized by magnetoencephalography for localization of a primary epileptogenic region. *Journal of Neurosurgery, 96,* 724–730.

Jasper, H., Kershman, J., & Elvidge, A. (1940). Electroencephalographic studies of injury to the head. *Archives of Neurology, 44,* 328.

Kaltenhäuser, M., Rampp, S., Ehrenfried, T., Heers, M., & Stefan, H. (2010). MEG slow wave dipole density (SWDD) in presurgical evaluation of epilepsy patients: Preliminary results of a prospective study. In S. Supek & A. Sušac (Eds.), 17th International Conference on Biomagnetism Advances in Biomagnetism—Biomag2010. *IFMBE Proceedings* (Vol. 28). Berlin, Heidelberg: Springer.

Kaltenhäuser, M., Scheler, G., Rampp, S., Paulini, A., & Stefan, H. (2007). Spatial intralobar correlation of spike and slow wave activity localisations in focal epilepsies: A MEG analysis. *Neuroimage, 34,* 1466–1472.

Kamada, K., Möller, M., Saguer, M., Ganslandt, O., Kaltenhäuser, M., Kober, H., & Vieth, J. (2001). A combined study of tumor-related brain lesions using MEG and proton MR spectroscopic imaging. *Journal of Neurological Science, 186,* 13–21.

Knake, S., Halgren, E., Shiraishi, H., Hara, K., Hamer, H. M., Grant, P. E., . . . Stufflebeam, S. M. (2006). The value of multichannel MEG and EEG in the presurgical evaluation of 70 epilepsy patients. *Epilepsy Research, 69,* 80–86.

Koutroumanidis, M., Martin-Miguel, C., Hennessy, M. J., Akanuma, N., Valentin, A., Alarcon, G., . . . Polkey, C. E. (2004). Interictal temporal delta activity in temporal lobe epilepsy: Correlations with pathology and outcome. *Epilepsia, 45,* 1351–1367.

Kreidenhuber, R., Demarchi, G., Kalss, G., Leitinger, M., Winkler, P. A., Trinka, E., & Rampp, S. (2018). Benefit of magnetic source localization in challenging refractory epilepsies. *Zeitschrift fur Epileptologie, 31,* 179–184.

Krishnan, B., Vlachos, I., Wang, Z. I., Mosher, J., Najm, I., Burgess, R., . . . Alexopoulos, A. V. (2015). Epileptic focus localization based on resting state interictal MEG recordings is feasible irrespective of the presence or absence of spikes. *Clinical Neurophysiology, 126*, 667–674.

Lee, R. R., & Huang, M. (2014). Magnetoencephalography in the diagnosis of concussion. *Progress in Neurological Surgery, 28*, 94–111.

Lin, Y., Zhang, Z., Zhang, X., Yang, Y., Huang, Z., Zhu, Y., . . . Wang, U. (2018). Lateralization value of low frequency band beamformer magnetoencephalography source imaging in temporal lobe epilepsy. *Frontiers in Neurology, 9*, 829.

Mălîia, M. D., Meritam, P., Scherg, M., Fabricius, M., Rubboli, G., Mîndruţă, I., & Beniczky, S. (2016). Epileptiform discharge propagation: Analyzing spikes from the onset to the peak. *Clinical Neurophysiology, 127*, 2127–2133.

Modarres, M., Kuzma, N. N., Kretzmer, T., Pack, A. I., & Lim, M. M. (2016). EEG slow waves in traumatic brain injury: Convergent findings in mouse and man. Neurobiology of Sleep and Circadian Rhythm, 1, S24519944163000025.

Mohanraj, R., & Brodie, M. J. (2006). Diagnosing refractory epilepsy: Response to sequential treatment schedules. *European Journal of Neurology 13*, 277–282.

Mu, J., Rampp, S., Carrette, E., Roessler, K., Sommer, B., Schmitt, F. C., . . . Stefan, H. (2014). Clinical relevance of source location in frontal lobe epilepsy and prediction of postoperative long-term outcome. *Seizure, 23*, 553–559.

Normand, M. M., Wszolek, Z. K., & Klass, D. W. (1995). Temporal intermittent rhythmic delta activity in electroencephalograms. *Journal of Clinical Neurophysiology, 12*, 280–284.

Oshino, S., Kato, A., Wakayama, A., Taniguchi, M., Hirata, M., & Yoshimine, T. (2007). Magnetoencephalographic analysis of cortical oscillatory activity in patients with brain tumors: Synthetic aperture magnetometry (SAM) functional imaging of delta band activity. *Neuroimage, 34*, 957–964.

Pallud, J., Capelle, L., & Huberfeld, G. (2013). Tumoral epileptogenicity: How does it happen? *Epilepsia, 54*, 30–34.

Rampp, S., Kakisaka, Y., Shibata, S., Wu, X., Rössler, K., Buchfelder, M., et al. (2018). Normal variants in magnetoencephalography. *Journal of Clinical Neurophysiology*.

Rampp, S., Kaltenhäuser, M., Weigel, D., Buchfelder, M., Ingmar Blümcke, I., Dörfler, A., & Stefan, H. (2010). MEG correlates of epileptic high gamma oscillations in invasive EEG. *Epilepsia, 51*, 1638–1642.

Rampp, S., & Stefan, H. (2007). Magnetoencephalography in presurgical epilepsy diagnosis. *Expert Review of Medical Devices, 4*, 335–347.

Reiher, J., Beaudry, M., & Leduc, C. P. (1989). Temporal intermittent rhythmic delta activity (TIRDA) in the diagnosis of complex partial epilepsy: Sensitivity, specificity and predictive value. *Canadian Journal of Neurological Science,16*, 398–401.

Rockstroh, B. S., Wienbruch, C., Ray, W. J., & Elbert, T. (2007). Abnormal oscillatory brain dynamics in schizophrenia: a sign of deviant communication in neural network? *BMC Psychiatry, 7*, 44.

Rosenow, F., & Lüders, H. (2001). Presurgical evaluation of epilepsy. *Brain, 124*, 1683–1700.

Schönherr, M., Stefan, H., Hamer, H., Rössler, K., Buchfelder, M., & Rampp, S. (2017). The delta between postoperative seizure freedom and persistence: Automatically detected focal slow waves after epilepsy surgery. *NeuroImage: Clinical, 13*, 256–263.

Stefan, H., Hummel, C., Scheler, G., Genow, A., Druschky, K., Tilz, C., . . . Römstock, J. (2003). Magnetic brain source imaging of focal epileptic activity: A synopsis of 455 cases. *Brain, 126*, 2396–405.

Stefan, H., Wu, X., Buchfelder, M., Rampp, S., Kasper, B., Hopfengärtner, R., . . . Weigel, D. (2011). MEG in frontal lobe epilepsies: Localization and postoperative outcome. *Epilepsia, 52*, 2233–2238.

Vadera, S., Jehi, L., Burgess, R. C., Shea, K., Alexopoulos, A. V., Mosher, J., . . . Bingaman, W. (2013). Correlation between magnetoencephalography-based "clusterectomy" and postoperative seizure freedom. *Neurosurgical Focus, 34*, E9.

van Klink, N., Hillebrand, A., & Zijlmans, M. (2016). Identification of epileptic high frequency oscillations in the time domain by using MEG beamformer-based virtual sensors. *Clinical Neurophysiology, 127*: 197–208.

Vanrumste, B., Jones, R. D., Bones, P. J., & Carroll, G. J. (2005). Slow-wave activity arising from the same area as epileptiform activity in the EEG of paediatric patients with focal epilepsy. *Clinical Neurophysiology, 116*, 9–17.

von Ellenrieder, N., Pellegrino, G., Hedrich, T., Gotman, J., Lina, J. M., Grova, C., & Kobayashi, E. (2016). Detection and magnetic source imaging of fast oscillations (40–160 Hz) recorded with magnetoencephalography in focal epilepsy patients. *Brain Topography, 29*, 218–231.

Walter, W. (1936). The location of cerebral tumors by electroencephalography. *Lancet, 2*, 305.

Watemberg, N., Linder, I., Dabby, R., Blumkin, L., & Lerman-Sagie, T. (2007). Clinical correlates of occipital intermittent rhythmic delta activity (OIRDA) in children. *Epilepsia, 48,* 330–334.

Xiang, J., Liu, Y., Wang, Y., Kirtman, E. G., Kotecha, R., Chen, Y., et al. (2009). Frequency and spatial characteristics of high-frequency neuromagnetic signals in childhood epilepsy. *Epileptic Disorders, 11,* 113–25.

SECTION IV

SOMATOSENSORY, MOTOR, AND LANGUAGE MAPPING

15

CLINICAL MOTOR MAPPING WITH MAGNETOENCEPHALOGRAPHY

HISTORICAL APPROACHES, CHALLENGES, AND RECOMMENDATIONS FOR BEST PRACTICE

William Gaetz, Christos Papadelis, and Tony W. Wilson

15.1. WHAT IS MOTOR MAPPING?

Motor cortex functional mapping procedures were first conducted by neurosurgeons who famously stimulated their patient's exposed brain during surgery and then systematically documented (i.e., "mapped") the responses observed from the activated muscles of the body (Penfield & Rasmussen, 1957). Numerous neuroimaging-based functional mapping techniques followed, such as functional magnetic resonance imaging (fMRI), transcranial magnetic stimulation (TMS), high-density electroencephalography (HD-EEG), and magnetoencephalography (MEG), which are currently used to map the motor areas in relation to isolated volitional movements. Compared with the other methods, MEG presents a unique set of significant advantages,

particularly for vulnerable populations like children: (a) preparation is faster and easier than fMRI or HD-EEG; (b) MEG signals, unlike HD-EEG, are reference-free and not distorted by skull conductivity; and (c) recordings are passive without requiring the application of a magnetic field that implies possible risks (i.e., generation of seizures in the case of TMS) (Papadelis, Harini, Ahtam, Doshi, Grant, & Okada, 2013). The *clinical goal* of MEG motor mapping is to identify eloquent areas of the primary motor cortex in close proximity to the planned surgical cortical areas and determine the central sulcus used to orient the surgeon by defining the somatosensory and motor gyri. The delineation of the eloquent cortex is critical in order to limit possible postsurgical motor functional deficits. Once identified and confirmed (by electrical stimulation), these

William Gaetz, Christos Papadelis, and Tony W. Wilson, *Clinical Motor Mapping With Magnetoencephalography: Historical Approaches, Challenges, and Recommendations for Best Practice* In: *Fifty Years of Magnetoencephalography*. Edited by: Andrew C. Papanicolaou, Timothy P. L. Roberts, and James W. Wheless, Oxford University Press (2020). © Oxford University Press. DOI: 10.1093/oso/9780190935689.003.0015.

eloquent motor areas can also be used as sites for intraoperative monitoring, where surgeons continually monitor the connectivity between a cortical motor site and the corresponding muscles of the body throughout the course of surgery (Cedzich, Taniguchi, Schäfer, & Schramm, 1996; Korvenoja et al., 2006), or as seed points for delineation and further sparing of the associated descending white matter tracts through diffusion tensor imaging (DTI) (Gaetz et al., 2010b; Kamada et al., 2003).

15.2. CHALLENGES OF MAGNETOENCEPHALOGRAPHY MOTOR MAPPING

Motor mapping presents many practical and technical challenges that separate it methodologically from conventional functional mapping of sensory modalities such as vision, audition, and somatosensation. Whereas it is relatively trivial to stimulate a targeted primary sensory cortical area by presenting a peripheral stimulus such as a tone, a flash of light, or a tactile stimulus (thus producing a time-locked evoked response from the brain area of interest), motor cortical function cannot be activated with the same temporal precision. Indeed, early electroencephalography (EEG)-based demonstrations showed that the movement-related slow cortical responses associated with transient (i.e., ballistic) finger movements emerge several seconds before a self-paced movement is performed (Kornhuber & Deecke, 1965). Motor cortical responses also occur in close proximity to the homologous somatosensory responses, which receive proprioceptive feedback from movement-related somatosensory activity. So, even a perfectly controlled transient finger movement, for example, will produce additional sources of correlated activity in close spatial and temporal proximity to the primary motor cortical source of interest. Methods to address these technical challenges are detailed in the sections that follow.

15.3. BACKGROUND: MOVEMENT-RELATED EVOKED POTENTIALS

The first EEG study of movement-related evoked potentials was conducted by Kornhuber and Deecke in 1965. In this study, subjects were asked to perform isolated self-paced voluntary movements followed by several seconds of rest. While no significant modulations were noted in the single-trial EEG recordings, Kornhuber and Deecke used a newly available Mnemotron CAT 400 computer (circa 1962) to compute an average of the single trial responses, which was aligned to electromyographic (EMG) onset, and thus improved the signal-to-noise (SNR) ratio. Using this technique, Kornhuber and Deecke (1965) observed a slow negative (DC) potential from central electrodes contralateral to movement, which grew in amplitude during the premovement period (the potential was termed *Bereitschaftspotential* [BP] or *readiness potential* [RP]). Subsequent studies further reported that the RP sharply increases in amplitude directly before (~200 ms) movement onset, with the peak of this evoked-response component termed the *motor potential* (MP) (Deecke, 1987; Deecke, Scheid, & Kornhuber, 1969; Kristeva, Keller, Deecke, & Kornhuber, 1979). Following this MP component, the response then consistently reversed polarity around movement onset (Deecke, Scheid, & Kornhuber, 1969; Kristeva, Keller, Deecke, & Kornhuber, 1979).

15.3.1. Magnetoencephalography Analogs

In the early 1960s, James Zimmerman developed a radiofrequency superconductive quantum interference device (RF-SQUID). MEG hardware incorporating this SQUID-based technology for measuring brain function became available in the early 1980s (Zimmerman, Thiene, & Harding, 1970). This was a significant technical advance because SQUID-based sensors were sensitive enough to detect the extremely faint magnetic fields emanating from the human brain. However, early MEG hardware designs were unfortunately constrained by housing only a single MEG sensor (Figure 15.1). To achieve comparable measures to the prior evoked potential reports of the day, early MEG studies measured evoked magnetic field recordings one sensor location at a time, and thus a complete replication of an experiment (routinely consisting of >40 trials) was required for each MEG sensor location of interest. Thus, hours of recording time were required per subject to measure the movement-related magnetic fields of interest (the magnetic analogs of the readiness potential [RP] and motor potential [MP]). Multichannel and whole-head MEG became increasingly available in the 1990s, with presently available hardware now consisting of whole-head coverage typically exceeding more than 200 sensors. Despite the early technological challenges, pioneering work first conducted by Deecke, Weinberg, and Brickett (1982) described the Bereitschaftsmagnetfeld

(the "readiness field" [RF]) using a single sensor CTF MEG recorded at the midline at three EEG locations (C3, C4, and Cz electrode locations; see Figure 15.1).

Soon after, Deecke, Boschert, Weinberg, and Brickett (1983) and Hari, Antervo, and Salmi (1983) defined the magnetic counterparts of both the RP and MP (i.e., RF and motor field [MF]) associated with limb movements of the hands and feet. Cheyne and Weinberg (1989) first reported that ballistic self-paced finger movements consistently produced both RF and MF components, as well a series of large movement-evoked field (MEF) components, immediately following EMG onset (Chiarenza, Cheyne, Kristeva, & Deecke, 1991; Cheyne & Weinberg, 1989; Hari, Karhu, & Tessore, 1991; Kristeva, Cheyne, & Deecke, 1991). The RF and MF (reflecting supplementary and primary motor areas, respectively) components were later confirmed using electrocorticography (ECoG) (Ikeda, Lüdors, Burgess, & Shibasaki, 1992). The clinical utility of presurgical functional mapping based on the MEF, which

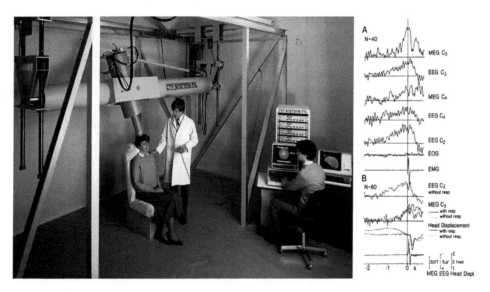

FIGURE 15.1 Single-channel magnetoencephalography (MEG): the Bereitschaftspotential. Averaged MEG and electroencephalography (EEG) recordings accompanying finger movement. Left precentral (C3) and right precentral (C4) recordings (average of 40 self-paced finger movements) are shown. (From Deecke, L., Weinberg, H., & Brickett, P. [1982]. Magnetic fields of the human brain accompanying voluntary movement: Bereitschaftsmagnetfeld. *Experimental Brain Research, 48*[1], 144–148. Photo courtesy of CTF MEG International Services LP.)

directly follows EMG onset and thus reflects movement-related somatosensory and proprioceptive feedback, was first reported by Ganslandt et al. in 1999 (Ganslandt et al., 1999; Kamada et al., 1999).

15.4. GENERAL CONSIDERATIONS FOR MEASURING MOVEMENT-EVOKED FIELDS

Clinical MEG guidelines have been published recently, including a variety of recommendations for clinical motor mapping (Burgess et al., 2011; Hari et al., 2018). Presently, however, a generally accepted "gold standard" motor mapping protocol for clinical or research purposes has not been articulated by the MEG community. Given that the general approaches tend to share some consistencies, we will focus on the more commonly shared approaches in this section.

Motor mapping starts with the goal of identifying and targeting a particular motor cortical representation for a specific body part. For upper limb motor representations, such as the fingers and hands, the motor task generally consists of pushing a button, finger flexion, or similar movement, isolating one body representation at a time. Early approaches typically used a "self-paced" transient finger movement paradigm whereby each finger movement occurred as a brief flexion and returned to rest, with an intermovement duration of several (~3–5) seconds (Deecke et al., 1982, 1983; Cheyne & Weinberg, 1989; Cheyne et al., 1991). While generally effective in adults, these protocols are difficult for young children, who have limited attention span or may not understand what is meant by a "self-paced" finger movement and consequently move much more frequently or infrequently than desired. In addition, these self-paced tasks tend to promote subvocal counting/pacing strategies, which are difficult to control for. More recently, a variety of visual cues have been used to prompt movement onset and control the movement rate (e.g., one movement every 3–5 seconds followed by a rest period) (Gaetz, Macdonald, Cheyne, & Snead, 2010a; Gaetz et al., 2009; Heinrichs-Graham et al., 2014; Wilson, Heinrichs-Graham, & Becker, 2014; Wilson et al., 2010, 2013) or protocols in which the subject continuously performs a motor task guided by visual stimuli (Jerbi et al., 2007; Papadelis et al., 2016). It is also important to collect enough trials to maximize the SNR; thus, most laboratories have each patient complete at least 100 repetitions of the target movement (or more) because some trials may be rejected because of excessive head motion or nonbrain "noise" sources (e.g., eye movements). While most researchers and technicians will agree that 100 trials is conventionally appropriate, there is little published literature to define the acceptable lower bound of trial number on these tasks. Typically, collecting 80 to 100 motor response trials is sufficient, depending on the interstimulus interval (ISI) and patient compliance (e.g., age, functional and cognitive ability). For methods that depend on beta rhythm event-related desynchrony (ERD; described in more detail later in this chapter), the age of the participant may be a more relevant parameter than the trial number (Gaetz et al., 2010a; Heinrichs-Graham et al., 2018b; Trevarrow et al., 2018).

Another critical methodological issue involves quantifying the movement onset precisely. This aspect is critical because all conventional analysis procedures epoch the data into trials using the movement onset as the defining event. Typically, movement onset is defined as time 0 seconds, which then allows the premovement and postmovement data segments to be evaluated separately. Different methods have been proposed to quantify the onset of the movement; the most common ones measure (a) the EMG signal (muscle belly to tendon montage) of the target muscle, (b) the stimulus-related movement cue (e.g., markers for visual cue onsets and offset), and (c) the physical movement itself (e.g., accelerometer, light trigger, force transducer, or button-press event marker). Together, these peripheral measures provide confirmation that the response of interest is produced consistently and done so in accordance with the presented movement cue.

After the MEG data have been acquired, the conventional approach is to conduct some form of noise reduction (e.g., signal-space separation), then exclude noisy channels, and then conduct trials using signal amplitude/power criteria and visual inspection. Often, artifacts can be corrected using specific algorithms like signal-space projection (SSP) (e.g., cardiac and eye blinks), but when in doubt it is generally better to exclude trials. Artifacts can include environmental disturbances (e.g., hospital elevators, local construction) and participant noise sources from the heart (e.g., electrocardiography [ECG]), eyes (e.g., blinking, moving), mouth (e.g., swallowing, talking), and neck (e.g., head movements) (Papadelis, AlHilani, & Pearl, 2018; Wilson, Heinrichs-Graham, Proskovec, & McDermott, 2016). After all of the artifacts have been addressed and are

ameliorated, the next step is to apply a source analysis procedure to determine the location in the brain likely generating the evoked response MF and MEF components.

Early source localization approaches for clinical motor mapping typically involve the application of ECD models of the MF and MEF evoked responses observed with respect to movement onset. Filter settings applied to the evoked response are typically DC to about 30 Hz (baselined using the premovement period). Ideally, the observed response would appear like that in Figure 15.2, with a slow increase in field strength (RF), peaking maximally just before movement onset (MF), and immediately followed by a polarity reversal (MEF) (Cheyne & Weinberg, 1989; Cheyne, Weinberg, Gaetz, & Jantzen, 1995; Oishi et al., 2003).

ECD source analysis is conducted to use a mathematical source model—a dipole, to represent the location, orientation, and amplitude of a source in the brain. The ECD model offers a reliable source localization approach

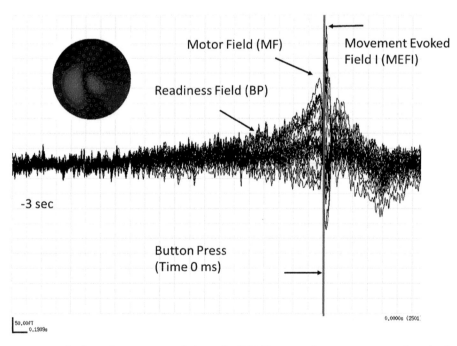

FIGURE 15.2 Multichannel magnetoencephalography (MEG): averaged response to 100 right index finger (visually cued button press). The readiness field (RF), motor field (MF), and movement-evoked fields (MEFs) are shown. A contour plot shows the field pattern for the peak MF response, with the individual sensors shown as *gray circles*.

with an accuracy of a few millimeters when the model fits the data extremely well (i.e., goodness-of-fit [GOF] >90%) and with spatial fidelity sufficient to allow for the interpretation of cytoarchitectonic representations (Papadelis, Eickhoff, Zilles, & Ioannides, 2011; Papadelis, Poghosyan, Fenwick, & Ioannides, 2009). Typically, an evoked response component (e.g., MF, MEF) peak latency is identified, and the topographic (dipolar) field pattern observed at the time point of the peak evoked response is modeled. With this procedure, one often improves GOF by restricting the channels to a subset of sensors covering both magnetic flux extrema. Then, using ECD software (e.g., Brainstorm, BESA), the objective is to iteratively derive the best possible location and orientation in the least-squares sense (Hämäläinen, Hari, Ilmoniemi, Knuutila, & Lounasmaa, 1993; Wilson, Leuthold, Lewis, Georgopoulos, & Pardo, 2005b) to reproduce the observed topography. ECD analysis is typically done on a single time point (i.e., the time when the largest (i.e., "peak") response amplitude is observed, to maximize the SNR), although it can also be computed on a window of data around the peak (i.e., a spatiotemporal dipole fit approach) (Mosher, Lewis, & Leahy, 1992; Papadelis et al., 2011; Papadelis, Leonardelli, Staudt, & Braun, 2012; Wilson, Leuthold, Lewis, Georgopoulos, & Pardo, 2005a). The resulting dipole models are then evaluated by their residual variance (i.e., GOF), confidence volume, and location relative to co-registered brain anatomy and proximity to somatosensory and motor cortices.

15.5. EARLY FINDINGS USING EQUIVALENT CURRENT DIPOLE: A CLEAR NEED FOR NEW SOURCE ANALYSIS METHODS

Early MEG motor mapping studies relied on ECD source analysis methods, and findings were somewhat controversial. Ganslandt et al. (1999) first reported good localization of the MEF component in a study including 50 patients with centrally located lesions (self-paced finger tapping, 3- to 5-second movement rate; ECD source modeling). However, Lin, Berger, and Nagarajan (2006) conducted presurgical motor mapping in 19 patients (same self-paced repetitive finger tapping protocol; 3- to 5-second movement rate) and compared the spatial distribution of MF and MEF dipoles in relation to those modeled for the somatosensory evoked field (SEF). Lin et al. (2006) reported that the motor source locations were not spatially distinct from the somatosensory dipoles, and thus the MF and MEF components were not sensitive enough for presurgical functional mapping (2006). These early observations highlighted the need for new methods, which were subsequently developed to address and improve localization of motor function with MEG.

15.5.1. Event-Related Beamformer

One problem with the ECD source analysis of motor function is that the approach only works (i.e., produces reliable source locations) when the evoked response is strong and the noise sources are trivial (i.e., high SNR). Thus, motor mapping in children presents a significant problem, given that evoked responses in children (measured using MEG hardware designed to accommodate adult head sizes) are typically much weaker than in adults, and the evoked response averages also typically contain more sources of contamination because blinks and other movement-related artifacts are common owing to limited cooperation in children (i.e., low SNR). To improve source localization performance in such cases, new source analysis methods were developed, such as the event-related beamformer method (Cheyne, Bostan, Gaetz, & Pang, 2007), which increases the sensitivity by projecting out of the data the correlated sources of noise identified in the data covariance. This approach has been used to identify MF and MEF components (Figure 15.3), both in healthy children and in clinical pediatric populations (Gaetz et al.,

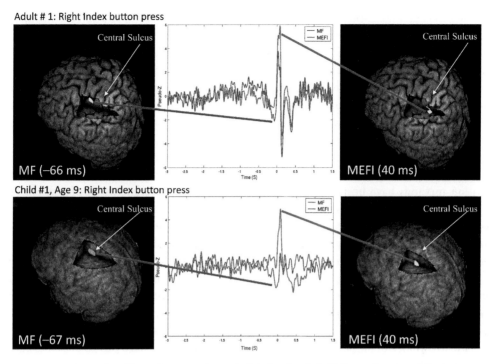

Adult # 1: Right Index button press

Central Sulcus

Central Sulcus

MF (−66 ms)

MEFI (40 ms)

Child #1, Age 9: Right Index button press

Central Sulcus

Central Sulcus

MF (−67 ms)

MEFI (40 ms)

FIGURE 15.3 Event-related beamformer analysis of adult (*top*) and child (*bottom*) motor evoked responses. Motor field (MF) timing is about 66 ms for both participants; and movement-evoked field I (MEFI) peak latency is identical (40 ms). Note that lower traces are weaker, likely owing to the increased distance from the source to sensor array.

2009, 2010b; Pang et al., 2008; Sutcliffe, Gaetz, Logan, Cheyne, & Fehlings, 2007).

15.5.2. New Methods for Motor Mapping: Differential Beamformer

As mentioned, low SNR is a significant problem for ECD source localization where one or both evoked-field components are not obvious in the evoked response average. This problem is common and can be attributed to numerous factors. One possible cause is variability in the active neural population used to perform the movement. While it seems likely that the target neural population is used for each performed movement, it may be that this population response varies (to some degree) from movement to movement and that this variability causes the magnetic signal (which is a product of superimposition of the ultra-tiny fields produced by smaller populations of cells) to vary in phase and/or time with each

motor response. Such variability, especially in phase, can cause large parts of the signal of interest to "average out" over trials when using time-domain averaging approaches. Beyond this, in young children, for example, there are the issues of compliance mentioned previously. For example, young children are unable to successfully follow the typical "cue/response" protocols that are used to elicit dozens of identical responses over minutes of recording. Moreover, these patients have relatively smaller heads and shorter necks than adults, which increases the distance between the sensors and the brain and thus reduces the SNR (Wilson et al., 2016). Finally, unlike the somatosensory cortex, eloquent motor function may shift to the ipsilateral hemisphere in the context of white matter tract lesion, and in such cases the actual response components can be so abnormal that they are basically unrecognizable from the time-domain average (Wilke et al., 2009). Even if these representations remain in the contralateral hemisphere, there may be gross differences in the timing or phase of their neural response from trial to trial (resulting at least partially from differences in the actual movement from trial to trial). In other patients, tumors and/or white matter tract lesions can produce weakness or motor functional deficits, rendering the ballistic motor responses difficult or impossible to reproduce. For these reasons and other complicating factors, new source localization methods have been developed that focus on modulating resting rhythms (e.g., mu rhythm 8–13 Hz; beta-band 15–30 Hz) of the sensorimotor cortex. Paramount among these methods is the differential beamformer approach, which involves defining passive and active periods and computing a difference image using one of multiple different flavors of beamforming. Key benefits of this approach include the irrelevance of phase differences from trial to trial and the tolerance of trial-to-trial variations in the timing of movements and thus the neural response. The latter is made possible by applying a time window with a duration typically capturing hundreds of milliseconds of data. The most common protocol is to first epoch the data into time segments spanning several seconds (e.g., ~3–6 s), with movement onset aligned to zero seconds. A baseline period can be defined as a period of premovement data (ideally capturing resting background brain activity) and placed several hundred milliseconds before movement onset (e.g., –1.0 to –0.5 s). A time–frequency decomposition is then performed on the MEG sensor-level signals, and the power per frequency bin is normalized using the premovement baseline period (Figure 15.4). The resulting spectrograms near sensorimotor cortex typically show a robust ERD, or decrease in the band-limited power relative to the baseline, in the beta range (15–30 Hz) that begins few hundred milliseconds before movement onset and continues through the duration of the movement.

This beta ERD response is often termed the *perimovement beta ERD* and has been repeatedly linked to motor planning and performance (Heinrichs-Graham, Arpin, & Wilson, 2016; Heinrichs-Graham, Hoburg, & Wilson, 2018a; Heinrichs-Graham & Wilson, 2015). The cortical origins of the response can be easily reconstructed using a differential beamformer: a baseline time-window (e.g., ~0.5 s duration; ~–1.5 to –1.0 s) premovement) is used in reference to an active time window covering the strongest features of the response (e.g., –0.2 to 0.3 s around movement onset). The results typically show two large clusters of desynchronous activity, with the strongest (most negative) response centered on the contralateral precentral and postcentral gyri and a weaker cluster near the ipsilateral homologue. Of note, in computing differential beamformer responses, it is important to ensure that the passive and active periods used in the computation are of equal duration and bandwidth. Otherwise, the power in the resulting image can be biased toward the period with more data (Wilson et al., 2016).

In addition to the perimovement beta ERD, there is generally a higher frequency response in roughly the same sensor-level spectrograms that coincides with movement onset and is relatively transient. Most commonly, this event-related synchronization (ERS) response, or increase in band-limited power relative to the baseline, is within the 60- to 90-Hz gamma range and begins around –0.1 second and extends about 0.2 second postmovement (see Figure 15.4) (Gaetz et al., 2010a; Heinrichs-Graham et al., 2018, 2018b; Trevarrow et al., 2018; Wilson et al., 2010). The differential beamformer approach can also be used to reconstruct this motor gamma-band response by focusing the active period on the peak ERS (e.g., –0.1 to 0.2 s) and adjusting the baseline accordingly. The output images typically show a tight cluster of activity centered on the contralateral precentral gyrus, with the maxima near the so-called motor hand knob in the case of finger movements (Heinrichs-Graham et al., 2018a). This movement-related gamma synchronization (MRGS) is known to be strongly lateralized to contralateral motor cortex and tightly aligned to the onset

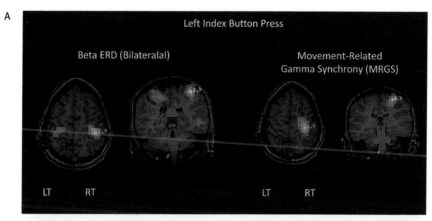

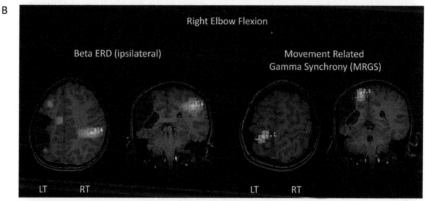

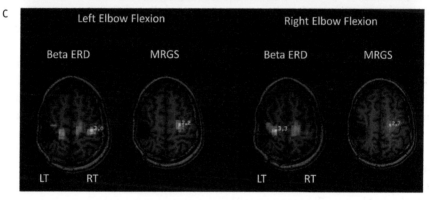

FIGURE 15.4   A group-averaged time–frequency response plot consisting of the average of 63 typically developing (TD) subjects (aged 8–24 years; right hand button-press) is shown. The time and frequency of beta event-related desynchrony (ERD) and movement-related gamma synchrony (MRGS) responses are highlighted.

of self-paced and cued transient movements (Cheyne, Bells, Ferrari, Gaetz, & Bostan, 2008; Muthukumaraswamy, 2010). On more complex cognitive tasks, premovement motor gamma amplitude is also modulated by cognitive tasks such as response interference and action selection (Bramson, Jensen, Toni, & Roelofs, 2018; Gaetz, Liu, Zhu, Bloy, & Roberts, 2013). As a result, MRGS likely represents the best candidate motor response for presurgical motor mapping. However, in cases in which the MRGS is not visible in the sensor-level spectrograms, beta ERD can be used because it is also a reliable marker of the sensorimotor cortices, albeit commonly bilateral. Prior studies have shown that motor gamma follows the expected somatotopic representations (Cheyne et al., 2008), and thus, revealing motor homuncular organization with MEG is likely only limited by the ability of the subject to perform transient movements with onset event markers that can be aligned consistently per trial.

15.6. CHALLENGING CLINICAL EXAMPLES

The previous sections described promising beamformer-based analysis methods for identifying motor function. However, these methods all rely on the patient to make numerous controlled responses of a specific body part (e.g., a finger, toe), which can be problematic for some patients. For example, motor weakness (i.e., paresis) is common in clinical populations, such as in patients with lesions that disrupt the corticospinal motor tracts (e.g., cerebral palsy, brain tumors in periventricular areas). For patients with paresis, the usual targets of distal limb movement (e.g., index fingers or large toes) are sensible starting points. If a patient cannot move the targeted body parts, or can, but only infrequently, the method of choice should allow the technician to switch the functional target to the next proximal joint in series (wrist or ankle flexion in this example), without consequence to subsequent analysis methods. Thus, in clinical settings, the *ideal* MEG motor mapping protocol needs to be *flexible* to anticipate and adapt to the wide variety of cognitive and functional abilities and limitations. The standard approaches that work reliably in research settings may not be practical objectives in a clinical setting.

We next present two challenging motor mapping cases: one without (5A) and one with (5B) lateralized lesions affecting motor function. For patient 5A, left index finger button-press responses produced strong, bilateral beta ERD (stronger contralaterally), whereas the MRGS for this patient was lateralized to contralateral primary motor cortex. As described previously, some patients may not be able to produce distal finger movements because of white matter lesions and hemiparesis. For such cases, we focus on the next viable proximal muscle that the patient can control (e.g., in this case, elbow flexion). Figure 15.5B contrasts beta ERD and MRGS for left and right elbow flexion. For left elbow flexion, beta ERD and MRGS were comparable to Figure 15.5A. However, for this patient, right elbow flexion (typically controlled by the affected left motor cortex) had shifted to the right motor cortex (see Figure 15.5B). A shift from contralateral to ipsilateral motor cortex is not uncommon. For this case, we confirmed the shift to ipsilateral motor control using transcranial magnetic stimulation.

15.7. SUMMARY

The use of MEG for presurgical functional mapping has become a standard component of clinical MEG practice. Knowledge regarding the location of eloquent MEG motor representations is valuable for presurgical planning and can improve outcomes by limiting the production of postsurgical deficits of motor function. Source localization challenges using ECD models have given way to newer methods, such as beamformer spatial filters, which have been validated clinically using electrical stimulation. Where patients can reliably execute transient movements, MRGS ("motor gamma") may be the best target for presurgical motor mapping. If patients have less precise control (such as those with paresis and cerebral palsy), differential beamformers focused on beta ERD would likely be more suitable to index functional markers for presurgical motor function. Finally, it should be noted that it is becoming increasingly evident that motor cortical oscillations are changing consistently over the life span (both in power and frequency), and thus consideration of the patient's age will likely aid the interpretation of results.

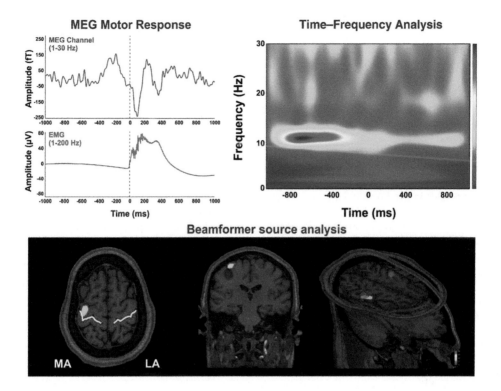

FIGURE 15.5 (A) Beta event-related desynchrony (ERD) and movement-related gamma synchrony (MRGS) responses to left hand button-press task in an 11-year-old epilepsy patient. Results show concordance between beta ERD and MRGS responses, which both localized to the contralateral motor cortex following left index finger-button presses. (B) Patient is a 16-year-old girl with right hand weakness due to prior resective epilepsy surgery of the left frontoparietal cortex. Left elbow flexion produced as expected bilateral beta ERD and contralateral MRGS responses. Right (affected) elbow flexion showed bilateral beta ERD and ipsilateral (right hemisphere MRGS; confirmed with transcranial magnetic stimulation).

REFERENCES

Bramson, B., Jensen, O., Toni, I., & Roelofs, K. (2018). Cortical oscillatory mechanisms supporting the control of human social-emotional actions. *Journal of Neuroscience, 38*(25), 5739–5749.

Burgess, R. C., Funke, M. E., Bowyer, S. M., Lewine, J. D., Kirsch, H. E., Bagic, A. I.,; ACMEGS Clinical Practice Guideline Committee. (2011). American Clinical Magnetoencephalography Society Clinical Practice guideline 2: Presurgical functional brain mapping using magnetic evoked fields. *Journal of Clinical Neurophysiology, 28*(4), 355–361.

Cedzich, C., Taniguchi, M., Schäfer, S., & Schramm, J. (1996). Somatosensory evoked potential phase reversal and direct motor cortex stimulation during surgery in and around the central region. *Neurosurgery, 38*(5), 962–970.

Cheyne, D., Bells, S., Ferrari, P., Gaetz, W., & Bostan, A. C. (2008). Self-paced movements induce high-frequency gamma oscillations in primary motor cortex. *Neuroimage, 42*(1), 332–342.

Cheyne, D., Bostan, A. C., Gaetz, W., & Pang, E. W. (2007). Event-related beamforming: A robust method for presurgical functional mapping using MEG. *Clinical Neurophysiology, 118*(8), 1691–1704.

Cheyne, D., Kristeva, R., & Deecke, L. (1991). Homuncular organization of human motor cortex as indicated by neuromagnetic recordings. *Neuroscience Letters, 122*(1), 17–20.

Cheyne, D., & Weinberg, H. (1989). Neuromagnetic fields accompanying unilateral finger movements: Pre-movement and movement-evoked fields. *Experimental Brain Research, 78*(3), 604–612.

Cheyne, D., Weinberg, H., Gaetz, W., & Jantzen, K. J. (1995). Motor cortex activity and predicting side of movement: Neural network and dipole analysis of pre-movement magnetic fields. *Neuroscience Letters, 188*(2), 81–84.

Chiarenza, G. A., Hari, R. K., Karhu, J. J., & Tessore, S. (1991). Brain activity associated with skilled finger movements: Multichannel magnetic recordings. *Brain Topography, 3*(4), 433–439.

Deecke, L., Boschert, J., Weinberg, H., & Brickett, P. (1983). Magnetic fields of the human brain (Bereitschaftsmagnetfeld) preceding voluntary foot and toe movements. *Experimental Brain Research, 52*(1), 81–86.

Deecke, L., Scheid, P., & Kornhuber, H. H. (1969). Distribution of readiness potential, pre-motion positivity, and motor potential of the human cerebral cortex preceding involuntary finger movements. *Experimental Brain Research, 7*, 158–168.

Deecke, L., Weinberg, H., & Brickett, P. (1982). Magnetic fields of the human brain accompanying voluntary movement: Bereitschaftsmagnetfeld. *Experimental Brain Research, 48*(1), 144–148.

Gaetz, W., Cheyne, D., Rutka, J. T., Drake, J., Benifla, M., Strantzas, J., . . . Pang, E. W. (2009). Presurgical localization of primary motor cortex in pediatric patients with brain lesions by the use of spatially filtered magnetoencephalography. *Neurosurgery, 64*(3 Suppl), ons177–185; discussion ons186.

Gaetz, W., Liu, C., Zhu, H., Bloy, L., & Roberts, T. P. (2013). Evidence for a motor gamma-band network governing response interference. *Neuroimage, 74*, 245–253.

Gaetz, W., Macdonald, M., Cheyne, D., & Snead, O. C. (2010a). Neuromagnetic imaging of movement-related cortical oscillations in children and adults: Age predicts post-movement beta rebound. *Neuroimage, 51*(2), 792–807.

Gaetz, W., Scantlebury, M. Widjaja, E., Rutka, J., Bouffet, E., Rockel, C., . . . Mabbott, D. (2010b). Mapping of the cortical spinal tracts using magnetoencephalography and diffusion tensor tractography in pediatric brain tumor patients. *Childs Nervous System, 26*(11), 1639–1645.

Ganslandt, O., Falbusch, R., Nimsky, C., Kober, H., Möller, M., Steinmeir, R., . . . Vieth, J. (1999). Functional neuronavigation with magnetoencephalography: Outcome in 50 patients with lesions around the motor cortex. *Neurosurgery Focus, 6*(3), e3.

Hämäläinen, M., Hari, R., Ilmoniemi, R. J., Knuutila, J., & Lounasmaa, O. V. (1993). Magnetoencephalography—theory, instrumentation, and applications to noninvasive studies of the working human brain. *Reviews of Modern Physics, 65*, 413.

Hari, R., Antervo, A., & Salmi, T. (1983). Slow EEG potentials preceding self-paced plantar flexions of hand and foot. *Acta Physiologica Scandinavica, 119*(1), 55–59.

Hari, R., Baillet, S., Barnes, G., Burgess, R., Forss, N., Gross, J., . . . Taulu, S. (2018). IFCN-endorsed practical guidelines for clinical magnetoencephalography (MEG). *Clinical Neurophysiology, 129*(8), 1720–1747.

Heinrichs-Graham, E., Arpin, D. J., & Wilson, T. W. (2016). Cue-related temporal factors modulate movement-related beta oscillatory activity in the human motor circuit. *Journal of Cognitive Neuroscience, 28*(7), 1039–1051.

Heinrichs-Graham, E., Hoburg, J. M., & Wilson, T. W. (2018a). The peak frequency of motor-related gamma oscillations is modulated by response competition. *Neuroimage, 165*, 27–34.

Heinrichs-Graham, E., McDermott, T. J., Mills, M. S., Weisman, A. I., Wang, Y. P., Stephen, J. M., . . . Wilson, T. W. (2018b). The lifespan trajectory of neural oscillatory activity in the motor system. *Developments in Cognitive Neuroscience, 30*, 159–168.

Heinrichs-Graham, E., & Wilson, T. W. (2015). Coding complexity in the human motor circuit. *Human Brain Mapping, 36*(12), 5155–5167.

Heinrichs-Graham, E., Wilson, T. W., Santamaria, P. M., Heithoff, S. K., Torres-Russotto, D., Hutter-Saunders, J. A., . . . Gendelman, H. E. (2014). Neuromagnetic evidence of abnormal movement-related beta desynchronization in Parkinson's disease. *Cerebral Cortex, 24*(10), 2669–2678.

Ikeda, A., Lüdors, H. O., Burgess, R. C., & Shibasaki, H. (1992). Movement-related potentials recorded from supplementary motor area and primary motor area: Role of supplementary motor area in voluntary movements. *Brain, 115*, 1017–1043.

Jerbi, K., Lachaux, J-P., N'Diaye, K., Pantazis, D., Leahy, R. M., Garnero, L., & Baillet, S. (2007). Coherent neural representation of hand speed in humans revealed by MEG imaging. *Proceedings of the National Academy of Science U S A, 104*(18), 7676–7681.

Kamada, K., Houkin, K., Takeuchi, F., Ishii, N., Ikeda, J., Sawamura, Y., . . . Iwasaki, Y. (2003). Visualization of the eloquent motor system by integration of MEG, functional, and aniso-tropic diffusion-weighted MRI in functional neuronavigation. *Surgical Neurology, 59*(5), 352–361; discussion 361–362.

Kamada, K., Möller, M., Saguer, M., Ganslandt, O., Kaltenhäuser, M., Kober, H., & Vieth, J. (1999). A combined study of tumor-related brain lesions by using magnetoencephalography and 1H magnetic resonance spectroscopic imaging. Technical note. *Neurosurgery Focus, 7*(5), ecp2.

Kornhuber, H. H., & Deecke, L. (1965). Hirnpotentialänderungen bei Willkürbewegungen und passiven Bewegungen des Menschen: Bereitschaftspotential und reafferente Potentiale. *Pflügers Archiv, 284*, 1–17.

Korvenoja, A., Kirveskari, E., Aronen, H. J., Avikainen, S., Brander, A., Huttunen, J., . . . Seppä, J. (2006). Sensorimotor cortex localization: Comparison of magnetoencephalography, functional MR imaging, and intraoperative cortical mapping. *Radiology, 241*(1), 213–222.

Kristeva, R., Cheyne, D., & Deecke, L. (1991). Neuromagnetic fields accompanying unilateral and bilateral voluntary movements: Topography and analysis of cortical sources. *Electroencephalography and Clinical Neurophysiology, 81*(4), 284–298.

Kristeva, R., Keller, E., Deecke, L., & Kornhuber, H. H. (1979). Cerebral potentials preceding unilateral and simultaneous bilateral finger movements. *Electroencephalography and Clinical Neurophysiology, 47*(2), 229–238.

Lin, P. T., Berger, M. S., & Nagarajan, S. S. (2006). Motor field sensitivity for preoperative localization of motor cortex. *Journal of Neurosurgery, 105*(4), 588–594.

Mosher, J. C., Lewis, P. S., & Leahy, R. M. (1992). Multiple dipole modeling and localization from spatio-temporal MEG data. *IEEE Transactions on Biomedical Engineering, 39*(6), 541–557.

Muthukumaraswamy, S. D. (2010). Functional properties of human primary motor cortex gamma oscillations. *Journal of Neurophysiology, 104*(5), 2873–2885.

Oishi, M., Fukuda, M., Kameyama, S., Kawaguchi, T., Masuda, H., & Tanaka, R. (2003). Magnetoencephalographic representation of the sensorimotor hand area in cases of intracerebral tumour. *Journal of Neurology, Neurosurgery, and Psychiatry, 74*(12), 1649–1654.

Pang, E. W., Drake, J. M., Otsubo, H., Martineau, A., Strantzas, S., Cheyne, D., & Gaetz, W. (2008). Intraoperative confirmation of hand motor area identified preoperatively by magnetoencephalography. *Pediatric Neurosurgery, 44*(4), 313–317.

Papadelis, C., AlHilani, M., & Pearl, P. L. (2018). Artifacts in pediatric and adult magnetoencephalography. In W. O. Tatum (Ed.), New York, NY: Demos.

Papadelis, C., Arfeller, C., Erla, S., Nollo, G., Cattaneo, L., & Braun, C. (2016). Inferior frontal gyrus links visual and motor cortices during a visuomotor precision grip force task. *Brain Research, 1650*, 252–266.

Papadelis, C., Eickhoff, S. B., Zilles, K., & Ioannides, A. A. (2011). BA3b and BA1 activate in a serial fashion after median nerve stimulation: Direct evidence from combining source analysis of evoked fields and cytoarchitectonic probabilistic maps. *Neuroimage, 54*(1), 60–73.

Papadelis, C., Harini, C., Ahtam, B., Doshi, C., Grant, E., & Okada, Y. (2013). Current and emerging potential for magnetoencephalography in pediatric epilepsy. *Journal of Pediatric Epilepsy, 2*, 73–85.

Papadelis, C., Leonardelli, E., Staudt, M., & Braun, C. (2012). Can magnetoencephalography track the afferent information flow along white matter thalamo-cortical fibers? *Neuroimage, 60*(2), 1092–1105.

Papadelis, C., Poghosyan, V., Fenwick, P. B. C., & Ioannides, A. A. (2009). MEG's ability to localise accurately weak transient neural sources. *Clinical Neurophysiology, 120*(11), 1958–1970.

Penfield, W., & Rasmussen, T. (1957). *The cerebral cortex of man: A clinical study of localization*. New York, NY: Macmillan.

Sutcliffe, T. L., Gaetz, W., Logan, W., Cheyne, D., & Fehlings, D. (2007). Cortical reorganization after modified constraint-induced movement therapy in pediatric hemiplegic cerebral palsy. *Journal of Child Neurology, 22*(11), 1281–1287.

Trevarrow, M. P., Kurz, M. J., McDermott, T. J., Weisman, A. I., Mills, M. S., Wang, Y. P., . . . Wilson, T. W. (2018). The developmental trajectory of sensorimotor cortical oscillations. *Neuroimage, 184*, 455–461.

Wilke, M., Staudt, M., Juenger, H., Grodd, W., Braun, C., & Krägeloh-Mann, I. (2009). Somatosensory system in two types of motor reorganization in congenital hemiparesis: Topography and function. *Human Brain Mapping, 30*(3), 776–788.

Wilson, T. W., Heinrichs-Graham, E., & Becker, K. M. (2014). Circadian modulation of motor-related beta oscillatory responses. *Neuroimage, 102*(Pt 2), 531–539.

Wilson, T. W., Heinrichs-Graham, E., Proskovec, A. L., & McDermott, T. J. (2016). Neuroimaging with magnetoencephalography: A dynamic view of brain pathophysiology. *Translational Research, 175*, 17–36.

Wilson, T. W., Heinrichs-Graham, E., Robertson, K. R., Sandkovsky, U., O'Neill, J., Knott, N. L., . . . Swindells, S. (2013). Functional brain abnormalities during finger-tapping in HIV-infected older adults: A magnetoencephalography study. *Journal of Neuroimmune Pharmacology, 8*(4), 965–974.

Wilson, T. W., Leuthold, A. C., Lewis, S. M., Georgopoulos, A. P., & Pardo, P. J. (2005a). The time and space of lexicality: A neuromagnetic view. *Experimental Brain Research, 162*(1), 1–13.

Wilson, T. W., Leuthold, A. C., Lewis, S. M., Georgopoulos, A. P., & Pardo, P. J. (2005b). Cognitive dimensions of orthographic stimuli affect occipitotemporal dynamics. *Experimental Brain Research, 167*(2), 141–147.

Wilson, T. W., Slason, E., Asherin, R., Kronberg, E., Reite, M. L., Teale, P. D., & Rojas, D. C. (2010). An extended motor network generates beta and gamma oscillatory perturbations during development. *Brain Cognition, 73*(2), 75–84.

Zimmerman, J. E., Thiene, P., & Harding, J. T. (1970). Design and operation of stable rf-biased superconducting point-contact quantum devices, and a note on the properties of perfectly clean metal contacts. *Journal of Applied Physics, 41,* 1572.

16

INVESTIGATIONS OF THE SOMATOSENSORY SYSTEM WITH MAGNETOENCEPHALOGRAPHY

FROM RESEARCH TO CLINICAL APPLICATIONS

Xavier De Tiège and Veikko Jousmäki

IN ANCIENT Greek, *sõma* refers to body and *aísthēsis* to perception by the intellect as well as the senses. Accordingly, the somesthesic or somatosensory system is involved in the perception of the body. It mediates a range of sensations such as touch, pressure, vibration, limb position (i.e., proprioception), balance, heat, cold, interoception, and pain transduced by a multitude of receptors disseminated within the body. Information is then conveyed to the brain through distinct central pathways.

This chapter reviews the historical contribution of magnetoencephalography (MEG) to the understanding of the functioning of the somatosensory system and how some achievements have been transferred to clinical research or routine to be integrated in clinical guidelines (Burgess et al., 2011; Hari et al., 2018). Considering the vast literature and the existence of comprehensive MEG review papers

on the topic (see, e.g., Hari & Forss, 1999; Hari & Puce, 2017b; Kakigi et al., 2000; Kakigi & Forss, 2010), we will here focus on pioneering or specific studies in a historical framework.

16.1. THE SOMATOSENSORY SYSTEM

Somatic sensations are conveyed by afferent nerve fibers whose peripheral processes ramify within the skin, joints, tendons, muscles, and viscera. All somatosensory information from the limbs and trunk is transmitted by spinal dorsal root ganglia neurons, while that from cranial structures is conveyed by trigeminal sensory neurons. These neurons are involved in stimulus transduction and transmission from the periphery to the brain. The terminals of the peripheral axonal branches are the only cell portions that are sensitive to natural stimuli (Gardner,

Xavier De Tiège and Veikko Jousmäki, *Investigations of the Somatosensory System With Magnetoencephalography: From Research to Clinical Applications* In: *Fifty Years of Magnetoencephalography*. Edited by: Andrew C. Papanicolaou, Timothy P. L. Roberts, and James W. Wheless, Oxford University Press (2020). © Oxford University Press. DOI: 10.1093/oso/9780190935689.003.0016.

Martin, & Jessell, 2000). These terminals may be free nerve endings for nociceptors (for pain sensation) and thermal receptors (for heat and cold sensations) or encapsulated for the numerous types of mechanoreceptors (for touch and proprioception). Information from nociceptors and thermal receptors is conveyed by small-diameter unmyelinated or thinly myelinated axons, which conduct encoded information rather slowly (<35 m/s). By contrast, information from mechanoreceptors is transmitted by large-diameter, myelinated axons conducting information more rapidly (from 35 to >100 m/s).

All submodalities of somatic sensations are transmitted to the neocortex using a three-neuron system relaying somatosensory information from the periphery through dedicated neural pathways within the thalamus (Gardner et al., 2000). Information from mechanoreceptors is conveyed by the dorsal column–medial lemniscal system, whereas those from nociceptors and thermal receptors are transmitted by the anterolateral system (Gardner et al., 2000). Of note, nociceptive stimuli are mediated by two different neuroanatomical pathways, one for the discriminative (i.e., location, intensity, and quality of the noxious stimulation) aspects of pain and another for the affective–motivational aspects of pain eliciting the unpleasant feeling, fear, and anxiety, as well as autonomic activation, that accompany pain (Gardner et al., 2000).

16.2. SOMATOSENSORY STIMULATORS

The somatosensory system is, in general, more difficult to study than auditory and visual systems using natural, highly controlled, and selective stimuli (Hari & Puce, 2017b; Jousmäki, Nishitani, & Hari, 2007). For example, the high sensitivity of MEG to magnetic fields complicates the development of stimulators eliciting natural body stimulation without generating high-amplitude artifacts. For a detailed description of somatosensory stimulations that can be used in the MEG setting, see Hari and Puce (2017a, 2017b).

Historically, brief (typically 0.1–0.2 ms duration) electric stimuli applied on the skin over the peripheral nerves (e.g., median or tibial nerves) have been used in seminal and subsequent large number of MEG studies aiming at unraveling the spatial, temporal, and spectral dynamics of neocortical activity to peripheral somatosensory stimulation. Such stimuli have the advantages of being precisely controlled and of eliciting robust neocortical somatosensory evoked fields (SEFs). Although electric stimuli are widely used, they are unnatural, often unpleasant, and unspecific in the sense that they activate a large number of afferent fibers with different conduction velocities.

To complement electric stimulation, different devices have been ingeniously developed to assess brain responses to natural mechanoreceptors stimulation. Natural tactile stimulations have been performed in the MEG setting using air puffs (Forss, Salmelin, & Hari, 1994b; Huttunen, 1986), vibrotactile stimuli (Jagow, Ribary, Lado, & Llinas, 1992; Jousmäki & Hari, 1999), moving tactile stimuli produced with a brush (Lin & Kajola, 2003), taps produced by compressed-air-driven small balloons (Hoshiyama et al., 1995) or balloon diaphragms (Mertens & Lutkenhoner, 2000; Nguyen, Inui, Hoshiyama, Nakata, & Kakigi, 2005; Nguyen, Tran, Hoshiyama, Inui, & Kakigi, 2004), or optic fiber bundle forming a small brush (Jousmäki et al., 2007).

Neuromagnetic responses to natural stimulation of spinocortical proprioceptive pathways have been explored using either active or passive movements of the fingers or toes in the corticokinematic coherence (CKC) framework (see Bourguignon et al., 2011, 2015; Piitulainen, Bourguignon, De Tiège, Hari, & Jousmäki, 2013b; Smeds, Piitulainen, Bourguignon, Jousmäki, & Hari, 2017). Passive movements were elicited either by an experimenter or by pneumatic artificial muscles (Piitulainen, Bourguignon, Hari, & Jousmäki, 2015; Smeds et al., 2017).

Nociceptive stimuli have been induced by surface electrical stimulation of peripheral (Kitamura et al., 1995, 1997) or trigeminal (Hari et al., 1983b) nerves, intracutaneous epidermal electrical stimulation (Howland et al., 1995; Inui & Kakigi, 2012), carbon dioxide (CO_2) gas applied to the nasal mucosa (Hari et al., 1997a; Huttunen et al., 1986), CO_2 (Kakigi et al., 1995; Watanabe, Kakigi, Koyama, Hoshiyama, & Kaneoke, 1998) or thulium (Ploner, Schmitz, Freund, & Schnitzler, 1999; Forss, Raij, Seppa, & Hari, 2005) laser pulses applied on the skin, or noxious heat stimulation induced by a contact heat evoked potential stimulator (CHEPS) (Adjamian et al., 2009; Gopalakrishnan, Machado, Burgess, & Mosher, 2013; Worthen et al., 2007). Compared with electrical stimulation, laser pulses can offer, depending on stimulation parameters, the possibility to selectively activate the thinly myelinated Aδ- and unmyelinated C fibers in the skin, which convey painful information at different velocities (Aδ fibers: 5–30 m/s; C fibers: 0.5–2 m/s) (Forss, Raij, Seppa, & Hari, 2005). This offers the unique opportunity to

investigate the brain responses to first and second pain (Forss et al., 2005). CHEPS stimulations are associated with high-amplitude artifacts requiring advanced methods of signal processing to uncover the neuromagnetic responses of interest (Worthen et al., 2007; Gopalakrishnan et al., 2013).

To the best of our knowledge, no MEG study has been published on brain responses elicited by nonpainful thermal (heat or cold) stimulation. This is probably due to the difficulty eliciting artifact-free, sharp-onset timely controlled repetitive thermal stimulation in the MEG setting.

16.3. SOMATOSENSORY EVOKED MAGNETIC FIELDS

Figure 16.1 illustrates the spatiotemporal dynamics of SEFs elicited by electrical median nerve stimulation.

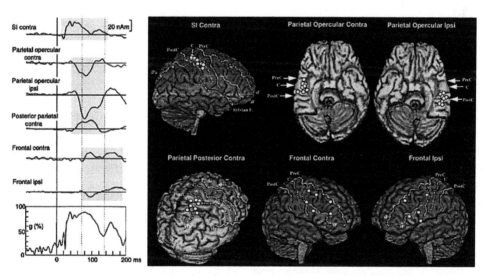

FIGURE 16.1   (*Left*) Time course of dipole activation following electrical (0.3-ms constant current pulses at motor threshold, random interstimulus interval [ISI] from 2.4 to 21.6 s) stimulation of the left median nerve obtained in one subject. Source strengths are plotted as a function of time. The lowest curve represents the goodness-of-fit value (g%) calculated over all channels. The *shaded areas* indicate the activation period for each source, and the area between the two *vertical dashed lines* corresponds to their overlap. (*Right*) Distribution of sources across the eight investigated subjects. Source locations for each subject are plotted on a brain magnetic resonance imaging (MRI) profile. Based on individual MRI studies, each source is reported on the three-dimensional MRI profile on the basis of its relative position to the fissures. The main sulci are indicated by *dashed lines*. C = central sulcus; iF = inferior frontal sulcus; iPa = intraparietal sulcus; preC = precentral sulcus; postC = postcentral sulcus; sF = superior frontal sulcus; Sylvian F = sylvian fissure. (Adapted from Mauguiere, F., Merlet, I., Forss, N., Vanni, S., Jousmäki, V., Adeleine, P., & Hari, R. [1997]. Activation of a distributed somatosensory cortical network in the human brain. A dipole modelling study of magnetic fields evoked by median nerve stimulation. Part I: Location and activation timing of SEF sources. *Electroencephalography and Clinical Neurophysiology, 104*[4], 281–289.)

The first SEF recordings performed in humans were carried out in 1978 using a single-channel device with a steady-state approach based on periodic electrical thumb and little finger stimulation (Brenner, Lipton, Kaufman, & Williamson, 1978). This study demonstrated that dipolar field patterns were about 2 cm more lateral for stimulation of the thumb than the little finger, consistent with the known somatotopy of the primary somatosensory (SI) cortex (Brenner et al., 1978). In the next decade, subsequent studies used electrical median (Hari et al., 1983a, 1984; Huttunen et al., 1987; Kaufman, Nishitani, & Hari, 1981; Okada, Kaufman, Brenner, & Williamson, 1981; Rossini et al., 1989; Sutherling et al., 1988; Tiihonen, Hari, & Hämäläinen, 1989a; Wood, Cohen, Cuffin, Yarita, & Allison, 1985), ulnar (Huttunen et al., 1987), or peroneal (Hari et al., 1984) nerve stimulations to characterize the spatiotemporal dynamics of SEFs. Overall, those seminal studies demonstrated that evoked responses at SI cortex (a) mainly originated from tangential area 3b sources (for a detailed discussion about the role of tangential versus radial S1 cortical sources on MEG and electroencephalography (EEG) evoked responses, see Hari & Puce, 2017b), (b) had latencies that were dependent on the traveling distance of action potentials from the periphery to Brodmann area 3b of S1 cortex, and (c) were organized in a somatotopic manner in accordance with the "homuncular" organization of S1 cortex (Penfield & Boldrey, 1937). Interestingly, MEG studies were also the first to differentiate in space and time responses from SI and secondary somatosensory (SII) cortices (Hari et al., 1983a, 1984; Teszner, Hari, Nicolas, & Varpula, 1983), before both direct cortical recordings and positron emission tomography (PET) studies (Hari & Puce, 2017b). Unilateral stimulations elicited SEFs at bilateral SII cortex, with longer latencies compared with S1 cortex responses, and with slightly longer latencies at ipsilateral than contralateral SII cortices (Hari et al., 1983a,

1984). Additionally, MEG allowed identification of significant phase-locking between responses of SI and SII cortices after electrical median nerve stimulation (Simoes, Jensen, Parkkonen, & Hari, 2003). It also contributed to the identification of weak SI cortex and strong left hemisphere dominant SII cortices magnetic responses following electrical dorsal penile nerve stimulation (Mäkelä et al, 2003).

Subsequent studies also demonstrated the existence of magnetic responses to electrical median nerve stimulation at the posterior parietal cortex (PPC) located median and posterior to SI cortex, presumably at Brodmann area 5 (Forss et al., 1994a; Mauguiere et al., 1997b). Timing of those PPC SEFs were similar to those of SII cortices.

Most of the first MEG studies that used natural tactile stimulations were done in the 1990s (Forss et al., 1994b; Gallen et al., 1994; Hashimoto, 1987; Hoshiyama et al., 1995; Huttunen, 1986; Rossini et al., 1996). They demonstrated weaker amplitudes and up to 20 to 40 ms longer latencies for SEFs at the SI cortex to natural tactile stimuli than to electrical stimulations. Amplitudes are weaker because natural tactile stimuli recruit more specifically cutaneous afferent fibers than do electrical stimuli, which recruit both proprioceptor and cutaneous fibers (Forss et al., 1994b; Rossini et al., 1996). Longer latencies are due to transduction time at the skin mechanoreceptors (Hoshiyama et al., 1995) or to longer time rise of natural tactile stimuli compared with the sharpness of electrical stimulations (Forss et al., 1994b). Importantly, the amplitude of SEFs elicited at PPC and SII cortices by natural tactile stimuli roughly corresponded to those obtained after electrical stimulation (Forss et al., 1994b). These findings suggested that the SI cortex encodes details about somatosensory stimuli, while responses at SII cortices and PCC are less sensitive to stimulus type and have more integrative features (Forss et al., 1994b). Similar observations have been made in patients with progressive myoclonic epilepsy, in whom "giant" SEFs have been

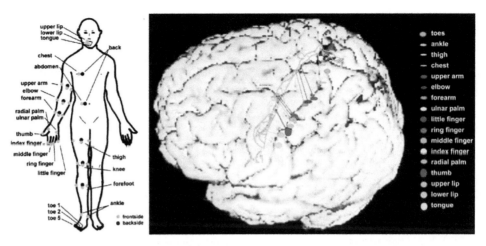

FIGURE 16.2 (*Left*) Location of the 43 points of the right body stimulated using air-puff-derived tactile stimulator providing a light, superficial pressure stimulus to the skin surface. *Gray circles* indicate stimulus points on the frontside of the body. *Black circles* indicate stimulus points on the backside of the body. In the case of arm and leg stimulations, lateral, medial anterior, and posterior points were stimulated. (*Right*) Detailed somatosensory receptive maps represented by magnetoencephalography. The three-dimensional brain magnetic resonance imaging (MRI) study was reconstructed using the MRI of one subject. The size of each *ellipse* reflects the presumed size of the activated cortical area. (Adapted from Nakamura, A., Yamada, T., Goto, A., Kato, T., Ito, K., Abe, Y., ... Kakigi, R. [1998]. Somatosensory homunculus as drawn by MEG. *Neuroimage, 7*[4 Pt 1], 377–386.)

observed at bilateral SI cortex but with normal responses at bilateral SII cortices (Forss, Silen, & Karjalainen, 2001).

Electrical and natural tactile stimuli were both used to investigate the somatotopic or "homuncular" organization of magnetic responses at the SI and SII cortices (for a detailed list of references, see Kakigi & Forss, 2010). Studies demonstrated a clear and reproductive somatotopic organization of the SI cortex magnetic responses compatible with the anatomy of the central sulcus and the Penfield's homunculus (see, e.g., Nakamura et al., 1998; Figure 16.2). By contrast, SII cortex showed some degree of somatotopy but with large interindividual differences and a differentiation of the different body parts that was less clear than those observed at the SI cortex (Hari et al., 1993; Maeda, Kakigi, Hoshiyama, & Koyama, 1999; Nguyen et al., 2005; Sakamoto, Nakata, & Kakigi, 2008). This latter finding is in line with the integrative role of the SII cortex for the somatosensory function.

Several studies have investigated the impact of interstimulus interval (ISI), stimulus intensity, and attention on the SEFs at the SI and SII cortices and PPC. Figure 16.3 summarizes findings from those MEG studies. They basically identified a significant effect of ISI on the amplitude of subcomponents (P35m and P60m) of the SI cortex responses and of bilateral SII cortices and PPC (Mauguiere et al., 1997a; Wikström et al., 1996). SEF amplitudes at those brain areas were significantly weaker (P35m, P60m) or even abolished (SII cortices and PPC) with decreasing ISI (typically, <1 s) (Mauguiere et al., 1997a; Wikström et al., 1996). Amplitude of the N20m response at SI cortex increased linearly with electrical stimulus intensity (from sensory, weak motor to strong motor thresholds), while it plateaued from weak motor threshold for bilateral SII cortices and PPC (Jousmäki & Forss, 1998). This finding is again in line with the role of SI cortex in informing about the details of somatosensory stimuli and the integrative role of SII cortices and PPC (Forss et al., 1994b; Jousmäki

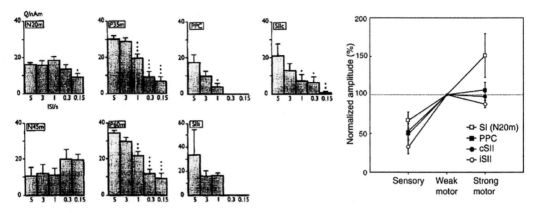

FIGURE 16.3   (*Left*) Average (± standard error of the mean) source strengths of the somatosensory evoked fields (SEFs) elicited by electrical (0.2-ms constant current pulses; motor threshold; interstimulus intervals [ISIs] of 0.15, 0.3, 1, 3, and 5 s) right median nerve stimulation in nine subjects. *$p < 0.05$; **$p < 0.005$; ***$p < 0.0005$. (Adapted from Wikström, H., Huttunen, J., Korvenoja, A., Virtanen, J., Salonen, O., Aronen, H., & Ilmoniemi, R. J. [1996]. Effects of interstimulus interval on somatosensory evoked fields (SEFs): A hypothesis concerning SEF generation at the primary sensorimotor cortex. *Electroencephalography and Clinical Neurophysiology, 100*[6], 479–487). (*Right*) Mean (± standard error of the mean) source strengths obtained in seven subjects after electrical (0.3-ms constant current pulses; ISI of 3 s; sensory, weak motor, strong motor thresholds) left median nerve stimulation. Source strengths have been normalized with respect to the strength of responses to weak motor stimuli (=100%). (Adapted from Jousmäki, V., & Forss, N. [1998]. Effects of stimulus intensity on signals from human somatosensory cortices. *Neuroreport, 9*[15], 3427–3431).

& Forss, 1998). Orienting spatial attention toward the site of stimulation or not (e.g., reading a book during the stimulation) had no substantial effect on SEFs elicited by electrical median nerve stimulation (Mauguiere et al., 1997a).

Taken together, all the SEF data have brought impressive novel insights into the spatiotemporal dynamics of brain responses to somatosensory stimulation. They have also contributed substantially to the understanding of the specific roles of the different somatosensory network nodes such as SI cortex, bilateral SII cortex, and PPC. Of note, later SEF studies confirmed some seminal findings (Hinkley, Krubitzer, Nagarajan, & Disbrow, 2007; Jones, Pritchett, Stufflebeam, Hamalainen, & Moore, 2007; Jousmäki et al., 2007; Theuvenet et al., 2005; Torquati et al., 2002).

16.4. SOMATOSENSORY EVOKED MAGNETIC FIELDS ELICITED BY CHANGE DETECTION

Detecting changes or unexpected sensory events is vital to evolve safely and adapt to an ever-changing environment. To do so, the human brain has to efficiently isolate salient sensory inputs from irrelevant stimuli by detecting as early as possible sensory changes within the environment.

The electrophysiological correlate of early sensory change detection corresponds to the mismatch negativity (MMN), which is typically observed when subtracting evoked responses to repeated sensory stimuli (standards) from those elicited by rare sensory stimuli (deviants). The MMN was initially described in 1978 and mainly studied using EEG for the auditory modality (for a review, see, e.g., Näätänen et al., 2011). Still, MMN responses have been described both using EEG and MEG for the somatosensory modality (sMMN for EEG, somatosensory mismatch fields [sMMF] for MEG). It typically peaks around 75 to 120 ms after deviant onset and mainly involves contralateral SII cortex (Naeije et al., 2018; Figure 16.4).

Several MEG studies contributed to a better understanding of the neural mechanisms involved in early somatosensory change detection, as indexed by sMMF responses.

Initially, SEFs similar to those involved in typical sMMF responses were first recorded at SII cortex using oddball paradigms with standards (electrical stimuli) presented to the thumb and deviants (10%) to the middle finger, or vice versa (Hari et al., 1990). SII cortex responses to deviants were almost three times as high in amplitude as those to standards (Hari et al., 1990). Still, similar amplitude enhancement was obtained when deviants were presented in the absence of intervening standards but with the same ISI than during oddballs (Hari et al., 1990). Based on this latter finding (reported in one subject only), SII cortex responses to deviants were interpreted as being not specific of stimulus change per se but rather as resulting from differences in stimulus repetition rates, leading to the "rate effect" hypothesis (Hari et al., 1990). Five years later, a second study that used rather similar oddball paradigms demonstrated that somatosensory deviants presented alone (i.e., without

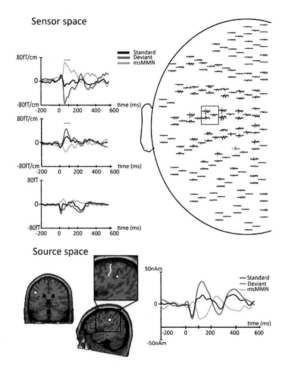

FIGURE 16.4   Grand-average results of the mismatch responses obtained at sensor and source levels in 16 subjects. Standards corresponded to pneumatic tactile stimulations applied to the right index fingertip, while deviants consisted of tactile stimulations applied to the middle phalange and another to the fingertip of the right index finger. (*Top, right*) Left part of the magnetoencephalography (MEG) sensor array viewed from top. (*Left*) Enlarged orthogonal planar gradiometers (*top, middle*) and magnetometer (*bottom*) signals showing evoked magnetic responses. *Green lines* indicate the timing of significant differences between standards and deviants disclosed by nonparametric cluster-based statistics performed at the sensor level (planar gradiometers only). Of note, in the sensor space, the polarity of the cortical responses may appear different from sensor to sensor because of different spatial sensitivity (i.e., lead field) of orthogonal planar gradiometers and magnetometers to right beneath or nearby neural sources. (*Bottom, left*) Coronal (*left*) and sagittal (*right, left hemisphere*) slices showing the location of the source (*white dot*; missmatch negativity (MNI) coordinates: [−43, −19, 21] mm) that best explains the magnetic field pattern at the magnetic somatosensory mismatch negativity (smMMN) response maximum amplitude. (*Right*) Source waveforms corresponding to standards (*black line*), deviants (*red line*), and msMMN (*blue line*). (Adapted from Naeije, G., Vaulet, T., Wens, V., Marty, B., Goldman, S., & De Tiège, X. [2016]. Multilevel cortical processing of somatosensory novelty: A magnetoencephalography study. *Frontiers in Human Neuroscience, 10*, 259.)

intervening standard) elicited higher SII cortex amplitude response than when presented among standards with similar rates of occurrence (Forss, Jousmäki, & Hari, 1995). This finding contradicted the initial "rate effect" hypothesis to explain the difference in SII cortex response between deviant and standard stimuli.

One MEG study relying on sequences of identical pneumatic tactile stimuli disclosed substantial attenuation of SII cortex responses after a first tactile stimulus (Popescu, Barlow, Venkatesan, Wang, & Popescu, 2013). This finding is in line with previous MEG studies that demonstrated significant effects of ISI on SII cortex responses, which were characterized by a substantial attenuation of response amplitude when the ISI is constant and less than 1 s (Mauguiere et al., 1997a; Wikström et al., 1996). These findings are in accordance with the "neural adaptation" theory (May & Tiitinen, 2010) proposed to explain MMN/MMF neural bases, which shares some features with the "rate effect" hypothesis. This theory postulates that MMN/MMF is a mere subtraction artifact between the attenuated response of feature-specific neurons to repeated standards and the response from sensory-specific neurons sensitive to deviants.

Still, amplitudes of magnetic SII cortex responses were demonstrated as being dependent not only on the magnitude of the change in stimulus intensity but also on the length of the conditioning stimulus before the change (Otsuru et al., 2011). These findings suggest that storage of prior tactile information before deviant occurrence is involved in generating SII cortex responses (Otsuru et al., 2011). They are thus in accordance with another hypothesis that has been proposed to explain the neural bases of MMN/MMF, which is the "model adjustment" theory (Näätänen, Paavilainen, Rinne, & Alho, 2007). In this theory, the MMN/MMF is considered to reflect the neural detection of a deviation from a sensory memory trace based on preceding standard stimuli. But, the existence of magnetic SII cortex activity in the context of "off responses," that is, SEFs elicited at SII cortices when abruptly stopping trains of electrical finger stimuli (Yamashiro, Inui, Otsuru, Kida, & Kakigi, 2009) contradicts this "model adjustment" theory.

Therefore, another theory to reconcile all these MEG findings is the "predictive coding" theory, which considers that the brain predicts incoming sensory information based on previous experience and discards expected information to allocate neural resources only to novel or surprising information (for a review, see, e.g., Friston, 2010). This theory has gained increasing interests because it allows combining the "neural adaptation" and the "model adjustment" theories for MMN genesis by considering (a) that the MMN is generated by specific neuronal error prediction units when a deviant incoming stimulus fails the prediction of higher level cortices for incoming stimuli (adjustment), and (b) that activity of such error prediction units is modulated by the reproducibility of incoming stimuli (adaptation) (for a review, see Garrido, Kilner, Stephan, & Friston, 2009). This theory might also explain why infrequent somatosensory deviants embedded among standards or presented alone with identical rates of occurrence (i.e., the "rate effect" hypothesis) might share similar levels of surprise or expectation. It could also explain why "off-responses" might generate SII cortex activity in the absence of any physical somatosensory stimulus. By showing that (a) in tactile oddball paradigms, the predictability of deviants occurrence modulates the amplitude of SII cortex sMMF responses (Naeije et al., 2016, 2018), (b) SII cortex responses are attenuated after a first tactile stimulation even if the second stimulation is different from the first one (Naeije et al., 2018), and (c) omission of expected tactile stimulus generates similar (or higher) SII cortex responses than preceding tactile stimuli (Andersen & Lundqvist, 2018; Mauguiere et al., 1997a; Naeije et al., 2018), MEG studies brought novel and robust empirical evidence supporting the involvement of predictive coding in the genesis of sMMN/

sMMF responses at SII cortex. One of those MEG studies also brought data in favor of a multilevel, hierarchical neocortical processing of somatosensory novelty, with early change detection responses (i.e., sMMF) occurring at SII cortex, and late (i.e., P300) responses related to the conscious detection of complex changes in a continuous stream of sensory inputs at bilateral temporoparietal junctions and supplementary motor area (SMA) (Naeije et al., 2016). It also demonstrated that progressive changes in expectation associated with each correct prediction of incoming sensory inputs was associated with a magnetic correlate of contingent negative variation response at SMA and PPC (Naeije et al., 2016).

16.5. SOMATOSENSORY EVOKED MAGNETIC FIELDS ELICITED BY NOCICEPTIVE STIMULI

Historically, MEG has provided the first evidence in humans that painful stimuli activate SII cortex (Hari et al., 1983b). This was obtained by stimulating electrically the dental pulp of six adult subjects (Hari et al., 1983b). Responses peaked at about 90 to 100 ms after stimulus at locations compatible with SII cortex (Hari et al., 1983b). Involvement of SII cortex in pain processing elicited by trigeminal nociceptive stimulation was confirmed in later MEG studies that investigated the cortical responses to CO_2 stimulation of the nasal mucosa (Hari et al., 1997a; Huttunen et al., 1986). Responses (a) had longer latencies (about 350–400 ms after stimulation) than those elicited by dental pulp nociceptive stimulation, probably owing to delay in nociceptor transduction (Hari et al., 1997a; Huttunen et al., 1986); (b) were modulated in amplitude by ISI (Hari et al., 1997a); and (3) predominated over the right hemisphere SII cortex (Hari et al., 1997a).

Two MEG studies demonstrated bilateral SII cortices (peaking at 150 ms and 250 ms after stimulation) and anterior cingulate cortices (ACC, peaking at 250 ms after stimulation) magnetic responses following nociceptive electrical stimulation of the right index finger and of the sural nerve with responses that did not depend on the stimulation site (Kitamura et al., 1995, 1997).

Implication of other areas than SII cortex was also evidenced using MEG and nociceptive intracutaneous epidermal electrical stimulation. Indeed, apart from SI and SII cortices, such painful stimuli elicited responses in the insula (peaking at about 160 ms after stimulation), in the ACC (peaking at 250 ms after stimulation), and possibly in the midtemporal region (amygdala or hippocampus, peaking at 250 ms after stimulation) (Inui et al., 2003a, 2003b).

Finally, several MEG studies used nociceptive stimuli elicited by CO_2 (Kakigi et al., 1995) or thulium (Forss et al., 2005; Ploner et al., 1999; Ploner, Schmitz, Freund, & Schnitzler, 2000) laser pulses applied on the skin. The use of laser pulses opened the possibility to selectively activate the thinly myelinated Aδ-fibers and unmyelinated C-fibers in the skin, which convey painful information at different velocities (Aδ-fibers: 5–30 m/s; C-fibers: <2 m/s). Indeed, most of the studies described previously reported cortical magnetic activations either to Aδ-fiber-mediated pain or to a combination of Aδ-fibers and C-fibers. The first MEG studies that investigated the brain areas involved in the processing of pain elicited by specific stimulation of C-fibers demonstrated the existence of a first response peaking at about 750 ms after stimulation in a network comprising contralateral SI, bilateral SII, and insular cortices (Qiu et al., 2004; Tran et al., 2002). A second response peaking at about 950 ms involved additional brain areas such as the ACC and medial temporal areas (Qiu et al., 2004; Tran et al., 2002). Similar findings were obtained by selective stimulation of C-fibers using intracutaneous epidermal electrical stimulation (Maihofner, Jesberger, Seifert, & Kaltenhauser, 2010; Motogi, Kodaira, Muragaki, Inui, & Kakigi, 2014). Another MEG study investigated using a thulium laser to selectively stimulate

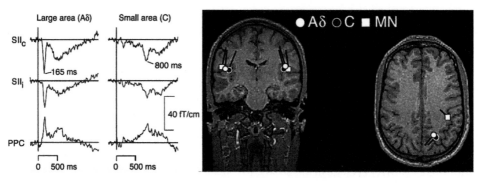

FIGURE 16.5 (*Left*) Grand averages of contralateral and ipsilateral SII and posterior parietal cortex (PPC) responses to Aδ-fiber (*left*) and C-fiber stimuli in eight subjects. (*Right*) Source locations in the SII cortices and PPC to Aδ-fiber (*white circle*) and C-fiber (*black circle*) and electrical median nerve (*white square*) stimuli superimposed on the magnetic resonance image of one subject. (Adapted from Forss, N., Raij, T. T., Seppa, M., & Hari, R. [2005]. Common cortical network for first and second pain. *Neuroimage, 24*[1], 132–142.)

the neuromagnetic responses of Aδ-fibers and C-fibers in adult subjects (Forss et al., 2005). Results showed that selective Aδ-fibers stimulation was associated with responses at bilateral SII cortices and contralateral PPC, peaking at about 160 ms after stimulation, while stimulation of C-fibers was associated with responses in a similar neocortical network but peaking at about 800 ms after stimulation (Forss et al., 2005; Figure 16.5). These findings were in agreement with the conduction velocities of the corresponding nerve fibers.

Overall, MEG studies investigating SEFs elicited by nociceptive stimuli demonstrated a clear and robust involvement of SII cortex in pain processing with varying (depending of nociceptive stimulation type and source reconstruction used) magnetic responses at SI cortex, ACC, midtemporal regions, and PPC.

16.6. OSCILLATORY ACTIVITIES INDUCED BY SOMATOSENSORY STIMULATION

Two main types of oscillatory activities have been described following stimulation of somatosensory pathways: a 600-Hz oscillatory burst at human SI cortex following electrical peripheral nerve stimulation as well as the event-related modulations of the Rolandic mu rhythm amplitude after electrical or natural tactile stimulation.

16.6.1. 600-Hz Responses

In the middle of the 1990s, bursts of high-frequency oscillations (HFOs) occurring at 600 Hz were described at the Brodmann area 3b of SI cortex about 20 ms after electrical median nerve stimulation (Curio et al., 1994). These HFOs occurred almost concomitantly to the first SI cortex evoked magnetic response, the N20m (Curio et al., 1994). During sleep, HFOs were drastically reduced in amplitude, while the N20m amplitude exhibited moderate increment (Hashimoto, Mashiko, & Imada, 1996). This different behavior of HFOs and N20m responses during the wake–sleep cycle suggested that they resulted from different neural generators (Hashimoto et al., 1996). HFOs were considered to be generated by GABAergic inhibitory interneurons located at layer 4 of Brodmann area 3b (Hashimoto et al., 1996). This hypothesis was supported by data obtained in rabbits, which demonstrated that those interneurons respond to thalamocortical inputs with a high-frequency (600–900 Hz) burst of short duration spikes (Swadlow, 1989). It was further supported in humans by the demonstration of reduced HFO amplitudes in patients with cervical dystonia (Inoue, K.,

Shimizu, Nakasato, Kumabe, & Yoshimoto, 2004). Indeed, cervical dystonia is presumed to be caused by deficient inhibition within SI and M1 cortices (Inoue, K., et al., 2004). Interestingly, the comparison of electrical median, ulnar, and tibial nerve stimulations demonstrated the existence of a somatotopic arrangement of the HFOs at SI cortex (Curio et al., 1997; Sakuma & Hashimoto, 1999a; Sakuma, Sekihara, & Hashimoto, 1999b). Of note, HFOs elicited by tibial nerve stimulation occurred concomitantly to the first SI cortex evoked magnetic response, the P37m (Sakuma & Hashimoto, 1999a).

16.6.2. Modulation of Mu Rhythm

At rest, the Rolandic mu rhythm is characterized by two main frequencies that have a nearly, but not exactly, harmonic relationship (Tiihonen, Kajola, & Hari, 1989b). These two frequency components appear to be related to separate functional networks: approximately 10 Hz reflects predominantly (but not exclusively) somatosensory cortical function, while the approximately 20-Hz rhythm is mainly associated with motor cortex function (for a review, see Hari & Salmelin, 1997b).

Evidence indicates that the amplitude of mu rhythm—visible in intracranial recordings, in scalp EEG, as well as in MEG—is suppressed during active or passive movements (Chatrian, Petersen, & Lazarte, 1959), movement preparation (Caetano, Jousmäki, & Hari, 2007), motor imagery (Schnitzler, Salenius, Salmelin, Jousmäki, & Hari, 1997), and action observation (Hari et al., 1998). Suppression is followed by enhancement of mu rhythm amplitude when the task has ceased during 0.5 to 2.5 s. Suppression of primary sensorimotor (SMI) cortex rhythmic activity is likely related to excitation of the cortex, while enhancement would reflect inhibitory control (Klimesch, Sauseng, & Hanslmayr, 2007), cortical stabilization (Caetano et al., 2007), or active immobilization (Salmelin, Hamalainen, Kajola, & Hari, 1995) of SM1 cortex activity.

Importantly, MEG studies have demonstrated modulations of both mu rhythm frequency components following electrical peripheral nerve (Hirata et al., 2002; Gaetz & Cheyne, 2003; Salenius, Schnitzler, Salmelin, Jousmaki, & Hari, 1997; Salmelin & Hari, 1994) and natural tactile (Cheyne et al., 2003; Gaetz & Cheyne, 2006; Salenius et al., 1997; Figure 16.6) stimulation. Typically, the SMI cortex rhythmic activity decreases about 100 to 200 ms after the stimulus and increases above prestimulus level within 0.3 to 0.5 s afterwards. The enhancement occurs 100 to 300 ms earlier for the 20-Hz than for the 10-Hz activity. Suppression and enhancement are strongest at contralateral SMI cortex for the 20-Hz activity, but not for the 10-Hz activity. Natural tactile finger/hand stimulations produce weaker mu rhythm modulations than electrical median nerve stimulations. Modulations of the 10-Hz rhythmic activity usually occur at postcentral gyrus, while those of the 20-Hz activity appear more focal and located at the hand knob of the precentral gyrus. Of note, there is a high degree of interindividual variations in the spatial, spectral, and temporal dynamics of event-related mu rhythm amplitude modulations after somatosensory stimulation (Cheyne et al., 2003).

16.7. INVESTIGATION OF PROPRIOCEPTIVE PATHWAYS USING CORTICOKINEMATIC COHERENCE

Seminal MEG studies found significant coupling between SMI cortex activity and the rhythmicity of finger movements performed actively (Gross et al., 2002; Jerbi et al., 2007; Kelso et al., 1998; O'Suilleabhain, Lagerlund, & Matsumoto, 1999; Pollok, Gross, Dirks, Timmermann, & Schnitzler, 2004; Pollok, Sudmeyer, Gross, & Schnitzler, 2005). This coupling phenomenon was later coined the CKC (Bourguignon et al., 2011).

In a typical CKC setting, participants perform repetitive flexion-extensions of the fingers or of the index finger at about 3 Hz for

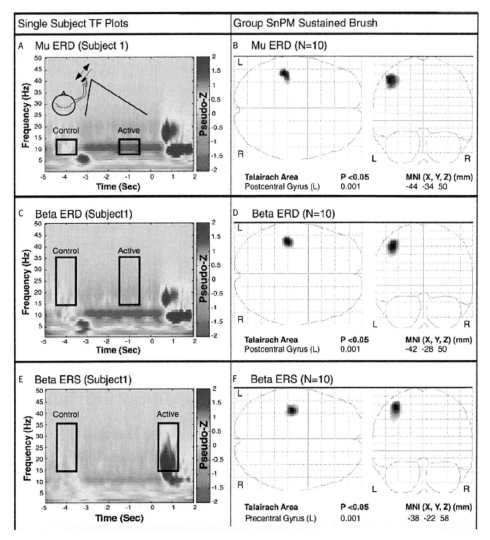

FIGURE 16.6   (*Left*) Time–frequency plots corresponding to responses elicited by transient brush stimulation from a single subject based on the observed virtual sensor peak locations for 10-Hz (mu event-related desynchrony [ERD]) and 20-Hz (beta ERD) suppressions, and for 20-Hz (beta ERS) enhancement. (*Right*) Grouped average (10 subjects) and statistically thresholded activity for the corresponding modulations of 10-Hz and 20-Hz rhythms. Note the different location for the different modulations of the mu rhythm. ERD = event-related desynchrony; ERS = event-related synchrony; MNI = Montreal Neurological Institute. (Adapted from Gaetz, W. C., & Cheyne, D. O. [2006]. Localization of sensorimotor cortical rhythms induced by tactile stimulation using spatially filtered MEG. *Neuroimage, 30,* 899–908.)

about 3 minutes, while their cortical signals are recorded with MEG and their finger kinematics is recorded with an accelerometer (Bourguignon et al., 2011, 2012). Coherence is then computed between MEG and acceleration signals (Figure 16.7). CKC typically peaks at movement frequency and its first harmonic, with its main cortical source located at the SMI hand area contralateral to finger movements (Bourguignon et al., 2011, 2012). CKC can also be estimated based on other kinetic, kinematics, and electromyography (EMG) signals (Piitulainen, Bourguignon, De Tiège, Hari, & Jousmäki, 2013a). Indeed, apart from acceleration or velocity signals, CKC has been reported based on (a) pressure, (b) force, and

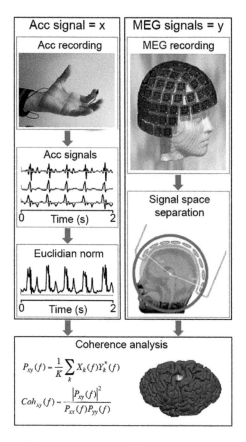

Acc signal = x	MEG signals = y
Acc recording	MEG recording
Acc signals 0 — Time (s) — 2	Signal space separation
Euclidian norm 0 — Time (s) — 2	

Coherence analysis

$$P_{xy}(f) = \frac{1}{K}\sum_k X_k(f)Y_k^*(f)$$

$$Coh_{xy}(f) = \frac{\left|P_{xy}(f)\right|^2}{P_{xx}(f)P_{yy}(f)}$$

FIGURE 16.7 Summary of the corticokinematic coherence pipeline using active repetitive finger flexion-extensions. (*Top, left*) The three-axis accelerometer (Acc) signals are bandpass-filtered and then combined into a single Acc signal using the Euclidian norm. (*Top, right*) Magnetoencephalography (MEG) signals are filtered using signal space separation (SSS) method to correct for head movements and subtract external interferences. (*Bottom*) Both signals are subsequently epoched to compute individual coherence maps. In the case of group-level analyses, individual coherence maps are thereafter normalized to standard MNI space and used to compute a group-level coherence map. (Adapted from Bourguignon, M., Jousmäki, V., Op de Beeck, M., Van Bogaert, P., Goldman, S., & De Tiège, X. [2012]. Neuronal network coherent with hand kinematics during fast repetitive hand movements. *Neuroimage*, 59[2], 1684–1691.)

(c) rectified EMG signals (Piitulainen et al., 2013a). CKC can therefore be investigated with typical surface EMG electrodes that are available in most of the MEG settings. Of note,

CKC has also been demonstrated during goal-directed hand action tasks (Jerbi et al., 2007; Marty et al., 2015a) and for slower finger movement rates (at ~1 Hz and ~2 Hz) (Marty et al., 2015b).

CKC is observed at SMI cortex in a somatotopic manner during passive movements of the fingers or toes (i.e., when participants' limb is moved by an experimenter or a PAM stimulator), with similar (or higher) coherence level and source location compared with active tasks (Piitulainen et al., 2013b, 2015). This finding brought major insights into the understanding of the neurophysiological basis of the CKC phenomenon. Indeed, the comparison of active and passive index finger movements with various tactile input levels, as well as the assessment of coupling directionality (with renormalized partial directed coherence [rPDC]), demonstrated that CKC is mainly driven by proprioceptive inputs to contralateral SMI cortex (Bourguignon, Piitulainen, De Tiège, Jousmäki, & Hari, 2015; Piitulainen et al., 2013b). Indeed, CKC and rPDC levels are independent of the motor output, while rPDC levels are influenced by the amount of tactile afferences (i.e., increased afferent coupling with increasing tactile input) but not CKC levels. These findings are in agreement with the fact that both SI (Brodmann areas 3a and 2) and MI cortices receive proprioceptive feedback during both active and passive hand movements (Goldring & Ratcheson, 1972).

Studies demonstrated that CKC (a) is detectable in most investigated subjects, with a high level of coherence compared with, for example, corticomuscular coherence (CMC), which is detectable in about 60 to 70% of subjects (Pohja, Salenius, & Hari, 2005); (b) shows a high degree of intersession reproducibility at the individual level (Piitulainen, Illman, Laaksonen, Jousmäki, & Forss, 2018); and (c) is robust against artifacts associated with implanted ferro-magnetic materials provided that the temporal signal space separation method is used to subtract the artifact from raw MEG signals (Bourguignon et al., 2016).

Apart from spinocortical proprioceptive pathways, significant but weaker (about one-third of the CKC levels observed at SM1 cortex) coupling has also been described during repetitive finger movements between cerebellar neuromagnetic signals and movement kinematics (Marty et al., 2018). This coupling occurs only at movement frequency at the posterior cerebellar lobe (presumably cerebellar lobule VIII) ipsilateral to finger movements, with no influence of movement frequency on coupling levels (Marty et al., 2018). Assessment of coupling directionality using rPDC demonstrated that this coupling is mainly driven by spinocerebellar, presumably, proprioceptive pathways with no contribution of corticocerebellar or cerebellocortical pathways (Marty et al., 2018).

CKC is therefore a robust noninvasive method to investigate spinocortical and spinocerebellar pathways in humans.

16.8. CLINICAL APPLICATIONS

The interest in using MEG for clinical applications has paralleled the development of MEG from its early phase in the 1970s (Hughes et al., 1977). Since then, despite intense clinical research and impressive developments of MEG instruments as well as of signal processing methods, identification of epileptic zones (see section 2) and localization of eloquent cortices (see also section 4) in neurosurgical patients remain, to date, the only recognized clinical indications of MEG worldwide.

In this general context, investigations of the somatosensory system have valuably contributed to the noninvasive localization of SMI cortex in neurosurgical patients who have to undergo resective surgery due to a lesion at the central sulcus. The aim of the functional MEG mapping procedure in such patients is typically to determine as precisely as possible the anatomical relationship between SMI cortices and the brain lesion in order to optimally tailor the surgical resection, assess related functional risks, and contribute to the decision-making process. In specialized clinical centers, the guidance of noninvasive (e.g., transcranial magnetic stimulation; Neggers et al., 2004) and invasive (e.g., electrical epidural cortex stimulation; Pirotte et al., 2005) SMI cortex stimulation procedures can be considered an additional clinical indication for MEG to provide accurate stimulation targets in patients with or without brain lesions. Also, results of functional SMI cortex mapping can be integrated into stereotactic radiosurgery planning systems to minimize the radiation dose applied on SMI cortices and reduce undesirable radiosurgery-related side effects (Conti et al., 2013; Pantelis et al., 2010; Stancanello et al., 2007). For practical guidelines regarding the use of MEG in this clinical indication, see Burgess et al. (2011) and Hari et al. (2018).

Several methods have been validated to identify the SMI cortex using MEG regardless of the source reconstruction methods used (i.e., equivalent current dipole modeling, minimum norm estimate, spatial filtering approaches): electrical peripheral nerve stimulation (Bourguignon et al., 2013; Cheyne, Bostan, Gaetz, & Pang, 2007; Kober et al., 2001; Korvenoja et al., 2006; Mäkelä et al., 2001; Solomon, Boe, & Bardouille, 2015; Vitikainen et al., 2009; Willemse et al., 2007; Willemse, Hillebrand, Ronner, Vandertop, & Stam, 2016), tactile stimulation (Roberts & Rowley, 1997; Schiffbauer et al., 2002), readiness and motor evoked fields (Gaetz et al., 2009; Kamada et al., 2003; Kober et al., 2001; Lin, Berger, & Nagarajan, 2006; Willemse et al., 2016), Rolandic mu rhythm suppression (alpha or beta band) (Bourguignon et al., 2013; Nagarajan et al., 2008; Willemse et al., 2010, 2016), corticomuscular coherence (CMC) (Bourguignon et al., 2013; Mäkelä et al., 2001), and CKC (Bourguignon et al., 2011, 2013). Among those, electrical peripheral nerve stimulation is often used because of its easiness, the robustness of the elicited SEF at the individual level, and the fact that simple source reconstruction methods such as equivalent current dipole modeling can be used to localize the cortical sources at the origin of the recorded SEFs. Also, some studies demonstrated that functional MEG mapping based on electrical median nerve stimulation may be superior to functional magnetic resonance imaging (fMRI) in some patients with unclear fMRI localization to locate the central sulcus (Inoue, T., Shimizu, Nakasato, Kumabe, & Yoshimoto, 1999; Kober et al., 2001; Korvenoja et al., 2006; Morioka et al., 1995a, 1995b; Roberts & Rowley, 1997; Shimizu, Nakasato, Mizoi, & Yoshimoto, 1997). MEG presents an additional key strength over fMRI, which is the ability to investigate in one single MEG session different neurophysiological processes (i.e., evoked magnetic responses, induced magnetic responses, coupling between peripheral and cortical signals) that can be altered or affected differently by brain disorders or patients' clinical status. Thus, MEG provides the unique opportunity to acquire several MEG "functional localizers" in a reasonable time for the patients. Here, a "functional localizer" is defined as a given validated MEG method to identify the SMI cortex (i.e., electrical peripheral nerve stimulation, tactile stimulation, readiness and motor evoked fields, Rolandic mu rhythm suppression (alpha or beta band), CMC, and CKC). The anatomical convergence of the different MEG functional localizers at the central sulcus has been demonstrated in healthy subjects and contributes to the assessment of the confidence level in functional mapping results (compared with a unimodal or bimodal approach) and to determine the clinical need to undergo further intracranial mapping procedures (Bourguignon et al., 2013). Such an approach also increases the yield of MEG in the case of failure, inaccurate or atypical localization of one MEG functional localizer, or fMRI mapping (Bourguignon et al., 2013).

Apart from presurgical functional SM1 cortex mapping, numerous MEG investigations of the somatosensory system have been performed in the context of clinical research to better understand the pathophysiology of various brain disorders. Describing all these clinical research data here would be out of the scope of this chapter. Interested readers can refer to Kakigi et al. (2010) for some detailed information.

16.9. CONCLUSION

Thanks to its noninvasiveness and excellent temporal and good spatial resolutions, MEG has substantially contributed in the past 50 years to the characterization of the spatial, temporal, and spectral dynamics of somatosensory system activity. It has brought a tremendous amount of novel insights into the neural mechanisms at the basis of body perception. The methods developed for this purpose appeared useful in clinical routine and also in clinical research to investigate the pathophysiology of various brain disorders.

ACKNOWLEDGMENTS

We would like to thank Professor Riitta Hari for her helpful comments and suggestions on this chapter.

REFERENCES

Adjamian, P., Worthen, S. F., Hillebrand, A., Furlong, P. L., Chizh, B. A., Hobson, A. R., . . . Barnes, G. R. (2009). Effective electromagnetic noise cancellation with beamformers and synthetic gradiometry in shielded and partly shielded environments. *Journal of Neuroscientific Methods, 178*(1), 120–127.

Andersen, L. M., & Lundqvist, D. (2018). Somatosensory responses to nothing: An MEG study of expectations during omission of tactile stimulations. *Neuroimage, 184,* 78–89.

Bourguignon, M., De Tiège, X., Op de Beeck, M., Pirotte, B., Van Bogaert, P., Goldman, S., . . . Jousmäki, V. (2011). Functional motor-cortex mapping using corticokinematic coherence. *Neuroimage, 55*(4), 1475–1479.

Bourguignon, M., Jousmäki, V., Marty, B., Wens, V., Op de Beeck, M., Van Bogaert, P., . . . De Tiège, X. (2013). Comprehensive functional mapping scheme for non-invasive primary sensorimotor cortex mapping. *Brain Topography, 26*(3), 511–523.

Bourguignon, M., Jousmäki, V., Op de Beeck, M., Van Bogaert, P., Goldman, S., & De Tiège, X. (2012).

Neuronal network coherent with hand kinematics during fast repetitive hand movements. *Neuroimage, 59*(2), 1684–1691.

Bourguignon, M., Piitulainen, H., De Tiège, X., Jousmäki, V., & Hari, R. (2015). Corticokinematic coherence mainly reflects movement-induced proprioceptive feedback. *Neuroimage, 106*, 382–390.

Bourguignon, M., Whitmarsh, S., Piitulainen, H., Hari, R., Jousmäki, V., & Lundqvist, D. (2016). Reliable recording and analysis of MEG-based corticokinematic coherence in the presence of strong magnetic artifacts. *Clinical Neurophysiology, 127*(2), 1460–1469.

Brenner, D., Lipton, J., Kaufman, L., & Williamson, S. J. (1978). Somatically evoked magnetic fields of the human brain. *Science, 199*(4324), 81–83.

Burgess, R. C., Funke, M. E., Bowyer, S. M., Lewine, J. D., Kirsch, H. E., Bagic, A. I., & ACMEGS Clinical Practice Guideline Committee. (2011). American Clinical Magnetoencephalography Society clinical practice guideline 2: Presurgical functional brain mapping using magnetic evoked fields. *Journal of Clinical Neurophysiology, 28*(4), 355–361.

Caetano, G., Jousmäki, V., & Hari, R. (2007). Actor's and observer's primary motor cortices stabilize similarly after seen or heard motor actions. *Proceedings of the National Academy of Science U S A, 104*(21), 9058–9062.

Chatrian, G. E., Petersen, M. C., & Lazarte, J. A. (1959). The blocking of the Rolandic wicket rhythm and some central changes related to movement. *Electroencephalography and Clinical Neurophysiology, 11*(3), 497–510.

Cheyne, D., Bostan, A. C., Gaetz, W., & Pang, E. W. (2007). Event-related beamforming: A robust method for presurgical functional mapping using MEG. *Clinical Neurophysiology, 118*(8), 1691–1704.

Cheyne, D., Gaetz, W., Garnero, L., Lachaux, J. P., Ducorps, A., Schwartz, D., & Varela, F. J. (2003). Neuromagnetic imaging of cortical oscillations accompanying tactile stimulation. *Brain Research: Cognitive Brain Research, 17*(3), 599–611.

Conti, A., Pontoriero, A., Ricciardi, G. K., Granata, F., Vinci, S., Angileri, F. F., . . . Tomasello, F. (2013). Integration of functional neuroimaging in CyberKnife radiosurgery: Feasibility and dosimetric results. *Neurosurgical Focus, 34*(4), E5.

Curio, G., Mackert, B. M., Burghoff, M., Koetitz, R., Abraham-Fuchs, K., & Harer, W. (1994). Localization of evoked neuromagnetic 600 Hz activity in the cerebral somatosensory system. *Electroencephalography and Clinical Neurophysiology, 91*(6), 483–487.

Curio, G., Mackert, B. M., Burghoff, M., Neumann, J., Nolte, G., Scherg, M., & Marx, P. (1997). Somatotopic source arrangement of 600 Hz oscillatory magnetic fields at the human primary somatosensory hand cortex. *Neuroscience Letters, 234*(2–3), 131–134.

Forss, N., Hari, R., Salmelin, R., Ahonen, A., Hämäläinen, M., Kajola, M., . . . Simola, J. (1994a). Activation of the human posterior parietal cortex by median nerve stimulation. *Experiments in Brain Research, 99*(2), 309–315.

Forss, N., Jousmäki, V., & Hari, R. (1995). Interaction between afferent input from fingers in human somatosensory cortex. *Brain Research, 685*(1–2), 68–76.

Forss, N., Raij, T. T., Seppa, M., & Hari, R. (2005). Common cortical network for first and second pain. *Neuroimage, 24*(1), 132–142.

Forss, N., Salmelin, R., & Hari, R. (1994b). Comparison of somatosensory evoked fields to airpuff and electric stimuli. *Electroencephalography and Clinical Neurophysiology, 92*(6), 510–517.

Forss, N., Silen, T., & Karjalainen, T. (2001). Lack of activation of human secondary somatosensory cortex in Unverricht-Lundborg type of progressive myoclonus epilepsy. *Annals of Neurology, 49*(1), 90–97.

Friston, K. (2010). The free-energy principle: A unified brain theory? *Nature Reviews Neuroscience, 11*(2), 127–138.

Gaetz, W. C., & Cheyne, D. O. (2003). Localization of human somatosensory cortex using spatially filtered magnetoencephalography. *Neuroscience Letters, 340*(3), 161–164.

Gaetz, W. C., & Cheyne, D. O. (2006). Localization of sensorimotor cortical rhythms induced by tactile stimulation using spatially filtered MEG. *Neuroimage, 30*, 899–908.

Gaetz, W., Cheyne, D., Rutka, J. T., Drake, J., Benifla, M., Strantzas, S., . . . Pang, E. W. (2009). Presurgical localization of primary motor cortex in pediatric patients with brain lesions by the use of spatially filtered magnetoencephalography. *Neurosurgery, 64*(3 Suppl), ons177–185; discussion ons186.

Gallen, C. C., Schwartz, B., Rieke, K., Pantev, C., Sobel, D., Hirschkoff, E., & Bloom, F. E. (1994). Intrasubject reliability and validity of somatosensory source localization using a large array biomagnetometer. *Electroencephalography and Clinical Neurophysiology, 90*(2), 145–156.

Gardner, E. P., Martin, J. H., & Jessell, T. M. (2000). The bodily senses. In E. R. Kandel, J. H. Schwartz, & M. J. Jessell (Eds.), *Principles of neural science* (pp. 430–450). New York, NY: McGraw-Hill.

Garrido, M. I., Kilner, J. M., Stephan, K. E., & Friston, K. J. (2009). The mismatch negativity: A review of underlying mechanisms. *Clinical Neurophysiology, 120*(3), 453–463.

Goldring, S., & Ratcheson, R. (1972). Human motor cortex: Sensory input data from single neuron recordings. *Science, 175*(4029), 1493–1495.

Gopalakrishnan, R., Machado, A. G., Burgess, R. C., & Mosher, J. C. (2013). The use of contact heat evoked potential stimulator (CHEPS) in magnetoencephalography for pain research. *Journal of Neuroscientific Methods, 220*(1), 55–63.

Gross, J., Timmermann, L., Kujala, J., Dirks, M., Schmitz, F., Salmelin, R., & Schnitzler, A. (2002). The neural basis of intermittent motor control in humans. *Proceedings of the National Academy of Science U S A, 99*(4), 2299–2302.

Hari, R., Baillet, S., Barnes, G., Burgess, R., Forss, N., Gross, J., . . . Taulu, S. (2018). IFCN-endorsed practical guidelines for clinical magnetoencephalography (MEG). *Clinical Neurophysiology, 129*(8), 1720–1747.

Hari, R., & Forss, N. (1999). Magnetoencephalography in the study of human somatosensory cortical processing. *Philosophical Transactions of the Royal Society B, 354*(1387), 1145–1154.

Hari, R., Forss, N., Avikainen, S., Kirveskari, E., Salenius, S., & Rizzolatti, G. (1998). Activation of human primary motor cortex during action observation: A neuromagnetic study. *Proceedings of the National Academy of Science U S A, 95*(25), 15061–15065.

Hari, R., Hämäläinen, H., Hämäläinen, M., Kekoni, J., Sams, M., & Tiihonen, J. (1990). Separate finger representations at the human second somatosensory cortex. *Neuroscience, 37*(1), 245–249.

Hari, R., Hämäläinen, M., Kaukoranta, E., Reinikainen, K., & Teszner, D. (1983a). Neuromagnetic responses from the second somatosensory cortex in man. *Acta Neurologica Scandinavica, 68*(4), 207–212.

Hari, R., Karhu, J., Hamalainen, M., Knuutila, J., Salonen, O., Sams, M., & Vilkman, V. (1993). Functional organization of the human first and second somatosensory cortices: A neuromagnetic study. *European Journal of Neuroscience, 5*(6), 724–734.

Hari, R., Kaukoranta, E., Reinikainen, K., Huopaniemie, T., & Mauno, J. (1983b). Neuromagnetic localization of cortical activity evoked by painful dental stimulation in man. *Neuroscience Letters, 42*(1), 77–82.

Hari, R., Portin, K., Kettenmann, B., Jousmäki, V., & Kobal, G. (1997a). Right-hemisphere preponderance of responses to painful CO_2 stimulation of the human nasal mucosa. *Pain, 72*(1-2), 145–151.

Hari, R., & Puce, A. (2017a). Instrumentation for MEG and EEG. In R. Hari & A. Puce (Eds.), *MEG–EEG primer* (pp. 47–76). New York, NY: Oxford University Press.

Hari, R., & Puce, A. (2017b). Somatosensory responses. In R. Hari & A. Puce (Eds.), *MEG–EEG primer* (pp. 227–241). New York, NY: Oxford University Press.

Hari, R., Reinikainen, K., Kaukoranta, E., Hamalainen, M., Ilmoniemi, R., Penttinen, A., . . . Teszner, D. (1984). Somatosensory evoked cerebral magnetic fields from SI and SII in man. *Electroencephalography and Clinical Neurophysiology, 57*(3), 254–263.

Hari, R., & Salmelin, R. (1997b). Human cortical oscillations: A neuromagnetic view through the skull. *Trends in Neuroscience, 20*(1), 44–49.

Hashimoto, I. (1987). Somatosensory evoked potentials elicited by air-puff stimuli generated by a new high-speed air control system. *Electroencephalography and Clinical Neurophysiology, 67*(3), 231–237.

Hashimoto, I., Mashiko, T., & Imada, T. (1996). Somatic evoked high-frequency magnetic oscillations reflect activity of inhibitory interneurons in the human somatosensory cortex. *Electroencephalography and Clinical Neurophysiology, 100*(3), 189–203.

Hinkley, L. B., Krubitzer, L. A., Nagarajan, S. S., & Disbrow, E. A. (2007). Sensorimotor integration in S2, PV, and parietal rostroventral areas of the human sylvian fissure. *Journal of Neurophysiology, 97*(2), 1288–1297.

Hirata, M., Kato, A., Taniguchi, M., Ninomiya, H., Cheyne, D., Robinson, S. E., . . . Yoshimine, T. (2002). Frequency-dependent spatial distribution of human somatosensory evoked neuromagnetic fields. *Neuroscience Letters, 318*(2), 73–76.

Hoshiyama, M., Kakigi, R., Koyama, S., Kitamura, Y., Shimoio, M., & Watanabe, S. (1995). Somatosensory evoked magnetic fields after mechanical stimulation of the scalp in humans. *Neuroscience Letters, 195*(1), 29–32.

Howland, E. W., Wakai, R. T., Mjaanes, B. A., Balog, J. P., & Cleeland, C. S. (1995). Whole head mapping of magnetic fields following painful electric finger shock. *Brain Research: Cognitive Brain Research, 2*(3), 165–172.

Hughes, J. R., Cohen, J., Mayman, C. I., Scholl, M. L., & Hendrix, D. E. (1977). Relationship of the magnetoencephalogram to abnormal activity in the electroencephalogram. *Journal of Neurology, 217*(2), 79–93.

Huttunen, J. (1986). Magnetic cortical responses evoked by tactile stimulation of the middle finger in man. *Pflugers Archiv, 407*(2), 129–133.

Huttunen, J., Hari, R., & Leinonen, L. (1987). Cerebral magnetic responses to stimulation of ulnar and median nerves. *Electroencephalography and Clinical Neurophysiology, 66*(4), 391–400.

Huttunen, J., Kobal, G., Kaukoranta, E., & Hari, R. (1986). Cortical responses to painful CO2 stimulation of nasal mucosa; a magnetoencephalographic study in man. *Electroencephalography and Clinical Neurophysiology, 64*(4), 347–349.

Inoue, K., Hashimoto, I., Shirai, T., Kawakami, H., Miyachi, T., Mimori, Y., & Matsumoto, M. (2004). Disinhibition of the somatosensory cortex in cervical dystonia-decreased amplitudes of high-frequency oscillations. *Clinical Neurophysiology, 115*(7), 1624–1630.

Inoue, T., Shimizu, H., Nakasato, N., Kumabe, T., & Yoshimoto, T. (1999). Accuracy and limitation of functional magnetic resonance imaging for identification of the central sulcus: Comparison with magnetoencephalography in patients with brain tumors. *Neuroimage, 10*(6), 738–748.

Inui, K., & Kakigi, R. (2012). Pain perception in humans: Use of intraepidermal electrical stimulation. *Journal of Neurology, Neurosurgery, and Psychiatry, 83*(5), 551–556.

Inui, K., Tran, T. D., Qiu, Y., Wang, X., Hoshiyama, M., & Kakigi, R. (2003a). A comparative magnetoencephalographic study of cortical activations evoked by noxious and innocuous somatosensory stimulations. *Neuroscience, 120*(1), 235–248.

Inui, K., Wang, X., Qiu, Y., Nguyen, B. T., Ojima, S., Tamura, Y., . . . Kakigi, R. (2003b). Pain processing within the primary somatosensory cortex in humans. *European Journal of Neuroscience, 18*(10), 2859–2866.

Jagow, R., Ribary, U., Lado, F., & Llinas, R. (1992). A new sensory stimulator for the MEG environment: The Piezo Undulative Multifrequency Apparatus (PUMA). In M. Hoke, S. N. Erne, Y. C. Okada, & G. L. Romani (Eds.), *Biomagnetism: Clinical aspects. Proceedings of the 8th International Conference on Biomagnetism* (pp. 891–894). New York, NY: Excerpta Medica.

Jerbi, K., Lachaux, J. P., N'Diaye, K., Pantazis, D., Leahy, R. M., Garnero, L., & Baillet, S. (2007). Coherent neural representation of hand speed in humans revealed by MEG imaging. *Proceedings of the National Academy of Science U S A, 104*(18), 7676–7681.

Jones, S. R., Pritchett, D. L., Stufflebeam, S. M., Hamalainen, M., & Moore, C. I. (2007). Neural correlates of tactile detection: A combined magnetoencephalography and biophysically based computational modeling study. *Journal of Neuroscience, 27*(40), 10751–10764.

Jousmäki, V., & Forss, N. (1998). Effects of stimulus intensity on signals from human somatosensory cortices. *Neuroreport, 9*(15), 3427–3431.

Jousmäki, V., & Hari, R. (1999). Somatosensory evoked fields to large-area vibrotactile stimuli. *Clinical Neurophysiology, 110*(5), 905–909.

Jousmäki, V., Nishitani, N., & Hari, R. (2007). A brush stimulator for functional brain imaging. *Clinical Neurophysiology, 118*(12), 2620–2624.

Kakigi, R., & Forss, N. (2010). Somatosensory and motor function. In P. C. Hansen, M. L. Kringelbach, & R. Salmelin (Eds.), *MEG: An introduction to methods* (pp. 300–345). New York, NY: Oxford University Press.

Kakigi, R., Hoshiyama, M., Shimojo, M., Naka, D., Yamasaki, H., Watanabe, S., . . . Nakamura, A. (2000). The somatosensory evoked magnetic fields. *Progress in Neurobiology, 61*(5), 495–523.

Kakigi, R., Koyama, S., Hoshiyama, M., Kitamura, Y., Shimojo, M., & Watanabe, S. (1995). Pain-related magnetic fields following painful CO2 laser stimulation in man. *Neuroscience Letters, 192*(1), 45–48.

Kamada, K., Houkin, K., Takeuchi, F., Ishii, N., Ikeda, J., Sawamura, Y., . . . Iwasaki, Y. (2003). Visualization of the eloquent motor system by integration of MEG, functional, and anisotropic diffusion-weighted MRI in functional neuronavigation. *Surgical Neurology, 59*(5), 352–361; discussion 361–352.

Kaufman, L., Okada, Y., Brenner, D., & Williamson, S. J. (1981). On the relation between somatic evoked potentials and fields. *International Journal of Neuroscience, 15*(4), 223–239.

Kelso, J. A., Fuchs, A., Lancaster, R., Holroyd, T., Cheyne, D., & Weinberg, H. (1998). Dynamic cortical activity in the human brain reveals motor equivalence. *Nature, 392*(6678), 814–818.

Kitamura, Y., Kakigi, R., Hoshiyama, M., Koyama, S., Shimojo, M., & Watanabe, S. (1995). Pain-related somatosensory evoked magnetic fields. *Electroencephalography and Clinical Neurophysiology, 95*(6), 463–474.

Kitamura, Y., Kakigi, R., Hoshiyama, M., Koyama, S., Watanabe, S., & Shimojo, M. (1997). Pain-related somatosensory evoked magnetic fields following lower limb stimulation. *Journal of the Neurological Sciences, 145*(2), 187–194.

Klimesch, W., Sauseng, P., & Hanslmayr, S. (2007). EEG alpha oscillations: The inhibition-timing hypothesis. *Brain Research Reviews, 53*(1), 63–88.

Kober, H., Nimsky, C., Moller, M., Hastreiter, P., Fahlbusch, R., & Ganslandt, O. (2001). Correlation of sensorimotor activation with functional magnetic resonance imaging and magnetoencephalography in presurgical functional imaging: A spatial analysis. *Neuroimage, 14*(5), 1214–1228.

Korvenoja, A., Kirveskari, E., Aronen, H. J., Avikainen, S., Brander, A., Huttunen, J., . . . Seppa, M. (2006). Sensorimotor cortex localization: Comparison of magnetoencephalography, functional MR imaging, and intraoperative cortical mapping. *Radiology, 241*(1), 213–222.

Lin, P. T., Berger, M. S., & Nagarajan, S. S. (2006). Motor field sensitivity for preoperative localization of motor cortex. *Journal of Neurosurgery, 105*(4), 588–594.

Lin, Y. Y., & Kajola, M. (2003). Neuromagnetic somatosensory responses to natural moving tactile stimulation. *Canadian Journal of Neurological Sciences, 30*(1), 31–35.

Maeda, K., Kakigi, R., Hoshiyama, M., & Koyama, S. (1999). Topography of the secondary somatosensory cortex in humans: A magnetoencephalographic study. *Neuroreport, 10*(2), 301–306.

Maihofner, C., Jesberger, F., Seifert, F., & Kaltenhauser, M. (2010). Cortical processing of mechanical hyperalgesia: A MEG study. *European Journal of Pain, 14*(1), 64–70.

Mäkelä, J. P., Illeman, M., Jousmäki, V., Numminen, J., Lehecka M., Salenius, S., . . . Hari, R. (2003). Dorsal penile nerve stimulation elicits left-hemisphere dominant activation in the second somatosensory cortex. *Human Brain Mapping, 18*(2), 90–99.

Mäkelä, J. P., Kirveskari, E., Seppa, M., Hämäläinen, M., Forss, N., Avikainen, S., . . . Hari, R. (2001). Three-dimensional integration of brain anatomy and function to facilitate intraoperative navigation around the sensorimotor strip. *Human Brain Mapping, 12*(3), 180–192.

Marty, B., Bourguignon, M., Jousmäki, V., Wens, V., Op de Beeck, M., Van Bogaert, P., . . . De Tiège, X. (2015a). Cortical kinematic processing of executed and observed goal-directed hand actions. *Neuroimage, 119,* 221–228.

Marty, B., Bourguignon, M., Op de Beeck, M., Wens, V., Goldman, S., Van Bogaert, P., . . . De Tiège, X. (2015b). Effect of movement rate on corticokinematic coherence. *Neurophysiology Clinics, 45*(6), 469–474.

Marty, B., Wens, V., Bourguignon, M., Naeije, G., Goldman, S., Jousmäki, V., & De Tiège, X. (2018).

Neuromagnetic cerebellar activity entrains to the kinematics of executed finger movements. *Cerebellum, 17*(5), 531–539.

Mauguiere, F., Merlet, I., Forss, N., Vanni, S., Jousmäki, V., Adeleine, P., & Hari, R. (1997a). Activation of a distributed somatosensory cortical network in the human brain: A dipole modelling study of magnetic fields evoked by median nerve stimulation. Part II: Effects of stimulus rate, attention and stimulus detection. *Electroencephalography and Clinical Neurophysiology, 104*(4), 290–295.

Mauguiere, F., Merlet, I., Forss, N., Vanni, S., Jousmäki, V., Adeleine, P., & Hari, R. (1997b). Activation of a distributed somatosensory cortical network in the human brain. A dipole modelling study of magnetic fields evoked by median nerve stimulation. Part I: Location and activation timing of SEF sources. *Electroencephalography and Clinical Neurophysiology, 104*(4), 281–289.

May, P. J., & Tiitinen, H. (2010). Mismatch negativity (MMN), the deviance-elicited auditory deflection, explained. *Psychophysiology, 47*(1), 66–122.

Mertens, M., & Lutkenhoner, B. (2000). Efficient neuromagnetic determination of landmarks in the somatosensory cortex. *Clinical Neurophysiology, 111*(8), 1478–1487.

Morioka, T., Mizushima, A., Yamamoto, T., Tobimatsu, S., Matsumoto, S., Hasuo, K., . . . Fukui, M. (1995a). Functional mapping of the sensorimotor cortex: Combined use of magnetoencephalography, functional MRI, and motor evoked potentials. *Neuroradiology, 37*(7), 526–530.

Morioka, T., Yamamoto, T., Mizushima, A., Tombimatsu, S., Shigeto, H., Hasuo, K., . . . Fukui, M. (1995b). Comparison of magnetoencephalography, functional MRI, and motor evoked potentials in the localization of the sensory-motor cortex. *Neurology Research, 17*(5), 361–367.

Motogi, J., Kodaira, M., Muragaki, Y., Inui, K., & Kakigi, R. (2014). Cortical responses to C-fiber stimulation by intra-epidermal electrical stimulation: An MEG study. *Neuroscience Letters, 570,* 69–74.

Näätänen, R., Kujala, T., Kreegipuu, K., Carlson, S., Escera, C., Baldeweg, T., & Ponton, C. (2011). The mismatch negativity: An index of cognitive decline in neuropsychiatric and neurological diseases and in ageing. *Brain, 134*(Pt 12), 3435–3453.

Näätänen, R., Paavilainen, P., Rinne, T., & Alho, K. (2007). The mismatch negativity (MMN) in basic research of central auditory processing: A review. *Clinical Neurophysiology, 118*(12), 2544–2590.

Naeije, G., Vaulet, T., Wens, V., Marty, B., Goldman, S., & De Tiège, X. (2016). Multilevel cortical processing of somatosensory novelty: A magnetoencephalography study. *Frontiers in Human Neuroscience, 10,* 259.

Naeije, G., Vaulet, T., Wens, V., Marty, B., Goldman, S., & De Tiège, X. (2018). Neural basis of early somatosensory change detection: A magnetoencephalography study. *Brain Topography, 31*(2), 242–256.

Nagarajan, S., Kirsch, H., Lin, P., Findlay, A., Honma, S., & Berger, M. S. (2008). Preoperative localization of hand motor cortex by adaptive spatial filtering of magnetoencephalography data. *Journal of Neurosurgery, 109*(2), 228–237.

Nakamura, A., Yamada, T., Goto, A., Kato, T., Ito, K., Abe, Y., . . . Kakigi, R. (1998). Somatosensory homunculus as drawn by MEG. *Neuroimage, 7*(4 Pt 1), 377–386.

Neggers, S. F., Langerak, T. R., Schutter, D. J., Mandl, R. C., Ramsey, N. F., Lemmens, P. J., & Postma, A. (2004). A stereotactic method for image-guided transcranial magnetic stimulation validated with fMRI and motor-evoked potentials. *Neuroimage, 21*(4), 1805–1817.

Nguyen, B. T., Inui, K., Hoshiyama, M., Nakata, H., & Kakigi, R. (2005). Face representation in the human secondary somatosensory cortex. *Clinical Neurophysiology, 116*(6), 1247–1253.

Nguyen, B. T., Tran, T. D., Hoshiyama, M., Inui, K., & Kakigi, R. (2004). Face representation in the human primary somatosensory cortex. *Neuroscience Research, 50*(2), 227–232.

Okada, Y. C., Kaufman, L., Brenner, D., & Williamson, S. J. (1981). Application of a SQUID to measurement of somatically evoked fields: Transient responses to electrical stimulations of the median nerve. In S. N. Erne, H. D. Hahlbohm, & H. Lubbig (Eds.), *Biomagnetism.* Berlin, Germany: Walter de Gruyter.

O'Suilleabhain, P. E., Lagerlund, T. D., & Matsumoto, J. Y. (1999). Cortical potentials at the frequency of absolute wrist velocity become phase-locked during slow sinusoidal tracking movements. *Experimental Brain Research, 126*(4), 529–535.

Otsuru, N., Inui, K., Yamashiro, K., Urakawa, T., Keceli, S., & Kakigi, R. (2011). Effects of prior sustained tactile stimulation on the somatosensory response to the sudden change of intensity in humans: An magnetoencephalography study. *Neuroscience, 182,* 115–124.

Pantelis, E., Papadakis, N., Verigos, K., Stathochristopoulou, I., Antypas, C., Lekas, L., . . . Salvaras, N. (2010). Integration of functional MRI and white matter tractography in stereotactic radiosurgery clinical practice. *International Journal*

of Radiation Oncology, Biology, Physics, 78(1), 257–267.

Penfield, W., & Boldrey, E. (1937). Somatic motor and sensory representation in the cerebral cortex of man as studied by electrical stimulation. *Brain, 60,* 389–443.

Piitulainen, H., Bourguignon, M., De Tiège, X., Hari, R., & Jousmäki, V. (2013a). Coherence between magnetoencephalography and hand-action-related acceleration, force, pressure, and electromyogram. *Neuroimage, 72,* 83–90.

Piitulainen, H., Bourguignon, M., De Tiège, X., Hari, R., & Jousmäki, V. (2013b). Corticokinematic coherence during active and passive finger movements. *Neuroscience, 238,* 361–370.

Piitulainen, H., Bourguignon, M., Hari, R., & Jousmäki, V. (2015). MEG-compatible pneumatic stimulator to elicit passive finger and toe movements. *Neuroimage, 112,* 310–317.

Piitulainen, H., Illman, M., Laaksonen, K., Jousmäki, V., & Forss, N. (2018). Reproducibility of corticokinematic coherence. *Neuroimage, 179,* 596–603.

Pirotte, B., Voordecker, P., Neugroschl, C., Baleriaux, D., Wikler, D., Metens, T., . . . Levivier, M. (2005). Combination of functional magnetic resonance imaging-guided neuronavigation and intraoperative cortical brain mapping improves targeting of motor cortex stimulation in neuropathic pain. *Neurosurgery, 56*(2 Suppl), 344–359; discussion 344–359.

Ploner, M., Schmitz, F., Freund, H. J., & Schnitzler, A. (1999). Parallel activation of primary and secondary somatosensory cortices in human pain processing. *Journal of Neurophysiology, 81*(6), 3100–3104.

Ploner, M., Schmitz, F., Freund, H. J., & Schnitzler, A. (2000). Differential organization of touch and pain in human primary somatosensory cortex. *Journal of Neurophysiology, 83*(3), 1770–1776.

Pohja, M., Salenius, S., & Hari, R. (2005). Reproducibility of cortex-muscle coherence. *Neuroimage, 26*(3), 764–770.

Pollok, B., Gross, J., Dirks, M., Timmermann, L., & Schnitzler, A. (2004). The cerebral oscillatory network of voluntary tremor. *Journal of Physiology, 554*(Pt 3), 871–878.

Pollok, B., Sudmeyer, M., Gross, J., & Schnitzler, A. (2005). The oscillatory network of simple repetitive bimanual movements. *Brain Research: Cognitive Brain Research, 25*(1), 300–311.

Popescu, E. A., Barlow, S. M., Venkatesan, L., Wang, J., & Popescu, M. (2013). Adaptive changes in the neuromagnetic response of the primary and association somatosensory areas following repetitive tactile hand stimulation in humans. *Human Brain Mapping, 34*(6), 1415–1426.

Qiu, Y., Inui, K., Wang, X., Nguyen, B. T., Tran, T. D., & Kakigi, R. (2004). Effects of distraction on magnetoencephalographic responses ascending through C-fibers in humans. *Clinical Neurophysiology, 115*(3), 636–646.

Roberts, T. P., & Rowley, H. A. (1997). Mapping of the sensorimotor cortex: Functional MR and magnetic source imaging. *AJNR American Journal of Neuroradiology, 18*(5), 871–880.

Rossini, P. M., Deuschl, G., Pizzella, V., Tecchio, F., Pasquarelli, A., Feifel, E., ... Lucking, C. H. (1996). Topography and sources of electromagnetic cerebral responses to electrical and air-puff stimulation of the hand. *Electroencephalography and Clinical Neurophysiology, 100*(3), 229–239.

Rossini, P. M., Narici, L., Romani, G. L., Peresson, M., Torrioli, G., & Traversa, R. (1989). Simultaneous motor output and sensory input: Cortical interference site resolved in humans via neuromagnetic measurements. *Neuroscience Letters, 96*(3), 300–305.

Sakamoto, K., Nakata, H., & Kakigi, R. (2008). Somatotopic representation of the tongue in human secondary somatosensory cortex. *Clinical Neurophysiology, 119*(9), 2125–2134.

Sakuma, K., & Hashimoto, I. (1999a). High-frequency magnetic oscillations evoked by posterior tibial nerve stimulation. *Neuroreport, 10*(2), 227–230.

Sakuma, K., Sekihara, K., & Hashimoto, I. (1999b). Neural source estimation from a time-frequency component of somatic evoked high-frequency magnetic oscillations to posterior tibial nerve stimulation. *Clinical Neurophysiology, 110*(9), 1585–1588.

Salenius, S., Schnitzler, A., Salmelin, R., Jousmaki, V., & Hari, R. (1997). Modulation of human cortical Rolandic rhythms during natural sensorimotor tasks. *Neuroimage, 5*(3), 221–228.

Salmelin, R., Hamalainen, M., Kajola, M., & Hari, R. (1995). Functional segregation of movement-related rhythmic activity in the human brain. *Neuroimage, 2*(4), 237–243.

Salmelin, R., & Hari, R. (1994). Spatiotemporal characteristics of sensorimotor neuromagnetic rhythms related to thumb movement. *Neuroscience, 60*(2), 537–550.

Schiffbauer, H., Berger, M. S., Ferrari, P., Freudenstein, D., Rowley, H. A., & Roberts, T. P. (2002). Preoperative magnetic source imaging for brain tumor surgery: A quantitative comparison with intraoperative sensory and motor mapping. *Journal of Neurosurgery, 97*(6), 1333–1342.

Schnitzler, A., Salenius, S., Salmelin, R., Jousmaki, V., & Hari, R. (1997). Involvement of primary motor

cortex in motor imagery: Neuromagnetic study. *Neuroimage, 6*(3), 201–208.

Shimizu, H., Nakasato, N., Mizoi, K., & Yoshimoto, T. (1997). Localizing the central sulcus by functional magnetic resonance imaging and magnetoencephalography. *Clinical Neurology and Neurosurgery, 99*(4), 235–238.

Simoes, C., Jensen, O., Parkkonen, L., & Hari, R. (2003). Phase locking between human primary and secondary somatosensory cortices. *Proceedings of the National Academy of Science U S A, 100*(5), 2691–2694.

Smeds, E., Piitulainen, H., Bourguignon, M., Jousmäki, V., & Hari, R. (2017). Effect of interstimulus interval on cortical proprioceptive responses to passive finger movements. *European Journal of Neuroscience, 45*(2), 290–298.

Solomon, J., Boe, S., & Bardouille, T. (2015). Reliability for non-invasive somatosensory cortex localization: Implications for pre-surgical mapping. *Clinical Neurology and Neurosurgery, 139*, 224–229.

Stancanello, J., Cavedon, C., Francescon, P., Causin, F., Avanzo, M., Colombo, F., ... Uggeri, F. (2007). BOLD fMRI integration into radiosurgery treatment planning of cerebral vascular malformations. *Medical Physics, 34*(4), 1176–1184.

Sutherling, W. W., Crandall, P. H., Darcey, T. M., Becker, D. P., Levesque, M. F., & Barth, D. S. (1988). The magnetic and electric fields agree with intracranial localizations of somatosensory cortex. *Neurology, 38*(11), 1705–1714.

Swadlow, H. A. (1989). Efferent neurons and suspected interneurons in S-1 vibrissa cortex of the awake rabbit: Receptive fields and axonal properties. *Journal of Neurophysiology, 62*(1), 288–308.

Teszner, D., Hari, R., Nicolas, P., & Varpula, T. (1983). Somatosensory evoked magnetic fields: Mapping and the influence of stimulus repetition rate. *Nuovo Cimento D, 2*, 429–437.

Theuvenet, P. J., van Dijk, B. W., Peters, M. J., van Ree, J. M., Lopes da Silva, F. L., & Chen, A. C. (2005). Whole-head MEG analysis of cortical spatial organization from unilateral stimulation of median nerve in both hands: No complete hemispheric homology. *Neuroimage, 28*(2), 314–325.

Tiihonen, J., Hari, R., & Hämäläinen, M. (1989a). Early deflections of cerebral magnetic responses to median nerve stimulation. *Electroencephalography and Clinical Neurophysiology, 74*(4), 290–296.

Tiihonen, J., Kajola, M., & Hari, R. (1989b). Magnetic mu rhythm in man. *Neuroscience, 32*(3), 793–800.

Torquati, K., Pizzella, V., Della Penna, S., Franciotti, R., Babiloni, C., Rossini, P. M., & Romani, G. L. (2002). Comparison between SI and SII responses as a function of stimulus intensity. *Neuroreport, 13*(6), 813–819.

Tran, T. D., Inui, K., Hoshiyama, M., Lam, K., Qiu, Y., & Kakigi, R. (2002). Cerebral activation by the signals ascending through unmyelinated C-fibers in humans: A magnetoencephalographic study. *Neuroscience, 113*(2), 375–386.

Vitikainen, A. M., Lioumis, P., Paetau, R., Salli, E., Komssi, S., Metsahonkala, L., . . . Gaily, E. (2009). Combined use of non-invasive techniques for improved functional localization for a selected group of epilepsy surgery candidates. *Neuroimage, 45*(2), 342–348.

Watanabe, S., Kakigi, R., Koyama, S., Hoshiyama, M., & Kaneoke, Y. (1998). Pain processing traced by magnetoencephalography in the human brain. *Brain Topography, 10*(4), 255–264.

Wikström, H., Huttunen, J., Korvenoja, A., Virtanen, J., Salonen, O., Aronen, H., & Ilmoniemi, R. J. (1996). Effects of interstimulus interval on somatosensory evoked magnetic fields (SEFs): A hypothesis concerning SEF generation at the primary sensorimotor cortex. *Electroencephalography and Clinical Neurophysiology, 100*(6), 479–487.

Willemse, R. B., de Munck, J. C., van't Ent, D., Ris, P., Baayen, J. C., Stam, C. J., & Vandertop, W. P. (2007). Magnetoencephalographic study of posterior tibial nerve stimulation in patients with intracranial lesions around the central sulcus. *Neurosurgery, 61*(6), 1209–1217; discussion 1217–1208.

Willemse, R. B., de Munck, J. C., Verbunt, J. P., van 't Ent, D., Ris, P., Baayen, J. C., . . . Vandertop, W. P. (2010). Topographical organization of mu and Beta band activity associated with hand and foot movements in patients with perirolandic lesions. *Open Neuroimaging Journal, 4*, 93–99.

Willemse, R. B., Hillebrand, A., Ronner, H. E., Vandertop, W. P., & Stam, C. J. (2016). Magnetoencephalographic study of hand and foot sensorimotor organization in 325 consecutive patients evaluated for tumor or epilepsy surgery. *Neuroimage: Clinical, 10*, 46–53.

Wood, C. C., Cohen, D., Cuffin, B. N., Yarita, M., & Allison, T. (1985). Electrical sources in human somatosensory cortex: Identification by combined magnetic and potential recordings. *Science, 227*(4690), 1051–1053.

Worthen, S. F., Adjamian, P., Hobson, A. R., Aziz, Q., Chizh, B. A., & Furlong, P. L. (2007). Investigating the neural correlates of thermal and electrical stimulation following successful stimulus-artefact removal: A MEG study. *Clinical Neurophysiology, 118*, e182.

Yamashiro, K., Inui, K., Otsuru, N., Kida, T., & Kakigi, R. (2009). Somatosensory off-response in humans: An MEG study. *Neuroimage, 44*(4), 1363–1368.

17

LANGUAGE MAPPING WITH MAGNETOENCEPHALOGRAPHY

CLINICAL AND RESEARCH APPLICATIONS

Panagiotis G. Simos, Susan M. Bowyer, and Kyousuke Kamada

17.1. THEORETICAL CONSIDERATIONS

The auditory and the temporal association cortices, as well as parts of the parietal and frontal cortices, are implicated in the language production and perception functions. Several different hypotheses as to the precise nature of specialization of each cortical region for particular aspects of linguistic processing have emerged over the years, from observation of the effects of focal lesions and, more recently, from functional neuroimaging data. These differ because the lesion data are rarely clear enough to support, unequivocally, a particular hypothesis because lesions vary across patients in severity, extent, and other aspects and because the interpretation of functional neuroimaging data is hampered by a number of unresolved technical problems. Although there is very little agreement regarding which cortical regions

are necessary for what specific linguistic operations, some exceptions do exist. First, it is universally acknowledged that acoustic processing of both speech and nonspeech stimuli is mediated by the auditory cortex in the midportion of the superior temporal gyrus (STG) in the left and right hemispheres equally. Second, that the inferior frontal gyrus (IFG), comprising pars opercularis and pars triangularis, is necessary for production of speech in general. There is also considerable agreement that IFG may be necessary for comprehension of sentences, that is, for syntactic processing of linguistic input, although its contribution may not be necessary for comprehension of isolated words (Mesulam, Thompson, Weintraub, & Rogalski, 2015).

Beyond these points of agreement, most other hypotheses regarding cortical organization for language vary among theorists.

Panagiotis G. Simos, Susan M. Bowyer, and Kyousuke Kamada, *Language Mapping With Magnetoencephalography: Clinical and Research Applications* In: *Fifty Years of Magnetoencephalography*. Edited by: Andrew C. Papanicolaou, Timothy P. L. Roberts, and James W. Wheless, Oxford University Press (2020). © Oxford University Press. DOI: 10.1093/oso/9780190935689.003.0017.

According to the "canonical" model that has emerged over the years, mostly from consideration of the effects of focal cortical lesions, phonological processing of linguistic input requires the contribution of the posterior part of STG (pSTG) of only the left hemisphere (Rauschecker & Scott, 2009). This view has been recently challenged, however, especially by Hickok and Poeppel (2015) on the basis of results of some focal lesion studies (Rogalsky & Hickok, 2011) and on some functional neuroimaging data (Price, 2012; Schirmer, Fox, & Grandjean, 2012; Turkeltaub & Coslett, 2010). They have proposed a "dual-route" model, which predicts that, in tasks requiring perception of speech sounds, both the left and the right pSTG are active, although the contribution of the anterior STG cannot be ruled out (see, e.g., Narain et al., 2003; Scott, Blank, Rosen, & Wise, 2000; Spitsyna, Warren, Scott, Turkheimer, & Wise, 2006). On the basis of this model, it is further expected that electrical stimulation in either the left or the right pSTG (and/or the anterior STG) would not result in interference with phonemic perception, based on lesion data suggesting that the unaffected STG of either hemisphere should suffice in mediating phoneme perception tasks (Wolmetz, Poeppel, & Rapp, 2011).

With respect to semantic processing required for comprehension of individual words, the canonical view since the time of Wernicke's first publication on this issue (Wernicke, 1874/1969) is that this linguistic operation is mediated by the region that encompasses the pSTG, a portion of the middle temporal gyrus (MTG), as well as the angular and supramarginal gyri (AG and SMG, respectively) of the left cerebral hemisphere (known as Wernicke's area), in most people. This view has been widely supported by clinical data indicating that lesions in that area appear to disrupt comprehension of both words and sentences (Turken & Dronkers, 2011). But this view has also been challenged by findings in patients with dementia (Hurley, Paller, Rogalski, & Mesulam, 2012; Jefferies &

Lambon Ralph, 2006; Mesulam et al., 2013) and acquired focal lesions (Schwartz et al., 2009), indicating that whereas Wernicke's area may appear to be necessary for both phonological and semantic analysis of linguistic input, it is actually only necessary for phonological analysis, resulting in the derivation of the word-form (i.e., an activation pattern coding the phonological profile of words; see, e.g., Pulvermüller, 2013). In the context of this alternative view, its disruption would be expected not only to affect phonological analyses but also to interfere with word and sentence comprehension because the latter assumes phonological analysis and not because the area mediates semantic operations. Semantic processing, according to this alternative view, relies heavily on the left anterior temporal lobe (ATL), but the precise role of the ATL is not clear. According to one hypothesis (Mesulam et al., 2015), the ATL is necessary for mediating the activation of semantic circuits distributed throughout the cortex on the basis of word-form–related input that it receives from Wernicke's region, or for activating word-form circuits on the basis of input from semantic circuits as in object-naming tasks (Mesulam et al., 2013; Schwartz et al., 2009). Therefore, according to this alternative to the canonical model, disruption of the left ATL by electrical stimulation would be expected to interfere with word comprehension (consequently also sentence comprehension) tasks and/or performance of object-naming tasks, whereas increased activation during word comprehension tasks should be found in both the left ATL and Wernicke's area, especially the pSTG. Lesion data have further suggested that cortex in the inferior temporal gyrus as well as the ATL may be critically involved in word comprehension (Gorno-Tempini et al., 2004).

But the results of some cortical stimulation mapping (CSM) studies (Lüders et al., 1991) have pointed to the conclusion that the left fusiform gyrus (rather than the left ATL) is necessary for word and sentence comprehension, leading to the expectation that during performance of word and sentence comprehension tasks, increased activation should be observed in this region. The basal temporal language area (BTLA) has been found to be active during a verb generation with concrete nouns (Bowyer et al., 2005a). In view of the fact that most words used in that study were concrete nouns, and in view of the known involvement of this area in object recognition, its contribution to word comprehension may be limited to that word category and to sentences that contain names of objects.

As mentioned previously, there is general agreement as far as the role of the left IFG in production of speech (whether of phonemes, words, or sentences), as well as in the comprehension of sentences is concerned. It is, however, disputed whether it suffices for the latter task because, according to the dual route model, cortex in the parietotemporal junction is necessary (Hickok & Poeppel, 2015).

17.2. A REVIEW OF THE MAGNETOENCEPHALOGRAPHY TECHNIQUES FOR LANGUAGE LATERALIZATION AND LOCALIZATION

Magnetoencephalography (MEG) recordings performed for the purpose of determining the location and extent of cortex mediating language functions require that the function under investigation be repeated several times, while the magnetic flux over the head is sampled at regular intervals. Each segment of recorded activity, beginning a few milliseconds before and extending up to approximately 1,000 ms after each repetition of the stimulus is stored separately as a MEG epoch. The resulting averaged event-related field (ERF) consists of both early components (50–200 ms after stimulus onset) that correspond to activation of the sensory cortex specific to the stimulus modality and late components (200–~1,000 ms after stimulus onset), which reflect activation of the association cortex or higher functions.

The final step in the analysis of MEG data entails computing a viable model of the anatomic layout (location and extent) of the intracranial sources producing the observed magnetic flux recordings. A variety of algorithms have been developed in order to obtain an accurate mapping of recorded neuromagnetic activity onto underlying electrical cortical current sources. Most of these algorithms treat intracranial generators of magnetic flux as electrical dipoles representing the coherent activity of tens to hundreds of thousands of neurons. The best solution to this "inverse problem" in source localization is achieved using residual variance minimization algorithms. Key differences among the different approaches concern the number of dipolar sources that can be modeled simultaneously and the geometric characteristics of the model of the brain used. The single equivalent current dipole (ECD) method permits identification of one relatively independent and spatially distinct point source at each point in time. Typically, single ECD approaches do not take into account the anatomy of the person's brain (with the exception of the local curvature of the brain) in estimating the characteristics of the underlying source (location and strength of the electrical dipole). After estimates of the coordinates of such sources are made in the MEG coordinate system, they are co-registered with a set of structural images of the patient's brain (using magnetic resonance imaging [MRI]) in order to determine the anatomical location of each source. This approach has been adapted for mapping of more than one cortical source of concurrent neuromagnetic activity by using subsets of contiguous sensors (typically 30–37) to estimate the location and strength of each source. As long as concurrently active sources generate spatially distinct maps of neuromagnetic activity at the sensor level, up to three such sources can be reliably estimated in each hemisphere. The degree of regional cortical engagement in the activation task may be indexed by the current strength of the modeled intracranial source and/or the duration of successfully modeled dipolar activity in a given brain region.

Conversely, multisource or extended-source modeling algorithms operate on a geometric model of the cortical surface, which is partitioned into several thousand potential sources (cortical patches containing populations of pyramidal neurons that can produce detectable magnetic flux). There are two main classes of extended-source modeling algorithms: those that attempt to model instantaneous current distribution on the cortical surface and those that operate in the time–frequency domain and use beamforming algorithms originally developed for telecommunication applications and involve some type of spatial filtering. The most common current distribution modeling techniques are minimum-norm estimate (MNE; Ilmoniemi, 1993) and multiresolution focal underdetermined system solver (MR-FOCUSS; Moran, Bowyer, & Tepley, 2005). These methods use the amplitude distribution of recorded neuromagnetic signals over the entire sensor array and are thus inherently more sensitive to weaker or less extensive cortical sources of activity than the ECD method, perhaps at the expense of spatial specificity. MR-FOCUSS (Moran et al., 2005) has been used successfully to image cortical areas involved in language processing (Bowyer et al., 2004, 2005a, 2005b). This method produces a time sequence of whole-brain images of both focal and extended source structures for a model of cortical gray matter consisting of x-, y-, and z-oriented current dipoles located at 4,000 cortical sites. MR-FOCUSS uses a recursively adapted sparse wavelet representation of cortical activity where the least-squares solution replaces the weighted minimum-norm technique in the FOCUSS iterative algorithm (Gorodnitsky, George, & Rao, 1995). For statistical robustness against initialization bias, random amplitudes are incorporated in source initialization, and 20 solutions are generated and averaged for each time slice of MEG data, at each latency.

Common beamformer techniques include synthetic aperture magnetometry (SAM) and linearly constrained minimum variance (LCVM) (Hillebrand & Barnes, 2005). These spatial filtering algorithms decompose the recorded signal into frequency bands and project modeled sources of each band onto the cortical surface. Using spatial filtering variants, several groups have documented systematic reduction in event-related power in the beta band (12–30 Hz) in perisylvian areas during performance of language tasks (Findlay et al., 2012; Hirata et al., 2004). For instance, Findlay et al. (2012) recorded ERFs in response to spoken nouns in the context of a verb-generation task. Beta power was found to be significantly reduced in the inferior frontal region between approximately 250 and 350 ms after stimulus onset followed by a similar reduction in the vicinity of Wernicke's area, which was, in turn, followed by beta power reduction in the inferior frontal region lasting up to approximately 250 ms before vocalization (production of the verb that corresponded to the noun). The degree of regional reduction in beta power was greater in the left than the right hemisphere in patients who were left hemisphere dominant for language. In a manner similar to the adapted ECD methods described previously, this approach has produced reliable indices of the degree of engagement of language-related brain regions in each hemisphere based on indices of the duration of suprathreshold activity during late portions of the evoked magnetic response to linguistic stimuli.

Recording of late ERFs has two main clinical indications: (a) to establish the profile of hemispheric involvement in the mechanism that supports basic language functions (hemispheric dominance) and (b) to identify the location and extent of functionally intact cortex involved in language functions in relation to the area to be resected (epileptogenic zone or mass lesion).

17.3. CLINICAL APPLICATIONS: ESTABLISHING HEMISPHERIC DOMINANCE FOR LANGUAGE

Using MEG as a method of functional imaging, several groups have verified that MEG assessments of hemispheric dominance for language are concordant with those based on the Wada procedure. Using a 148-channel whole-head MEG system, one group established a protocol for eliciting and modeling neuromagnetic activity associated with word-level receptive language functions. Early studies reported excellent concordance with hemispheric dominance estimates provided by the Wada procedures in pediatric and adult patients (Breier et al., 1999b; Breier, Simos, Wheless, Constantinou, & Papanicolaou, 2001). The activation protocol consisted of an auditory, continuous word recognition task involving six blocks of 40 abstract nouns, and the patient is instructed to detect words repeated across blocks (75% of total). The degree of language-specific activity was indexed by the number of consecutive sources (modeled as ECDs) in perisylvian brain areas. Only late-component activity sources (i.e., between 200 and 600 ms after stimulus onset) that were observed with a high degree of spatial and temporal overlap in two "split-half" data sets were used to compute the MEG laterality index. Pooling data from 85 consecutive surgical candidates with intractable epilepsy aged 8 to 56 years, Papanicolaou et al. (2005) reported a high degree of concordance (87%) between independent clinical judgments based on MEG and Wada data. MEG laterality judgments had an overall sensitivity of 0.98 and a selectivity of 0.83 because of the fact that MEG detected more activity in the nondominant hemisphere than would be predicted on the basis of the results of the Wada procedure. Using identical stimulation and analysis procedures, Doss, Zhang, Risse, and Dickens (2009) obtained sensitivity and specificity values of 0.80 and 1.00, respectively, in determining whether the hemisphere to be treated was critical for language functions in a series of 35 consecutive patients with epilepsy or tumors. Excellent concordance between MEG and the Wada results has also been reported by Maestú et al. (2002) using a Spanish adaptation of the continuous word recognition task in eight Spanish-speaking patients.

Notably, this activation and analysis protocol may be suitable for uncooperative patients tested under sedation as yielding percentages of left hemisphere dominant cases similar to those obtained in unsedated patients (Rezaie et al., 2014). This finding implies that activation of auditory association regions, especially in the language-dominant hemisphere, may not require conscious control. Two other groups have used the same analysis method for estimating hemispheric dominance in the context of different activation tasks. Using a silent reading and a naming task, agreement with the Wada procedure was noted in 81% of 11 patients with tumors or vascular lesions (and partial agreement in the remaining patients). More recently, Kamada et al. (2007) combined laterality estimates obtained with MEG (in the context of an abstract/concrete categorization task with printed stimuli) and functional magnetic resonance imaging (fMRI) (using a verb-generation task) to obtain perfect prediction of hemispheric dominance in a series of 87 surgical candidates suffering from epilepsy or tumors.

Comparable concordance rates regarding hemispheric dominance for speech have been obtained between the results of invasive methods and MEG using a variety of activation tasks and extended-source modeling techniques. In studies relying on spatial filtering algorithms (involving a total of 98 patients with epilepsy, tumors, or arteriovenous malformation), estimates of complete agreement with the Wada test ranged from 83% (verb generation; Findlay et al., 2012) to 85% (silent word reading task; Hirata et al., 2004), although the likelihood of obtaining usable data was as low as 51%. In smaller samples of patients with epilepsy (total of 43), minimum-norm algorithms have also been applied to model extended patches of cortex that became electrophysiologically active during semantic categorization of printed words (McDonald et al., 2009; Tanaka et al., 2013). The aggregate concordance rate with Wada results in these studies was 88%. Finally, a concordance rate higher than

90% ($N = 24$ patients with epilepsy) has been reported using another extended-source modeling algorithm (MR-FOCUSS) in the context of a verb-generation and a picture-naming task (Bowyer et al., 2005b).

17.4. CLINICAL APPLICATIONS: FUNCTIONAL MAPPING OF THE RECEPTIVE AND EXPRESSIVE LANGUAGE-RELATED CORTEX

Few studies have systematically examined the clinical utility of MEG activation and analysis protocols designed to identify the location and extent of cortical patches critically involved in receptive language functions (i.e., Wernicke's area). Using the protocol described in section 3 (Papanicolaou et al., 2004), one group defined the language-specific cortex as the regions where systematic overlap was found in the activation maps associated with two or more within-session replications of the same continuous auditory word recognition task. This method typically reveals one or two sites in the temporal lobe and/or temporoparietal junction of the dominant hemisphere that display consistent activity represented by a series of successive ECDs (source clusters) during the late portion of the event-related neuromagnetic epoch. In cases of bilateral language representation, sites demonstrating consistent late activation are typically found in both temporal lobes. The accuracy of these estimates has been verified against the results of invasive intraoperative or extraoperative electrocortical stimulation (ECS) mapping (Castillo et al., 2005; Simos et al., 1999a,b). Specifically, electrical stimulation of the cortical surface corresponding to these ECD clusters reliably impaired repetition of aurally presented sentences.

More recently, spatial filtering has been used to localize receptive language–related brain activity in 47 patients who later underwent ECS (Castillo et al., 2005; Figure 17.1). A total of 63 language-specific cortical sites were identified by MEG; 55 of these sites (87%) were verified using ECS (within ~1 cm). Verification between MEG and ECS was based

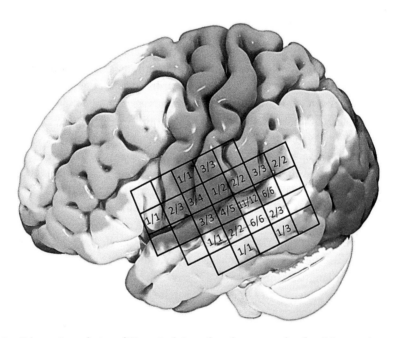

FIGURE 17.1 Schematic rendering of 63 cortical sites where language-related activity was detected by magnetoencephalography and verified by electrocortical stimulation (ECS) in 47 patients (based on data from Castillo et al., 2005). The number of cases displaying activity within a given sector is given in the denominator, and the number of cases confirmed through ECS in the same sector is shown in the numerator.

most commonly on repetition errors (78%), followed by naming errors (37%). Other groups have been successful in eliciting reliable activation of temporal lobe sites in the vicinity of Wernicke's area using extended-source modeling algorithms, for example, using silent reading, object-naming tasks, spatial filtering (Kober et al., 2001), and object naming using the MR-FOCUSS source localization technique (Bowyer et al., 2004). The precise location of cortical sites identified using these methods awaits verification by the results of electrocortical stimulation.

Several groups have thus far reported success in eliciting frontal magnetic activity in the vicinity of Broca's area associated with the performance of a variety of expressive language tasks. For instance, Kober et al.'s (2001) spatial localization and time course results were consistent with the Wernicke-Geschwind model of language organization. Moreover, they showed a high degree of concordance between results from spatial filtering and single ECD modeling. More recently, promising results were reported by Hirata et al. (2010) using spatial filtering to model activity in the beta band recorded during performance of a silent word reading task in 12 patients with epilepsy or tumors. They reported an average distance of 6.0 ± 7.1 mm between the intraoperative stimulation sites associated with speech arrest and the cortical patches that displayed significant activation in the inferior or middle frontal gyri.

17.5. MAGNETOENCEPHALO-GRAPHY MEASURES AS PROBES OF CORTICAL LANGUAGE FUNCTION IN THE INTACT BRAIN

17.5.1. The Early Portion of the Event-Related Field

Most studies have focused on the most prominent early magnetic response, which peaks at approximately 100 ms after stimulus onset (M100), the amplitude of which is known to be affected by simple acoustic parameters in both speech and nonspeech sounds (such as stimulus intensity). Systematic variations in M100 amplitude and/or latency have been shown to parallel perceptual categorization boundaries for both speech and nonspeech stimuli (Makela, Alku, May, Makinen, & Tiitinen, 2005; Obleser, Lahiri, & Eulitz, 2004; Peoppel et al., 1997; Shestakova, Brattico, Soloviev, Klucharev, & Huotilainen, 2004). Similar evidence in favor of the sensitivity of the M100 component to the phenomenon of *categorical perception* has been reported for consonants varying on the acoustic parameter (known as voice-onset-time, or VOT) that speakers of most languages use to differentiate between voiced (e.g., /b/, /d/, /g/) and voiceless (/p/, /t/, /k/) consonants (Simos et al., 1998a, 1998b, 1998c).

An alternative experimental technique is to use higher presentation rates (at least one stimulus per second) and series of stimuli that contain a majority of identical tokens (the standard stimulus), some of which are followed by a different token (the deviant or oddball stimulus). The ERF elicited by the latter contains an amplified segment compared with the ERF elicited by standard (frequent) stimuli. This segment, known as the mismatch magnetic field (MMF), occurs during and immediately after the resolution of the M100 response and originates from the auditory cortex (usually slightly anterior to the cortical patch that generates the peak of the M100 response). There is evidence that the magnitude of the MMF parallels the perceptual discriminability of the standard and deviant stimuli (Näätänen et al., 1997; Pihko et al., 2005).

Although earlier reports regarding hemisphere asymmetries in the amplitude (or estimated source current strength) of the early components of the ERF (e.g., Zouridakis, Simos, & Papanicolaou, 1998) were inconclusive, a recent systematic comparison of auditory and visual event-related responses to a variety of linguistic and nonlinguistic stimuli modeled using a minimum-norm algorithm indicated the presence of left lateralization of early activity in primary auditory and visual cortices (Papanicolaou et al., 2017).

17.5.2. The Late Portion of the Event-Related Field

A different pattern of activity is produced in the processing of more complex and meaningful, or potentially meaningful, spoken utterances (isolated real words and pseudowords). Initially, within the first 200 ms or so after stimulus onset, neurophysiological processes involved in the analysis of spoken words take place in and around the primary auditory cortex, bilaterally, regardless of the particular task demands. The spatial layout of cortical activity within the next 500 ms depends largely on the type of verbal stimulus used and the task that participants are asked to perform. When the task explicitly required analysis of spoken words into their constituent phonemes, activity can be found primarily among neuronal populations in the left STG. Sustained neurophysiological activity was particularly prominent in the regions surrounding the primary auditory cortex, which are coextensive with Brodmann's area 22 (auditory association cortex; Castillo et al., 2001a). This finding agrees with prior knowledge (acquired independently of functional imaging) regarding the location of Wernicke's area, which is specialized for high-level analysis of verbal input. Permanent damage or transient inactivation of this region severely impairs the ability to perceive spoken words as linguistic entities and to read meaningless letter strings (Boatman et al., 1995; Phillips & Farmer, 1990; Simos et al., 2000c). Neuromagnetic activity localized in the posterior dorsolateral prefrontal cortices was also found to be significantly increased during a task that involved phonological judgments on line drawings of common objects peaking between 500 and 600 ms after stimulus onset (Vihla, Laine, & Salmelin, 2006).

When the experimental task requires access to stored lexical/semantic representations,

neurophysiological processes engaged the posterior portion of the left posterior MTG and mesial temporal cortex (Castillo et al., 2001a). Nonword stimuli that obey the phonotactic rules of the English language are associated with significantly reduced activation of these regions. Several independent sources of evidence, including noninvasive functional imaging investigations and lesion studies, suggest the involvement of the MTG in lexical/semantic analysis (Damasio & Damasio, 1989; Hart et al., 2000; Kuperberg et al., 2000; Mummery et al., 1998).

The studies reviewed thus far in this section involve presentation of isolated meaningful (words) or meaningless spoken utterances (vowels, consonant–vowel syllables, or multisyllabic pseudowords). An alternative approach to investigating brain regions involved in phonological or lexical/semantic analysis involves presenting entire spoken sentences and asking participants to monitor each sentence for an inappropriate ending. Inappropriate or mismatching stimuli elicit stronger magnetic fields between approximately 300 and 600 ms after stimulus onset compared with appropriate or matching stimuli. The augmented portion of the ERF is referred to as the N400m response. Overall, source locations cluster around the superior temporal sulcus, including the ventral bank of the superior temporal gyrus and the dorsal bank of the middle temporal gyrus (Halgren et al., 2002; Kwon et al., 2005; Simos, Basile, & Papanicolaou, 1997; Vartiainen et al., 2009). Exactly what type of process this response reflects (phonological or lexical/semantic) is still under debate.

Finally, performance on tasks that exemplify expressive language functions (overt or silent reading, picture-naming, and word-generation or fluency tasks) is invariably associated with activation in posterior prefrontal areas of the dominant hemisphere (in the vicinity of Broca's area: Billingsley et al., 2004; Bowyer et al., 2004; Castillo et al., 2001b; Kober et al., 2001; Salmelin et al., 1994; Vihla, Laine, & Salmelin, 2006). Typically, activity in Wernicke's area is observed within the first 200 to 500 ms after stimulus onset, followed by activity in Broca's area, which in turn precedes activity in motor cortices.

Analyses of the late portion of the ERF in response to spoken words have been used to document postoperative intrahemispheric and interhemispheric language reorganization. In one of the few large patient series reported (Pataraia et al., 2004), it was found that patients with medically intractable epilepsy arising from the left temporal lobe showed significantly higher frequency of atypical lateralization of language (either right hemisphere dominance or bilateral language representation) compared with patients sustaining focal lesions (43% vs. 13%, respectively). In fact, the majority of patients who experienced early seizure onset (before age 5 years) showed atypical lateralization of language. In contrast, the precise location of cortex involved in language comprehension within the dominant hemisphere was found to be atypical (outside of Wernicke's area) in 30% of patients with focal lesions but only 14% of the epilepsy patients (who also showed significant degeneration of the mesial temporal lobe. These findings indicate that there is an increased probability of reorganization of the brain mechanism responsible for language comprehension to the nondominant hemisphere in patients with mesial temporal sclerosis (MTS). In a subsequent study, reorganization of brain mechanisms for language comprehension as a result of resection of the anterior portion of the left temporal lobe was investigated (Pataraia et al., 2005). Patients with atypical (bilateral) language lateralization (according to both the Wada procedure and preoperative MEG) were significantly more likely than patients with left hemisphere dominance to show a shift in language representation toward greater right hemispheric activity after surgery. Conversely, patients with left hemispheric dominance preoperatively were more likely to show intrahemispheric changes involving a slight inferior shift of the putative location of Wernicke's area. Patients with bilateral representation tended to perform worse on neuropsychological test measures before and after surgery (see also Breier et al., 2005).

In addition to the identity of brain regions involved in specific language processes, the outline of the mechanisms responsible for language functions requires data on the dynamics of corticocortical interactions. This information can be procured through various computational approaches, collectively referred to as "connectivity analyses."

17.6. BRAIN CONNECTIVITY ASSESSED THROUGH NEUROMAGNETIC DATA

During language processing, brain activity is characterized by bursts of information flow and correlated network activity. These bursts of focal brain activity can be viewed as "nodes" within a functional network of brain regions interconnected through functional links or "vertices" (Varela, Lachaux, Rodriguez, & Martinerie, 2001). These regions (nodes) show transient increases in neurophysiological activity, a portion of which represents locally generated and transmitted signals (i.e., within and across cortical layers), and the remaining entails neuronal signals transmitted to other regions (i.e., corticocortical signaling; Towle et al., 2007). The latter can in turn be modeled mathematically to produce indices of "functional connectivity," which entails computing a variety of measures of association between neuromagnetic signals at the sensor-source (e.g., Dimitriadis et al., 2013) or cortical-source level (e.g., Clarke, Taylor, & Tyler, 2011).

Applications of functional connectivity analyses to MEG data vary on such features as the time scale on which functional associations are estimated and the type of association that is targeted. The time scale of functional connectivity varies between tens or hundreds of milliseconds to the millisecond range. In the formal case, the question addressed is whether the degree of increased cortical activity in one region within a given time window (e.g., 100–150 ms after stimulus onset) correlates with the degree of increased activity in a different region estimated at a subsequent time window (e.g., 200–250 ms; Sideridis, Simos, Papanicolaou, & Fletcher, 2014; Simos, Rezaie, Fletcher, & Papanicolaou, 2013). Along the same lines, the degree of association in signal power at a given sensor (or brain region) within a specific time window and frequency band with signal power in the same frequency band recorded from a different sensor (or brain region) within a later time window can be quantified through the power correlation envelope (O'Neill, Barratt, Hunt, Tewarie, & Brookes, 2015).

Corticocortical signal associations can be estimated at an even smaller time-scale by computing measures of phase synchrony between neuronal oscillations at specific frequency bands. Coherence and phase synchrony are common mathematical methods for quantifying frequency-dependent corticocortical signaling (Bowyer, 2014). Coherence analysis supplies information on the degree of synchrony of brain activity at different locations for each frequency, independent of power, and is more suitable for long time series because it relies on the assumption that associations between two signals are relatively stable in time. However, individual time points with large amplitudes are more highly weighted in the fast Fourier transform and subsequently in coherence calculations. This is in contrast to phase synchrony, which uses instantaneous measurements of only the phase differences between signals, typically indexed by the *phase locking value*. In a recent study, connectivity during language was assessed using MEG coherence source imaging. In this framework, a total of 1,431 possible pairs of functionally connected sources can be modeled in response to images of objects (picture-naming task) or spoken words (word-identification task). As expected from previous studies contrasting activation maps to meaningful auditory versus visual stimuli (printed words, pictures), a more extensive and, therefore, complex network of

interconnected areas was found in the latter compared with the former case (Bowyer et al., unpublished data). This finding may reflect the recruitment of the dorsal pathways for processing of visual stimuli as contrasted to the engagement of the ventral pathway for auditory processing.

17.7. LIMITATIONS OF MAGNETOENCEPHALOGRAPHY AND FEATURE DIRECTIONS

Applications of MEG to the study of the brain mechanisms for language functions face most of the limitations that characterize brain imaging techniques relying on hemodynamic measures. Perhaps the most fundamental of these limitations concerns the degree of specificity of results: Activation profiles feature brain regions that may not be indispensable for a particular target function. This problem is particularly serious in the case of language mapping and to a lesser degree in motor cortex mapping. Replication studies in the same patients may help in this context by reducing (or eliminating) activations attributed to nonsystematic sources of variability in the recorded signals (e.g., certain components of extraneous noise and activity attributable to temporal variations in the realization of language processes involved). Although it is extremely helpful in this respect, within-session replication of the activation task is limited by time constraints and depends heavily on the patient's level of cooperation, fatigue, and habituation to the task. Employing variations of the activation task (e.g., presenting stimuli in a different modality) may help in this direction.

Sensitivity of results is equally important clinically, although it appears to be less of an issue in MEG applications targeting receptive language functions. Sensitivity of MEG protocols is considerably reduced in motor cortex and expressive language mapping (applications that are also associated with the lowest success rates for obtaining clinically useful MEG test results). In these applications, the nature of the phenomenon being targeted (limb movement or speech) is inherently more difficult to image with MEG than somatic sensation and recognition of an aurally presented word. This difficulty is related to the averaging procedure that MEG entails, whereby several epochs of neuromagnetic activity are recorded, each to one of several repetitions of the same (or a similar) event. For the averaged ERF to accurately represent the neurophysiological activity elicited by each event, the temporal characteristics of this activity have to be identical (or at least very similar) across its successive repetitions. This requirement is met to a large degree in the case of stimulation and processing of somatic and language stimuli and much less in tasks involving planning, programming, and execution of motor acts (Bourguignon, 2014).

The external validity and therefore interpretation of MEG results depend heavily, as in the case of fMRI, on the approach used to model the recorded signals. Each modeling technique bears characteristic advantages and disadvantages, with the capacity of each to approximate the inverse problem being the most fundamental. Specific approaches bear specific positive and negative features. For instance, methods that operate in the frequency domain may be more suitable in capturing fine-grained corticocortical interactions that may rely on phase synchrony. These methods, however, have yet to produce a convincing account of the functional role of event-related reductions or increases of power in specific frequency bands. Maps of regional cortical activation derived from such indices, which are commonly referred to as event-related synchronization and event-related desynchronization, may lead to very diverse conclusions regarding the involvement of specific brain regions (such as the inferior frontal cortex) in language functions (e.g., Pammer et al., 2004). Combining results from MEG and fMRI may present a solution to this problem, as has been demonstrated in one large-scale study thus far, although activation and analysis protocols ensuring efficient and

meaningful integration of data from the two modalities are yet to be established.

Despite these limitations, language mapping with MEG has proved helpful in presurgical estimates of the location and extent of language-related cortex as well as in the intraoperative identification of these cortical patches. In fact, in several neurosurgical centers around the world, such assessments are part of the protocol of surgical interventions, especially in the case of epilepsy. Moreover, MEG alone or in combination with other imaging methods, such as fMRI and transcranial magnetic stimulation, is extensively used for the testing of alternative models of cortical organization for language in normal populations.

REFERENCES

Billingsley-Marshall, R. L., Simos, P. G., & Papanicolaou, A. C. (2004). Reliability and validity of functional neuroimaging techniques for identifying language-critical areas in children and adults. *Developmental Neuropsychology, 26*, 541–563.

Boatman, D., Lesser, R., & Gordon, B. (1995). Auditory speech processing in the left temporal lobe: an electrical interference study. *Brain and Language, 51*, 269–290.

Bourguignon, N. J. (2014). A rostro-caudal axis for language in the frontal lobe: The role of executive control in speech production. *Neuroscience and Biobehavioral Review, 47*, 431–444.

Bowyer, S. M. (2014). Connectivity measurements for network imaging. *Current Topics in Behavioral Neuroscience, 21*, 315–330.

Bowyer, S. M., Fleming, T., Greenwald, M. L., Moran, J. E., Mason, K. M., Weiland, B. J., . . . Tepley, N. (2005a). Magnetoencephalographic localization of the basal temporal language area. *Epilepsy Behavior, 6*(2), 229–234.

Bowyer, S. M., Moran, J. E., Mason, K. M., Constantinou, J. E., Smith, B. J., Barkley, G. L., & Tepley, N. (2004). MEG localization of language-specific cortex utilizing MR-FOCUSS. *Neurology, 62*, 2247–2255.

Bowyer, S. M., Moran, J. E., Weiland, B. J., Mason, K. M., Greenwald, M. L., Smith, B. J., . . . Tepley, N. (2005b). Language laterality determined by MEG mapping with MR-FOCUSS. *Epilepsy Behavior, 6*(2), 235–241.

Breier, J. I., Castillo, E. M., Simos, P. G., Billingsley-Marshall, R. L., Pataraia, E., Sarkari, S., et al. (2005). Atypical language representation in patients with chronic seizure disorder and achievement deficits with Magnetoencephalography. *Epilepsia, 46,* 540–548.

Breier, J. I., Simos, P. G., Wheless, J. W., Constantinou, J. E. C., & Papanicolaou, A. C. (2001). Hemispheric language dominance in children determined by magnetic source imaging. *Journal of Child Neurology, 16,* 124–130.

Breier, J. I., Simos, P. G., Zouridakis, G., Wheless, J. W., Willmore, L. J., Constantinou, J. E., . . . Papanicolaou, A. C. (1999b). Language dominance determined by magnetic source imaging: A comparison with the Wada procedure. *Neurology, 53,* 938–945.

Castillo, E. M., Breier, J. I., Wheless, J. W., Slater, J. D., Tandon, N., Baumgartner, J. E., & Papanicolaou, A. C. (2005). Contributions of direct cortical stimulation and MEG recordings to identify "essential" language cortex. *Epilepsia, 46,* 324.

Castillo, E. M., Simos, P. G., Davis, R. N., Breier, J. I., Fitzgerald, M., & Papanicolaou, A. C. (2001a). Levels of word processing and incidental memory: dissociable mechanisms in the temporal lobe. *Neuroreport, 12,* 3561–3566.

Castillo, E. M., Simos, P. G., Venkataraman, V., Breier, J. I., Wheless, J. W., & Papanicolaou, A. C. (2001b). Mapping of expressive language cortex using Magnetic Source Imaging. *Neurocase, 7,* 419–422.

Clarke, A., Taylor, K. I., & Tyler, L. K. (2011). The evolution of meaning: Spatio-temporal dynamics of visual object recognition. *Journal of Cognitive Neuroscience, 23*(8), 1887–1899.

Damasio, H., & Damasio, A. (1989). *Lesion Analysis in Neuropsychology.* New York: Oxford University Press.

Dimitriadis, S. I., Laskaris, N. A., Simos, P. G., Micheloyannis, S., Fletcher, J. M., Rezaie, R., & Papanicolaou, A. C. (2013). Altered temporal correlations in resting-state connectivity fluctuations in children with reading difficulties detected via MEG. *Neuroimage, 83,* 307–317.

Doss, R. C., Zhang, W., Risse, G. L., & Dickens, D. L. (2009). Lateralizing language with magnetic source imaging: Validation based on the Wada test. *Epilepsia, 50,* 2242–2248.

Findlay, A. M., Ambrose, J. B., Cahn-Weiner, D. A., Houde, J. F., Honma, S., Hinkley, L. B., . . . Kirsch, H. E. (2012). Dynamics of hemispheric dominance for language assessed by magnetoencephalographic imaging. *Annals of Neurology, 71,* 668–686.

Gorno-Tempini, M. L., Dronkers, N. F., Rankin, K. P., Ogar, J. M., Phengrasamy, L., Rosen, H. J., . . . Miller, B. L. (2004). Cognition and anatomy in three variants of primary progressive aphasia. *Annals of Neurology, 55,* 335–346.

Gorodnitsky, I. F., George, J. S., & Rao, B. D. (1995). Neuromagnetic source imaging with FOCUSS: A recursive weighted minimum norm algorithm. *Electroencephalography and Clinical Neurophysiology, 95,* 231–251.

Halgren, E., Dhond, R. P., Christensen, N., Van Petten, C., Marinkovic, K., Lewine, J. D., et al. (2002). N400-like magnetoencephalography responses modulated by semantic context, word frequency, and lexical class in sentences. *NeuroImage, 17,* 1101–1116.

Hart, J., Jr, Kraut, M. A., Kremen, S., Soher, B., & Gordon, B. (2000). Neural substrates of orthographic lexical access as demonstrated by functional brain imaging. *Neuropsychiatry Neuropsychology Behavioral Neurology, 13,* 1–7.

Hickok, G., & Poeppel, D. (2015). Neural basis of speech perception. In M. J. Aminoff, F. Boller, & D. F. Swaab (Eds.), *Handbook of clinical neurology* (3rd ed., pp. 149–160). Oxford, UK: Elsevier.

Hillebrand, A., & Barnes, G. R. (2005). Beamformer analysis of MEG data. *International Review of Neurobiology, 68,* 149–171.

Hirata, M., Goto, T., Barnes, G., Umekawa, Y., Yanagisawa, T., Kato, A., . . . Yoshimine, T. (2010). Language dominance and mapping based on neuromagnetic oscillatory changes: Comparison with invasive procedures. *Journal of Neurosurgery, 112*(3), 528–538.

Hirata, M., Kato, A., Taniguchi, M., Saitoh, Y., Ninomiya, H., Ihara, A., . . . Yoshimine, T. (2004). Determination of language dominance with synthetic aperture magnetometry: Comparison with the Wada test. *Neuroimage, 23,* 46–53.

Hurley, R. S., Paller, K. A., Rogalski, E. J., & Mesulam, M. M. (2012). Neural mechanisms of object naming and word comprehension in primary progressive aphasia. *Journal of Neuroscience, 32,* 4848–4855.

Ilmoniemi, R. J. (1993). Models of source currents in the brain. *Brain Topography, 5*(4), 331–336.

Jefferies, E., & Lambon Ralph, M. A. (2006). Semantic impairment in stroke aphasia versus semantic dementia: A case-series comparison. *Brain, 129,* 2132–2147.

Kamada, K., Sawamura, Y., Takeuchi, F. Kuriki, A., Kawai, K., Morita, A., & Todo, T. (2007). Expressive and receptive language areas determined by a non-invasive reliable method using functional magnetic resonance imaging and magnetoencephalography. *Neurosurgery, 60,* 296–305.

Kober, H., Moller, M., Nimsky, C., Vieth, J., Fahlbusch, R., & Ganslandt, O. (2001). New approach to localize speech relevant brain areas and hemispheric dominance using spatially filtered magnetoencephalography. *Human Brain Mapping, 14,* 236–250.

Kuperberg, G. R., McGuire, P. K., Bullmore, E. T., Brammer, M. J., Rabe-Hesketh, S., Wright, I. C., et al. (2000). Common and distinct neural substrates for pragmatic, semantic, and syntactic processing of spoken sentences: An fMRI study. *Journal of Cognitive Neuroscience, 12,* 321–341.

Kwon, H., Kuriki, S., Kim, J. M., Lee, Y. H., Kim, K., & Nam, K. (2005). MEG study on neural activities associated with syntactic and semantic violations in spoken Korean sentences. *Neuroscience Research, 51,* 349–357.

Lüders, H., Lesser, R. P., Hahn, J., Dinner, D. S., Morris, H. H., Wyllie, E., & Godoy, J. (1991). Basal temporal language area. *Brain, 114*(Pt 2), 743–754.

Maestu, F., Ortiz, T., Fernandez, A., Amo, C., Martin, P., Fernandez, S., & Sola, R. G. (2002). Spanish language mapping using MEG: A validation study. *Neuroimage, 17,* 1579–1586.

Makela, A. M., Alku, P., May, P. J., Makinen, V., & Tiitinen, H. (2005). Left-hemispheric brain activity reflects formant transitions in speech sounds. *Neuroreport, 16,* 549–553.

McDonald, C. R., Thesen, T., Hagler, D. J., Jr., Carlson, C., Devinksy, O., Kuzniecky, R., . . . Halgren, E. (2009). Distributed source modeling of language with magnetoencephalography: Application to patients with intractable epilepsy. *Epilepsia, 50,* 2256–2266.

Mesulam, M. M., Thompson, C. K., Weintraub, S., & Rogalski, E. J. (2015). The Wernicke conundrum and the anatomy of language comprehension in primary progressive aphasia. *Brain, 138,* 2423–2437.

Mesulam, M. M., Wieneke, C., Hurley, R., Rademaker, A., Thompson, C. K., Weintraub, S., & Rogalski, E. J. (2013). Words and objects at the tip of the left temporal lobe in primary progressive aphasia. *Brain, 136,* 601–618.

Moran, J. E., Bowyer, S. M., & Tepley, N. (2005). Multi-resolution FOCUSS: A source imaging technique applied to MEG data. *Brain Topography, 18*(1), 1–17.

Mummery, C. J., Patterson, K., Hodges, J. R., & Price, C. J. (1998). Functional neuroanatomy of the semantic system: divisible by what? *Journal of Cognitive Neuroscience, 10,* 766–777.

Narain, C., Scott, S. K., Wise, R. J., Rosen, S., Leff, A., Iversen, S. D., & Matthews, P. M. (2003). Defining a left-lateralized response specific to intelligible speech using fMRI. *Cerebral Cortex, 13,* 1362–1368.

Näätänen, R., Lehtokoski, A., Lennes, M., Cheour, M., Huotilainen, M., Livonen, A., et al. (1997). Language-specific phoneme representations revealed by electric and magnetic responses. *Nature, 385,* 432–433.

Obleser, J., Eulitz, C., & Lahiri, A. (2004). Magnetic brain response mirrors extraction of phonological features from spoken vowels. *Journal of Cognitive Neuroscience, 16,* 31–39.

O'Neill, G. C., Barratt, E. L., Hunt, B. A., Tewarie, P. K., & Brookes, M. J. (2015). Measuring electrophysiological connectivity by power envelope correlation: A technical review on MEG methods. *Physics in Medicine and Biology, 60*(21), R271–R295.

Pammer, K., Hansen, P. C., Kringelbach, M. L., Holliday, I., Barnes, G., Hillebrand, A., . . . Cornelissen, P. L. (2004). Visual word recognition: The first half second. *Neuroimage, 22*(4), 1819–1825.

Papanicolaou, A. C., Kilintari, M., Rezaie, R., Narayana, S., & Babajani-Feremi, A. (2017). The Role of the Primary Sensory Cortices in Early Language Processing. *Journal of Cognitive Neuroscience, 29*(10), 1755–1765.

Papanicolaou, A. C., Pataraia, E., Billingsley-Marshall, R., Castillo, E. M., Wheless, J. W., Swank. P., . . . Simos, P. G. (2005). Toward the substitution of invasive electroencephalography in epilepsy surgery. *Journal of Clinical Neurophysiology, 22,* 231–237.

Papanicolaou, A. C., Simos, P. G., Castillo, E. M., Breier, J. I., Sarkari, S., Pataraia, E., . . . Maggio, W. W. (2004). Magnetoencephalography: A noninvasive alternative to the Wada procedure. *Journal of Neurosurgery, 100,* 867–876.

Pataraia, E., Simos, P. G., Castillo, E. M., Billingsley-Marshall, R. L., McGregor, A. L., Breier, J. I., et al. (2004). Reorganization of language-specific cortex in patients with lesions or mesial temporal epilepsy. *Neurology, 63*(10), 1825–1832.

Phillips, D. P., & Farmer, M. E. (1990). Acquired word deafness, and the temporal grain of sound representation in the primary auditory cortex. *Behavioural Brain Research, 40*(2), 85–94.

Pihko, E., Kujala, T., Mickos, A., Antell, H., Alku, P., Byring, R., et al. (2005). Magnetic fields evoked by speech sounds in preschool children. *Clinical Neurophysiology, 116,* 112–119.

Poeppel, D., Phillips, C., Yellin, E., Rowley, H. A., Roberts, T. P. L., & Marantz, A. (1997). Processing of vowels in supratemporal auditory cortex. *Neuroscience Letters, 221,* 145–148.

Price, C. J. (2012). A review and synthesis of the first 20 years of PET and fMRI studies of heard speech, spoken language and reading. *Neuroimage, 62,* 816–847.

Pulvermüller, F. (2013). How neurons make meaning: Brain mechanisms for embodied and abstract-symbolic semantics. *Trends in Cognitive Science, 17,* 458–470.

Rauschecker, J. P., & Scott, S. K. (2009). Maps and streams in the auditory cortex: Nonhuman primates illuminate human speech processing. *Nature Neuroscience, 12,* 718–724.

Rezaie, R., Narayana, S., Schiller, K., Birg, L., Wheless, J. W., Boop, F. A., & Papanicolaou, A. C. (2014). Assessment of hemispheric dominance for receptive language in pediatric patients under sedation using magnetoencephalography. *Frontiers in Human Neuroscience, 8,* 657.

Rogalsky, C., & Hickok, G. (2011). The role of Broca's area in sentence comprehension. *Journal of Cognitive Neuroscience, 23,* 1664–1680.

Salmelin, R., Hari, R., Lounasmaa, O. V., et al. (1994). Dynamics of brain activation during picture naming. *Nature, 368,* 463–465.

Schirmer, A., Fox, P. M., & Grandjean, D. (2012). On the spatial organization of sound processing in the human temporal lobe: A meta-analysis. *Neuroimage, 63,* 137–147.

Schwartz, M. F., Kimberg, D. Y., Walker, G. M., Fasyitan, O., Brecher, A., Dell, G. S., & Coslettt, H. B. (2009). Anterior temporal involvement in semantic word retrieval: Voxel-based lesion-symptom mapping evidence from aphasia. *Brain, 132,* 3411–3427.

Scott, S. K., Blank, C. C., Rosen, S., & Wise, R. J. (2000). Identification of a pathway for intelligible speech in the left temporal lobe. *Brain, 123,* 2400–2406.

Shestakova, A., Brattico, E., Soloviev, A., Klucharev, V., & Huotilainen, M. (2004). Orderly cortical representation of vowel categories presented by multiple exemplars. *Brain Research. Cognitive Brain Research, 21,* 342–350.

Sideridis, G., Simos, P., Papanicolaou, A., & Fletcher, J. (2014). Using structural equation modeling to assess functional connectivity in the brain: Power and sample size considerations. *Educational and Psychological Measurement, 74*(5), 733–758.

Simos, P. G., Basile, L. F. H., & Papanicolaou, A. C. (1997). Source localization of the N400 response in a sentence-reading paradigm using evoked magnetic fields and magnetic resonance imaging. *Brain Research, 762,* 29–39.

Simos, P. G., Breier, J. I., Maggio, W. W., Gormley, W. B., Zouridakis, G., Willmore, L. J., . . . Papanicolaou, A. C. (1999a). Atypical temporal lobe language representation: MEG and intraoperative stimulation mapping correlation. *Neuroreport, 10,* 139–142.

Simos, P. G., Breier, J. I., Wheless, J. W., Maggio, W. W., Fletcher, J. M., Castillo, E. M., & Papanicolaou, A. C. (2000c). Brain mechanisms for reading: The role of the superior temporal gyrus in word and pseudoword naming. *Neuroreport, 11,* 2443–2447.

Simos, P. G., Breier, J. I., Zouridakis, G., & Papanicolaou, A. C. (1998a). MEG correlates of categorical-like temporal cue perception in humans. *Neuroreport, 9,* 2475–2479.

Simos, P. G., Breier, J. I., Zouridakis, G., & Papanicolaou, A. C. (1998b). Magnetic fields elicited by a tone onset time continuum in humans. *Cognitive Brain Research, 6,* 285–294.

Simos, P. G., Diehl, R., Breier, J. I., Molis, M., Zouridakis, G., & Papanicolaou, A. C. (1998c). MEG correlates of categorical perception of a voice onset continuum in humans. *Cognitive Brain Research, 7,* 215–219.

Simos, P. G., Rezaie, R., Fletcher, J. M., & Papanicolaou, A. C. (2013). Time-constrained functional connectivity analysis of cortical networks underlying phonological decoding in typically developing school-aged children: A magnetoencephalography study. *Brain Language, 125*(2), 156–164.

Spitsyna, G., Warren, J. E., Scott, S. K., Turkheimer, S. W., & Wise, R. J. (2006). Converging language streams in the human temporal lobe. *Journal of Neuroscience, 26,* 7328–7336.

Tanaka, N., Liu, H., Reinsberger, C., Madsen, J. R., Bourgeois, B. F., Dworetzky, B. A., . . . Stufflebeam, S. M. (2013). Language lateralization represented by spatiotemporal mapping of magnetoencephalography. *American Journal of Neuroradiology, 34,* 558–563.

Towle, V. L., Hunter, J. D., Edgar, J. C., Chkhenkeli, S. A., Castelle, M. C., Frim, D. M., . . . Hecox, K. E. (2007). Frequency domain analysis of human subdural recordings. *Journal of Clinical Neurophysiology, 24*(2), 205–213.

Turkeltaub, P. E., & Coslett, H. B. (2010). Localization of sublexical speech perception components. *Brain Language, 114,* 1–15.

Turken, A. U., & Dronkers, N. F. (2011). The neural architecture of the language comprehension network: Converging evidence from lesion and connectivity analyses. *Frontiers in Systems Neuroscience, 5,* 1.

Varela, F., Lachaux, J. P., Rodriguez, E., & Martinerie, J. (2001). The brainweb: Phase synchronization and large-scale integration. *Nature Reviews Neuroscience, 2*(4), 229–239.

Vartiainen, J., Parviainen, T., & Salmelin, R. (2009). Spatiotemporal convergence of semantic processing in reading and speech perception. *Journal of Neuroscience, 29,* 9271–9280.

Vihla, M., Laine, M., & Salmelin, R. (2006). Cortical dynamics of visual/semantic vs. phonological analysis in picture confrontation. *Neuroimage, 33*(2), 732–738.

Wernicke, C. (1874/1969). The symptom complex of aphasia: A psychological study on an anatomical basis. In R. S. Cohen & M. W. Wartofsky (Eds.), *Boston studies in the philosophy of science* (pp. 34–97). Dordrecht, The Netherlands: D. Reidel.

Wolmetz, M., Poeppel, D., & Rapp, B. (2011). What does the right hemisphere know about phoneme categories? *Journal of Cognitive Neuroscience, 23*(3), 552–569.

Zouridakis, G., Simos, P. G., & Papanicolaou, A. C. (1998). Multiple bilaterally asymmetric cortical sources account for the auditory N1m component. *Brain Topography, 10,* 183–189.

SECTION V

EXPLORING THE BRAIN MECHANISMS OF COGNITION

18

READING, READING ACQUISITION, AND READING DISABILITY (DYSLEXIA)

Panagiotis G. Simos

18.1. THE NEUROBIOLOGICAL SUBSTRATE OF READING IN CHILDREN AND ADULTS

A useful conceptual view of the brain mechanisms supporting skilled word recognition specifies that access to word-like representations of printed stimuli relies heavily on a ventral circuit, consisting primarily of ventral occipitotemporal regions and the middle temporal gyrus, when the stimulus is familiar and task demands are appropriate (Pugh et al., 2000). Notably, activity in ventral association areas takes place early during reading (Simos et al., 2009; Tarkiainen, Helenius, Hansen, Cornelissen, & Salmelin, 1999). Conversely, the mechanism that supports reading may rely more heavily on a dorsal system (consisting of the superior temporal, supramarginal, and angular gyri) and an anterior component (in the inferior frontal gyrus), when the printed material is novel or low frequency (Pugh et al.,

2000). This functional differentiation within the brain mechanism for reading parallels the classical dual route notion that was developed to account for reading behavior (Coltheart, Rastle, Perry, Langdon, & Ziegler, 2001).

Behavioral studies have characterized critical cognitive processes necessary to acquire fluent reading and how these processes are altered in struggling readers. The core difficulty in word level reading disability (RD, the most common kind of reading disorder; Fletcher, Lyon, Fuchs, & Barnes, 2007) manifests as a deficiency within the language system and, in particular, a deficiency at the level of phonological analysis. To learn to read words, a child must first develop an appreciation of the segmental nature of speech and come to realize that spoken words are composed of small segments, or phonemes. This appreciation of the segmental nature of speech is termed *phonemic awareness*. Subsequently, the beginning

Panagiotis G. Simos, *Reading, Reading Acquisition, and Reading Disability (Dyslexia)* In: *Fifty Years of Magnetoencephalography.* Edited by: Andrew C. Papanicolaou, Timothy P. L. Roberts, and James W. Wheless, Oxford University Press (2020). © Oxford University Press.
DOI: 10.1093/oso/9780190935689.003.0018.

reader must understand that written words possess an internal phonological structure that can be deciphered based on their understanding of the internal structures of the spoken word, a skill known as phonological decoding. It is phonemic awareness and the understanding that the constituents of a printed word—its letters—bear a relationship to phonemes that allows the reader to connect printed words to the corresponding words in his/her speech lexicon. As many studies have shown, phonemic awareness and phonological decoding are deficient in RD children and adults who, as a consequence, have difficulty mapping the alphabetic characters of print onto the spoken word (Fletcher et al., 2007). With experience, word reading becomes automatic, and decoding occurs without conscious effort as the proficient reader develops representations of words at a neural level. There is extensive evidence that even severe and persistent phonological processing deficits can be remediated through instruction delivered in small-group formats (i.e., Torgesen et al., 2001), which may enable students to continue to make adequate progress in reading without extensive long-term support. While highly individualized, intensive intervention programs focusing on phonological processing skills have proved very effective in small-scale studies, current research and practice are focusing on multistep programs that focus on word-level reading skills as well as phonological processing abilities and can be implemented in schools to meet the needs of the vast majority of RD students (Denton, Fletcher, Simos, Papanicolaou, & Anthony, 2007).

Neuroimaging relying on hemodynamic methods such as functional magnetic resonance imaging (fMRI) and magnetoencephalography (MEG) has been instrumental in establishing brain activation profiles during a variety of reading tasks through the phases of acquisition of reading skills. Importantly, both methods have contributed to establishing associations between individual profiles of reading-related brain activity and specific reading skills. More

recently, MEG studies have even attempted to account for individual differences of response to educational interventions. This chapter includes a conceptual review of the quite extensive literature of MEG studies on reading and is organized in the following subsections: studies examining the mature outline of the brain circuits for reading; developmental studies of typical reading acquisition; investigations of the activation profiles associated with reading in children manifesting difficulties in learning to read and in adults with a history of reading disability; and studies on the effects of reading interventions on reading-related neuromagnetic activity.

18.2. MAGNETOENCEPHALO-GRAPHY STUDIES ON THE BRAIN CIRCUITS FOR READING IN ADULT, FLUENT READERS

Regions that show increased levels of activation consistently, both within and across individuals, include the following: the primary visual cortex, ventral and lateral temporo-occipital areas (association visual cortex), the posterior portion of the superior temporal gyrus extending posteriorly into the supramarginal gyrus, the posterior portion of the middle temporal gyrus, and posterior dorsolateral prefrontal cortices (inferior frontal gyrus; Helenius, Salmelin, Service, & Connolly, 1998; Salmelin, Service, Kiesila, Uutela, & Salonen, 1996; Simos et al., 2009; Tarkiainen et al., 1999).

18.2.1. Processing Letter Strings in Visual Association Cortex

Activity in ventral temporo-occipital areas is detectable as early as 150 ms after the onset of any type of printed stimulus (letters, syllables, and symbol strings). Activity in the right hemisphere appears to be sensitive primarily to visual stimulus characteristics, so that it increased in magnitude with increasing image noise level (Tarkiainen et al., 1999). Conversely, activity in the left hemisphere was delayed and reduced in magnitude with increasing visual noise levels and was greater in magnitude in response to letter strings compared with symbol strings. This early neuromagnetic response does not appear to vary with stimulus lexicality (six-letter words vs. six-letter consonants; Cornelissen, Tarkiainen, Helenius, & Salmelin, 2003).

18.2.2. Brain Circuits for Word-Level Reading Skills

Other studies focused on linguistic characteristics of the printed stimuli such as lexicality. According to dual-process models of reading, the brain mechanism for reading words that require assembled phonology (i.e., involving sublexical processing), in experienced readers, is different from the mechanism for reading words that do not. To address these questions, activation profiles were obtained during reading of three types of print: exception words (relying more on addressed phonology and having meaning), pseudohomophones (requiring assembled phonology and also having meaning), and pseudowords (requiring assembled phonology but having no meaning; Simos et al., 2002b). While all subjects showed activity in the posterior portion of the left superior temporal gyrus (Brodmann's area [BA] 22) in all three conditions, a prominent feature of the activation profile associated with reading aloud both exception words and pseudohomophones involved the posterior middle temporal gyrus (BA 21) and mesial temporal regions (in 14 of 16 participants). The significant correlation between onset of activity in the left BA 21 and naming latency of exception words indicated that the earlier the engagement of this area, following word presentation, the faster the pronunciation of the printed stimuli. The fact that activity in BA 21 did not predict pronunciation speed for pseudohomophones (or pseudowords) suggests that engagement of this area may be a byproduct of phonological access achieved through the assembled route for nonwords that sound like real words. Direct evidence supporting the critical role of the dorsal

system, at least for sublexical phonological analysis, comes from an electrocortical stimulation study (Simos et al. 2000a), in which it was seen that electrical interference with a small portion of the posterior superior temporal gyrus consistently impaired the patients' ability to decode pseudowords.

An alternative experimental paradigm employed to induce cortical activity reflecting access to a word-like stored representation involves incongruity detection. In the original version of the task, stimuli are sequentially presented single words that form a sentence. The final word in the sentence can be either semantically appropriate or inappropriate (i.e., incongruous), yielding a highly reliable and therefore easily identified and measured electrical and magnetic response peaking at approximately 400 ms after the onset of this word (N400/N400m; Kutas & Hillyard, 1980). In variations of this task, the type (semantic, orthographic, phonological) and level of incongruity can be systematically manipulated, so that the brain areas that participate in the evaluation of contextual congruity can be mapped. In the earliest MEG study, the N400m response elicited by semantically incongruous sentence endings was larger in field strength, as well as in the strength of its estimated dipole source, compared with the response elicited by congruous endings (Simos, Basile, & Papanicolaou, 1997). In every case, N400m sources (modeled as equivalent current dipoles [ECDs]) were localized in posterior temporal lobe cortex, including neocortical areas on the lateral surface of the left hemisphere (near the temporoparietal junction and in the middle temporal gyrus) and medial temporal paleocortical and archicortical regions, that is, in the vicinity of the hippocampus and the parahippocampal gyrus. Using a similar task, enriched with a syntactic incongruity condition and a whole-head neuromagnetometer system, N400m sources (also modeled as ECDs) were localized in the vicinity of the superior temporal sulcus (posterior middle and superior temporal gyri, predominantly in the left hemisphere; Service, Helenius, Maury, & Salmelin, 2007). Moreover, ECD strength was significantly higher in response to semantic compared with syntactic sentence-ending violations. Similar latencies and source locations for the N400m peak were found in response to the final word of four-word lists that was either phonologically or semantically dissimilar to the previous three words (Vartiainen, Parviainen, & Salmelin, 2009).

18.2.3. Individual Differences in the Outline of Activity

Although the presence of systematic individual differences in the activation profiles associated with performance of a given reading task is recognized (e.g., Seghier & Price, 2018; Van Horn, Grafton, & Miller, 2008), it remains customary to present functional activation maps as group averages. The distribution of cases demonstrating detectable activity in specific regions of the brain circuit for reading has often reported, even in smaller-scale normative studies (e.g., Vartiainen et al., 2009). Equally important is the need to establish intrasubject reproducibility of regional activation. In one such attempt, ECD-derived activation profiles were reconstructed from eight split-data sets obtained in response to printed words in a lexical decision task (Simos et al., 2009). Identification of patches of cortex that showed reliable neurophysiological activity across all eight data sets was performed blindly with the aid of a clustering algorithm. All participants reliably showed ECDs in the posterior portion of the middle and superior temporal gyri and in motor/premotor cortex in the left hemisphere. There was, however, a notable systematic variation in the precise location of systematic occipitotemporal activity: 12 of 17 participants demonstrated activity in the posterior portion of the middle temporal gyrus near its border with BA 37, and five of 17 persons showed ECDs in posterior ventral occipitotemporal cortices. Such individual differences may in part account for discrepancies in activation

observed in parieto-occipital and temporo-occipital areas across different brain imaging studies during the performance of single-word reading tasks, as described previously (e.g., Horwitz, Rumsey, & Donohue, 1998; Joubert et al., 2004; Turkeltaub et al., 2002).

18.2.4. Prefrontal Activity During Reading

Neuromagnetic activity in posterior prefrontal cortices during silent reading tasks has not been as consistently reported. For instance, inferior prefrontal sources (mainly in the left hemisphere) were modeled as ECDs during passive word reading after 300 to 400 ms (Salmelin et al., 1996; Tarkiainen et al., 1999). In general, it appears that the ECD approach is not the method of choice to reveal prefrontal sources, even when more than one temporally overlapping dipolar sources can be modeled in each hemisphere. Minimum-norm estimate (MNE) models and synthetic aperture magnetometry (SAM) may be more suitable in this task. In a more recent study, activation profiles associated with printed words in the context of a lexical decision task were obtained using ECDs and MNE, supporting the aforementioned conclusion (Simos et al., 2009). When MNE-derived peak latencies of regional activity were considered, there was a clear temporal progression of activation from occipitotemporal to motor/premotor cortex, then to the posterior portion of the superior temporal gyrus, and finally to the inferior frontal gyrus. The train of regional activity took place, on average, more than 450 ms after stimulus onset, culminating in the participant's manual response, which occurred between 530 and 580 ms. It is important to note that the regular progression of activity from occipitotemporal to lateral temporal and subsequently to inferior frontal cortices is in agreement with results from electrocorticographic recordings in the gamma band (Mainly et al., 2008). There is, however, some debate as to the latency of the earliest detectable activity in the Inferior

Frontal Gyrus (IFG), with studies relying on SAM presenting evidence of cortical activation (in the form of event-related synchronization or event-related desynchronization in the 10- to 20-Hz range) that was practically concurrent with occipitotemporal activity (Cornelissen et al., 2009).

A further emerging trend in the study of the brain circuits involved in reading that has not been addressed in this chapter involves analyses of effective corticocortical connectivity for which MEG is uniquely suited. In one study, dynamic imaging of coherent sources (DICS) was used to estimate phase coupling in the alpha range between left hemisphere cortical nodes associated with reading of rapidly presented words in context (Kujala et al., 2007). Granger causality was then employed to determine feed-forward interactions from occipitotemporal and cerebellar nodes toward posterior temporal, precentral, and dorsolateral prefrontal regions. An alternative approach to establish effective connectivity profiles employs regression analyses applied to source-current density waveforms (obtained using MNE). Using this approach on data from a sample of 58 typical, school-aged readers, it was shown that activity in left hemisphere temporoparietal regions was largely driven by feed-forward input from occipitotemporal areas, whereas activity in the former regions determines to a large extent the degree of subsequent activity in the inferior frontal gyrus (Simos, Rezaie, Fletcher, & Papanicolaou, 2013).

18.3. DEVELOPMENT OF BRAIN CIRCUITS FOR READING

In the earliest cross-sectional study, age-related changes in spatiotemporal brain activation profiles associated with printed word recognition and phonological decoding (pseudoword reading) were examined in 27 adults and 22 children without reading problems (Simos et al., 2001). Adults showed a distinct spatiotemporal profile during reading of both types of print, consisting of bilateral activation of occipital

cortices, followed by strongly left-predominant activation of basal temporal regions and, finally, left hemisphere temporoparietal (including the angular gyrus) and inferior frontal activation. Children lacked the clear temporal distinction in the engagement of basal and temporoparietal areas and displayed significantly weaker activation of the left inferior frontal gyrus. In addition, the consistent hemispheric asymmetries in the degree of activation of basal temporal areas that were present in the adult readers were not apparent in the children. In contrast, the strong left hemisphere preponderance in the degree of activation of temporoparietal areas was present in children as well as adults, regardless of the type of print they were asked to read. The data suggest that the degree of specialization of cortical regions for reading, as well as the pattern of regional interactions that supports this specialization, may change with age.

Activity in occipitotemporal and temporoparietal cortices during performance of a visual detection tasks involving letter strings and symbol strings embedded in varying levels of visual names was recorded in 18 typical readers who were 7- to 8 years old (Parviainen, Helenius, Poskiparta, Niemi, & Salmelin, 2006). In agreement with Simos et al. (2001), the occipitotemporal response to letter strings was strongly left-lateralized and significantly delayed compared with the adult readers, although the temporal distinction between the peaks of the occipitotemporal and posterior temporal responses was preserved in this task.

In a subsequent longitudinal study of 17 kindergarten students who showed typical acquisition of reading skills in grade 1, the brain mechanism that supports phonological decoding appeared to be rather stable during the initial stages of reading acquisition (Simos et al., 2005). There were no apparent changes in the degree (or total duration) of activity in regions that constitute major components of the reading circuit for either group of nonimpaired readers. The most notable developmental changes were those concerning the *temporal* features of the brain mechanism for reading featuring a reduction in the onset latency of activity in occipitotemporal regions and a corresponding increase in the onset latency in inferior frontal regions. The former change can probably be viewed as reflecting increased "efficiency" of the ventral component of the reading mechanism with reading experience. The latter change could reflect the declining role of neurophysiological processes hosted by inferior frontal cortices. This change is consistent with reports of unusually early frontal activity in adults with persisting reading disability (Salmelin et al., 1996).

18.4. ABERRANT PATTERNS OF BRAIN ACTIVITY ASSOCIATED WITH READING DIFFICULTIES AND DYSLEXIA

MEG studies on impaired reading function have been conducted with children who had been either diagnosed with reading disability (RD; dyslexia) or presented with significant underperformance on standardized reading tests, as well as with adults who had a history of reading difficulties.

The earliest MEG study of reading compared activation profiles of six adults with a childhood diagnosis of reading disability with those of eight fluent adult readers performing silent reading of various types of print (real concrete and abstract words, pronounceable and unpronounceable nonwords; Salmelin et al., 1996). Results indicated significantly attenuated neuromagnetic activity in the former group in the left occipitotemporal and posterior temporal regions (middle and superior temporal gyri) across stimulus types. Using a similar source reconstruction method (relying on single, successive ECDs) and a task involving silent reading of words embedded in various levels of visual noise in adults with a childhood diagnosis of reading disability, the early occipitotemporal response was absent in the majority of cases (eight of 10 participants; Helenius, Tarkiainen, Cornelissen, Hansen,

& Salmelin, 1999). Moreover, the response peaking at approximately 300 ms in the left superior temporal gyrus was present in eight of 12 fluent readers but in only five of 10 of the participants with RD.

Studies with school-aged children have revealed clear functional differences between typical and RD readers with regard to several components of the brain mechanism for reading. Based on results obtained using the single equivalent current dipole model, the most prominent finding in RD children is reduced activation of the left superior temporal and inferior parietal cortices, especially in tasks in which phonological processing demands are high (Simos, Breier, Fletcher, Bergman, & Papanicolaou, 2000b; Simos et al., 2000c, 2002a). Evidence for reduced engagement of additional components of the brain mechanism, which normally supports reading, is also found, albeit less consistently in RD children. These include the angular gyrus and the ventral occipitotemporal region (Simos et al., 2007a).

Reduced activity in left hemisphere circuits for reading is typically accompanied by increased activity in brain areas that are not typically indispensable components of the reading mechanism, namely right temporoparietal regions and the inferior frontal gyrus bilaterally. Although frontal activity is observed in typical readers as well, it can be distinguished from the activity that is typically found in RD readers because it is disproportionate in magnitude to the (already reduced) activation in temporoparietal regions and occurs much earlier during stimulus processing than in non-reading impaired (NI) readers (Simos et al., 2007a, 2007b). The aberrant profile of brain activation associated with decoding is detectable as early as the end of kindergarten in children who have not reached important milestones in learning to read (Simos et al., 2005).

Further insight into the organization of the neural circuits underlying reading ability has been gained through more recent MEG studies of NI and RD students, with emphasis on the adoption of distributed source modeling techniques (MNE), adequate sample diversity (in terms of socioeconomic status, general intelligence, and attention-deficit/hyperactivity disorder comorbidity), and modifications in task demands. For example, a recent study (Rezaie et al., 2011a) included a large, representative sample of typical (*n* = 40) and struggling readers (*n* = 44) matched on age, gender, ethnic background, and general cognitive ability. MEG recordings were obtained during a continuous visual word recognition task (involving silent reading). Relative to the strong lateralized differences reported in earlier MEG studies, findings from this larger scale investigation found that children with RD showed decreased degree of neurophysiological activity in the posterior temporal lobe regions (superior and middle temporal gyri) bilaterally, during late phases of word reading (Figure 18.1).

Moreover, while a previously reported bilateral increase in activation of the prefrontal cortex was replicated in this larger and more diverse sample, we also detected overactivation of the mesial and ventral occipitotemporal regions in the RD group. Increased activation in ventral occipitotemporal cortices could be associated with the need to maintain orthographic representations of target words throughout task performance, reflecting greater reliance on a visual/orthographic strategy for encoding and recognition of the printed word stimuli. Importantly, the degree of activity in left posterior temporal regions was a significant positive predictor of reading and spelling skill among NI readers, but this relation was absent in RD children. Instead, this group displayed a significant negative association between degree of activity in right hemisphere homologous areas and prefrontal regions, and achievement scores. When participants from the same cohort were engaged in tasks varying on explicit phonological decoding demands (letter-naming and pseudoword reading), children with RD exhibited markedly reduced activation in the left inferior parietal region (supramarginal and angular gyri), relative to the NI readers (Simos et al., 2011a). These effects were restricted to the more demanding pseudoword reading task and were more prominent during late stages of stimulus processing. Activity–performance

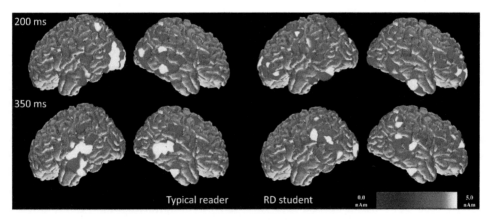

FIGURE 18.1   Brain activation snapshots associated with printed word processing and recognition in two representative elementary school students: a typically achieving (*left-hand set of images*) and an RD student (*right-hand set of images*). Images in the *top row* were obtained near the peak of activity in the left ventral occipitotemporal cortex (at 200 ms), and in the posterior temporal cortices (superior and middle temporal gyrus at 350 ms) in the *lower row*. (Data adapted from Rezaie, R., Simos, P. G., Fletcher, J. M., Juranek, J., Cirino, P., Li, Z., Passaro, A. D., & Papanicolaou, A. C. [2011]. The timing and strength of regional brain activation associated with word recognition in children with reading difficulties. *Frontiers in Behavioral Neuroscience, 5*[45], 1–12.)

correlational analyses revealed that good decoding ability was predicted by high levels of neurophysiological activity in *left* hemisphere superior temporal, inferior parietal, inferior frontal, and ventral occipitotemporal regions. In sharp contrast, high levels of activity in *right* hemisphere homologous regions appeared to be detrimental to decoding ability among RD individuals. Interestingly, underactivation of the temporoparietal cortex (supramarginal gyrus [SMG]) bilaterally has been found in RD students performing a silent passage reading tasks (i.e., when phonological decoding demands were minimized; Simos, Rezaie, Fletcher, Juranek, & Papanicolaou, 2011b).

18.5. CHANGES IN BRAIN ACTIVITY ASSOCIATED WITH READING INTERVENTIONS

If the left occipitotemporal and temporoparietal regions play a key role in normal reading acquisition, and atypical engagement of these regions accounts, at least in part, for pervasive reading difficulties in the majority of RD cases, one would predict that successful remedial instruction would affect the timing and/or degree of activation. This issue has been examined in several MEG studies.

In the earliest study (Simos et al., 2002a), eight children with very severe reading difficulties underwent a brief but intensive remediation program, focusing on the development of phonological awareness and decoding skills. The intervention was performed on a one-to-one basis for 2 months (approximately 80 hours of instruction). The most salient change observed on a case-by-case basis was a several-fold increase in the apparent engagement of the left temporoparietal region, accompanied by a moderate reduction in the activation of the right temporoparietal area. Although results confirmed the prediction regarding the critical role of left temporoparietal cortices in acquiring adequate decoding skills in RD, the

relatively small surface–spatial sampling capacity of the neuromagnetometer used the study, in conjunction with the limitations of the ECD model of magnetic source localization, precluded a more thorough evaluation of intervention-related changes in additional components of the reading mechanism.

These initial findings were extended to a larger group of 15 children who showed severe difficulties in reading despite adequate exposure to the alphabetic principle in the regular classroom (Simos et al., 2007a). In this study, brain activation profiles were obtained with a higher density neuromagnetometer that afforded greater sensitivity for detecting less prominent activity sources (such as those in the angular gyrus and inferior frontal cortex). MEG scans were registered during performance of an oral reading task involving three-letter pseudowords (i.e., KAK), placing explicit demands for phonological decoding. Each participant was assessed three times: (a) baseline, (b) following completion of an 8-week small-group remedial program focusing on the development of phonological awareness and decoding skills (Phono-Graphix administered for 2 hours daily; McGuinness, McGuinness, & McGuinness, 1996), and (c) at the end of a subsequent 8-week program targeting reading fluency (based on the Read Naturally program; Ihnot, Mastoff, Gavin, & Hendrickson, 2001) administered for 1 hour each day of the week. Baseline scores on standardized reading tests showed group mean performance that was at least 1 standard deviation below average on measures of word and pseudoword reading accuracy and efficiency. At baseline, participants showed brain activation profiles typical of RD children, consisting of early activity in occipitotemporal regions, followed by activity in bilateral dorsolateral prefrontal and premotor regions. Activity in temporoparietal regions was noted much later (typically between 500 and 700 ms after stimulus onset), which either lasted longer in the right hemisphere or was bilaterally symmetric in duration (or degree). The 16-week intervention resulted in significant improvement in word recognition and decoding, fluency, and comprehension for eight children ("adequate responders"), demonstrating a mean improvement on the Basic Reading Composite of 15 ± 3 points (range: 11–19.5 points). The remaining seven students demonstrated smaller gains (4 ± 3 points on average: "inadequate responders"). Brain activation profiles of inadequate responders were essentially identical to those obtained at baseline. For adequate responders, postintervention results were consistent with both normalizing and compensatory changes in the brain activation profiles. Normalizing changes consisted of an increase in the degree of activity in left temporoparietal regions, a parallel reduction in the onset latency of activity in the same region, and an increase in the onset latency of activity in inferior frontal regions. Following these latency changes, the relative timing of activity in the left temporoparietal area and inferior frontal cortex became similar to that observed in NI readers. Compensatory changes, consisting of smaller scale increases in right superior temporal and bilateral inferior frontal activity, were observed less consistently across participants (in 30 and 60% of cases, respectively).

Spatiotemporal profiles from the same group of participants during an externally paced word reading task (Simos et al., 2007b) were also obtained at each of the three testing sessions described previously. The stimuli were high-frequency words of the sort that most students are regularly exposed as sight words. At baseline, the spatiotemporal profiles of activity preceding the pronunciation of sight words featured, again, early activation of occipitotemporal regions followed by prominent activity in the right middle temporal gyrus and dorsolateral prefrontal and premotor cortices, bilaterally. Activity was observed last in the superior temporal gyrus bilaterally and in the left middle temporal gyrus. Because our word-reading task did not make significant demands on phonological decoding, increased relative activation of the middle temporal gyrus

compared with the superior temporal and supramarginal gyri was expected (Damasio & Damasio, 1989; Fiebach, Friederici, Muller, & von Cramon, 2002; Hagoort et al., 1999; Roux et al., 2004; Simos et al., 2002b, 2009; Turkeltaub, Eden, Jones, & Zeffiro, 2002). Significant changes in the duration and relative timing of regional activity following intervention consisted of (a) increased degree (or total duration) of neurophysiological activity in the posterior portion of the middle temporal gyrus bilaterally, (b) decreased onset latency of activity in the left middle temporal gyrus and in the right occipitotemporal region, and (c) increased onset latency of activity in dorsolateral prefrontal and premotor regions. The combined changes in frontal and temporal lobe onset latencies resulted in activation profiles resembling those typically found in average readers. It is of particular interest that systematic individual variability in the duration and onset of activity in brain regions "normally" involved in the circuit for reading was again a positive predictor of reading accuracy measures: the greater the duration of neurophysiological activity in the posterior portion of the middle temporal gyrus in the left hemisphere and the earlier the onset of activity in visual association areas, the higher the reading performance following intervention. Conversely, earlier onset of activity in "compensatory" components of the brain circuit for reading (inferior frontal regions) was associated with lower the performance on these measures. The aforementioned results are in general agreement with fMRI findings (Eden et al., 2004; Meyler, Keller, Cherkassky, Gabrieli, & Just, 2008; Shaywitz et al., 2004; Temple et al., 2003) showing that completion of an intensive instruction program focusing on the development of phonological awareness and decoding skills was accompanied by increased neurophysiological activity in temporoparietal cortices in the left hemisphere. Importantly, results provided additional support to the crucial role of left temporoparietal regions in reading acquisition by showing that increased activity in this area accompanies successful remediation of RD. Increased activity in other areas following such training are sometimes observed, but do not appear to be sufficient to support the development of an effective brain mechanism capable of supporting skilled reading. Another important conclusion that stems from recent MEG studies on reading and RD is that the precise nature of aberrant features of the activation profile in RD depends to a certain extent on specific task demands.

Further studies addressed possible differences in brains of children who respond adequately and inadequately to reading interventions, in view of preliminary fMRI evidence of higher, preintervention activation in the left inferior parietal region for responders compared with nonresponders (Odegard, Ring, Smith, Biggan, & Black, 2008). To address this issue, neuromagnetic activity was recorded from 27 students in grades 6 and 7 experiencing reading difficulties during performance of a pseudoword-naming task (Rezaie et al., 2011b). Students were subsequently enrolled in small-group school-based reading remediation programs focusing on word-level skills and were classified as adequate responders (n = 16) if they showed significant gains in word-level reading skills after 6 to 8 months of intervention and as inadequate responders if they did not show such gains. Neurophysiological activity was modeled by a distributed source estimation algorithm (MNE). Adequate responders' activation profiles featured increased activity in several posterior temporal, inferior parietal, occipitotemporal, and anterior frontal regions compared with inadequate responders. Importantly, the degree of activity in temporoparietal regions accounted for a substantial portion of variability (50%) in postintervention improvement on reading fluency scores, mainly among adequate responders. In the same cohort of students, a neuromagnetic predictor of intervention gains, obtained during performance of a silent word-recognition task, was increased degree of activity in the middle temporal gyrus and ventral occipitotemporal cortex in the left hemisphere (Rezaie et al., 2011c; Figure 18.2).

18.6. CONCLUSIONS, LIMITATIONS, AND FUTURE DIRECTIONS

As a functional brain mapping technique, MEG represents a viable alternative to neuroimaging methods that rely on hemodynamic correlates of brain activity for the purposes of outlining the spatial and temporal characteristics of cerebral mechanisms that mediate mature and developing reading skills, and as such are potentially involved in the pathophysiology of reading disability and may mediate the behavioral effects of educational interventions.

MEG is a technique that holds great value for developmental neuroscience. Brain function in children as young as 5 years can be studied reliably with MEG, yielding results of both theoretical and practical significance. The sensitivity of MEG to both developmental and intervention-related changes in brain function highlights its potential to be used, along with cognitive assessments, to determine which children may be at greatest risk for reading impairment later in development, and who may benefit most from remediation.

As a complementary method to hemodynamic imaging, however, MEG has certain limitations, including the indeterminacy of the inverse problem and the related difficulty in applying voxel-based analyses on source-reconstructed data. It should also be noted that with very few exceptions MEG studies on reading have employed single-word tasks; therefore, reading words in context has not been investigated properly.

Future investigations should examine additional factors that may influence response to intervention. These studies should involve larger samples of children that better represent the skill profiles and possible etiologies suspected in the population of children with reading problems. Another issue that deserves closer scrutiny concerns the type of intervention (in

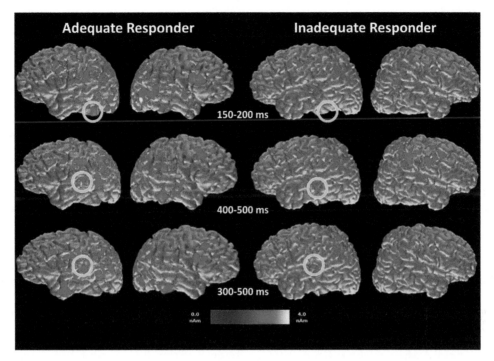

FIGURE 18.2   Preintervention brain activation snapshots associated with printed word processing and recognition in two representative elementary school students: a student who later showed significant progress in word-level reading skills in response to intervention ("adequate responder"), and a student who demonstrated minimal progress ("inadequate responder"). Significant group differences were found in the left occipitotemporal cortex (150–250 ms), the left middle temporal gyrus (400–500 ms), and the left superior temporal gyrus (300–500 ms) after the onset of the printed words. (Data adapted from Rezaie, R., Simos, P. G., Fletcher, J. M., Cirino, P., Vaughn, S., & Papanicolaou, A. C. [2011]. Engagement of temporal lobe regions predicts response to educational interventions in adolescent struggling readers. *Developmental Neuropsychology, 36,* 869–888.)

terms of intensity, duration, and content) associated with permanent changes in brain activation profiles capable of sustaining lasting and clinically significant improvement in reading performance.

REFERENCES

Coltheart, M., Rastle, K., Perry, C., Langdon, R., & Ziegler, J. (2001). DRC: A dual route cascaded model of visual word recognition and reading aloud. *Psychological Review, 108*(1), 204–256.

Cornelissen, P. L., Kringelbach, M. L., Ellis, A. W., Whitney, C., Holliday, I. E., & Hansen, P. C. (2009). Activation of the left inferior frontal gyrus in the first 200 ms of reading: Evidence from magnetoencephalography (MEG). *PLoS One, 4*(4), e5359.

Cornelissen, P., Tarkiainen, A., Helenius, P., & Salmelin, R. (2003). Cortical effects of shifting letter position in letter strings of varying length. *Journal of Cognitive Neuroscience, 15,* 731–746.

Damasio, H., & Damasio, A. (1989). *Lesion analysis in neuropsychology.* New York, NY: Oxford University Press.

Denton, C. A., Fletcher, J. M., Simos, P. G., Papanicolaou, A. C., & Anthony, J. (2007). An implementation of a tiered intervention model: Reading outcomes and neural correlates. In D. Haager, S. Vaughn, & J. K. Klingner (Eds.), *Validated reading practices for three tiers of intervention.* Baltimore, MD: Paul H. Brookes.

Eden, G. F., Jones, K. M., Cappell, K., Gareau, L., Wood, F. B., Zeffiro, T. A., … Flowers, D. L. (2004). Neural changes following remediation in adult developmental dyslexia. *Neuron, 44*(3), 411–422.

Fiebach, C. J., Friederici, A. D., Muller, K., & von Cramon, D. Y. (2002). fMRI evidence for dual routes to the mental lexicon in visual word recognition. *Journal of Cognitive Neuroscience, 14*(1), 11–23.

Fletcher, J. M., Lyon, G. R., Fuchs, L. S., & Barnes, M. A. (2007). *Learning disabilities: From identification to intervention.* New York, NY: The Guildford Press.

Hagoort, P., Indefrey, P., Brown, C., Herzog, H., Steinmetz, H., & Seitz, R. J. (1999). The neural circuitry involved in the reading of German words and pseudowords: A PET study. *Journal of Cognitive Neuroscience, 11*, 383–398.

Helenius, P., Salmelin, R., Service, E., & Connolly, J. F. (1998). Distinct time courses of word and context comprehension in the left temporal cortex. *Brain, 121*, 1133–1142.

Helenius, P., Tarkiainen, A., Cornelissen, P., Hansen, P. C., & Salmelin, R (1999). Dissociation of normal feature analysis and deficient processing of letter strings in dyslexic adults. *Cerebral Cortex, 9*, 476–483.

Horwitz, B., Rumsey, J. M., & Donohue, B. C. (1998). Functional connectivity of the angular gyrus in normal reading and dyslexia. *Proceedings of the National Academy of Sciences U S A, 95*(15), 8939–8944.

Ihnot, C., Mastoff, J., Gavin, J., & Hendrickson, L. (2001). *Read naturally.* St. Paul, MN: Read Naturally.

Joubert, S., Beauregard, M., Walter, N., Bourgouin, P., Beaudoin, G., Leroux, J. M., . . . Lecours, A. R. (2004). Neural correlates of lexical and sublexical processes in reading. *Brain & Language, 89*(1), 9–20.

Kujala, J., Pammer, K., Cornelissen, P., Roebroeck, A., Formisano, E., & Salmelin, R. (2007). Phase coupling in a cerebro-cerebellar network at 8-13 Hz during reading. *Cerebral Cortex, 17*(6), 1476–1485.

Kutas, M., & Hillyard, S. A. (1980). Reading senseless sentences: Brain potentials reflect semantic incongruity. *Science, 207*, 203–205.

McGuinness, C., McGuinness, D., & McGuinness, G. (1996). Phono-Graphix: A new method for remediation reading difficulties. *Annals of Dyslexia, 46*, 73–96.

Meyler, A., Keller, T. A., Cherkassky, V. L., Gabrieli, J. D., & Just, M. A. (2008). Modifying the brain activation of poor readers during sentence comprehension with extended remedial instruction: A longitudinal study of neuroplasticity. *Neuropsychologia, 46*(10), 2580–2592.

Odegard, T. N., Ring, J., Smith, S., Biggan, J., & Black, J. (2008). Differentiating the neural response to intervention in children with developmental dyslexia. *Annals of Dyslexia, 58*, 1–14.

Parviainen, T., Helenius, P., Poskiparta, E., Niemi, P., & Salmelin, R. (2006). Cortical sequence of word perception in beginning readers. *Journal of Neuroscience, 26*(22), 6052–6061.

Pugh, K. R., Mencl, W. E., Jenner, A. R., Katz, L., Frost, S. J., Lee, J. R., . . . Shaywitz, B. A. (2000). Functional neuroimaging studies of reading and reading disability (developmental dyslexia). *Mental Retardation and Developmental Disabilities Research Reviews, 6*(3), 207–213.

Rezaie, R., Simos, P. G., Fletcher, J. M., Cirino, P., Vaughn, S., & Papanicolaou, A. C. (2011c). Engagement of temporal lobe regions predicts response to educational interventions in adolescent struggling readers. *Developmental Neuropsychology, 36*, 869–888.

Rezaie, R., Simos, P. G., Fletcher, J. M., Cirino, P., Vaughn, S., & Papanicolaou, A. C. (2011b). Temporo-parietal brain activity as a longitudinal predictor of response to educational interventions among middle school struggling readers. *Journal of the International Neuropsychological Society, 17*, 875–885.

Rezaie, R., Simos, P. G., Fletcher, J. M., Juranek, J., Cirino, P., Li, Z., Passaro, A. D., & Papanicolaou, A. C. (2011a). The timing and strength of regional brain activation associated with word recognition in children with reading difficulties. *Frontiers in Behavioral Neuroscience, 5*(45), 1–12.

Roux, F. E., Lubrano, V., Lauwers-Cances, V., Tremoulet, M., Mascott, C. R., & Demonet, J. F. (2004). Intra-operative mapping of cortical areas involved in reading in mono- and bilingual patients. *Brain, 127*(Pt 8), 1796–1810.

Salmelin, R., Service, E., Kiesila, P., Uutela, K., & Salonen, O. (1996). Impaired visual word processing in dyslexia revealed with magnetoencephalography. *Annals of Neurology, 40*, 157–162.

Seghier, M. L., & Price, C. J. (2018). Interpreting and utilising intersubject variability in brain function. *Trends in Cognitive Science, 22*(6), 517–530.

Service, E., Helenius, P., Maury, S., & Salmelin, R. (2007). Localization of syntactic and semantic brain responses using magnetoencephalography. *Journal of Cognitive Neuroscience, 19*(7), 1193–1205.

Shaywitz, B. A., Shaywitz, S. E., Blachman, B. A., Pugh, K. R., Fulbright, R. K., Skudlarski, P., . . . Gore, J. C. (2004). Development of left occipitotemporal systems for skilled reading in children after a phonologically- based intervention. *Biological Psychiatry, 55*(9), 926–933.

Simos, P. G., Basile, L. F. H., & Papanicolaou, A. C. (1997). Source localization of the N400 response in a sentence-reading paradigm using evoked magnetic fields and magnetic resonance imaging. *Brain Research, 762,* 29–39.

Simos, P. G., Breier, J. I., Fletcher, J. M., Bergman, E., & Papanicolaou, A. C. (2000b). Cerebral mechanisms involved in word reading in dyslexic children: A magnetic source imaging approach. *Cerebral Cortex, 10*(8), 809–816.

Simos, P. G., Breier, J. I., Fletcher, J. M., Foorman, B. R., Bergman, E., Fishbeck, K., & Papanicolaou, A. C. (2000c). Brain activation profiles in dyslexic children during non-word reading: A magnetic source imaging study. *Neuroscience Letters, 290*(1), 61–65.

Simos, P. G., Breier, J. I., Fletcher, J. M., Foorman, B. R., Mouzaki, A., & Papanicolaou, A. C. (2001). Age-related changes in regional brain activation during phonological decoding and printed word recognition. *Developmental Neuropsychology, 19*(2), 191–210.

Simos, P. G., Breier, J. I., Fletcher, J. M., Foorman, B. R., Castillo, E. M., & Papanicolaou, A. C. (2002b). Brain mechanisms for reading words and pseudowords: An integrated approach. *Cerebral Cortex, 12*(3), 297–305.

Simos, P. G., Breier, J. I., Wheless, J. W., Maggio, W. W., Fletcher, J. M., Castillo, E. M., & Papanicolaou, A. C. (2000a). Brain mechanisms for reading: The role of the superior temporal gyrus in word and pseudoword naming. *Neuroreport, 11*(11), 2443–2447.

Simos, P. G., Fletcher, J. M., Bergman, E., Breier, J. I., Foorman, B. R., Castillo, E. M., & Papanicolaou, A. C. (2002a). Dyslexia-specific brain activation profile becomes normal following successful remedial training. *Neurology, 58*(8), 1203–1213.

Simos, P. G., Fletcher, J. M., Sarkari, S., Billingsley, R. L., Francis, D. J., Castillo, E. M., . . . Papanicolaou, A. C. (2005). Early development of neurophysiological processes involved in normal reading and reading disability: A magnetic source imaging study. *Neuropsychology, 19*(6), 787–798.

Simos, P. G., Fletcher, J. M., Sarkari, S., Billingsley, R. L., Denton, C., & Papanicolaou, A. C. (2007a). Altering the brain circuits for reading through intervention: A magnetic source imaging study. *Neuropsychology, 21*(4), 485–496.

Simos, P. G., Fletcher, J. M., Sarkari, S., Billingsley-Marshall, R., Denton, C. A., & Papanicolaou, A. C. (2007b). Intensive instruction affects brain magnetic activity associated with oral word reading in children with persistent reading disabilities. *Journal of Learning Disabilities, 40*(1), 37–48.

Simos, P. G., Pugh, K., Mencl, E., Frost, S., Fletcher, J. M., Sarkari, S., & Papanicolaou, A. C. (2009). Temporal course of word recognition in skilled readers: A magnetoencephalography study. *Behavior Brain Research, 197*(1), 45–54.

Simos, P. G., Rezaie, R., Fletcher, J. M., Juranek, J., Passaro, A. D., Li, Z., Cirino, P., & Papanicolaou, A. C. (2011a). Functional disruption of the brain mechanism for reading: Effects of comorbidity and task difficulty among children with developmental learning problems. *Neuropsychology, 24,* 520–534.

Simos, P. G., Rezaie, R., Fletcher, J. M., Juranek, J., & Papanicolaou, A. C. (2011b). Neural correlates of sentence reading in children with reading difficulties. *Neuroreport, 22,* 674–678.

Simos, P. G., Rezaie, R., Fletcher, J. M., & Papanicolaou, A. C. (2013). Time-constrained functional connectivity analysis of cortical networks underlying phonological decoding in typically developing school-aged children: A magnetoencephalography study. *Brain & Language, 125,* 156–164.

Tarkiainen, A., Helenius, P., Hansen, P. C., Cornelissen, P. L., & Salmelin, R. (1999). Dynamics of letter string perception in the human occipitotemporal cortex. *Brain, 122,* 2119–2132.

Temple, E., Deutsch, G. K., Poldrack, R. A., Miller, S. L., Tallal, P., Merzenich, M. M., & Gabrieli, J. D. E. (2003). Neural deficits in children with dyslexia ameliorated by behavioral remediation: Evidence from functional MRI. *Proceedings of the National Academy of Science U S A, 100*(5), 2860–2865.

Torgesen, J. K., Alexander, A. W., Wagner, R. K., Rashotte, C. A., Voeller, K. K., & Conway, T. (2001). Intensive remedial instruction for children with severe reading disabilities: Immediate and long-term outcomes from two instructional approaches. *Journal of Learning Disabilities, 34,* 33–58.

Turkeltaub, P. E., Eden, G. F., Jones, K. M., & Zeffiro, T. A. (2002). Meta-analysis of the functional neuroanatomy of single-word reading: Method and validation. *Neuroimage, 16,* 765–780.

Van Horn, J. D., Grafton, S. T., & Miller, M. B. (2008). Individual variability in brain activity: A nuisance or an opportunity? *Brain Imaging & Behavior, 2,* 327–334.

Vartiainen, J., Parviainen, T., & Salmelin, R. (2009). Spatiotemporal convergence of semantic processing in reading and speech perception. *Journal of Neuroscience, 29,* 9271–9280.

19

DECODING COGNITIVE FUNCTION WITH MAGNETOENCEPHALOGRAPHY

Dimitrios Pantazis

19.1. DECODING PATTERNS IN NEUROIMAGING

Multivariate methods enable us to study content-based processing in the human brain through pattern-based analysis of neuronal data. That is, we can establish a direct link between mental representations and the corresponding multivariate activity patterns. We can decode considerable information about mental states from noninvasive measures of human brain activity. We can reveal what the person is seeing, perceiving, and remembering (Tong & Pratte, 2012). We can investigate how the brain encodes complex visual scenes or abstract semantic information.

Multivariate methods are now replacing univariate methods in many research areas, in part owing to the higher sensitivity afforded by these techniques (Hebart & Baker, 2018). Traditional *univariate* methods in neuroimaging

treat each variable as an independent piece of data, using statistical tests to determine whether, for example, a single MEG sensor or a single source voxel responds more under one experimental condition compared with another (Friston et al., 1994; Pantazis & Leahy, 2010). When exploring effects in hundreds of MEG sensors or tens of thousands of source voxels, the typical analysis strategy becomes marginal or "massively univariate," involving a large number of univariate statistical tests where data for each variable are independently fit to the same model (Luo & Nichols, 2003). By contrast, *multivariate* methods extract the information contained in distributed patterns of activity across multiple variables (Cichy & Pantazis, 2017; Haynes, 2015). Multivariate analyses are designed to test whether two (or more) experimental conditions can be distinguished from each other on the basis of activity

Dimitrios Pantazis, *Decoding Cognitive Function With Magnetoencephalography* In: *Fifty Years of Magnetoencephalography*. Edited by: Andrew C. Papanicolaou, Timothy P. L. Roberts, and James W. Wheless, Oxford University Press (2020). © Oxford University Press.
DOI: 10.1093/oso/9780190935689.003.0019.

patterns observed in a set of measurement variables (Tong & Pratte, 2012). A multivariate (as opposed to mass-univariate) framework is able to characterize the full information contained in distributed neuronal patterns.

In computational neuroscience, the analysis of multivariate data almost exclusively relies on the use of models called *classifiers*. Thus, in this chapter we interchangeably use the terms *multivariate methods, multivariate pattern analysis, multivariate classification,* and *multivariate decoding* to refer to methods that apply classifiers to multivariate data.

19.1.1. The Motivation Behind Using Multivariate Methods

The motivation behind the use of multivariate methods in neuroscience is based on a mathematically well-formulated theory, neural population coding (Averbeck, Latham, & Pouget, 2006). According to population coding, information about the outside world and plans for motor action are represented in the brain by the joint activation patterns of distributed groups of neurons. Thus, to reliably distinguish between different behaviorally relevant conditions that are present in the world, we should build a model that samples and analyzes patterns of activity from distributed neuronal populations (Meyers & Kreiman, 2011).

Cross-validation is an excellent approach for assessing the reliability of such a model. We train the model, such as a support vector machine (SVM) (Duda, Hart, & Stork, 2000) or linear discriminant analysis (LDA) classifier (Fisher, 1936), to discriminate between experimental conditions using only part of the data, the *training data*. The remaining data, constituting the *test data*, are left out and used to validate whether the model has indeed learned to discriminate between experimental conditions. This is repeated across different splits of training and testing data, and the performance is quantified in the form of *classification accuracy* (decoding accuracy), which is the fraction of correctly classified test data (Allefeld & Haynes, 2014). Such a cross-validation procedure affords strong inferences. First, by training the model using a subset of the data, then showing that it performs well in held-out data, we obtain a high degree of confidence that neural activity can reliably distinguish between conditions (Meyers & Kreiman, 2011). Second, we demonstrate that our model can successfully capture this neuronal information. Third, if we show that the same model can generalize to a different but related set of conditions, we can infer that the brain represents information in a way that is invariant to the exact set of conditions used to build the model. And fourth, the type and format of information that can be captured by the model can provide insight into what is represented in the brain.

19.1.2. Spatial Scale of Decodable Information

The theory of neural population coding postulates that populations of neurons jointly encode information about the outside world, and thus directly motivates multivariate methods in cell recordings. However, the precise basis of why multivariate techniques also work for macroscopic measurements is less clear and, in fact, has been a topic of a longstanding debate ever since two seminal studies showed that the orientation of a grating stimulus can be reliably decoded from functional magnetic resonance imaging (fMRI) activation patterns (Haynes & Rees, 2005; Kamitani & Tong, 2005). These findings were significant because different orientations are not represented in distant brain areas, but rather within narrow cortical columns of about 800 μm in diameter each (Yacoub, Harel, & Ugurbil, 2008). If fMRI can decode information from such fine spatial scales, then perhaps it is also sensitive to other neuronal signals at submillimeter scales, and may even provide informational content comparable to single-unit recordings in nonhuman primates (Stokes, Wolff, & Spaak, 2015).

With the spatial scale of orientation cortical columns much smaller than the 3-mm wide fMRI voxels, how can fMRI capture these patterns? While there are a number of possible confounds (Alink, Krugliak, Walther, & Kriegeskorte, 2013; T. Carlson, Tovar, & Kriegeskorte, 2013; Cichy, Ramirez, & Pantazis, 2015; Sasaki et al., 2006), a prevailing explanation in the fMRI community has been the biased sampling account, which states that random local variations in cortical organization may lead to weak orientation biases in individual fMRI voxels (Kamitani & Tong, 2005; Kriegeskorte, Cusack, & Bandettini, 2010). For example, some voxels may sample more cells coding for horizontal orientations, whereas others may sample more cells coding for vertical orientations. As a result, individual voxels may activate more strongly for preferred orientations, depending on the distribution of cells with different tuning properties within the voxel. Although such biases may be weak at single voxels, by pooling the information available from many independent voxels, a pattern classifier may robustly differentiate the activation patterns of different stimulus orientations (Tong & Pratte, 2012).

More recently, it was shown that orientation information can also be decoded from magnetoencephalography (MEG) and electroencephalography (EEG) using multivariate pattern analysis (Cichy et al., 2015; Ramkumar, Jas, Pannasch, Hari, & Parkkonen, 2013; Wolff, Ding, Myers, & Stokes, 2015). The proposed bases for decoding stimulus orientations in MEG is in some respect analogous to fMRI. That is, MEG can differentiate stimulus orientation due to variable sampling of orientation columns caused by the folding of the cortical manifold, analogous to the way that fMRI variably samples the orientation columns within each voxel (Stokes et al., 2015). In detail, the elemental model sources of MEG signals are current dipoles oriented normally to the cortex, and neighboring current dipoles are too close to be resolved if they are parallel to one another. However, because of the highly convoluted nature of the cortical manifold, neighboring current dipoles are rotated in space, thus producing distinct magnetic fields (Hari et al., 1996). Two activation patterns on cortex that differ on the scale of orientation columns would therefore give rise to different magnetic field topographies outside the head. Orientation information represented on the scale of orientation columns might, as a result, be resolvable with multivariate MEG methods, given the complex folding pattern of cortex. This result has wide implications for the interpretation of studies using MEG multivariate pattern classification, suggesting that any type of information encoded in the human brain at the level of cortical columns may be accessible by MEG (Cichy et al., 2015).

The precise basis for decoding multivariate information in macroscopic fMRI, MEG, and EEG measurements is still under debate, in part because even diligent investigations with empirical data and theoretical modeling cannot conclusively exclude unknown confounding factors (Cichy et al., 2015). Multivariate methods in neuroimaging may be able to access information encoded in fine spatial scales at the level of orientation columns, as the previous studies have argued, or only in much coarser spatial scales. Regardless, the robustness of multivariate techniques in capturing neuronal information from macroscopic activation patterns has been decisively demonstrated in multiple studies (Cichy & Pantazis, 2017; Contini, Wardle, & Carlson, 2017; Haynes & Rees, 2005; Hebart, Bankson, Harel, Baker, & Cichy, 2018; Kamitani & Tong, 2005; J.-R, King, Pescetelli, & Dehaene, 2016; Kriegeskorte, Goebel, & Bandettini, 2006). In MEG, both sensor and source measurements have been shown to contain stimulus information accessible with multivariate techniques (T. Carlson et al., 2013; Cichy, Pantazis, & Oliva, 2014; Cichy et al., 2015; Dobs, Isik, Pantazis, & Kanwisher, 2019; Isik, Meyers, Leibo, & Poggio, 2014; Mohsenzadeh, Mullin, Oliva, & Pantazis, 2019; Pantazis et al., 2018; Ramkumar et al., 2013) (Figure 19.1).

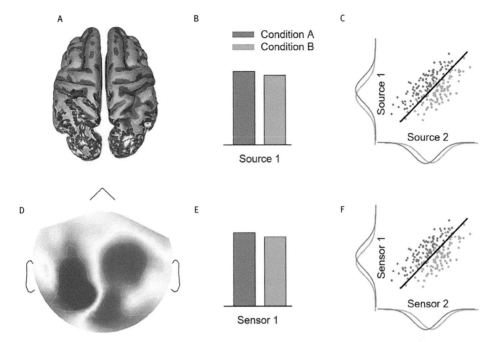

FIGURE 19.1 Multivariate pattern analysis can offer higher sensitivity than univariate analysis in both source and sensor data. (A) A brain activation map reconstructed from magnetoencephalography (MEG) data has highly variable spatial patterns, in part owing to the convoluted nature of the cortical manifold. (B) A hypothetical single source with similar response amplitude in two experimental conditions does a poor job in resolving experimental effects. (C) Two hypothetical sources with correlated responses can jointly separate the two experimental conditions. The scatterplot shows the response amplitude of each source in each experimental condition, with the dividing line indicating a decision threshold estimated by a support vector machine classifier. The density plots in the margins indicate the distribution of responses to the two conditions for each source considered in isolation. (D) Topography of magnetic field with spatially varying patterns. (E and F) Same as parts B and C, but for sensor measurements. MEG sensors yield highly variable spatial patterns that can also discriminate the two conditions.

19.1.3. Activation-Based Versus Information-Based Imaging

Since their introduction, multivariate classification methods have had a transformative influence in cognitive neuroscience. They are now increasingly complementing traditional univariate methods for the analysis of neuroimaging data. The significance of multivariate classification methods becomes clear by the juxtaposition of *activation-based* and *information-based* imaging, adapted from Kriegeskorte and Bandettini (2007). Activation-based imaging typically involves averaging activity across patches of cortex to yield a single measure of overall regional activation, which is then correlated with experimental conditions. By contrast, information-based imaging looks for statistical dependencies between spatial patterns of activity and experimental conditions. What distinguishes the two approaches is whether they are sensitive to spatial patterns of regional brain activity. Information-based imaging measures the information contained in distributed patterns of activity using multivariate tools, whereas activation-brain imaging obscures this information by analyzing spatially averaged patterns using univariate tools. If we accept the population coding dictum that neural representations in the form of distributed patterns of activity are the true information currency in the brain, that is, they play a functional role in the brain based on the information that they carry, then information-based (multivariate) approaches have a distinct advantage over activation-based (univariate) approaches. For example, mean fMRI activity and the evoked response of a single MEG sensor are not signals that the brain itself processes. In contrast, if the brain uses population codes to represent information, then studying spatial patterns of activation implies that we are sensitive to the actual informational content processed by the brain (Ritchie, Kaplan, & Klein, 2019).

19.1.4. Applications of Multivariate Methods in Neuroimaging

Although multivariate methods have been applied before, the pioneering work of Haxby et al. (2001) directly linked multivoxel activation patterns to experimental conditions in fMRI. Using a correlation-based classifier, they showed that activity patterns in the ventral temporal lobe could accurately discriminate between multiple object categories of visual stimuli. A few years later, Kriegeskorte et al. (2006) introduced the *searchlight approach* that performs multivariate analysis using sphere-shaped groups of voxels centered on each brain voxel in iteration. This method has been seen as a mass-multivariate counterpart to the standard mass-univariate analysis in fMRI.

In MEG and EEG, multivariate pattern classification tools have been used for the detection and monitoring of disease (Lehmann et al., 2007; Maestú et al., 2015), for brain computer interfaces (Besserve et al., 2007; Schlögl, Lee, Bischof, & Pfurtscheller, 2005), and for neuroimaging-based lie detection (Matsuda, Nittono, & Allen, 2013; Sugata et al., 2012). In the majority of these applications, the source of information was not necessarily of interest, as long as the prediction was successful in the corresponding application. However, recently there have been a growing number of MEG/EEG studies aiming to interpret and understand brain function. Multivariate pattern classification methods have been used to study simple visual features (T. A. Carlson, Hogendoorn,

Kanai, Mesik, & Turret, 2011; Cichy et al., 2015; Groen, Silson, & Baker, 2017; Pantazis et al., 2018; Ramkumar et al., 2013; Wardle, Kriegeskorte, Grootswagers, Khaligh-Razavi, & Carlson, 2016), complex visual patterns (Barragan-Jason, Cauchoix, & Barbeau, 2015; T. Carlson et al., 2013; Cauchoix, Barragan-Jason, Serre, & Barbeau, 2014; Cichy et al., 2014; Cichy, Pantazis, & Oliva, 2016; Clarke, Devereux, Randall, & Tyler, 2015; Dima, Perry, Messaritaki, Zhang, & Singh, 2018; Grootswagers, Cichy, & Carlson, 2018; Hebart et al., 2018; Isik et al., 2014; Kaneshiro, Perreau Guimaraes, Kim, Norcia, & Suppes, 2015; Mohsenzadeh, Cichy, Oliva, & Pantazis, 2017), auditory representations (J. R. King et al., 2013; J-R. King & Dehaene, 2014; Teng, Sommer, Pantazis, & Oliva, 2017), and temporal maintenance of information and working memory (T. A. Carlson et al., 2011; Cichy et al., 2014; Isik et al., 2014; J-R. King & Dehaene, 2014; Spaak, Watanabe, Funahashi, & Stokes, 2017). Their application in brain disorders is also expected to grow because they can characterize the information contained in distributed MEG neural patterns in both the normal and abnormal brain. Language abnormalities in dyslexia, atypical brain function in autism, and phantom auditory perception in tinnitus are example cases that can be investigated with decoding techniques.

19.2. ANALYSIS OF MAGNETOENCEPHALOGRAPHY SIGNAL PATTERNS

Applying decoding analysis in MEG is conceptually a straightforward idea. Consider the simple case of a visual experiment presenting different image stimuli across several trials. The goal of the experiment is to test whether the MEG activity patterns elicited in response to the different stimuli can be differentiated. We first need to decide the format in which the data create multivariate patterns. The simplest case is to consider the spatial patterns of magnetic fields measured by the MEG sensor array

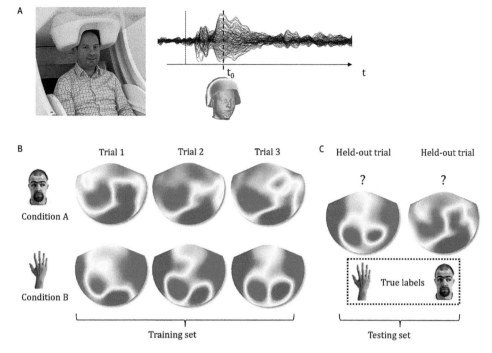

FIGURE 19.2 Conceptual framework of decoding information from magnetoencephalography (MEG) signals. (A) At each time point, the MEG sensors capture a snapshot of patterned brain activity that contains rich information about the underlying neuronal processes. (B) Hypothetical patterns of magnetic fields, at a given time point ($t = t_0$) from stimulus onset, evoked by the presentation of two different images over multiple trials. (C) A human observer trained to separate the two stimuli from the previous patterns has no difficulty in predicting the correct stimulus labels from patterns in new (held out) trials.

at each time point separately (Figure 19.2A). Whenever we present a face image (condition A), it is reasonable to expect similar activation patterns in the sensors, and the same holds true for a hand image (condition B). Figure 19.2B shows such hypothetical patterns over different trials for a given time point t_0 from stimulus onset. These patterns are very robust and consequently can be easily differentiated by a human observer. When new trials become available (held-out trials), the same human observer can correctly infer the true identity of the stimuli that generated these data. The correct label for the first pattern is the hand image, and for the second pattern is the face image (see Figure 19.2C). When all predictions agree with the true labels, classification accuracy is 100%. If, instead, the patterns were extremely noisy, the human observer could only offer random guesses of the image labels, in which case

performance would tend to be at 50% chance level like a coin toss.

The previous paradigm exemplified MEG decoding with a human observer, but analysis proceeds the same way with a machine classifier. We will illustrate with the same hypothetical experiment that measures MEG data while participants view different image stimuli over a number of trials. It is useful to separate multivariate decoding into two distinct steps.

19.2.1. Feature Selection

The first step is *feature selection*, which involves choosing the format of the multivariate patterns that will enter the classifier. MEG data span a multidimensional space comprising spatial, temporal, and possibly spectral dimensions. As a first choice, one may consider it safe to use all available data to generate multivariate patterns, so that the classifier has access to the full information. But this approach suffers from the curse of dimensionality; that is, we have a small number of samples (trials) and a high number of variables (the entire spatio-temporal or spatiotemporal-spectral space), which easily leads to spurious correlations that will inflate the classifier performance. Further, such approach will not inform on how information is encoded in the MEG data across the different dimensions. A better choice is to create multivariate patterns from subsets of data. The most common choice is to perform *time-resolved* decoding, which constructs multivariate patterns for a given time point with respect to the trial onset. In this case, multivariate patterns can be spatial data from whole-head sensor measurements. If the sensor array comprises m sensors, then the measurements are concatenated into a $m \times 1$ pattern vector (Figure 19.3A). If source maps are available, multivariate patterns can be the activity of all sources within a particular region of interest (ROI) in the cortex. In both sensor and ROI cases, multivariate pattern vectors comprise a few hundred variables. The advantage of

time-resolved decoding is that the decoding procedure can be repeated for each time point separately, yielding a decoding time series that describes how the brain processes information over time. When the experimental design includes spectral responses, we can perform *frequency-resolved* decoding, which constructs multivariate patterns for a given frequency point and repeats the decoding procedure over all frequencies to yield a decoding frequency curve. Depending on the experimental design, other approaches may be appropriate, including combined time- and frequency-resolved decoding or constructing multivariate patterns from time and frequency bands. In all cases, the multivariate patterns are arranged into pattern vectors or feature vectors.

19.2.2. Feature Classification

The second step is *feature classification*, which measures the discriminability of multivariate patterns elicited from different experimental conditions. For example, in our hypothetical experiment, we want to determine whether patterns of sensor measurements from different

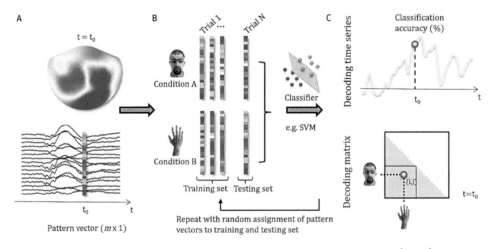

FIGURE 19.3   Time-resolved decoding of information from magnetoencephalography (MEG) sensor patterns using machine classifiers. (A) At a given time point t_0 from stimulus onset, the MEG data are arranged in the form of an $m \times 1$ pattern vector, where m is the number of sensors. (B) Decoding two image stimuli from MEG pattern vectors using a leave-one-out cross-validation procedure with a support vector machine (SVM) classifier. (C) Repeating the entire procedure across all time points results in a decoding time series. Repeating the entire procedure across all pairs of stimuli results in a time-resolved decoding matrix indexed by the different stimuli.

images can be distinguished from one another. The multivariate patterns are assigned labels indicating the condition under which they were acquired. In our hypothetical experiment, the labels are the stimulus images, such as a "face image" or a "hand image." In general, labels can denote properties of sensory stimuli (e.g., the category of an image stimulus), cognitive state (e.g., level of attention), or movement (e.g., direction of hand movement). Classification problems where the labels are known and imposed by the experimenter are referred to as *supervised learning*.

Feature classification proceeds by employing machine learning classifiers, which treat each element in the pattern vector as a separate dimension, or "feature," in a high-dimensional space. The aim of the classifier is to transform this high-dimensional space into a new space where the patterns associated with each condition are separated by a decision boundary. Consider the simple case of patterns based on activity of only two sensors. Each pattern can be thought of as a point on a plane, where the activity of each sensor determines one of the coordinates. One way to classify these patterns is by a line that separates the patterns belonging to condition A from the patterns belonging to condition B. For more than two sensors, the plane becomes a higher dimensional space, and the decision line generalizes to a decision hyperplane (Mur & Kriegeskorte, 2011). Two common classifiers that estimate linear decision boundaries are linear SVMs (Duda et al., 2000) and LDA (Fisher, 1936). They differ in the criterion used to compute the decision hyperplane. SVM maximizes the margin, that is, the distance between the decision hyperplane and the nearest data point on either side. LDA maximizes the between-conditions to within-condition variance. In certain cases, linear decision boundaries may not be sufficient to separate patterns between conditions. Because nonlinear classifiers produce more complicated boundaries, they may improve performance. However, they are prone to overfitting the data and thus do not generalize

well. Because of their complexity, they may also decode information in ways that are not biologically interpretable.

19.2.3. Cross-Validation Procedure

Classification involves separating the data into two disjoint sets: a training set and a testing set (see Figure 19.3B). The training set is used to estimate the classification function (decision boundary), and the testing set is used to evaluate the performance of the classifier. This is commonly done with a *k-fold cross-validation* procedure, which involves splitting the data into k equal-sized subsamples. Training is done on $k - 1$ subsamples, and the remaining single subsample is retained as the validation data for testing the model. The cross-validation process is then repeated k times, with each of the k subsamples used exactly once as the validation data. The k results are then averaged to produce a single estimation of classification accuracy. The advantage of this method over repeated random subsampling is that all observations are used for both training and validation, and each observation is used for validation exactly once. Ten-fold cross-validation is commonly used, but in general k remains an unfixed parameter. When implementing the cross-validation procedure, it is important to guarantee that there is no overlap between the training and the testing set; otherwise, the classifier will overfit and produce spurious results.

Because of the high temporal resolution of MEG, time-resolved decoding is the most common classification approach. We construct multivariate patterns and apply the k-fold cross-validation procedure separately for each time point, yielding a single averaged decoding accuracy for that time point. Repeating the procedure across all time points results in a *decoding time series*. Alternatively, for experiments involving several conditions, we can repeat the procedure across all pairs of conditions. This results in a time-resolved *decoding matrix* indexed by the experimental conditions (see Figure 19.3C). For example, if an experiment involves 92 image stimuli and we conduct all pairwise discriminations between all images, we will obtain a 92 × 92 decoding matrix for each time point (Cichy et al., 2014). Such matrices are useful to study the brain's internal representations and to compare them against hypothetical models or behavioral response matrices using representational similarity analysis (Kriegeskorte, Mur, & Bandettini, 2008).

19.2.4. Statistical Assessment of Decoding Results

At the end of the classification procedure, it is important to assess whether the classifier can extract information from the data above a chance level. In the case of two alternative categories, the chance decoding accuracy is 0.5 (or 50%), and in the case of n categories, it is $1/n$. Because a classifier has some internal variability in decoding accuracies, it is important to test whether a given decoding accuracy is *statistically* above chance. Statistical inference commonly relies on nonparametric permutation tests that have been proved to be valid and have only weak distributional assumptions on the data (Maris & Oostenveld, 2007; Nichols & Holmes, 2002; Pantazis, Nichols, Baillet, & Leahy, 2005). The procedure works by randomly permuting the assignment of labels to the data samples. Under the null hypothesis of no condition-specific experimental effects, the permuted data are statistically equivalent to the original data. We repeat this procedure iteratively to create new instances of the label-permuted data, each time running the full decoding procedure, eventually obtaining the empirical distribution of chance-level decoding accuracy. By comparing the decoding accuracy of the original data to the empirical distribution, we obtain the p value of the decoding accuracy of the original data. When the statistics involve multiple tests, such as decoding time series that include one decoding accuracy per time point, statistical inference must control for multiple comparisons using, for example, false discovery rate (Benjamini & Hochberg, 1995)

or cluster-size inference (Hayasaka, Phan, Liberzon, Worsley, & Nichols, 2004).

If the experiment involves multiple participants, multivariate classification is typically performed separately per participant because multivariate patterns do not align well across participants. In such cases, we obtain one decoding result per participant. For random-effects inference, permutation samples must be generated at the level of participants. This is achieved by subtracting the nominal chance level accuracy from the decoding accuracies and then randomly multiplying the data of each participant with +1 or −1.

19.3. EXAMPLES OF MAGNETOENCEPHALOGRAPHY DECODING

We demonstrate MEG decoding with a simple visual experiment presenting grating stimuli of different orientations (Pantazis et al., 2018). We focus on vision for three reasons. First, the visual system is the most extensively studied part of the brain, and we have a reasonably good understanding of its functional organization. Second, most methodological innovations in multivariate pattern analysis were driven by the field of vision. And third, multivariate decoding was popularized in the field of vision. Our example narrowly focuses on how stimulus orientation information is encoded in MEG brain signals, but the same techniques readily generalize to studies of perception and cognition in brain disorders. Language abnormalities in dyslexia and phantom auditory perception in tinnitus are example cases that can be investigated with decoding techniques.

In our case study, the stimulus set comprised six stationary square-wave Cartesian gratings with orientations 0 to 150 degrees with respect to vertical, in steps of 30 degrees (Figure 19.4A). This enabled the evaluation of brain responses to orientations differing by as little as 30 degrees, thus establishing a measure of sensitivity in disambiguating orientations. It also allowed the comparison of specific

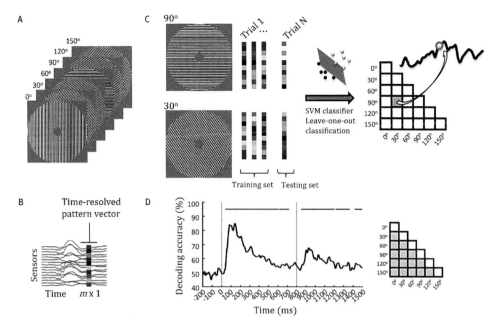

FIGURE 19.4   Example of magnetoencephalography (MEG) time-resolved decoding. (A) The stimulus set comprised six Cartesian square-wave gratings with orientations 0 to 150 degrees with respect to vertical, in steps of 30 degrees. (B) Construction of time-resolved pattern vectors comprising MEG sensor data arranged in $m \times 1$ vectors, where m is the number of sensors. (C) Multivariate pattern analysis. For each time point t, a support vector machine (SVM) was trained to discriminate pairs of stimuli (here excmplified for 90 and 30 degrees), and the resulting pairwise decoding accuracies populated the elements of a time-resolved 6 × 6 decoding matrix. (D) Decoding time series from evoked responses, averaged across all pairs of stimuli. *Gray vertical lines* indicate stimulus onset and offset; lines above plots indicate significant time points; *shaded region* in decoding matrix indicates which decoding values were averaged ($N = 14$; one-sided sign permutation test; $p < 0.05$ cluster defining threshold; $p < 0.05$ cluster threshold).

orientation combinations, namely cardinal (0, 90 degrees) versus oblique (30, 60, 120, 150 degrees). The gratings had black/white maximum contrast with a frequency of three cycles per degree, which is known to elicit strong evoked responses and induced narrow-band gamma oscillations in the early visual cortex (Adjamian et al., 2004; Koelewijn, Dumont, Muthukumaraswamy, Rich, & Singh, 2011). Images appeared in random order for 800 ms with an interstimulus interval (ISI) of 1,000 ms. The experiment presented a total of 352 trials per stimulus.

MEG data were recorded from 14 healthy volunteers using a 306-channel Elekta Triux system. We extracted peristimulus data from −200 ms to +1,500 ms with respect to stimulus onset. The data of each sensor were baseline-corrected by subtracting the mean and dividing by the standard deviation of the prestimulus baseline signal of that sensor. The purpose of this normalization is to scale the sensors to the same numerical range and avoid sensors with greater overall values dominating the decoding results. Finally, the sensor time series were smoothed with a 30-Hz low-pass filter for evoked analyses, or a 200-Hz low-pass filter for induced response analyses.

Using this MEG dataset, we explicate multivariate analyses methods of time-resolved decoding, combined time- and frequency-resolved decoding, temporal generalization, and representational similarity analysis. We demonstrate multivariate pattern analyses using the linear SVM classifier implemented in the LIBSVM software (Chang & Lin, 2011).

19.3.1. An Example of Magnetoencephalography Time-Resolved Decoding

To determine the time series with which MEG evoked responses discriminate orientation information, we performed SVM decoding separately for each subject in a time-resolved manner. In particular, for each time point t (from −200 ms to 1,500 ms in 1-ms steps), we extracted pattern vectors by concatenating the 306 MEG sensor measurements into 306-dimensional pattern vectors, resulting in 352 pattern vectors for each stimulus (condition) (see Figure 19.4B). For each pairwise combination of conditions separately, we assessed the performance of the classifier in discriminating between conditions using leave-one-out cross-validation: 351 vectors were randomly assigned to the training set, and the left-out vector to the testing set to evaluate the classifier decoding accuracy. The pairwise classification was repeated by assigning a different trial to the testing set in iteration, and the resulting decoding accuracies were averaged over iterations. This yielded a 6 × 6 decoding matrix for each time point t, indexed in rows and columns by the classified stimuli. This decoding matrix is symmetric and has an undefined diagonal (no classification within condition) (see Figure 19.4C). Finally, for every time point, we averaged all elements of the MEG decoding matrix, yielding a grand total decoding time series averaged across all condition pairs (see Figure 19.4D).

MEG evoked responses robustly resolved orientation information. The decoding time series reached significance at 38 ms (95% confidence interval, 37–39 ms), peaked at 141 ms (83–145 ms), and then progressively declined over time. Statistical inference procedures are detailed by Pantazis et al. (2018).

19.3.2. An Example of Magnetoencephalography Time- and Frequency-Resolved Decoding

Grating stimuli are known to elicit strong induced gamma activity in the visual cortex (Adjamian et al., 2004; Friedman-Hill, Maldonado, & Gray, 2000). Here we investigated whether induced gamma activity encodes grating orientation information. Induced responses were obtained by subtracting the evoked response (trial average) of each condition from individual trials, computing time–frequency power maps in the 50- to 58-Hz range using complex Morlet wavelets, and finally normalizing with average baseline power to compute event-related synchronization/desynchronization (ERS/ERD) responses.

SVM analysis was performed in a time- and frequency-resolved manner. In particular, for each time point t (from −200 ms to 1,500 ms in 1-ms steps) and frequency value f (from 50 Hz to 58 Hz in 1-Hz steps), we extracted pattern vectors by concatenating the sensor measurements into 306-dimensional pattern vectors (Figure 19.5A). Pairwise SVM classification proceeded similarly to the previously described time-resolved decoding, but this time we obtained a 6 × 6 decoding matrix for each time point t and frequency point f. Finally, for every time point, we aggregated all elements of the MEG decoding matrix over all 50- to 58-Hz frequencies, yielding a grand total decoding time series averaged across all condition pairs (see Figure 19.5D).

MEG 50- to 58-Hz induced responses robustly resolved orientation information. The decoding time series reached significance at 68 ms (95% confidence interval, 64–70 ms), peaked at 134 ms (122–154 ms), and then plateaued for an extended time until stimulus offset.

19.3.3. An Example of Temporal Generalization of Decoding

Temporal generalization of decoding analysis enables us to disambiguate transient from persistent neuronal representations (Cichy et al., 2014; J-R. King & Dehaene, 2014; Isik et al., 2014). The decoding procedure is generalized across time by training the SVM classifier at a given time point t, as before, but then testing across all other time points. Intuitively, if

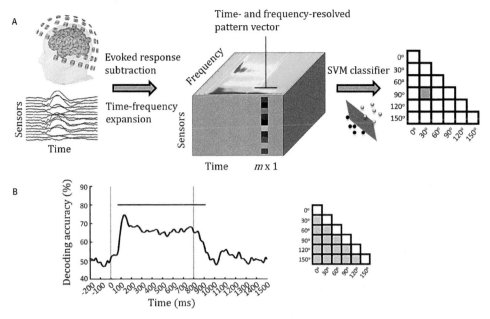

FIGURE 19.5 Example of MEG time- and frequency-resolved decoding. (A) Construction of time- and frequency-resolved pattern vectors. Following removal of the evoked response, single trial MEG data were expanded in time–frequency components using complex Morlet wavelets. The resulting data were concatenated in $m \times 1$ dimensional time- and frequency-resolved pattern vectors. For each time and frequency point, the pattern vectors were subjected to multivariate classification analysis analogous to Figure 19.4, resulting in time- and frequency-resolved decoding matrices. (B) Decoding time series from induced responses at 50 to 58 Hz, averaged across all pairs of stimuli. *Gray vertical lines* indicate stimulus onset and offset; lines above plots indicate significant time points; *shaded region* in decoding matrix indicates which decoding values were averaged ($N = 14$; one-sided sign permutation test; $p < 0.05$ cluster defining threshold; $p < 0.05$ cluster threshold). SVM = support vector machine.

representations are stable over time, the classifier should successfully discriminate signals not only at the trained time t but also over extended periods of time that share the same neural representation of orientation information. Since we train and test the classifier at different pairs of time points, the result is not a decoding time series, but rather a two-dimensional decoding matrix, with the x-axis indexed by training time and the y-axis by testing time. The diagonal of the decoding matrix is identical to the decoding time series because this corresponds to training and testing at the same time.

The results of the temporal generalization analysis revealed that 50- to 58-Hz induced responses carry the same orientation information throughout the 800-ms stimulus presentation (Figure 19.6B and D). The significance maps formed square shapes for the 50- to 58-Hz

responses, a signature pattern of sustained neuronal activity (J-R. King & Dehaene, 2014). By contrast, the evoked response maps showed an early narrow diagonal that subsequently broadened considerably, consistent with an early transient and then sustained pattern of activity (see Figure 19.6A and C).

Taken together, the evoked and induced responses had distinct temporal dynamics. The temporal generalization of the evoked response, with a rapid evolution of neuronal activity early and a greater generalization relatively late after stimulus onset, matched in shape corresponding results from other studies despite using diverse types of stimuli (T. Carlson et al., 2013; Cichy et al., 2014; Isik et al., 2014). In contrast, induced responses were predominantly sustained and generalized equally well throughout the neuronal activity.

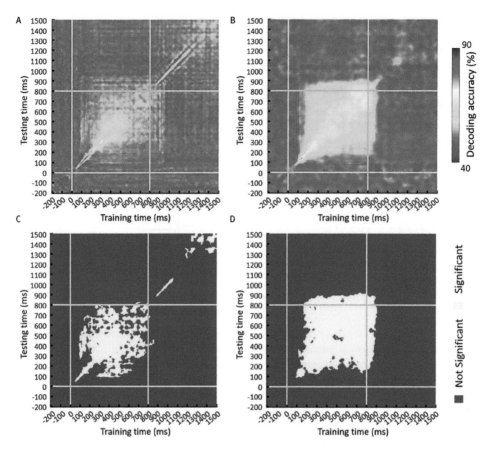

FIGURE 19.6 Example of temporal generalization of decoding. A support vector machine classifier was trained with MEG brain responses at any given time point *t* (x-axis) and tested against all other time points (y-axis). (A) Temporal generalization map from evoked responses. Decoding accuracy is averaged across all pairs of stimuli and subjects. (B) Temporal generalization map from 50- to 58-Hz induced responses. (C and D) Statistical significance maps for corresponding temporal generalization matrices ($N = 14$; one-sided sign-permutation test; $p < 0.005$ cluster defining threshold; $p < 0.05$ cluster threshold). *Gray vertical* and *horizontal lines* indicate stimulus onset and offset.

19.3.4. An Example of Representational Similarity Analysis

A MEG multivariate pattern associated with each experimental condition can been interpreted as a brain *representation*. By comparing the patterns associated with each pair of conditions, we obtain a *representational dissimilarity matrix* (RDM) (Kriegeskorte et al., 2008). RDMs serve as signatures of representations in the brain.

The advantage of performing decoding across all pairs of stimuli is that the resulting decoding matrices can be considered as brain RDMs.[1] Thus, the 6×6 MEG decoding matrices computed previously serve as signatures of how the brain represents orientation information in each time point.

To evaluate how the brain represents orientation information, we devised two models reflecting hypothesized representational formats (Figure 19.7A). The cardinal model had representational distance 2 for pairs of stimuli, with at least one of them cardinal, and 1 for pairs of

---

1. Decoding accuracy is a dissimilarity measure in that stimulus pairs with similar neural patterns are harder to discriminate and thus have lower decoding accuracies.

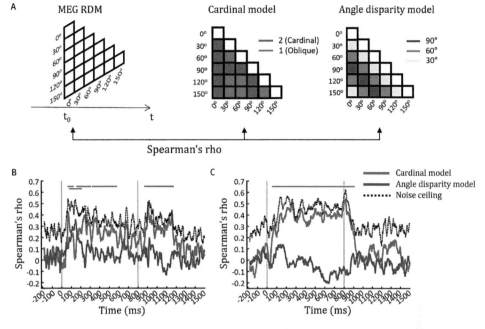

FIGURE 19.7 Example of representational similarity analysis. (A) For each time point, MEG representational dissimilarity matrices (RDMs) are compared (Spearman's correlation) to hypothesized models of orientation encoding a cardinal and an angle disparity model. (B) Representational similarity of the MEG evoked responses with the two models. *Black dashed lines* denote the noise ceiling; *gray vertical lines* indicate stimulus onset and offset; lines above plots indicate significant time points, color-coded as in decoding curves (*N* = 14; one-sided sign permutation test; $p < 0.05$ cluster defining threshold; $p < 0.05$ cluster threshold).

stimuli with both oblique. This model evaluated a categorical relationship between cardinal and oblique stimuli. The angle disparity model had representational distance equal to the angle disparity $\Delta\theta$ between the corresponding pairs of stimuli. This model thus assumed an ordinal relationship between angle disparities and neuronal representations, with higher angle disparities associated with increasingly different neuronal representations. We then used *representational similarity analysis* to compare (using Spearman's rho to capture ordinal relationships) the two models with the time-resolved MEG RDMs of the evoked response and the 50- to 58-Hz induced response. This resulted in time courses of representational similarity between the models and MEG data.

In all cases, the cardinal model predominantly explained the MEG data. Importantly, its performance was close to noise ceiling, that is, the highest possible correlation attained by the

(unknown) true model, given the inherent noise in the MEG data (Nili et al., 2014). Conversely, the angle disparity model proved a poor candidate model, with weak overall correlations.

19.3.5. Summary

Taken together, a variety of multivariate decoding tools provided a detailed view of orientation information processing in the human brain. Time-resolved decoding revealed the time series of orientation information encoded in MEG evoked responses. Combined time- and frequency-resolved decoding revealed robust orientation information in 50- to 58-Hz induced responses. Temporal generalization analysis revealed transient representation in evoked responses and sustained representation in induced responses. Representational similarity analysis informed us that a cardinal model predominantly explains the MEG data.

19.4. CHALLENGES IN THE INTERPRETATION OF DECODING RESULTS

Traditionally, decoding approaches in MEG have been employed in the context of prediction in real-world applications, such as brain–machine interfaces, detection and monitoring of brain disorders, or lie detection. The source of information is not necessarily of interest in these applications, as long as prediction is successful and generalizes to other data sets (Hebart & Baker, 2018). Recently, however, there has been a growing interest in using multivariate decoding for interpretation of brain function. Multivariate pattern analysis makes it possible to investigate a person's subjective mental states in unprecedented ways. Pattern analysis of brain activity can perform feats of mind-reading by revealing what a person is seeing, perceiving, attending to, or remembering (Tong & Pratte, 2012). Using decoding to interpret the neural substrate of these processes raises important conceptual and methodological issues that need to be handled with care.

19.4.1. What Is Being Decoded?

Classifier algorithms are extremely robust and powerful in discovering patterns in the data. They are designed to leverage any information available in the data to make successful predictions on experimental conditions, mental states, or behavioral responses (Tong & Pratte, 2012). When decoding accuracy is statistically above chance level, it confirms that information is latent in neural patterns. But this does not necessarily imply that this information is used by the brain. Decoding can also pick up on information that is computationally unused by the brain.

In reality, the information measured from the data (expressed in the form of decoding accuracy) intersects with the true information used by the brain. There are cases in which the observed decoding accuracy may *overestimate* the information that is used by the brain. One example is the award-winning entry (Olivetti, Sona, & Veeramachaneni, 2016) in the 2006 Pittsburgh Brain Activity Interpretation Competition, which assessed the ability to predict events from the time series of fMRI data collected while participants watched movie segments. The winning model achieved high decoding accuracy but relied mainly on fMRI signals from the brain's ventricles. These signals carried no meaningful measure of neural function, but rather physiological noise artifacts related to movement artifacts when participants experienced humorous movie segments. Consequently, the results of this competition did little to advance our understanding of the brain (Hebart & Baker, 2018; Tong & Pratte, 2012; Woo, Chang, Lindquist, & Wager, 2017). Another example of overestimating the information used by the brain is decoding signals from early visual areas. Since information in the retina and early visual cortex is stored in a pixel-like manner, in principle any visual information can be recovered from these areas using a sufficiently robust classifier, such as a convolutional neural network. However, decoding high-level object information from early visual cortex is possible only because of the pervasiveness of low-level differences between object categories, and not because object information is truly represented in this region.

There are also cases in which the observed decoding accuracy may *underestimate* the information that is used by the brain. Failure to decode information does not mean that this information is not contained in the neural populations. Instead, it may be present in distributed populations that generate weak macroscopic measurements to be picked up by MEG. Other causes for MEG false-negative results may include the limited sensitivity of MEG to deep sources, simultaneous activation of cortical regions with opposing currents that cancel the overall magnetic field, or cortical activity with currents in the radial direction that produce zero outside magnetic fields.

Consequently, poor decodability does not necessarily entail the absence of information.

19.4.2. Selection of a Classifier

A critical decision in multivariate pattern classification is the selection of a linear or nonlinear classifier. Linear classifiers restrict solutions to linear decision boundaries to discriminate experimental conditions, whereas nonlinear classifiers allow more complicated and potentially more powerful decision boundaries. If the aim is to make predictions in real-world applications, such as the detection of Alzheimer disease (Maestú et al., 2015) or estimation of movement in brain-computer interfaces (Schlögl et al., 2005), then nonlinear classifiers may yield higher decoding accuracies, and are thus encouraged in these applications.

By contrast, if the aim is to understand the neural processes that carry discriminative information, then the community consensus is to recommend linear classifiers (Hebart & Baker, 2018; Ritchie et al., 2019; Tong & Pratte, 2012). This is understood by making the distinction between *implicit* and *explicit* information. A neural representation is deemed explicit if it is amenable to a biologically plausible readout in a single step. It is generally assumed in the field that linear decodability suffices to reveal an explicit representation because a single neuron that receives the pattern as a input has direct access to this information. Thus, a linear classifier can reveal the information that is explicitly represented in the brain (although there are challenges to this view; see Ritchie et al., 2019). On the other hand, the performance of a nonlinear classifier applied to a brain region may reflect computations performed by the classifier, rather than the brain itself. As a result, a nonlinear classifier may tap into implicit information that is not directly accessible by the brain. Since brain processes are series of nonlinear computations transforming information to progressively more complex patterns, it is important to not introduce additional nonlinearities to characterize the information

available at each step. Consider, for example, two computational perspectives of the problem of visual recognition. Visual recognition can be viewed as a single-step problem of finding a complex decision boundary that operates on retinal image representation. Alternatively, it can be viewed as a sequence of steps that hierarchically transform signals into more complex visual representations in the ventral pathway (DiCarlo & Cox, 2007). Even though a nonlinear classifier can implement the former in one step, a linear classifier can detect the information emerging at each hierarchical step in the ventral pathway.

The choice among the different types of linear classifiers is not critical because recent studies have shown that several linear classifiers, such as SVM, LDA, regularized least squares (RLS), and Gaussian naïve Bayes (GNB) perform largely the same in MEG data (Guggenmos, Sterzer, & Cichy, 2018; Isik et al., 2014).

19.4.3. Interpreting Decoding Accuracies

Comparing decoding accuracies across conditions is not trivial because classification performance depends on several factors: the selection of the classifier, the cross-validation scheme, the degree of separation between the two classes, the number of data samples available for analysis, the number and selection of variables to construct multivariate patterns, the structure of noise and application of noise whitening (Tong & Pratte, 2012). Since any of these factors can drastically change the decoding results, it is important to keep the decoding parameters constant when comparing decoding accuracies across conditions.

For the same reason, low decoding accuracies should not be automatically discarded as weak experimental results of a small effect size. While decoding accuracy is linked to effect size, it does not reflect a standardized measure of effect size, such as Cohen's d, and low but statistically significant decoding accuracies may still reveal information truly represented in the brain (Hebart & Baker, 2018).

19.4.4. Interpreting Decoding Weights

After a classifier successfully discriminates experimental conditions, it is common to study the decoding weights to localize the source of information. The weights of each variable (e.g., MEG sensor, or source) are jointly plotted as a weight map, with the value in each location reflecting the contribution of that variable to the classification result. However, a decoding weight does not reflect the discriminability power of each variable in isolation, but collectively in the context of all other variables in the classification analysis. This can lead to wrong conclusions regarding the spatial (or temporal) extent of the neural signal of interest. For example, sensors that are not informative on their own may contribute to decoding by removing global noise effects in unspecified ways. Consider the case in which one MEG sensor contains signal with discriminative information plus noise statistically independent to this signal (e.g., heartbeat). A second MEG sensor is contaminated by identical noise, but contains no signal. The signal of interest can be completely recovered by taking the difference between the two channels, which is equivalent with multiplying the two sensor measurements with a weight vector $[1 -1]$. Even though the classifier assigns equally strong weights to the two sensors, only the first sensor contains signal of interest. Thus, strong weights do not conclusively imply the presence of discriminative signal, but they may also serve to suppress noise and thereby extract signal with high signal-to-noise ratio.

Specifically in the case of linear classifiers, Haufe et al. (2014) offer a clever way to achieve interpretability of the model parameters. This is accomplished by acknowledging the distinction between decoding and encoding models, and proposing a transformation that converts weight maps (filters) into interpretable pattern maps.

19.4.5. What Goes Into the Classifier?

Cross-validation requires training the classifier to discriminate between experimental conditions using only part of the data, the *training set*, and evaluating its performance using the remaining data, the *testing set*. There are different cross-validation schemes depending on the selection of the training and testing sets. In the typical *cross-trial* validation scheme, the training and testing sets consist of data from different MEG trials (Figure 19.8A). A *cross-examplar* validation scheme allows more powerful inferences by showing that the same model can generalize to a different but related set of stimuli. For example, we can train the classifier to discriminate human faces versus bodies using MEG data related to one set of image stimuli, and test using MEG data related to a different set of image stimuli (see Figure 19.8A). A *cross-condition* validation scheme allows even more powerful inferences by showing that the same model can generalize to a different but related set of conditions, such as training the classifier on a task measuring responses to human faces vs. bodies, and evaluating its performance on the related animal faces versus bodies task (see Figure 19.8B). In *cross-time* decoding, the classifier is trained and tested on MEG data from different time points, yielding temporal generalization results (see Figure 19.8c; also see Figure 19.6).

19.4.6. Best Practice

We listed earlier several conceptual issues and challenges in interpreting decoding results. The most critical concern is that decoding can only confirm that information is latent in neural patterns but does not prove that this information is actually used by the brain. We recommend several strategies to address this issue. One approach to determine the functional

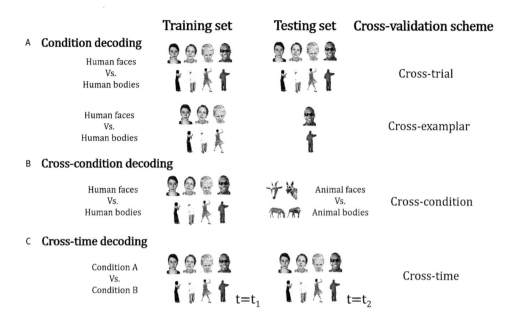

	Training set	Testing set	Cross-validation scheme

A Condition decoding

Human faces
Vs.
Human bodies

Cross-trial

Human faces
Vs.
Human bodies

Cross-examplar

B Cross-condition decoding

Human faces
Vs.
Human bodies

Animal faces
Vs.
Animal bodies

Cross-condition

C Cross-time decoding

Condition A
Vs.
Condition B

$t=t_1$

$t=t_2$

Cross-time

FIGURE 19.8   Different cross-validation schemes, exemplified with visual stimuli of faces and bodies of humans and animals. (A) In condition decoding, the training and testing sets can consist of data from different trials, or different exemplars. (B) In cross-condition decoding, the classifier is trained to distinguish two conditions, and tested in related but different conditions. (C) In cross-time decoding, the classifier is trained to distinguish two conditions at a given time point t_1, and tested at a different time point t_2 (also known as *temporal generalization*).

relevance of decoding results is to establish a link between behavioral and decoding performance. Demonstrating that decoding is higher for correct than incorrect trials, conscious than unconscious perception trials, and demonstrating that decoding accuracy is correlated with reaction time are examples of such an approach. Another good practice is to investigate decoding across a large number of stimuli, to show that inferences abstract from low-level features and carry high-level semantic content. Representational similarity analysis is an excellent framework to construct and compare representations across multiple conditions (see Figure 19.7). Importantly, one can show that decoding performance generalizes to novel and very different stimuli, using a cross-exemplar or cross-condition validation scheme. Finally, it is recommended to use a linear classifier in order to capture information that is potentially accessible by the brain, rather than classifier-specific nonlinear information, which is potentially inaccessible by the brain.

19.5. CONCLUSION

In this chapter, we motivated multivariate pattern classification techniques, provided examples of analyses methods that are particularly suitable for MEG data, and highlighted challenges in interpreting decoding results. In recent years, MEG pattern classification has led to advances in many areas of cognitive neuroscience, including the study of simple visual features, complex visual patterns, auditory representations, temporal maintenance of information, and working memory. Extension of these methods to real-world applications could lead to advances in understanding the neurobiological bases of brain disorders and the development of clinically actionable imaging biomarkers.

REFERENCES

Adjamian, P., Holliday, I. E., Barnes, G. R., Hillebrand, A., Hadjipapas, A., & Singh, K. D. (2004). Induced visual illusions and gamma oscillations in human primary visual cortex. *European Journal of Neuroscience, 20*(2), 587–592.

Alink, A., Krugliak, A., Walther, A., & Kriegeskorte, N. (2013). fMRI orientation decoding in V1 does not require global maps or globally coherent orientation stimuli. *Frontiers in Psychology, 4*, 493–493.

Allefeld, C., & Haynes, J.-D. (2014). Searchlight-based multi-voxel pattern analysis of fMRI by cross-validated MANOVA. *NeuroImage, 89*, 345–357.

Averbeck, B. B., Latham, P. E., & Pouget, A. (2006). Neural correlations, population coding and computation. *Nature Reviews Neuroscience, 7*(5), 358–366.

Barragan-Jason, G., Cauchoix, M., & Barbeau, E. J. (2015). The neural speed of familiar face recognition. *Neuropsychologia, 75*, 390–401.

Benjamini, Y., & Hochberg, Y. (1995). Controlling the false discovery rate: A practical and powerful approach to multiple testing. *Journal of the Royal Statistical Society: Series B (Methodological), 57*(1), 289–300.

Besserve, M., Jerbi, K., Laurent, F., Baillet, S., Martinerie, J., & Garnero, L. (2007). Classification methods for ongoing EEG and MEG signals. *Biological Research, 40*(4).

Carlson, T. A., Hogendoorn, H., Kanai, R., Mesik, J., & Turret, J. (2011). High temporal resolution decoding of object position and category. *Journal of Vision, 11*(10), 9.

Carlson, T., Tovar, D. A., & Kriegeskorte, N. (2013). Representational dynamics of object vision : The first 1000 ms. *Journal of Vision, 13*, 1–19.

Cauchoix, M., Barragan-Jason, G., Serre, T., & Barbeau, E. J. (2014). The neural dynamics of face detection in the wild revealed by MVPA. *Journal of Neuroscience, 34*(3), 846–854.

Chang, C.-C., & Lin, C.-J. (2011). LIBSVM: A library for support vector machines. *ACM Transactions on Intelligent Systems and Technology, 2*(3), 1–27.

Cichy, R. M., & Pantazis, D. (2017). Multivariate pattern analysis of MEG and EEG: A comparison of representational structure in time and space. *NeuroImage, 158*, 441–454.

Cichy, R. M., Pantazis, D., & Oliva, A. (2014). Resolving human object recognition in space and time. *Nature Neuroscience, 17*, 455–462.

Cichy, R. M., Pantazis, D., & Oliva, A. (2016). Similarity-based fusion of MEG and fMRI reveals spatio-temporal dynamics in human cortex during visual object recognition. *Cerebral Cortex, 26*(8), 3563–3579.

Cichy, R. M., Ramirez, F. M., & Pantazis, D. (2015). Can visual information encoded in cortical columns be decoded from magnetoencephalography data in humans? *NeuroImage, 121*, 193–204.

Clarke, A., Devereux, B. J., Randall, B., & Tyler, L. K. (2015). Predicting the time course of individual objects with MEG. *Cerebral Cortex, 25*(10), 3602–3612.

Contini, E. W., Wardle, S. G., & Carlson, T. A. (2017). Decoding the time-course of object recognition in the human brain: From visual features to categorical decisions. *Neuropsychologia, 105*, 165–176.

DiCarlo, J. J., & Cox, D. D. (2007). Untangling invariant object recognition. *Trends in Cognitive Sciences, 11*(8), 333–341.

Dima, D. C., Perry, G., Messaritaki, E., Zhang, J., & Singh, K. D. (2018). Spatiotemporal dynamics in human visual cortex rapidly encode the emotional content of faces. *Human Brain Mapping, 39*(10), 3993–4006.

Dobs, K., Isik, L., Pantazis, D., & Kanwisher, N. (2019). How face perception unfolds over time. *Nature Communications, 10*(1), 1258.

Duda, R., Hart, P., & Stork, D. (2000). *Pattern classification* (2nd ed.). Wiley-Interscience.

Fisher, R. A. (1936). The use of multiple measurements in taxonomic problems. *Annals of Eugenics, 7*(2), 179–188.

Friedman-Hill, S., Maldonado, P. E., & Gray, C. M. (2000). Dynamics of striate cortical activity in the alert macaque: I. Incidence and stimulus-dependence of gamma-band neuronal oscillations. *Cerebral Cortex, 10*(11), 1105–1116.

Friston, K. J., Holmes, A. P., Worsley, K. J., Poline, J.-P., Frith, C. D., & Frackowiak, R. S. J. (1994). Statistical parametric maps in functional imaging: A general linear approach. *Human Brain Mapping, 2*(4), 189–210.

Groen, I. I. A., Silson, E. H., & Baker, C. I. (2017). Contributions of low- and high-level properties to neural processing of visual scenes in the human brain. *Philosophical Transactions of the Royal Society B: Biological Sciences, 372*(1714), 20160102.

Grootswagers, T., Cichy, R. M., & Carlson, T. A. (2018). Finding decodable information that can be read out in behaviour. *NeuroImage, 179*, 252–262.

Guggenmos, M., Sterzer, P., & Cichy, R. M. (2018). Multivariate pattern analysis for MEG: A comparison of dissimilarity measures. *NeuroImage, 173*, 434–447.

Hari, R., Nagamine, T., Nishitani, N., Mikuni, N., Sato, T., Tarkiainen, A., & Shibasaki, H. (1996). Time-varying activation of different cytoarchitectonic areas of the human SI cortex after tibial nerve stimulation. *NeuroImage, 4*(2), 111–118.

Haufe, S., Meinecke, F., Görgen, K., Dähne, S., Haynes, J.-D., Blankertz, B., & Bießmann, F. (2014). On the interpretation of weight vectors of linear models in multivariate neuroimaging. *NeuroImage, 87*, 96–110.

Haxby, J. V., Gobbini, M. I., Furey, M. L., Ishai, A., Schouten, J. L., & Pietrini, P. (2001). Distributed and overlapping representations of faces and objects in ventral temporal cortex. *Science, 293*(5539), 2425–2430.

Hayasaka, S., Phan, K. L., Liberzon, I., Worsley, K. J., & Nichols, T. E. (2004). Nonstationary cluster-size inference with random field and permutation methods. *NeuroImage, 22*(2), 676–687.

Haynes, J.-D. (2015). A primer on pattern-based approaches to fMRI: Principles, pitfalls, and perspectives. *Neuron, 87*(2), 257–270.

Haynes, J.-D., & Rees, G. (2005). Predicting the orientation of invisible stimuli from activity in human primary visual cortex. *Nature Neuroscience, 8*(5), 686–691.

Hebart, M. N., & Baker, C. I. (2018). Deconstructing multivariate decoding for the study of brain function. *NeuroImage, 180*(Pt A), 4–18.

Hebart, M. N., Bankson, B. B., Harel, A., Baker, C. I., & Cichy, R. M. (2018). The representational dynamics of task and object processing in humans. *ELife, 7*.

Isik, L., Meyers, E. M., Leibo, J. Z., & Poggio, T. (2014). The dynamics of invariant object recognition in the human visual system. *Journal of Neurophysiology, 111*(1), 91–102.

Kamitani, Y., & Tong, F. (2005). Decoding the visual and subjective contents of the human brain. *Nature Neuroscience, 8*(5), 679–685.

Kaneshiro, B., Perreau Guimaraes, M., Kim, H.-S., Norcia, A. M., & Suppes, P. (2015). A representational similarity analysis of the dynamics of object processing using single-trial EEG classification. *PLoS One, 10*(8), e0135697.

King, J.-R., & Dehaene, S. (2014). Characterizing the dynamics of mental representations: The temporal generalization method. *Trends in Cognitive Sciences, 18*(4), 203–210.

King, J. R., Faugeras, F., Gramfort, A., Schurger, A., El Karoui, I., Sitt, J. D., . . . Dehaene, S. (2013). Single-trial decoding of auditory novelty responses facilitates the detection of residual consciousness. *NeuroImage, 83*, 726–738.

King, J.-R., Pescetelli, N., & Dehaene, S. (2016). Brain mechanisms underlying the brief maintenance of seen and unseen sensory information. *Neuron, 92*(5), 1122–1134.

Koelewijn, L., Dumont, J. R., Muthukumaraswamy, S. D., Rich, A. N., & Singh, K. D. (2011). Induced and evoked neural correlates of orientation selectivity in human visual cortex. *NeuroImage, 54*(4), 2983–2993.

Kriegeskorte, N., & Bandettini, P. (2007). Analyzing for information, not activation, to exploit high-resolution fMRI. *NeuroImage, 38*(4), 649–662.

Kriegeskorte, N., Cusack, R., & Bandettini, P. (2010). How does an fMRI voxel sample the neuronal activity pattern: Compact-kernel or complex spatiotemporal filter? *NeuroImage, 49*(3), 1965–1976.

Kriegeskorte, N., Goebel, R., & Bandettini, P. (2006). Information-based functional brain mapping. *Proceedings of the National Academy of Sciences of the United States of America, 103*(10), 3863–3868.

Kriegeskorte, N., Mur, M., & Bandettini, P. (2008). Representational similarity analysis—connecting the branches of systems neuroscience. *Frontiers in Systems Neuroscience, 2*, 4–4.

Lehmann, C., Koenig, T., Jelic, V., Prichep, L., John, R. E., Wahlund, L.-O., . . . Dierks, T. (2007). Application and comparison of classification algorithms for recognition of Alzheimer's disease in electrical brain activity (EEG). *Journal of Neuroscience Methods, 161*(2), 342–350.

Luo, W.-L., & Nichols, T. E. (2003). Diagnosis and exploration of massively univariate neuroimaging models. *NeuroImage, 19*(3), 1014–1032.

Maestú, F., Peña, J.-M., Garcés, P., González, S., Bajo, R., Bagic, A., . . . Becker, J. T. (2015). A multicenter study of the early detection of synaptic dysfunction in mild cognitive impairment using magnetoencephalography-derived functional connectivity. *NeuroImage: Clinical, 9*, 103–109.

Maris, E., & Oostenveld, R. (2007). Nonparametric statistical testing of EEG- and MEG-data. *Journal of Neuroscience Methods, 164*(1), 177–190.

Matsuda, I., Nittono, H., & Allen, J. J. B. (2013). Detection of concealed information by P3 and frontal EEG asymmetry. *Neuroscience Letters, 537*, 55–59.

Meyers, E., & Kreiman, G. (2011). Tutorial on pattern classification in cell recordings. In Nikolaus Kriegeskorte, Gabriel Krieman (Eds.), *Visual population codes: Toward a common multivariate framework for cell recording and functional imaging* (1st ed., pp. 517–538). Cambridge, Massachusetts: The MIT Press.

Mohsenzadeh, Y., Cichy, R., Oliva, A., & Pantazis, D. (2017). *Similarity-based fusion of MEG and fMRI discerns early feedforward and feedback processing in the ventral stream*. Presented at the Computational and Mathematical Models of Vision.

Mohsenzadeh, Y., Mullin, C., Oliva, A., & Pantazis, D. (2019). The perceptual neural trace of memorable unseen scenes. *Scientific Reports, 9*(1), 6033.

Mur, M., & Kriegeskorte, N. (2011). Tutorial on pattern classification in functional imaging. In Nikolaus Kriegeskorte, Gabriel Krieman (Eds.),

Visual population codes: Toward a common multivariate framework for cell recording and functional imaging (1st ed., pp. 539–564). Cambridge, Massachusetts: The MIT Press.

Nichols, T. E., & Holmes, A. P. (2002). Nonparametric permutation tests for functional neuroimaging: A primer with examples. *Human Brain Mapping, 15*(1), 1–25.

Nili, H., Wingfield, C., Walther, A., Su, L., Marslen-Wilson, W., & Kriegeskorte, N. (2014). A toolbox for representational similarity analysis. *PLoS Computational Biology, 10*(4), e1003553–e1003553.

Olivetti, E., Sona, D., & Veeramachaneni, S. (2016). Gaussian process regression and recurrent neural networks for fMRI image classification. Presented at the 12th Meeting of the Organization for Human Brain Mapping.

Pantazis, D., Fang, M., Qin, S., Mohsenzadeh, Y., Li, Q., & Cichy, R. M. (2018). Decoding the orientation of contrast edges from MEG evoked and induced responses. *NeuroImage, 180*, 267–279.

Pantazis, D., & Leahy, R. (2010). Statistical inference in MEG distributed source imaging. In P. C. Hansen, M. L. Kringelbach, & R. Salmelin (Eds.), *MEG: An Introduction to Methods* (1st ed., pp. 245–272). New York, NY: Oxford University Press.

Pantazis, D., Nichols, T. E., Baillet, S., & Leahy, R. M. (2005). A comparison of random field theory and permutation methods for the statistical analysis of MEG data. *NeuroImage, 25*(2), 383–394.

Ramkumar, P., Jas, M., Pannasch, S., Hari, R., & Parkkonen, L. (2013). Feature-specific information processing precedes concerted activation in human visual cortex. *Journal of Neuroscience, 33*(18), 7691–7699.

Ritchie, J. B., Kaplan, D. M., & Klein, C. (2019). Decoding the brain: Neural representation and the limits of multivariate pattern analysis in cognitive neuroscience. *British Journal for the Philosophy of Science, 70*(2), 581–607.

Sasaki, Y., Rajimehr, R., Kim, B. W., Ekstrom, L. B., Vanduffel, W., & Tootell, R. B. H. (2006). The radial bias: A different slant on visual orientation sensitivity in human and nonhuman primates. *Neuron, 51*(5), 661–670.

Schlögl, A., Lee, F., Bischof, H., & Pfurtscheller, G. (2005). Characterization of four-class motor imagery EEG data for the BCI-competition 2005. *Journal of Neural Engineering, 2*(4), L14–L22.

Spaak, E., Watanabe, K., Funahashi, S., & Stokes, M. G. (2017). Stable and dynamic coding for working memory in primate prefrontal cortex. *Journal of Neuroscience, 37*(27), 6503–6516.

Stokes, M. G., Wolff, M. J., & Spaak, E. (2015). Decoding rich spatial information with high temporal resolution. *Trends in Cognitive Sciences, 19*(11), 636–638.

Sugata, H., Goto, T., Hirata, M., Yanagisawa, T., Shayne, M., Matsushita, K., . . . Yorifuji, S. (2012). Neural decoding of unilateral upper limb movements using single trial MEG signals. *Brain Research, 1468*, 29–37.

Teng, S., Sommer, V. R., Pantazis, D., & Oliva, A. (2017). Hearing scenes: A neuromagnetic signature of auditory source and reverberant space separation. *Eneuro, 4*(1), ENEURO.0007-17.2017.

Tong, F., & Pratte, M. S. (2012). Decoding patterns of human brain activity. *Annual Review of Psychology, 63*(1), 483–509.

Wardle, S. G., Kriegeskorte, N., Grootswagers, T., Khaligh-Razavi, S.-M., & Carlson, T. A. (2016). Perceptual similarity of visual patterns predicts dynamic neural activation patterns measured with MEG. *NeuroImage, 132*, 59–70.

Wolff, M. J., Ding, J., Myers, N. E., & Stokes, M. G. (2015). Revealing hidden states in visual working memory using electroencephalography. *Frontiers in Systems Neuroscience, 9*, 123.

Woo, C.-W., Chang, L. J., Lindquist, M. A., & Wager, T. D. (2017). Building better biomarkers: Brain models in translational neuroimaging. *Nature Neuroscience, 20*(3), 365–377.

Yacoub, E., Harel, N., & Ugurbil, K. (2008). High-field fMRI unveils orientation columns in humans. *Proceedings of the National Academy of Sciences of the United States of America, 105*(30), 10607–10612.

20

HOW BRAIN RHYTHMS REFLECT COGNITIVE PROCESSES

Joachim Gross

20.1. INTRODUCTION

Since its invention, magnetoencephalography (MEG) has been used to study cognitive function and dysfunction by capitalizing on its main strengths, namely the excellent temporal resolution combined with a good spatial resolution that can be obtained from source localization. Still, over the past 50 years, the field has seen a number of transitions and developments at the level of hardware, analysis methods, and conceptual approaches. Nowadays, state-of-the-art MEG systems feature about 300 superconducting quantum-interference device (SQUID) sensors that allow whole-scalp coverage. The development of optically pumped magnetometers (OPMs) progresses at a rapid pace, leading to the next generation of multi-channel MEG systems (Boto et al., 2018).

Analytical approaches have also changed considerably. Many studies now exploit the rich information content of MEG signals by performing single-trial analysis. This is motivated by the fact that behavioral and brain responses change considerably during repeated presentations of identical stimuli. The traditional approach that is based on the simplifying assumption that intertrial variability of brain responses can be treated as noise is no longer tenable. Instead, general linear model, multivariate regression, classification, and information theoretic approaches have been used to relate brain activity to behavior at the level of single trials (Gross, 2014).

Another conceptual development is a transition from activation to information. Standard MEG analysis would extract peak amplitudes of evoked components and compare them statistically across conditions. Novel analysis approaches go further and rather extract more specific information from MEG signals.

Joachim Gross, *How Brain Rhythms Reflect Cognitive Processes* In: *Fifty Years of Magnetoencephalography*. Edited by: Andrew C. Papanicolaou, Timothy P. L. Roberts, and James W. Wheless, Oxford University Press (2020). © Oxford University Press.
DOI: 10.1093/oso/9780190935689.003.0020.

Information theory can be used to identify brain areas where neural activity measured with MEG contains information about specific stimulus features (such as the eye in a visually presented face) (Schyns, Thut, & Gross, 2011). Multivariate analysis (such as representational similarity analysis) quantifies relationships in the correlation structure in stimulus space, behavior, and multiple imaging modalities and thereby affords the mapping of "representations" based on MEG signals (Guggenmos, Sterzer, & Cichy, 2018; Martin Cichy, Khosla, Pantazis, & Oliva, 2017).

A third transition in experimental and analysis approaches relates to stimulus material. Traditionally, identical and often simple stimuli were presented repeatedly to allow trial averaging. More recently, researchers started using naturalistic stimuli such as movies or continuous speech (Chang et al., 2015; Lankinen, Saari, Hari, & Koskinen, 2014; H. Park, Kayser, Thut, & Gross, 2016). This mode of stimulus presentation is particularly suited to analyzing brain oscillations because it does not rely on trial averaging. Instead, sample-by-sample dependencies between the continuous stimulus and continuous brain activity are analysed. Owing to its continuous nature, the approach makes efficient use of all the recorded samples.

In this chapter, I will review and discuss several applications of these developments, specifically focusing on brain rhythms and their importance for cognitive processes. While I largely make use of examples from the field of cognitive neuroscience, most of the topics discussed here have direct or indirect clinical applications that will be pointed out.

I will start with a general introduction to brain rhythms and then provide an overview of specific spectral signatures that can be consistently observed in rest and during tasks. The best-studied task in this context is attention, which will form the basis of section 4. Finally, I will present some recent approaches that allow more detailed decoding of these spectral signatures or fingerprints.

20.2. BRAIN RHYTHMS

In humans, brain rhythms—rhythmic fluctuations in neural population dynamics that are ubiquitous across the brain—are closely related to many cognitive processes and even prominently evident in spontaneous brain activity (Schnitzler & Gross, 2005; Thut, Miniussi, & Gross, 2012; Wang, 2010). A large number of electrophysiological studies have demonstrated that these brain oscillations reflect brain states, encode stimulus and task-relevant information, are expressed by individual brain areas in a characteristic manner, and cause rhythms in action and perception (Thut et al., 2012). Furthermore, pathologically altered brain rhythms are associated with a variety of neurological and mental health disorders (Schnitzler & Gross, 2005; Uhlhaas et al., 2017). Altogether, the preeminent importance of brain rhythms for the efficient functioning of the brain is undisputed and rests on a large number of invasive and noninvasive studies in humans and animals.

Importantly, a common hallmark and requirement of oscillations (biological or physical, e.g., pendulum) is the existence of two opposing forces. For neuronal oscillations, these two forces are excitation and inhibition. Together—finely balanced and accurately timed with a specific delay—they lead to rhythmic changes in synchronized postsynaptic potentials (Fries, 2015) that can be recorded noninvasively with MEG. Depending on the exact physiological mechanisms and their respective time constants, these oscillations are expressed at frequencies ranging from below 1 Hz to above 150 Hz (Buzsáki & Draguhn, 2004; Buzsáki, Logothetis, & Singer, 2013; Wang, 2010).

Although brain rhythms are dynamically changing, they are naturally constrained and shaped by structural properties of the brain (H.-J. Park & Friston, 2013; Wang, 2010). Relevant structural properties are both local (cell types, neurotransmitters, time constants, local connectivity) and global (such as anatomical connectivity between cortical and subcortical areas). In the following section, I will explore the structure of these brain rhythms in rest.

20.3. SPECTRAL FINGERPRINTS DURING REST

Human electrophysiological brain activity during rest has been studied since 1929, when Hans Berger performed the first human electro-encephalography (EEG) recordings (Berger, 1929). He discovered prominent rhythmic fluctuations in the signal at a rate of about 10 per second. We now know that this so-called alpha oscillation dominates resting-state activity, is strongest over occipital brain areas, and reflects excitability changes in the underlying neuronal populations (Romei et al., 2008).

A vast number of MEG/EEG studies have been performed to investigate resting-state activity in healthy participants and patients (Cabral, Kringelbach, & Deco, 2017; Engels et al., 2017; Mandal, Banerjee, Tripathi, & Sharma, 2018; Uhlhaas, Grent-'t-Jong, & Gross, 2018).

Recently, Keitel and coworkers characterized the structure of these brain rhythms in a novel way (Keitel & Gross, 2016). Instead of simply computing a single power spectrum to describe the oscillatory activity over several minutes' recordings, they computed and analyzed power spectra for every 1-s segment of data separately for each anatomically defined brain area. This approach better accounts for the dynamic nature of brain rhythms. Subsequently, they normalized these power spectra by the global mean to emphasise local deviations and then performed a two-stage dimensionality reduction using k-means clustering and Gaussian mixture models. This resulted in a set of normalized power spectra that reflected a low-dimensional approximation of the local spectral profile. This set of spectra can be seen as a spectral profile, signature, or fingerprint (Figure 20.1). Indeed, further analysis revealed that this profile is characteristic for a given brain areas; that is, the identity of an anatomical brain area can be derived from its

resting-state activity in a way that generalizes across participants. This characteristic functional profile likely originates from the characteristic anatomical substrate and specific anatomical connectivity structure of each area (Mars, Passingham, & Jbabdi, 2018).

Indeed, this anatomical connectivity leads to functional correlations between brain areas that have been reported as resting-state networks in functional magnetic resonance imaging (fMRI) studies (H.-J. Park & Friston, 2013). The correlated activity in these fMRI networks has an electrophysiological correlate—resting-state amplitude correlations, especially in the alpha and beta frequency band, that can be observed in MEG/EEG recordings (Brookes et al., 2011; de Pasquale et al., 2012; Hipp, Hawellek, Corbetta, Siegel, & Engel, 2012). One standard method to identify these networks has been proposed by Brookes et al. (2011). Beamforming is used to compute time series of activation for individual voxels from bandpass-filtered resting-state data. Independent components analysis (ICA) is performed on the amplitude envelopes of the band-limited voxel time series to identify independent temporal components with corresponding spatial maps. Alternatively, ICA can be used as a first step to decompose the signal into statistically independent components that often correspond to different types of artifacts (e.g., eye blinks and cardiac artefacts) and different activated brain areas (Makeig et al., 2002). In a second step, neural generators of nonartifactual components are localized using standard source localization techniques such as minimum norm or beamforming methods (de Pasquale et al., 2012). The time series at any voxel in the brain is then computed from the summation of IC time courses weighted by the amplitude of their source reconstruction at that voxel. A bandpass filter is then applied, and the amplitude envelope is computed as the absolute value of the Hilbert transform of the filtered signal. Amplitude correlations are computed between a seed voxel and all other voxels.

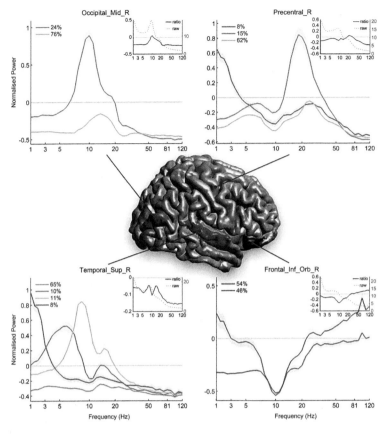

FIGURE 20.1   Regionally specific spectral fingerprints. Power spectra were computed for 1-s segments of source-localized data. Dimensionality reduction leads to spectral fingerprints for each anatomically defined brain area. Spectral fingerprints are defined as a small number of power spectra that best describe the spectral structure in the resting-state recordings across all participants. Here, four examples are presented. (From Keitel, A., & Gross, J. [2016]. Individual human brain areas can be identified from their characteristic spectral activation fingerprints. *PLoS Biology, 14*[6], e1002498.)

A typical problem with correlation approaches in MEG is the spurious correlation between two time series that is caused by leakage (Schoffelen & Gross, 2009). Therefore, it is important to account for these leakage effects when performing resting-state connectivity analysis. Current state-of-the-art analysis pipelines use an orthogonalization approach to remove components that are common in both time series with zero delay—the hallmark of leakage-related components (Hipp et al., 2012). These resting-state methods typically use amplitude correlations based on downsampled amplitude envelopes. However, recently, large-scale resting-state connectivity

has been additionally characterized using a phase-based connectivity measure (Hillebrand et al., 2016). This study showed spectrally specific directed connectivity from posterior to anterior brain areas for 8- to 30-Hz frequencies and predominantly from anterior to posterior at frequencies below 8 Hz.

More recently, the concept of spectral fingerprints in rest has been significantly extended. Vidaurre et al. (2018) use hidden Markov models (HMMs) to describe resting-state MEG data as a sequence of a finite number of states. These states correspond to brain networks with specific spectral properties (power spectra) but also to specific functional connectivity quantified with phase-locking. The study shows that HMM analysis leads to networks that are consistent with fMRI resting-state networks. State transitions were found on relatively fast time scales of about 100 to 200 ms. Together with the previously discussed study, this suggests that resting-state brain activity recorded with MEG shows a regionally specific organization in spectral power and spectral connectivity that can be characterized by a finite number of states. This begs the question of how these spectrotemporal signatures of resting-state activity shape human behavior and are in turn modulated by behavior. Arguably, spatial attention is the cognitive process that has been most studied in this context.

20.4. SPECTRAL FINGERPRINTS IN ATTENTION

The functional relevance of brain rhythms relies critically on the fact that they represent rhythmic excitability changes of neuronal populations. Neuronal firing rates are modulated by the phase of local field potential (LFP) oscillations (Lakatos, Chen, O'Connell, Mills, & Schroeder, 2007; Montemurro, Rasch, Murayama, Logothetis, & Panzeri, 2008; Panzeri, Macke, Gross, & Kayser, 2015) and the dynamic evolution of phase contains complementary information compared with information in spike trains (Kayser, Montemurro, Logothetis, & Panzeri, 2009). The cyclic excitability changes make brain rhythms a suitable mechanism for supporting information processing tasks that require accurate temporal coordination—a prerequisite for any form of human behavior. Buzsaki et al. (2013) summarize this nicely by stating that brain oscillations "form a hierarchical system that offers a syntactical structure for the spike traffic within and across circuits at multiple time scales." This dynamic functional structure complements the more static anatomical structure and allows the flexible task-dependent routing and gating of information flow within anatomically constrained networks. It is therefore not

surprising that brain oscillations and their task-dependent modulations have been linked to a wide range of cognitive tasks such as working memory, attention, perception, and language (Buzsáki & Draguhn, 2004; Schnitzler & Gross, 2005; Thut et al., 2012; Wang, 2010).

One of the best-studied cognitive processes in this context is spatial attention. This is often studied with the classical "Posner paradigm"—a cued target detection paradigm (Posner, Snyder, & Davidson, 1980). Typically, participants fixate a central fixation cross throughout the trial (Figure 20.2). A symbolic cue (e.g., visually presented small arrow, word, or tone) instructs the participant to covertly shift attention to the left or right visual hemifield while fixating a central cross. After a delay period (often between 500 and 1,500 ms), a target is presented in the left or right hemifield. Behavioral performance is better for targets presented in the attended hemifield. A number of variations of this classical paradigm exist. The validity of the cue stimulus can be changed (i.e., targets are presented in the uncued hemifield with a certain probability), participants can be instructed to respond (or not) to targets presented in the uncued hemifield, and distractors can be presented at the same time as the target stimulus in the attended or unattended hemifield. The task may involve the detection of near-threshold targets or the identification of a specific target stimulus.

Already, in a simple target detection task, the state of brain oscillations at stimulus presentation is related to target detection performance. Performance is higher when stimuli are presented when the amplitude of "alpha" (about 10 Hz) oscillations is low in parietal-occipital brain areas compared with when it is high. Recently, it has been shown that this is caused by a change in subjective perception (Iemi & Busch, 2018). Other studies suggest that not only the amplitude of alpha oscillations but also their phase at time of stimulus presentation are important for behavioral performance (Busch, Dubois, & VanRullen,

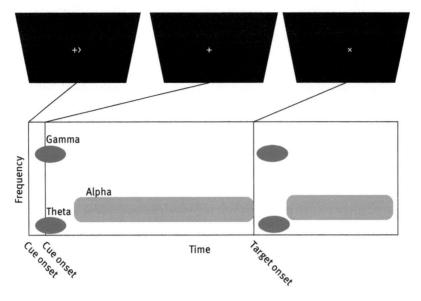

FIGURE 20.2   Spectral fingerprints associated with spatial attention. A cue instructs participants to covertly shift spatial attention to one visual hemifield (right hemifield in this example). Cue onset is associated with transient increases in theta (ca. 3–8 Hz) and gamma (ca. 40–90 Hz) activity in MEG/EEG recordings (displayed here as a schematic time–frequency representation). Even after cue offset and in the absence of any change in visual stimulation, a sustained suppression (relative to baseline) is observed in the alpha band (ca. 7–13 Hz). This typically lasts until target onset ("x" in this case). Target processing is again characterized by transient activity increases in theta and gamma band and a more sustained suppression of alpha band activity.

2009). In general, this leads to the conclusion that the brain state as it is reflected in ongoing brain oscillations determines the fate of a near-threshold stimulus (seen vs. not seen). The mechanistic model explaining these findings is based on the relationship between alpha amplitude (and phase) and neuronal excitability (Haegens, Nácher, Luna, Romo, & Jensen, 2011; Romei, Rihs, Brodbeck, & Thut, 2008).

These findings are further corroborated and extended in spatial attention studies. Here, the spectral signature that can be observed involves three frequency bands: theta (3–7 Hz), alpha (7–13 Hz), and gamma (40–90 Hz). The onset of the cue leads to transient amplitude increase in theta band (related to the evoked component) and the gamma band. Importantly, the alpha band shows a sustained modulation long after cue offset that lasts until target onset. This therefore reflects the sustained spatial attention to the left or right hemifield that the participant is instructed to perform in the absence of eye movements. Interestingly, the lateralization of

the sustained alpha modulation is sensitive to the spatial focus of attention. Attention to the left hemifield leads to stronger alpha suppression in the right hemisphere, whereas attention to the right hemifield leads to stronger alpha suppression in the left hemisphere. This is suggested to lead to preferred processing of stimuli in the attended hemifield.

Another important mechanism by which attention optimizes stimulus processing in the human brain is the suppression of unattended sensory input. Preventing task-irrelevant information from reaching higher processing stages optimizes the use of limited processing resources and avoids interference or competition between irrelevant and relevant information. Ideally, irrelevant information should be blocked at the earliest possible stage, that is, in early sensory areas. Importantly, several studies report an upregulation of alpha oscillations contralateral to the *unattended* hemifield, consistent with a suppression of the visual hemisphere that is less likely to receive target information (Capilla, Schoffelen, Paterson, Thut, & Gross, 2014; Siegel, Donner, Oostenveld, Fries, & Engel, 2008). Furthermore, the amount of alpha modulation in this type of paradigm seems to correlate with behavioral performance, indicating a functional role of alpha oscillations in the gating of target stimuli. It is important to note here that it is the single-trial alpha power in the cue–target interval (before presentation of the target) that correlates with subsequent target processing performance. This is consistent with the notion that alpha power reflects the anticipatory attentional bias of location-specific neural populations. However, it remains unclear to what extent this correlation holds for the inhibitory aspect of alpha oscillations. In fact, Capilla et al. (2014) found a correlation between anticipatory alpha power and behavior only for the alpha suppression contralateral to the attended hemifield and not for the alpha increase (thought to reflect suppression) contralateral to the unattended hemifield. Other studies have only looked at the lateralization of alpha power in occipitoparietal EEG electrodes (Kelly, Gomez-Ramirez, & Foxe, 2009; Thut, Nietzel, Brandt, & Pascual-Leone, 2006).

The correspondence between alpha modulation and shifts of visual attention has been generalized to more complex (and ecologically valid) scenarios. Tan, Leuthold, and Gross (2013) showed that during a dynamic action observation task, alpha modulation spatially coded for the predicted movement endpoint of the behaviorally relevant stimulus feature (in this case, the moving hand of an actor performing a pointing movement). After movement onset, participants dynamically predicted the endpoint of the pointing movement. The outcome of this prediction was reflected in hemisphere-specific occipitoparietal alpha modulations several hundred milliseconds before the observed movement was finished.

Similarly, the amount of alpha lateralization has been shown to correlate with cue validity (Gould, Rushworth, & Nobre, 2011).

Interestingly, these findings generalize across other sensory modalities as well as intermodal attention. The correspondence between visuospatial attention and alpha oscillations has been replicated in the somatosensory domain for painful stimuli by May et al. (2012). The authors report lateralized anticipatory alpha modulation in primary somatosensory cortex similar to attention-related modulations in visual cortex. However, it is important to note that while the pattern of alpha lateralization was identical to the visual domain (relatively more alpha suppression contralateral to attended side), there was no evidence of alpha power increasing relative to baseline. This is in agreement with results of a study of tactile attention that also reported lateralized alpha (and beta) modulation in anticipation of a tactile target stimulus but similarly failed to find alpha power increase as a sign of active inhibition (van Ede, de Lange, Jensen, & Maris, 2011).

However, another group reported a significant alpha increase in ipsilateral somatosensory cortex that contributed significantly to discrimination performance when distractors were introduced opposite to the attended side (Haegens, Luther, & Jensen, 2012). The lack of alpha increases in the previously mentioned studies could simply result from the fact that suppression was unnecessary because no distractors were presented. Therefore, these studies further support the notion of alpha oscillations playing a role in suppressing task-irrelevant information.

Other studies investigated the inhibitory role of alpha oscillations in intermodal attention tasks based on the Posner paradigm. Targets could be presented in the auditory or visual modality with a preceding cue instructing participants to focus attention on one of these two sensory modalities (Fu et al., 2001). Instructing participants to attend to auditory stimuli resulted in increased alpha power over visual brain areas, indicating inhibition of the irrelevant sensory modality. But no increase in auditory areas was reported when attending to the visual domain.

Taken together, there is now considerable evidence for an at least partially inhibitory role of alpha oscillations. Furthermore, there is even direct evidence for a *causal* involvement of alpha oscillations in the suppression of irrelevant stimuli. In one study, a short train of transcranial magnetic stimulation (TMS) pulses at individual alpha frequency (obtained from MEG data during Posner task) was applied to parieto-occipital cortex while EEG was recorded simultaneously. Interestingly, EEG signals at the stimulated site revealed a transient increase in the amplitude of local alpha oscillations indicative of progressive synchronization of underlying alpha generators (Thut et al., 2011). Another study revealed that this protocol indeed leads to a significant change in behavioral performance (Romei, Gross, & Thut, 2010). Specifically, stimulation of right parieto-occipital cortex transiently increases the amplitude of alpha oscillations and leads to reduced behavioral performance for target detection in the contralateral hemifield. Again, this is consistent with the inhibitory role of alpha oscillations.

However, as mentioned previously, the Posner task not only leads to a change in amplitude of alpha oscillations but also modulates other frequencies such as the gamma band. Over the last years, we have learned how different frequencies reflect different aspects of the processing of predicted stimuli. One study contributing to this discussion has been conducted by Bauer, Stenner, Friston, and Dolan (2014). Importantly, they temporally separated visual stimulus presentation from the onset of the task-relevant feature (both coincide in the classical Posner paradigm). The visual stimuli were contracting circles, and participants were asked to identify a change in motion speed. This change could occur at different delays relative to stimulus onset. Since the hazard rate of the speed change increased over time, it allowed the authors to identify oscillatory components that reflect prediction precision. Interestingly, the suppression of alpha

power before speed change correlated with prediction precision. In contrast, gamma band power (40–100 Hz) increased transiently after speed change and reflected the mismatch between prediction and sensory stimulus. This demonstrates that specific frequency bands represent specific aspects of prediction (Arnal & Giraud, 2012).

Sedley, Gander et al. (2016) studied these spectral signatures of prediction invasively in the auditory cortex of epilepsy patients. They presented auditory tone sequences of varying pitch and quantified the statistical structure of these sequences to study the neural correlates of the precision of predictions, prediction error, surprise, and the updating of predictions. Prediction error and surprise are correlated but not identical. Prediction error is related to the mismatch between prediction and sensory evidence. Surprise captures in addition the precision of the prediction that is violated. A mismatch of a more precise prediction leads to stronger surprise. Consistent with Bauer et al. (2014), they reported that transient stimulus-induced changes in gamma power reflected prediction error and surprise. Differentiating between both, they showed that gamma power changes are more closely related to surprise than prediction error. Importantly, alpha power changes were related to the precision of prediction, again consistent with Bauer et al. (2014). Prediction errors are known to lead to an updating of prediction. In this study, this process was related to changes in the beta band (12–30 Hz). This is in line with a recent study that aimed to identify the oscillatory correlates of sensory attenuation—the suppression of the M100 response to auditory tones that are caused by one's own action (e.g., button press) compared with a passively presented tone (Cao, Thut, & Gross, 2017). Interestingly, the tone onset was followed by changes of beta band oscillations that can be interpreted as indicating an updating of the internal forward model that is optimized to predict the sensory consequences of one's actions, similar to the role of beta oscillations in the previously mentioned study by Sedley, Gander et al (2016).

Together, these studies seem to provide converging evidence for spectral signatures of distinct prediction processes in distinct frequency bands.

Other studies suggest that this functional segregation of frequency bands has an anatomical basis. Anatomical connectivity between brain areas can be described as top-down or bottom-up based on the laminar distribution of anatomical connections. This approach capitalizes on the fact that feedforward projections typically start in supragranular layers and terminate in layer 4, whereas feedback projections predominantly start in infragranular layers and terminate in layers other than layer 4. This allows the construction of cortical hierarchies based on the "feedforwardness" of anatomical connectivity between pairs of areas (Figure 20.3). Some studies have compared how directed functional connectivity between pairs of areas is affected by their respective "feedforwardness" (Bastos et al., 2015; Gross, 2016; Michalareas et al., 2016; van Kerkoerle et al., 2014). Interestingly, spectral fingerprints emerge here that are consistent with the results described in the visuospatial attention literature and discussed earlier. Overall, connections that are anatomically more related to feedforward processing show stronger Granger connectivity in higher frequencies (gamma band). In contrast, connections that are anatomically more related to feedback processing show stronger Granger connectivity in lower frequencies (alpha/beta band). Also, within cortical areas, low-frequency (alpha, beta) rhythmic synchrony seems to be stronger in deeper layers compared with superficial layers, whereas the opposite is the case for higher frequency (gamma) activity. Since feedforward projections typically start in supragranular and feedback projections in deep layers, it seems plausible that this leads to the observed spectral asymmetry in

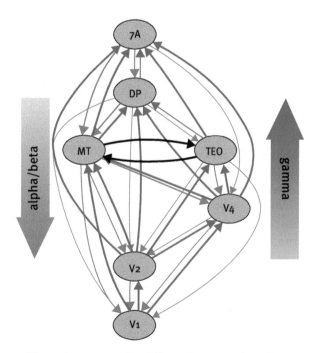

FIGURE 20.3   Functional hierarchies expressed in different frequency channels. Anatomically defined hierarchies (see Michalareas et al., 2016) can be reconstructed based on frequency-specific Granger causality between brain areas. Granger causality in the gamma frequency band is stronger for anatomical feedforward connections, and alpha/beta Granger causality is stronger for feedback connections.

interareal-directed connectivity where feedforward signaling is mediated through gamma rhythms and feedback signaling is mediated through alpha/beta rhythms. This model of frequency-specific communication channels suggests that directed connectivity might be used as a functional "marker" to disambiguate feedforward and feedback processes that often occur simultaneously and are notoriously difficult to separate—especially in noninvasively recorded data. Overall, the empirical anatomical and functional data largely support a computational model that builds on predictions and prediction errors in a hierarchically organized neural architecture (Bastos et al., 2012; Friston, Bastos, Pinotsis, & Litvak, 2015). In this predictive coding model, higher levels communicate predictions to lower level areas (feedback). In turn, lower level areas send prediction errors to higher levels (feedforward). The model posits segregated pathways for feedforward and feedback signals. This seems to be implemented in a functional and anatomical manner. In contrast to anatomical routes, functional communication channels and resulting hierarchies can be dynamically reconfigured faster and more flexibly than their anatomical counterparts. Taken together, these studies reveal spectral fingerprints related to different aspects of prediction that are supported by anatomical pathways.

This has important implications for our understanding of pathological mechanisms underlying various neurological and mental health disorders (Parr, Rees, & Friston, 2018; Seth & Friston, 2016). Within this predictive coding model, it has been suggested that pathological changes in the precision of predictions or the processing of predictions or prediction errors can possibly explain symptoms observed in autism (Friston, Stephan, Montague, & Dolan, 2014; Lawson, Rees, & Friston, 2014), schizophrenia (Limongi, Bohaterewicz, Nowicka, Plewka, & Friston, 2018), chronic pain (Ploner, Sorg, & Gross, 2017), and tinnitus (Sedley, Friston, Gander, Kumar, & Griffiths, 2016).

20.5. DECODING SPECTRAL FINGERPRINTS

In the previous sections, I have discussed the characteristics of spectral fingerprints in rest and during tasks requiring allocation of attention to stimulus features or spatial locations. Several studies have gone further with the aim of extracting even more specific stimulus features from frequency-resolved brain activity. This section focuses on approaches using information theory. Other techniques, such as multivariate pattern classification, are discussed in the following chapter. Information theory has been used extensively in neuroscience, but only recently has it become more common in MEG research (Brookes et al., 2015; Ince et al., 2017; Panzeri et al., 2015; Quian Quiroga & Panzeri, 2009; Silverstein, Wibral, & Phillips, 2017). While it provides versatile and powerful tools that can be applied in various ways, I focus here on the decoding of spectral fingerprints. This decoding is typically based on two related principal measures used in information theory, namely, entropy and mutual information (Cover & Thomas, 2006). Entropy is a measure of uncertainty of a random variable quantified from the probability distribution. Low entropy indicates less uncertainty, and high entropy indicates high uncertainty. Mutual information, instead, quantifies the statistical dependency between two random variables and is computed from entropies. It is sensitive to both linear and nonlinear dependencies between both variables. Mutual information is defined as the reduction of uncertainty of one variable conveyed by the knowledge of the other variable. This leads to interesting applications for fundamental and clinical MEG research. Dependencies between continuous or discrete stimuli and brain activity can be quantified precisely. Examples for this approach based on continuous stimuli have used natural auditory and/or visual speech (Cogan & Poeppel, 2011; Gross et al., 2013; H. Park et al., 2016) to study statistical dependencies between these stimuli and brain activity. This allows identification of brain areas and frequency bands with significant dependency on the stimulus. In the context of speech processing, this approach has revealed, for example, the representation of syllable rate in regionally specific brain activity (Keitel, Gross, & Kayser, 2018). The approach can be further extended for the case of dependencies between three variables—called partial information decomposition (PID) (Kay & Ince, 2018)—with one target variable (e.g., brain activity) and two predictor variables (e.g., audio and visual speech signals). PID is based on the decomposition of total information into unique information conveyed by each variable and redundancy (describing whether information conveyed by the two variables is the same) and synergy (measuring whether both variables convey more information when they are observed simultaneously). Again, this has been applied to decode cortical representations of auditory and visual speech and has led to the identification of two independent audio and visual integration mechanisms in the brain (H. Park, Ince, Schyns, Thut, & Gross, 2018).

Other approaches use mutual information to decode specific stimulus features from brain activity. One of these approaches has been successfully applied to study the dynamics of face processing in the brain. Each stimulus (e.g., a happy face or a sad face) is presented many times, and at each presentation it is degraded in a controlled way by a mixture of Gaussian apertures (called "bubbles"; Schyns, Bonnar, & Gosselin, 2002) that only make available randomly selected parts of the face. Participants are instructed to identify the gender or emotion of the face on each trial. Computing mutual information between behavioral performance and pixel values across trials reveals the position of pixels in the face image that contain relevant information for correct categorization of gender or emotion (e.g., to identify a happy face, the pixels representing the smiling mouth are highly informative). The use of mutual information quantifies informativeness in units of bits.

The clinical applications are obvious. For example, the approach has been used to quantify feature-selective impairments of face processing in participants with autism (Spezio, Adolphs, Hurley, & Piven, 2007). This novel use of mutual information can be easily extended to MEG/EEG data, where it is useful to decode task-relevant features from the data (Schyns et al., 2011). For example, mutual information between brain activity and the values of a given pixel over trials quantifies to what extent this pixel is represented in brain activity. Interestingly, this computation can be performed on source-localized MEG data (Ince et al., 2015) and also across time after stimulus onset and for phase and amplitude of different frequencies (Schyns et al., 2011) (Figure 20.4). This approach has revealed that the eyes of a visually presented face are specifically represented in contralateral hemisphere at about 160 ms following stimulus onset predominantly at a frequency of 12 Hz.

In general, tools from information theory are powerful and versatile and allow investigations into connectivity, linear and nonlinear brain–behavior relationships, and feature-specific stimulus representations in the brain (Ince et al., 2016, 2017; H. Park, Ince, Schyns, Thut, & Gross, 2015; Quian Quiroga & Panzeri, 2009).

20.6. CONCLUSION

MEG recordings from humans during rest and task performance show a complex, puzzling, and intriguing structure across individuals, space (brain areas), frequency, and time. We are only beginning to uncover the fundamental mechanisms shaping this structure. But we have learned that the intricate structure of brain oscillations is shaped by anatomical connectivity, neurotransmitters and genes, physiological time constants, and conduction delays (Buzsáki & Draguhn, 2004; Buzsáki et al., 2013; Salmela et al., 2016; Wang, 2010). Therefore, pathological changes in these parameters associated with neurological or mental health disorders are often reflected in

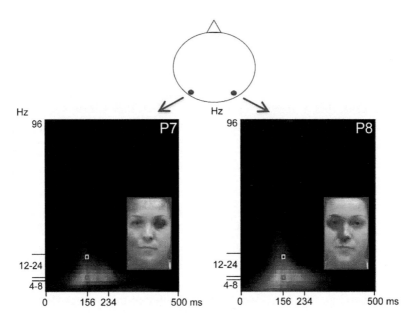

FIGURE 20.4   Reconstruction of specific stimulus features from MEG/EEG data. Mutual information was used to identify dependencies of time–frequency specific brain activity on features of the visually presented faces. Both the left EEG electrode (P7) and right EEG electrode (P8) show sensitivity of brain activity at about 156 ms after stimulus onset at a frequency of about 12 Hz to the contralateral eye (right eye for left electrode P7 and left eye for right electrode P8). (Modified from Schyns, P. G., Thut, G., & Gross, J. [2011]. Cracking the code of oscillatory activity. *PLoS Biology, 9*[5], e1001064.)

brain oscillations. This has prompted numerous studies aiming to identify spectral fingerprints of specific disorders that could assist with early diagnosis and the quantitative assessment of therapeutic performance (Schnitzler & Gross, 2005; Uhlhaas et al., 2018; van Diessen et al., 2015). The large interindividual variability and the "nonstationarity" of brain rhythms are still significant obstacles. However, we are seeing exciting developments in the field that try to address these problems. New analysis approaches quantify brain rhythms in novel ways and relate them to pathophysiology (Cole et al., 2017; Cole & Voytek, 2017; Keitel & Gross, 2016), while new computational models take into consideration the individual anatomical connectivity to model brain rhythms (Jobst et al., 2017; Schirner, McIntosh, Jirsa, Deco, & Ritter, 2018). Together, these might lead in the future to a comprehensive taxonomy of brain rhythms in health and disease.

REFERENCES

Arnal, L. H., & Giraud, A.-L. (2012). Cortical oscillations and sensory predictions. *Trends in Cognitive Sciences, 16*(7), 390–398.

Bastos, A. M., Usrey, W. M., Adams, R. A., Mangun, G. R., Fries, P., & Friston, K. J. (2012). Canonical microcircuits for predictive coding. *Neuron, 76*(4), 695–711.

Bastos, A. M., Vezoli, J., Bosman, C. A., Schoffelen, J.-M., Oostenveld, R., Dowdall, J. R., . . . Fries, P. (2015). Visual areas exert feedforward and feedback influences through distinct frequency channels. *Neuron, 85*(2), 390–401.

Bauer, M., Stenner, M.-P., Friston, K. J., & Dolan, R. J. (2014). Attentional modulation of alpha/beta and gamma oscillations reflect functionally distinct processes. *Journal of Neuroscience, 34*(48), 16117–16125.

Berger, H. (1929). On the EEG in humans. *Archiv Psychiatrie Nervenkr, 87*, 527–570.

Boto, E., Holmes, N., Leggett, J., Roberts, G., Shah, V., Meyer, S. S., . . . Brookes, M. J. (2018). Moving magnetoencephalography towards real-world applications with a wearable system. *Nature, 555*(7698), 657–661.

Brookes, M. J., Hall, E. L., Robson, S. E., Price, D., Palaniyappan, L., Liddle, E. B., . . . Morris, P. G. (2015). Complexity measures in magnetoencephalography: Measuring "disorder" in schizophrenia. *Plos One, 10*(4), e0120991.

Brookes, M. J., Woolrich, M., Luckhoo, H., Price, D., Hale, J. R., Stephenson, M. C., . . . Morris, P. G. (2011). Investigating the electrophysiological basis of resting state networks using magnetoencephalography. *Proceedings of the National Academy of Sciences of the United States of America, 108*(40), 16783–16788.

Busch, N. A., Dubois, J., & VanRullen, R. (2009). The phase of ongoing EEG oscillations predicts visual perception. *Journal of Neuroscience, 29*(24), 7869–7876.

Buzsáki, G., & Draguhn, A. (2004). Neuronal oscillations in cortical networks. *Science, 304*(5679), 1926–1929.

Buzsáki, G., Logothetis, N., & Singer, W. (2013). Scaling brain size, keeping timing: Evolutionary preservation of brain rhythms. *Neuron, 80*(3), 751–764.

Cabral, J., Kringelbach, M. L., & Deco, G. (2017). Functional connectivity dynamically evolves on multiple time-scales over a static structural connectome: Models and mechanisms. *Neuroimage, 160*, 84–96.

Cao, L., Thut, G., & Gross, J. (2017). The role of brain oscillations in predicting self-generated sounds. *Neuroimage, 147*, 895–903.

Capilla, A., Schoffelen, J.-M., Paterson, G., Thut, G., & Gross, J. (2014). Dissociated α-band modulations in the dorsal and ventral visual pathways in visuospatial attention and perception. *Cerebral Cortex, 24*(2), 550–561.

Chang, W.-T., Jääskeläinen, I. P., Belliveau, J. W., Huang, S., Hung, A.-Y., Rossi, S., & Ahveninen, J. (2015). Combined MEG and EEG show reliable patterns of electromagnetic brain activity during natural viewing. *Neuroimage, 114*, 49–56.

Cogan, G. B., & Poeppel, D. (2011). A mutual information analysis of neural coding of speech by low-frequency MEG phase information. *Journal of Neurophysiology, 106*(2), 554–563.

Cole, S. R., van der Meij, R., Peterson, E. J., de Hemptinne, C., Starr, P. A., & Voytek, B. (2017). Nonsinusoidal beta oscillations reflect cortical pathophysiology in Parkinson's disease. *Journal of Neuroscience, 37*(18), 4830–4840.

Cole, S. R., & Voytek, B. (2017). Brain oscillations and the importance of waveform shape. *Trends in Cognitive Sciences, 21*(2), 137–149.

Cover, T. M., & Thomas, J. A. (2006). *Elements of information theory* (2nd ed.). Hoboken, NJ: Wiley-Interscience.

de Pasquale, F., Della Penna, S., Snyder, A. Z., Marzetti, L., Pizzella, V., Romani, G. L., & Corbetta, M. (2012). A cortical core for dynamic integration of functional networks in the resting human brain. *Neuron, 74*(4), 753–764.

Engels, M. M. A., van der Flier, W. M., Stam, C. J., Hillebrand, A., Scheltens, P., & van Straaten, E. C. W. (2017). Alzheimer's disease: The state of the art in resting-state magnetoencephalography. *Clinical Neurophysiology, 128*(8), 1426–1437.

Fries, P. (2015). Rhythms for cognition: Communication through coherence. *Neuron, 88*(1), 220–235.

Friston, K. J., Bastos, A. M., Pinotsis, D., & Litvak, V. (2015). LFP and oscillations: What do they tell us? *Current Opinion in Neurobiology, 31*, 1–6.

Friston, K. J., Stephan, K. E., Montague, R., & Dolan, R. J. (2014). Computational psychiatry: The brain as a phantastic organ. *Lancet Psychiatry, 1*(2), 148–158.

Fu, K. M., Foxe, J. J., Murray, M. M., Higgins, B. A., Javitt, D. C., & Schroeder, C. E. (2001). Attention-dependent suppression of distracter visual input can be cross-modally cued as indexed by anticipatory parieto-occipital alpha-band oscillations. *Brain Research. Cognitive Brain Research, 12*(1), 145–152.

Gould, I. C., Rushworth, M. F., & Nobre, A. C. (2011). Indexing the graded allocation of visuospatial attention using anticipatory alpha oscillations. *Journal of Neurophysiology, 105*(3), 1318–1326.

Gross, J. (2014). Analytical methods and experimental approaches for electrophysiological studies of brain oscillations. *Journal of Neuroscience Methods, 228*, 57–66.

Gross, J. (2016). Let the rhythm guide you: Noninvasive tracking of cortical communication channels. *Neuron, 89*(2), 244–247.

Gross, J., Hoogenboom, N., Thut, G., Schyns, P., Panzeri, S., Belin, P., & Garrod, S. (2013). Speech rhythms and multiplexed oscillatory sensory coding in the human brain. *PLoS Biology, 11*(12), e1001752.

Guggenmos, M., Sterzer, P., & Cichy, R. M. (2018). Multivariate pattern analysis for MEG: A comparison of dissimilarity measures. *Neuroimage, 173*, 434–447.

Haegens, S., Luther, L., & Jensen, O. (2012). Somatosensory anticipatory alpha activity increases to suppress distracting input. *Journal of Cognitive Neuroscience, 24*(3), 677–685.

Haegens, S., Nácher, V., Luna, R., Romo, R., & Jensen, O. (2011). α-Oscillations in the monkey sensorimotor network influence discrimination performance by rhythmical inhibition of neuronal spiking. *Proceedings of the National Academy of*

Sciences of the United States of America, 108(48), 19377–19382.

Hillebrand, A., Tewarie, P., van Dellen, E., Yu, M., Carbo, E. W. S., Douw, L., . . . Stam, C. J. (2016). Direction of information flow in large-scale resting-state networks is frequency-dependent. *Proceedings of the National Academy of Sciences of the United States of America, 113*(14), 3867–3872.

Hipp, J. F., Hawellek, D. J., Corbetta, M., Siegel, M., & Engel, A. K. (2012). Large-scale cortical correlation structure of spontaneous oscillatory activity. *Nature Neuroscience, 15*(6), 884–890.

Iemi, L., & Busch, N. A. (2018). Moment-to-moment fluctuations in neuronal excitability bias subjective perception rather than strategic decision-making. *ENeuro, 5*(3).

Ince, R. A. A., Giordano, B. L., Kayser, C., Rousselet, G. A., Gross, J., & Schyns, P. G. (2017). A statistical framework for neuroimaging data analysis based on mutual information estimated via a Gaussian copula. *Human Brain Mapping, 38*(3), 1541–1573.

Ince, R. A. A., Jaworska, K., Gross, J., Panzeri, S., van Rijsbergen, N. J., Rousselet, G. A., & Schyns, P. G. (2016). The deceptively simple N170 reflects network information processing mechanisms involving visual feature coding and transfer across hemispheres. *Cerebral Cortex, 26*(11), 4123–4135.

Ince, R. A. A., van Rijsbergen, N. J., Thut, G., Rousselet, G. A., Gross, J., Panzeri, S., & Schyns, P. G. (2015). Tracing the flow of perceptual features in an algorithmic brain network. *Scientific Reports, 5*, 17681.

Jobst, B. M., Hindriks, R., Laufs, H., Tagliazucchi, E., Hahn, G., Ponce-Alvarez, A., . . . Deco, G. (2017). Increased stability and breakdown of brain effective connectivity during slow-wave sleep: Mechanistic insights from whole-brain computational modelling. *Scientific Reports, 7*(1), 4634.

Kay, J., & Ince, R. (2018). Exact partial information decompositions for Gaussian systems based on dependency constraints. *Entropy, 20*(4), 240.

Kayser, C., Montemurro, M. A., Logothetis, N. K., & Panzeri, S. (2009). Spike-phase coding boosts and stabilizes information carried by spatial and temporal spike patterns. *Neuron, 61*(4), 597–608.

Keitel, A., & Gross, J. (2016). Individual human brain areas can be identified from their characteristic spectral activation fingerprints. *PLoS Biology, 14*(6), e1002498.

Keitel, A., Gross, J., & Kayser, C. (2018). Perceptually relevant speech tracking in auditory and motor cortex reflects distinct linguistic features. *PLoS Biology, 16*(3), e2004473.

Kelly, S. P., Gomez-Ramirez, M., & Foxe, J. J. (2009). The strength of anticipatory spatial biasing predicts target discrimination at attended locations: A high-density EEG study. *European Journal of Neuroscience, 30*(11), 2224–2234.

Lakatos, P., Chen, C.-M., O'Connell, M. N., Mills, A., & Schroeder, C. E. (2007). Neuronal oscillations and multisensory interaction in primary auditory cortex. *Neuron, 53*(2), 279–292.

Lankinen, K., Saari, J., Hari, R., & Koskinen, M. (2014). Intersubject consistency of cortical MEG signals during movie viewing. *Neuroimage, 92*, 217–224.

Lawson, R. P., Rees, G., & Friston, K. J. (2014). An aberrant precision account of autism. *Frontiers in Human Neuroscience, 8*, 302.

Limongi, R., Bohaterewicz, B., Nowicka, M., Plewka, A., & Friston, K. J. (2018). Knowing when to stop: Aberrant precision and evidence accumulation in schizophrenia. *Schizophrenia Research, 197*, 386–391.

Makeig, S., Westerfield, M., Jung, T. P., Enghoff, S., Townsend, J., Courchesne, E., & Sejnowski, T. J. (2002). Dynamic brain sources of visual evoked responses. *Science, 295*(5555), 690–694.

Mandal, P. K., Banerjee, A., Tripathi, M., & Sharma, A. (2018). A comprehensive review of magnetoencephalography (MEG) studies for brain functionality in healthy aging and Alzheimer's disease (AD). *Frontiers in Computational Neuroscience, 12*, 60.

Mars, R. B., Passingham, R. E., & Jbabdi, S. (2018). Connectivity fingerprints: From areal descriptions to abstract spaces. *Trends in Cognitive Sciences, 22*(11), 1026–1037.

Martin Cichy, R., Khosla, A., Pantazis, D., & Oliva, A. (2017). Dynamics of scene representations in the human brain revealed by magnetoencephalography and deep neural networks. *Neuroimage, 153*, 346–358.

May, E. S., Butz, M., Kahlbrock, N., Hoogenboom, N., Brenner, M., & Schnitzler, A. (2012). Pre- and post-stimulus alpha activity shows differential modulation with spatial attention during the processing of pain. *Neuroimage, 62*(3), 1965–1974.

Michalareas, G., Vezoli, J., van Pelt, S., Schoffelen, J.-M., Kennedy, H., & Fries, P. (2016). Alpha-beta and gamma rhythms subserve feedback and feedforward influences among human visual cortical areas. *Neuron, 89*(2), 384–397.

Montemurro, M. A., Rasch, M. J., Murayama, Y., Logothetis, N. K., & Panzeri, S. (2008). Phase-of-firing coding of natural visual stimuli in primary visual cortex. *Current Biology, 18*(5), 375–380.

Panzeri, S., Macke, J. H., Gross, J., & Kayser, C. (2015). Neural population coding: Combining insights from microscopic and mass signals. *Trends in Cognitive Sciences, 19*(3), 162–172.

Park, H., Ince, R. A. A., Schyns, P. G., Thut, G., & Gross, J. (2015). Frontal top-down signals increase coupling of auditory low-frequency oscillations to continuous speech in human listeners. *Current Biology, 25*(12), 1649–1653.

Park, H., Ince, R. A. A., Schyns, P. G., Thut, G., & Gross, J. (2018). Representational interactions during audiovisual speech entrainment: Redundancy in left posterior superior temporal gyrus and synergy in left motor cortex. *PLoS Biology, 16*(8), e2006558.

Park, H., Kayser, C., Thut, G., & Gross, J. (2016). Lip movements entrain the observers' low-frequency brain oscillations to facilitate speech intelligibility. *ELife, 5.*

Park, H.-J., & Friston, K. (2013). Structural and functional brain networks: From connections to cognition. *Science, 342*(6158), 1238411.

Parr, T., Rees, G., & Friston, K. J. (2018). Computational neuropsychology and Bayesian inference. *Frontiers in Human Neuroscience, 12,* 61.

Ploner, M., Sorg, C., & Gross, J. (2017). Brain rhythms of pain. *Trends in Cognitive Sciences, 21*(2), 100–110.

Posner, M. I., Snyder, C. R., & Davidson, B. J. (1980). Attention and the detection of signals. *Journal of Experimental Psychology, 109*(2), 160–174.

Quian Quiroga, R., & Panzeri, S. (2009). Extracting information from neuronal populations: Information theory and decoding approaches. *Nature Reviews. Neuroscience, 10*(3), 173–185.

Romei, V., Gross, J., & Thut, G. (2010). On the role of prestimulus alpha rhythms over occipito-parietal areas in visual input regulation: Correlation or causation? *Journal of Neuroscience, 30*(25), 8692–8697.

Romei, V., Rihs, T., Brodbeck, V., & Thut, G. (2008). Resting electroencephalogram alpha-power over posterior sites indexes baseline visual cortex excitability. *Neuroreport, 19*(2), 203–208.

Salmela, E., Renvall, H., Kujala, J., Hakosalo, O., Illman, M., Vihla, M., ... Kere, J. (2016). Evidence for genetic regulation of the human parieto-occipital 10-Hz rhythmic activity. *European Journal of Neuroscience, 44*(3), 1963–1971.

Schirner, M., McIntosh, A. R., Jirsa, V., Deco, G., & Ritter, P. (2018). Inferring multi-scale neural mechanisms with brain network modelling. *ELife, 7.*

Schnitzler, A., & Gross, J. (2005). Normal and pathological oscillatory communication in the brain. *Nature Reviews Neuroscience, 6*(4), 285–296.

Schoffelen, J.-M., & Gross, J. (2009). Source connectivity analysis with MEG and EEG. *Human Brain Mapping, 30*(6), 1857–1865.

Schyns, P. G., Bonnar, L., & Gosselin, F. (2002). Show me the features! Understanding recognition from the use of visual information. *Psychological Science, 13*(5), 402–409.

Schyns, P. G., Thut, G., & Gross, J. (2011). Cracking the code of oscillatory activity. *PLoS Biology, 9*(5), e1001064.

Sedley, W., Friston, K. J., Gander, P. E., Kumar, S., & Griffiths, T. D. (2016). An integrative tinnitus model based on sensory precision. *Trends in Neurosciences, 39*(12), 799–812.

Sedley, W., Gander, P. E., Kumar, S., Kovach, C. K., Oya, H., Kawasaki, H., ... Griffiths, T. D. (2016). Neural signatures of perceptual inference. *ELife, 5,* e11476.

Seth, A. K., & Friston, K. J. (2016). Active interoceptive inference and the emotional brain. *Philosophical Transactions of the Royal Society of London. Series B, Biological Sciences, 371*(1708).

Siegel, M., Donner, T. H., Oostenveld, R., Fries, P., & Engel, A. K. (2008). Neuronal synchronization along the dorsal visual pathway reflects the focus of spatial attention. *Neuron, 60*(4), 709–719.

Silverstein, S. M., Wibral, M., & Phillips, W. A. (2017). Implications of information theory for computational modeling of schizophrenia. *Computational Psychiatry (Cambridge, MA), 1,* 82–101.

Spezio, M. L., Adolphs, R., Hurley, R. S. E., & Piven, J. (2007). Analysis of face gaze in autism using "bubbles." *Neuropsychologia, 45*(1), 144–151.

Tan, H.-R. M., Leuthold, H., & Gross, J. (2013). Gearing up for action: Attentive tracking dynamically tunes sensory and motor oscillations in the alpha and beta band. *Neuroimage, 82,* 634–644.

Thut, G., Miniussi, C., & Gross, J. (2012). The functional importance of rhythmic activity in the brain. *Current Biology, 22*(16), R658–R663.

Thut, G., Nietzel, A., Brandt, S. A., & Pascual-Leone, A. (2006). Alpha-band electroencephalographic activity over occipital cortex indexes visuospatial attention bias and predicts visual target detection. *Journal of Neuroscience, 26*(37), 9494–9502.

Thut, G., Veniero, D., Romei, V., Miniussi, C., Schyns, P., & Gross, J. (2011). Rhythmic TMS causes local entrainment of natural oscillatory signatures. *Current Biology, 21*(14), 1176–1185.

Uhlhaas, P. J., Grent-'t-Jong, T., & Gross, J. (2018). Magnetoencephalography and translational neuroscience in psychiatry. *JAMA Psychiatry, 75*(9), 969–971.

Uhlhaas, P. J., Liddle, P., Linden, D. E. J., Nobre, A. C., Singh, K. D., & Gross, J. (2017). Magnetoencephalography as a tool in psychiatric research: Current status and perspective. *Biological Psychiatry: Cognitive Neuroscience and Neuroimaging, 2*(3), 235–244.

van Diessen, E., Numan, T., van Dellen, E., van der Kooi, A. W., Boersma, M., Hofman, D., . . . Stam, C. J. (2015). Opportunities and methodological challenges in EEG and MEG resting state functional brain network research. *Clinical Neurophysiology, 126*(8), 1468–1481.

van Ede, F., de Lange, F., Jensen, O., & Maris, E. (2011). Orienting attention to an upcoming tactile event involves a spatially and temporally specific modulation of sensorimotor alpha- and beta-band oscillations. *Journal of Neuroscience, 31*(6), 2016–2024.

van Kerkoerle, T., Self, M. W., Dagnino, B., Gariel-Mathis, M.-A., Poort, J., van der Togt, C., & Roelfsema, P. R. (2014). Alpha and gamma oscillations characterize feedback and feedforward processing in monkey visual cortex. *Proceedings of the National Academy of Sciences of the United States of America, 111*(40), 14332–14341.

Vidaurre, D., Hunt, L. T., Quinn, A. J., Hunt, B. A. E., Brookes, M. J., Nobre, A. C., & Woolrich, M. W. (2018). Spontaneous cortical activity transiently organises into frequency specific phase-coupling networks. *Nature Communications, 9*(1), 2987.

Wang, X.-J. (2010). Neurophysiological and computational principles of cortical rhythms in cognition. *Physiological Reviews, 90*(3), 1195–1268.

SECTION VI

NEURONAL CORRELATES OF COGNITIVE AND AFFECTIVE DISORDERS

21

APPLICATIONS OF MAGNETOENCEPHALOGRAPHY TO AUTISM SPECTRUM DISORDER

Kristina Safar, Margot J. Taylor, Junko Matsuzaki, and Timothy P. L. Roberts

21.1. A BRIEF INTRODUCTION TO AUTISM SPECTRUM DISORDER AND THE OPPORTUNITY FOR MAGNETOENCEPHALOGRAPHY

Autism spectrum disorder (ASD) is a prevalent neurodevelopmental disorder affecting 1 to 2% of children and characterized by a cluster of symptoms in domains of social reciprocity, language and communication, and stereotypical/repetitive behaviors, often accompanied by an array of secondary conditions, including anxiety, sleep disorders, and even seizures (American Psychiatric Association [APA], 2013). Especially given the range of these impairments and the variation in their severity, ASD is also commonly associated with diagnosis of "comorbid" conditions such as attention-deficit hyperactivity disorder (ADHD) and epilepsy. It is likely that shared biological mechanisms in part underlie this apparent diagnostic overlap. Given the varying severity of each of these contributions, a dominant feature of ASD, and a great impediment to progress in its diagnosis and treatment, is its phenotypic heterogeneity.

While clinical diagnosis is made by observational behavioral assessment (often formalized by tailored neuropsychological instruments, questionnaires, etc.), a role exists for objective brain-based biomarkers, with potential utility not only for diagnostic purposes but also for combatting the disorder's phenotypic heterogeneity through biologically based stratification or subtyping. If a biologically based stratification can indeed be established, it seems likely that tailored interventions (both behavioral and pharmacological) can be more swiftly and effectively developed through clinical trial enrichment/ patient selection. Ultimately, it is our hope that this will pave the way for a precision medicine

Kristina Safar, Margot J. Taylor, Junko Matsuzaki, and Timothy P. L. Roberts, *Applications of Magnetoencephalography to Autism Spectrum Disorder*
In: *Fifty Years of Magnetoencephalography*. Edited by: Andrew C. Papanicolaou, Timothy P. L. Roberts, and James W. Wheless, Oxford University Press (2020). © Oxford University Press. DOI: 10.1093/oso/9780190935689.003.0021.

approach to ASD treatment: getting the *right* treatment to the *right* patient at the *right* time.

There are several features of electrophysiology, and in particular magnetoencephalography (MEG), that offer promise compared with conventional imaging (e.g., magnetic resonance imaging [MRI]). First, the high temporal resolution (submillisecond) of MEG recording and its intrinsic sensitivity to neuronal activity directly offer the ability to resolve subtle timing, or latency, anomalies that are inherently obscured in slower functional imaging techniques (such as functional MRI [fMRI]), limited (to approximately seconds) by either sampling rate (i.e., image acquisition time) or indirect physiology (i.e., hemodynamic response). High temporal resolution additionally offers the possibility of characterizing and resolving neural activity at different frequencies (e.g., alpha at 8–12 Hz or gamma at 30–80 Hz), where higher frequency oscillations clearly demand faster (approximately a few milliseconds) data collection sampling rates.

While this first property is largely shared with the (more available) sister technique of electroencephalography (EEG), a difference becomes apparent as analyses require more and more precise spatial source estimation, where MEG physics provides improved inverse model solutions compared with EEG, through its reduced dependency on intervening tissue properties and path differences. Both as a source of artifact rejection (spatial filtering) and as a means of identifying, and more precisely defining, discrete spatial loci participating in brain networks, the improved spatial resolution afforded by MEG offers attractive utility.

In this chapter, we review the extensive literature using MEG approaches to study ASD and highlight its areas of promise both for informing mechanistic neuroscience as well as providing biomarkers for clinical implementation. Since the majority of MEG studies of ASD have focused on the auditory and face processing systems, we address those in detail. Emerging studies of other sensory systems and inroads into cognitive functions as well as resting-state

analyses are appended to direct the interested reader to novel areas of MEG investigation.

21.2. MAGNETOENCEPHALOGRAPHY INVESTIGATIONS OF AUDITORY PROCESSING IN AUTISM SPECTRUM DISORDER

Since MEG is a noninvasive neuroimaging technique that provides a measure of cortical neural activity on a millisecond timescale with high spatial resolution, it has been used to study human auditory function almost since its earliest inception in the 1970s and 1980s. MEG is well-suited for the study of auditory function because of two major features (Tobimatsu et al., 2016). First, the MEG hardware (unlike MRI) does not make any sound during measurement, and thus researchers can measure brain neural activity in a background of silence. Second, the MEG can well-resolve signals produced by the auditory cortices located bilaterally in the temporal lobes, owing to the tangential orientation of neurons in the sulci of the superior temporal gyri.

In large part because of its high intrinsic temporal resolution, MEG has been adopted in the study of ASD since the late 1990s. Most earlier MEG studies of ASD were mainly focused on school-aged children or adults (Gage et al., 2003a, 2003b). However, since the development of dedicated "infant/small-child optimized hardware," such as the 76-channel babySQUID (Okada et al., 2006), 375-channel, whole-head MEG system "Baby MEG" (Okada et al., 2016), 64-channel whole-head MEG system (Johnson et al., 2010), 151-channel MEG system PQ 1151R, Yokogawa/KIT (RICOH, Kanazawa, Japan) (Kikuchi et al., 2010), and 123-channel whole-head MEG system Artemis 123 (Tristan Technologies, San Diego, CA) (Roberts et al., 2014) (Figure 21.1), all of which show the advantage of placing the head closer to the MEG sensors in infants and children, researchers have been able to focus on brain activity in all ages (including young children), which is especially significant

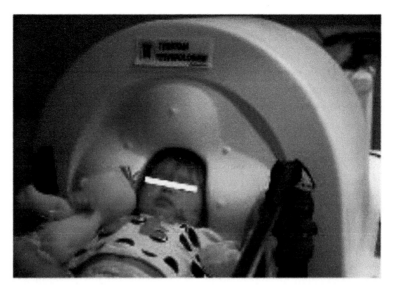

FIGURE 21.1   A 14-month -ld participant undergoing magnetoencephalography (MEG) recording in a dedicated (Artemis 123) infant/young child MEG device, in which the helmet is smaller than a conventional adult system, thus reducing the distance between the brain and sensors and improving signal detection sensitivity. (From Roberts, T. P. L., Paulson, D. N., Hirschkoff, E., Pratt, K., Mascarenas, A., Miller, P., . . . & Edgar, J. C. [2014]. Artemis 123: Development of a whole-head infant and young child MEG system. *Frontiers in Human Neuroscience, 8*[99].)

for ASD-related research, given the typical age of diagnosis of approximately 2 to 3 years.

Abnormal auditory cortical responses to auditory stimuli (e.g., tone, vowel, syllable, or word) in individuals with ASD have been studied as objective markers of autistic features (Gage et al., 2003a, 2003b; Oram Cardy et al., 2004; Roberts et al., 2010; Takahashi et al., 2016), language and communication ability (Edgar et al., 2014; Flagg et al., 2005; Roberts et al., 2011; Schmidt et al., 2009; Yoshimura et al., 2013), and abnormal sensory sensitivity (Matsuzaki et al., 2012; Orekhova et al., 2012). Most of the existing auditory MEG studies have focused on components of the early auditory evoked field (AEF; i.e., M50, M100), mismatch magnetic fields (MMFs), or gamma-band oscillatory activity in individuals with ASD.

21.2.1. Auditory M50/M100 Components in Autism Spectrum Disorder

Most of previous MEG studies have observed that verbal children who have ASD show prolonged/delayed early auditory processing compared with typically developing (TD) children (Demopoulos et al., 2017; Edgar et al., 2014; Gage et al., 2003a, 2003b; Oram Cardy et al., 2004; Roberts et al., 2010, 2013; Port et al., 2015). The M50 is analogous to the Pa/P1 complex of the EEG evoked responses; the M100 magnetic field is comparable to the N1 (Oram Cardy et al., 2004). In particular, delayed auditory responses have been observed for auditory response components around 50 ms (MEG: M50) and 100 ms (MEG: M100) and the responses primarily produced by neural activity from superior temporal gyrus (STG), including primary/association auditory cortex (Gage et al., 2003a, 2003b; Näätänen et al., 1987; Roberts et al., 2000). Of note, these findings have also been replicated using EEG (Brandwein et al., 2013), although this technique presents unique challenges due to the orientation of auditory cortex neurons and the need for source modeling to separate partially overlapping signals from bilateral generators.

In an early study in children with ASD, Gage et al. (2003a) reported maturational changes in cortical auditory systems in left (LH) and right (RH) hemispheres in children (8–16 years old) with ASD ($n = 15$) and controls ($n = 17$). The authors recorded auditory evoked responses over left and right temporal lobes during sinusoidal tones and found an estimate of the rate of latency change (ms/year) by hemisphere and subject group. M100 latency showed a tendency to vary with age in LH, decreasing at a rate of –4.6 ms/year. In this early study, M100 latency in RH appeared not to mature (actually increased slightly, at a rate of 0.8 ms/year) with age, in the age range studied, although this finding was contradicted in later, larger sample studies. In general, results provide support for a differential auditory system development in ASD children that may reflect abnormalities in cortical maturational processes in ASD.

Oram Cardy et al. (2004) investigated the M50 and M100 components of the AEF to explore further their changes during development. The authors measured MEG elicited by sinusoidal tones in adults (21–53 years old, $n = 10$) and two groups of TD ($n = 18$) or ASD (8–17 years old, $n = 10$) children and adolescents. M50 amplitude was larger in children than in adults, suggesting a developmental trajectory with M50 amplitude decreasing and M100 increasing with age. Child M50 and M100 latencies were prolonged relative to adults, as had previously been shown (e.g., Paetau et al., 1995). The M50 in relation to the M100 is a robust index of early auditory system maturation suitable for future developmental investigations. The authors also examined M50 and M100 latencies from children and adolescents (7–18 years old) controls, children with ASD ($n = 14$), children with Asperger syndrome ($n = 10$), and children with specific language impairment (SLI; $n = 5$) and reported that longer M50 latencies predicted impaired receptive language ability (Oram Cardy et al., 2008).

Roberts et al. (2010) also reported that the right STG M100 auditory response was delayed by approximately 10 ms in response to tone stimuli in children (8–12 years old) with ASD ($n = 25$) versus TD ($n = 17$) (Figure 21.2).

Findings implicating maturational changes in auditory pathway white matter as influencing conduction velocity in TD children and adolescents (6–18 years old) (Roberts et al., 2009) were not replicated in a cohort of children with ASD (whose M50 responses to sinusoidal tones were delayed), leading to the hypothesis that synaptic transmission may also influence auditory latency delay (Roberts et al., 2013). From the same laboratory, examining left and right STG activity, Edgar et al. (2015) reported delayed latency of left and right STG M50 and right STG M100 responses in children with ASD (6–14 years old, $n = 52$), again implicating maturational abnormalities in the development of primary/secondary auditory areas in children with ASD. The authors hypothesized that a longitudinal investigation of the maturation of auditory network activity will indicate delayed development of each component of the auditory processing system in ASD.

A few MEG studies have highlighted abnormal sensory abnormality in individuals with ASD. Orekhova et al. (2012) recorded magnetic field responses to a paired click paradigm in children (mean age, 10 years) with ASD ($n = 14$) and TD controls ($n = 15$). The "P100m" (analogue of adult M50) amplitude was rightward lateralized in the TD children, but not in the ASD children, who showed a tendency toward P100m reduction in the RH. The atypical P100m lateralization in the ASD subjects was associated with greater severity of sensory abnormalities as well as with auditory hypersensitivity during the first 2 years of life. The absence of RH predominance of the P100m and a tendency for its RH reduction in the ASD children suggest disturbance of the RH ascending reticular brainstem pathways and/or their thalamic and cortical projections, which in turn may contribute to abnormal arousal and attention, suggesting that reduced preattentive processing in the RH and/or its shift to the LH may contribute to abnormal sensory behaviour in ASD.

Matsuzaki et al. (2012) reported differential cortical responses of the primary auditory cortex during pure tone sound stimuli

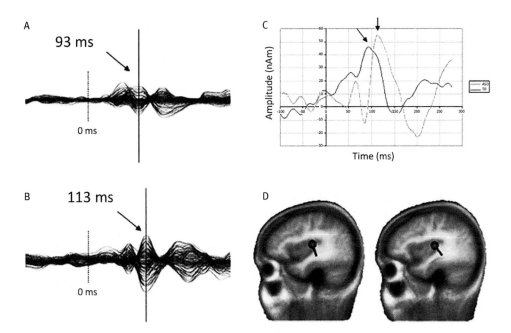

FIGURE 21.2   Auditory evoked response waveforms from representative individuals with (A) typical development (A) and with ASD (B) show pronounced latency delay of the M100 component (*arrows*) in autism spectrum disorder. (C) Source modeled waveforms confirm the delays in signals arising from sources (D) in superior temporal gyrus. (Adapted from Roberts, T. P. L., Khan, S. Y., Rey, M., Monroe, J. F., Cannon, K., Blaskey, L., ... Edgar, J. C. [2010]. MEG detection of delayed auditory evoked responses in autism spectrum disorders: Towards an imaging biomarker for autism. *Autism Research, 3*, 8–18.)

in children (8–10 years old) with ASD with or without abnormal auditory sensitivity (n = 18). ASD with abnormal auditory sensitivity showed significantly more delayed M50/M100 peak latencies than ASD without it or the TD (n = 12). M50 dipole moments in the sensitivity group were statistically larger than those in the other two groups. M50/M100 peak latencies were correlated with the severity of auditory sensitivity. The authors also reported M50 dipole moments were significantly increased during the time-course study only in the ASD subjects with auditory sensitivity compared with those for the other two groups (Matsuzaki et al., 2014). These findings suggested that auditory sensitivity in ASD is a characteristic response of the primary auditory cortex, possibly resulting from an abnormal sensory gating system, neurological immaturity, or dysfunction of inhibitory interneurons.

In a study using a dedicated "infants and toddlers" MEG system, Yoshimura et al. (2013)

examined the "P50m" (M50) component that was evoked through binaural auditory Japanese syllable sound stimulation in young children with ASD (n = 32) and TD (3–7 years old, n = 30) to examine differences in auditory cortex function that are associated with language development. The authors suggested that there is atypical brain function in the auditory cortex in young children with ASD, regardless of language development. Moreover, Kurita et al. (2016) used Omega complexity analysis and investigated the global coordination of AEFs in 3- to 8-year-old TD (n = 50) and ASD (n = 50) children in 50-ms time windows. Children with ASD displayed significantly higher Omega complexities compared with TD children, suggesting lower whole-brain synchronization in the early stage of the "P1m" (M50) component. The authors provided evidence of aberrant neural synchronization in young children with ASD by investigating auditory evoked neural responses to the Japanese human voice stimuli.

Edgar et al. (2015) also reported that maturation of auditory cortex responses in TD infants and toddlers is needed to later identify auditory processing abnormalities in infants (6–59 months old, $n = 29$) at risk for neurodevelopmental disorders. The authors found that strong early latencies (auditory response with a positive topography was observed at approximately 150 ms) decreased as a function of age, suggesting that age and latency associations, sensitivity to tone frequency, and good test–retest reliability support the viability of longitudinal infant MEG studies that include younger as well as older participants, as well as studies examining auditory processing abnormalities in infants at risk for neurodevelopmental disorders.

Taken together, these MEG studies have provided compelling evidence for atypical auditory sensory responses in ASD. These responses are characterized by atypical developmental trajectories, increasingly assessable through dedicated infant MEG hardware. Atypical courses of functional specialization revealed as lateralization differences are also evident. The implication of these differences and especially the evidence supporting atypical maturational processes raise the intriguing possibility that MEG might offer utility in identifying atypical auditory responses in very young children *before* a clinical ASD diagnosis. Such hypotheses are undergoing intense investigation at this time, particularly in cohorts of infants considered to be high risk for ASD, such as those with an older sibling already diagnosed.

21.2.2. Auditory Mismatch Magnetic Field Components in Autism Spectrum Disorders

The electrical mismatch negativity (MMN) and its magnetic analogue, the MMF, measured by MEG, describe the preattentive automatic neural discrimination response and serve as an indirect index of the ability of the auditory cortex to detect changes in a stimulus stream by presenting regularly occurring "standard " stimuli, occasionally interrupted with rare "deviant " stimuli (Näätänen et al., 1978, 2007). In general, MMN/

MMF peak latencies become shorter and/or amplitudes larger as the magnitude/salience of stimulus change increases (Näätänen et al., 1987; Rinne et al., 2000, 2006; Wolff & Schroger, 2001), reflecting the greater ease of auditory cortex to identify stimulus modifications.

The ability to detect an auditory change (e.g., pitch, frequency, and syllable) is an important neural processing feature and likely contributes to downstream language, communication skills, and abnormal sensory sensitivity in ASD (Berman et al., 2016; Matsuzaki et al., 2017, 2019; Oram Cardy et al., 2005; Roberts et al., 2011; Yoshimura et al., 2017). In an early study in children with ASD, Tecchio et al. (2003) reported that moderately to severely impaired verbal individuals with ASD (8–32 years old, $n = 11$) demonstrated a weak or absent MMF response compared with TD individuals ($n = 10$) during a tone burst oddball paradigm, and suggested that impaired auditory discrimination ability in preconscious cortical processing stages may hinder the development of more complex connections in ASD.

Oram Cardy et al. (2005) reported MMF elicited by changes in streams of vowels or spectrally matched tones in children and adolescents aged 8 to 17years with ASD ($n = 7$) relative to TD ($n = 9$) to explore whether impaired sound discrimination may contribute to language impairments in ASD. The authors recorded evoked neural activity to tones and vowels presented in an oddball paradigm with deviant stimuli (15%) occurring within a train of standards (85%). The MMF was robustly observed in both groups, but children with ASD demonstrated a significantly delayed MMF latency compared with TD children. The authors suggested that difficulty parsing transient differences in sounds may lead to impaired acoustic or phonological representations and subsequent language impairment in ASD. Roberts et al. (2011) reported auditory MMF abnormalities are frequently observed in ASD, and these abnormalities may have sequelae in terms of clinical language impairment (LI). This study assessed associations between LI and the amplitude and latency of the STG MMF in response to changes in an auditory stream of tones or vowels in children aged 6 to 15 years with ASD ($n = 52$) and TD ($n = 27$). The authors found delayed MMF latency in children with ASD compared with TD children. Furthermore, this delay was most pronounced (50 ms) in children with concomitant LI, with significant differences in latency between children with ASD with LI and those without. Receiver operator characteristic (ROC) analysis indicated a sensitivity of 82.4% and specificity of 71.2% for diagnosing LI based on MMF latency. Neural correlates of auditory change detection (the MMF) are significantly delayed in children with ASD, and especially those with concomitant LI, suggesting a neurobiological basis as well as a clinical biomarker for LI in ASD. Interestingly, the authors also found (Roberts et al., 2012) a similar MMF latency delay in children (7–11 years old, $n = 17$) with SLI (but not ASD)—suggesting a "trans-disorder" or domain-specific association (in line with the National Institute of Health Research Domain Criteria (RDoC) philosophy: see Insel et al., 2010).

Similarly, Berman et al. (2016) showed an association between MMF latency delay and language impairment in children with ASD ($n = 95$), as well as a corresponding relationship with microstructural diffusion tensor MRI of the arcuate fasciculus, supporting a white matter connectivity disruption hypothesis for the biological basis of observed MMF delays. In a recent study, in a new cohort of young children with ASD, we found a similar negative association between MMF latency and language ability after hierarchical regression to eliminate effects of age, token, and hemisphere in children with ASD ($n = 48$; Figure 21.3). These MMF anomalies appear to persist across spoken language because, although the previously mentioned studies applied English speech tokens to native English language speakers, in a Japanese population, Yoshimura et al. (2017) investigated the MMF evoked by a Japanese syllable oddball paradigm in 3- to 5-year-old TD ($n = 46$) and ASD ($n = 47$) children. The children with ASD exhibited significantly decreased MMF amplitude in the left STG compared with the TD children. When the authors classified the children with ASD according to the presence or absence of a speech onset delay (SOD) and compared these two groups with the TD children, both ASD groups exhibited decreased activation in the left STG compared with the TD children. In contrast, the ASD with SOD group exhibited increased activity in the left frontal cortex compared with the other groups. For all children with ASD, there was a significant negative correlation between the MMF amplitude in the left pars orbitalis and language performance. Matsuzaki et al. (2017) investigated alterations in MMFs in children with ASD ($n = 20$) and abnormal auditory sensitivity using pure tone oddball paradigm in children (8–10 years old) with ASD with abnormal auditory sensitivity, ASD without it, and TD ($n = 13$). The authors reported that MMF latencies were significantly longer only in children with ASD who had abnormal auditory sensitivity. In addition, prolonged MMF latencies were correlated with the severity of abnormal auditory sensitivity in both hemispheres. These findings suggest that children with ASD and abnormal auditory sensitivity may have atypical neural networks in the primary auditory area, as well as in brain areas associated with attention switching and inhibitory control processing.

Relatively little is known about MMF abnormalities in adults with ASD. Kasai et al. (2005) investigated duration discrimination of an oddball paradigm (pure tone, Japanese vowel, and vowel across-category change) in adults with ASD (27.2 ± 7.0 years old, $n = 9$) and TD (27.3 ± 7.0 years, $n = 19$). The authors reported no differences in MMF response amplitudes. However, the ASD group showed a left-biased latency prolongation of the MMF particularly under the across-phoneme change condition, and this latency delay was significantly associated with greater symptom severity. These results suggest that adults with ASD are associated with delayed processing for automatic change detection of speech sounds. Supporting this, Matsuzaki et al. (2019) examined

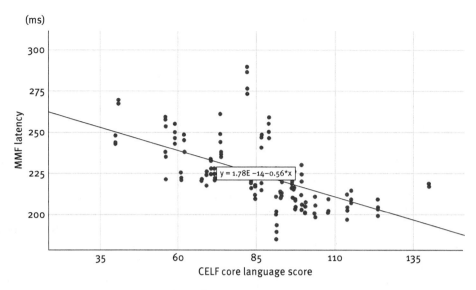

FIGURE 21.3   Mismatch magnetic field (MMF) latencies derived from an oddball paradigm with vowel stimuli in a cohort of children with autism spectrum disorder show a strong negative association with clinical language impairment (indexed by the core language score of the Clinical Evaluation of Language Fundamentals [CELF]; see Semel et al., 2003; Wiig et al., 2013), with longer latencies indicating lower language ability ($R^2 = 36\%$, $p < 0.05$).

neurophysiological mechanisms underlying auditory language discrimination during an auditory oddball paradigm with vowel stimuli in adults with ASD. The MMF was significantly delayed in adults with ASD (22.22 ± 5.74 years old, $n = 9$) compared with the TD participants (27.25 ± 6.63 years old, $n = 16$). Furthermore, whereas TD participants showed a leftward lateralization of MMF amplitude, participants with ASD showed an opposite (rightward) lateralization. Findings suggest that adults with ASD have hemispherically and temporally abnormal auditory discrimination processing.

Similar to the M50 and M100 findings, the previously discussed MMF studies provide significant support for atypical auditory processing in ASD. In general, however, the MMF findings show a more direct association with the degree of language impairment, perhaps attributable to the general use of language-related stimuli (vowels, consonant–vowel pairs), or perhaps reflecting the more sophisticated (higher order) auditory processing required to detect change in the auditory stream compared to simply identifying signal in the auditory stream. Thus, while M50 and M100 anomalies might be objective indices of ASD,

MMF differences may index abnormalities in the language domain, specifically.

21.2.3. Auditory Gamma-Band Activity in Autism Spectrum Disorder

MEG research has also revealed abnormal gamma-band oscillatory activity during task-evoked auditory processing in ASD (Gaetz et al., 2014; Gandal et al., 2010; Port et al., 2016; Tanigawa et al, 2018; Wilson et al., 2007;) and first-degree relatives of children with ASD (McFadden et al., 2012; Rojas et al., 2008).

Rojas et al. (2006) recorded auditory magnetic steady-state responses (SSRs) in 5-to 52-year-old ($n = 69$) healthy participants and reported gamma power significantly related to subject age in both hemispheres. Hemispheric asymmetry was observed for the anterior–posterior SSR source locations, suggestive of asymmetry similar to that previously described for the SSR and other auditory evoked magnetic field components.

In an ASD population, Wilson et al. (2007) examined integrity of local circuitry by focusing on gamma-band activity of auditory magnetic SSRs in children and adolescents (7–17 years old) with ASD (*n* = 10) and TD (*n* = 10). The study reported that the production and/or maintenance of LH gamma oscillations appeared abnormal in participants with ASD, suggesting that a lack of local inhibitory interneurons (Casanova et al., 2006) may be the neural mechanism underlying this impairment because of the known role of such cells in generating high-frequency activity. Gandal et al. (2010) assessed the translational potential of auditory evoked response endophenotypes of ASD in parallel mouse models and children with ASD (10.20 ± 2.15, *n* = 25) and TD (10.77 ± 2.15, *n* = 17) during pure tone stimuli. Children with ASD and valproic acid–exposed mice showed a similar 10% latency delay in the M100 evoked response and a reduction in gamma frequency (30–50 Hz) phase locking factor (a measure of phase synchrony, sometimes also referred to as *intertrial coherence*).

Examining first-degree relatives of children with ASD, Rojas et al. (2008) measured transient evoked and induced neuromagnetic gamma-band power and intertrial phase locking consistency during 1-kHz sine-wave stimuli in parents of children with ASD (42.64 ± 5.14 years old, *n* = 16), adults with ASD (31.46 ± 9.29 years old, *n* = 11), and control participants (43.14 ± 6.66 years old, *n* = 16). Induced gamma power at 40 Hz was significantly higher in the parent and autism groups than in controls, while evoked gamma-band power was reduced compared with the TD group. Furthermore, McFadden et al. (2012) also reported that the parent of a child with ASD (35.84 ± 9.99 years old, *n* = 23) showed increased evoked gamma activity, while controls (*n* = 28) had decreased evoked activity. Additionally, while both groups showed a reduction in total gamma power (commonly seen in language tasks), this reduction was more prominent in the control group. These findings suggest that gamma-band phase consistency and changes in induced power may be potentially useful endophenotypes for ASD, particularly given emerging molecular mechanisms concerning the generation of gamma-band signals.

Recently, Edgar et al. (2015) presented pure tones and assessed activity in STG auditory areas in children with ASD (*n* = 105) and TD (*n* = 36) aged 6 to 16 years and reported decreased early evoked gamma activity and intertrial coherence in children with ASD. These findings replicated previous findings (Rojas et al., 2008; Wilson et al., 2007); however, M100 latency and gamma abnormalities were unrelated. Port et al. (2016), studying children with ASD (6–11 years old, *n* = 27), showed perturbed auditory cortex neural activity during sinusoidal tones, as evident by M100 latency delays as well as reduced transient gamma-band activity. Despite evidence for maturation of these responses in ASD, the neural abnormalities in ASD persisted across time. The authors suggested that the auditory neural measures investigated in this study may serve as prognostic biomarkers, with further study needed to validate such findings. Moreover, Tanigawa et al. (2018) reported that adolescents with ASD (11–15 years old, *n* = 16) had an atypical gamma-band (25–40 Hz) network centered on the left ventral central sulcus (vCS) during Japanese auditory word comprehension task. This study suggested that impairments in the left vCS and gamma-band network activity play an important role in the pathophysiology of impaired auditory language processing in adolescents with ASD.

It has been proposed that ASD may arise from imbalances between excitatory and inhibitory neurotransmission (E/I imbalance). One neural process thought to be reliant on E/I balance is gamma-band activity, with support coming from observed correlations between gamma and underlying gamma-aminobutyric acid (GABA) concentrations in healthy adults. This hypothesis would be attractive in that it implicates a biochemical target for intervention. It remains to be established whether a subset of children with ASD can be defined in whom E/I imbalance is a defining feature. It has thus motivated concomitant investigation of GABA, primarily using magnetic resonance spectroscopy (MRS), as a part of a multimodal characterization of ASD.

Gaetz et al. (2014) investigated creatine-normalized GABA+ ratios (GABA+/Cr) in children with ASD (11.5 ± 2.7 years old, $n = 17$) and TD (13.3 ± 2.87 years old, $n = 17$) using MRS for auditory and other regions of interest (ROIs). MRS is a noninvasive neuroimaging technique that estimates the concentration of specific chemical metabolites and neurotransmitters in vivo (Jansen et al., 2006; Rudin & Sauter, 1992). The authors reported that the motor and auditory ROIs showed significantly reduced GABA+/Cr in ASD (but that visual areas did not). The mean deficiency in GABA+/Cr from the motor ROI was approximately 11%, and that in auditory ROI was approximately 22%. The findings support the model of regional differences in GABA+/Cr in the ASD brain, primarily in auditory and to a lesser extent motor but not visual areas.

Port et al. (2017) combined MEG during sinusoidal tones and edited MRS in TD individuals TD ($n = 27$) and those with ASD (6–40 years old, $n = 30$). Auditory cortex–localized phase locked gamma was compared with resting STG–relative cortical GABA concentrations for both children/adolescents and adults (Figure 21.4). These children/adolescents lacked the typical maturation of GABA+/Cr concentrations and gamma-band coherence. Furthermore, children/adolescents with ASD additionally failed to exhibit the typical GABA+/Cr to gamma-band coherence association. This altered coupling during childhood/adolescence may result in gamma decreases observed in the adults with ASD. Therefore, individuals with ASD may exhibit improper local neuronal circuitry maturation during a childhood/adolescence critical period, when GABA is involved in configuring such circuit functioning, with sequelae persisting into

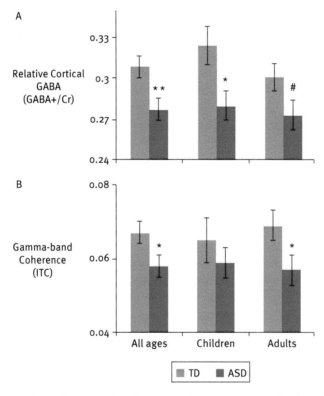

FIGURE 21.4   (A) Relative cortical GABA is reduced in autism spectrum disorder (ASD) compared with TD controls. (B) Deficits in the phase synchrony of gamma oscillations elicited by auditory stimuli are also observed in ASD, becoming more pronounced by adulthood. #, $p < 0.10$, *, $p < 0.05$; **, $p < 0.01$. (Adapted from Port, R. G., Gaetz, W., Bloy, L., Wang, D. J., Blaskey, L., Kuschner, E. S., . . . Roberts, T. P. L. [2017]. Exploring the relationship between cortical GABA concentrations, auditory gamma-band responses and development in ASD: Evidence for an altered maturational trajectory in ASD. *Autism Research, 10*, 593–607.)

adulthood. The authors suggested provocatively a novel line of treatment within a critical time window such that by increasing neural GABA levels in children/adolescents with ASD, proper local circuitry maturation may be restored, resulting in normalized gamma in adulthood. This hypothesis remains to be tested in trials of drugs such as the GABA-B agonist arbaclofen (Berry-Kravis et al., 2012, 2017; Erickson et al., 2014; Veenstra-VanderWeele et al., 2017).

21.3. MAGNETOENCEPHALO-GRAPHY STUDIES OF FACE PROCESSING

Another system of direct relevance to ASD that has undergone extensive MEG research is the area of face processing, as a proxy or probe, for the social impairments commonly experienced by individuals with ASD.

21.3.1. Typical Development of Face Processing

Faces convey an abundance of social signals that are necessary for successful social interactions (Bruce & Young, 1998). Invariant facial features offer information for rapid and accurate identity recognition, and the variant aspects of faces, such as facial expressions of emotion and eye gaze, inform our understanding about others' emotional, communicative, and behavioral intentions, and motivate approach–withdraw decisions (Haxby et al., 2000). Adults are experts at processing faces. The development of face and emotional face processing abilities emerges early in life, such that neonates show a preference for face-like compared with non-face-like stimuli (Goren et al., 1975), recognize familiar (e.g., mother's) compared with nonfamiliar faces (Bushnell et al., 2001), are sensitive to direct compared with averted eye gaze (Farroni et al., 2004), and discern happy, fearful, sad, and surprised facial expressions (Farroni et al., 2007; Field et al., 1982, 1983). Face recognition continues to improve gradually throughout childhood, reaching maturity in the adolescent period (Batty & Taylor,

2006; Carey et al., 1980; Diamond & Carey, 1977; Flin, 1980, 1985; Mondloch et al., 2006; Taylor et al., 2004—although see Crookes & McKone, 2009). Similarly, recognition of emotional faces undergoes a protracted development, with stepwise improvement at 11 years of age (Tonks et al., 2007) and maturation in late adolescence (Batty & Taylor, 2006; Kolb et al., 1992). Speed of processing and greater accuracy improve with age, particularly for negative emotions (De Sonneville et al., 2002; Thomas et al., 2007). Eye gaze direction also plays an important role in facilitating both face and emotional face processing (Adams & Kleck, 2003, 2005; Hood et al., 2003; Smith et al., 2006). In children and adults, direct compared with averted eye gaze boosts face encoding and recognition accuracy (Hood et al., 2003), with direct gaze face recognition accuracy improving with age in childhood (Smith et al., 2006). Eye gaze direction also differentially facilitates speed of emotion recognition depending on emotion type in adults (Adams & Kleck, 2003, 2005).

21.3.2. Face and Emotional Face Processing in Autism Spectrum Disorder

A key feature of ASD is an impairment in social interaction and communication (APA, 2013), thought to be associated with deficits in processing information from faces. Atypicalities in attention to faces are present early in life: high-risk infant siblings who later develop ASD show a lack of eye contact (Adrien et al., 1991; 1993; Clifford et al., 2007; Zwaigenbaum et al., 2005), decreased gaze monitoring (Bernabei et al., 1998), and less interest in faces, as indicated by reduced orienting (Bernabei et al., 1998; Osterling & Dawson, 1994; Werner et al., 2000). In addition, differences in high-risk ASD siblings compared with typical controls in expression of positive emotion (Adrien et al., 1993; Zwaigenbaum et al., 2005), as well as in the neural mechanisms underlying face and emotional face perception, have been reported (Fox et al., 2013). Face processing difficulties persist into child and adulthood. The majority of behavioral studies, although not all, indicate poorer face recognition accuracy and reduced facial memory accuracy in individuals with ASD compared with typical controls across a number of tasks (see Tang et al., 2015, for a review), as well as impairments in establishing eye contact during social interactions (Hobson & Lee, 1998) and in judging eye gaze direction (Wallace et al., 2006). Research on emotion recognition abilities in ASD are mixed, with a number of behavioral findings, including a meta-analysis indicating impaired recognition (Uljarevic & Hamilton, 2013), while others reveal no deficits (see Harms et al., 2010, for a review).

Results from fMRI studies have provided a further understanding of the neural mechanisms involved in face processing in ASD. The majority of these studies have outlined atypical neural activation in brain regions known to be part of the core and extended face processing network (Haxby et al., 2000, 2002) in individuals with ASD (Dalton et al., 2005; Deeley et al., 2007; Pierce et al., 2001; Pierce & Redcay, 2008; Schultz et al., 2000; see also Corbett et al., 2009; Critchley et al., 2000; Nomi & Uddin, 2015). For instance, abnormal activation in central face processing areas, including the inferior occipital gyri (Pierce et al., 2001, 2004), lateral fusiform gyri (Corbett et al., 2009; Critchley et al., 2000; Deeley et al., 2007; Pierce et al., 2001), and regions implicated in gaze processing such as superior temporal sulci (Pelphrey et al., 2005, 2007), have been reported in ASD compared with controls. Additionally, these studies have highlighted abnormal brain activity in the amygdalae (Ashwin, 2007; Baron-Cohen et al., 1999; Corbett et al., 2009; Dapretto et al., 2006; Pelphrey, et al., 2007; Pierce et al., 2001) and frontal areas, including orbitofrontal cortex, inferior frontal cortex, and anterior cingulate cortex (ACC), as well as the insular cortices (Ashwin et al., 2007; Dapretto et al., 2006; Di Martino et al., 2009; Hubl et al., 2003; Ogai et al., 2003), to emotional faces in ASD.

Fewer studies have used neurophysiological techniques, such as EEG and MEG, to explore face processing in ASD. EEG studies found a lack of sensitivity to different emotional face types (Wagner et al., 2013) or to inverted versus upright faces (an indication of face expertise; Webb et al., 2009), as well as attenuated and delayed neural components, particularly the P1—reflecting early global perceptual processing of faces (Halit et al., 2000), and N170—reflecting structural encoding specific to faces (Eimer, 2000), over occipital and occipital-temporal electrode areas involved in early perceptual processing of faces in ASD compared with controls (Apicella et al., 2013; Batty et al., 2011; McPartland et al., 2004; O'Connor et al., 2007; Webb et al., 2006). Only a small body of research has taken advantage of MEG, which offers a direct measure of neural activity, as well as excellent temporal resolution and high spatial accuracy (Hari & Puce, 2017; Hansen et al., 2010). Studies using MEG have greatly complemented and contributed to our understanding of the dynamics of neural activity underlying face and emotional processing in ASD. MEG research also sheds light on interregional differences in synchrony of neural oscillations, a key mechanism of brain communication, supporting social cognitive processes. In this section, we review the MEG studies highlighting temporal and spatial differences of neural activity, and alterations in patterns of functional connectivity underlying face and emotional processing in ASD compared with typical development. First, MEG studies of faces versus nonface stimuli, and the influence of eye gaze direction on neural responses and networks in ASD, will be described. Second, MEG work studying neural activation and functional connectivity during emotional face processing in ASD will be reviewed.

21.3.3. Magnetoencephalography Investigations of Face and Gaze Processing in Autism Spectrum Disorder

Only a handful of studies have used MEG to assess face and gaze processing in ASD (Bailey et al., 2005; Hasegawa et al., 2013; Kylliäinen et al., 2006; Sun et al., 2012). Bailey et al. (2005) investigated evoked responses in adults with (*n* = 12) and without (*n* = 22) ASD using a MEG sensor approach when presented with faces and nonface stimuli in two tasks, in which participants (a) categorized a target stimulus (either faces, motorbikes, animals, or dot patterns) and (b) identified whether sequentially presented pairs of stimuli (pairs of faces, mugs, or dot patterns) were the same or different. In both tasks, controls demonstrated greater activation mostly over the inferior occipital-temporal cortex at approximately 145 ms to faces compared with nonface stimuli. Specifically, in the first task, controls showed greater activation to faces than to animals, motorbikes, and dot patterns, and in the second task greater activation to faces than mugs. In contrast, responses to faces were attenuated in adults with ASD at 145 ms. In the first task, adults with ASD only showed greater activation to faces compared with motorbikes. Additionally, using equivalent dipole modeling, face-specific dipoles were laterally located in controls, while the location of dipoles in response to faces and nonface stimuli overlapped in ASD, indicating stimulus-nonspecific cortical localization for processing faces and nonface images. The authors suggested that in ASD, cortical regions involved in face processing may be involved additionally in processing nonface stimuli. Furthermore, in controls, stronger activation to the first versus the second face images was found at an early latency over right anterior temporal areas in the identification task. In ASD, the converse pattern of activation was found—second face images elicited greater activation than corresponding first face images in this early latency range. It was suggested that increased early activation to faces following the second image rather than the first may suggest atypical face processing strategies in ASD.

MEG research has also revealed abnormal gamma-band activation during face processing in ASD. Sun et al. (2012) examined sensor-level gamma-band spectral power and source-localized gamma-band activity in adults with (*n* = 13) and without (*n* =16) ASD during the perception of Mooney faces. Gamma-band oscillations are a key mechanism in synchronous neural spiking facilitating local circuitry related to perceptual processes and are implicated in face processing (Fries, 2009; Luo et al., 2007). At the sensor level, controls demonstrated an increase in low- and high-gamma-band power over parieto-occipital scalp regions (100–300 ms) following Mooney face presentation relative to baseline, as well as reduced low-gamma-band power over frontocentral areas. In ASD, a reduction in low- and high-gamma-band power over parieto-occipital regions was found. The source analyses revealed decreased activation in brain areas involved in face perception in ASD compared with controls, including the right fusiform, lingual, and superior temporal gyri, left hippocampal gyrus and precuneus, and bilateral supramarginal gyri in the high-gamma band, as well as the left inferior frontal gyrus and insula in the low-gamma band. When considering between-group differences in gamma activation to Mooney faces versus nonface stimuli, controls showed greater high-gamma-band activation among a frontoparietal network to faces compared with adults with ASD, whereas in ASD, increased high-gamma-band activation was found in visual areas. The results suggest that not only do adults with ASD show impaired gamma-band spectral power during visual processing/perceptual organization of faces, but they also engage a different neural circuit than controls.

Eye gaze processing in ASD, which is thought to contribute to difficulties in social cognition, was explored by Hasegawa et al. (2013). They investigated low- and high-level perceptual processes during gaze perception in adults with and without ASD (*n* = 12/group). MEG activity of the primary visual cortex (V1), superior temporal sulcus (STS), and fusiform gyrus were analyzed in an early (50–150 ms) and late (250–350 ms) time window following pairs of faces with a change (direct or averted) or no change in gaze direction. In adults with ASD, V1 amplitude was increased to averted gaze in the late time window, suggesting that individuals with ASD may exhibit atypical low-level visual processes. In controls, increased right posterior STS activation was found to direct gaze compared with avert gaze in the late latency window; this effect was absent in ASD. Because direct versus averted gaze serves as a social cue and engages the posterior STS in typical development, late V1 activation to averted gaze in ASD was thought to reflect featural part-based processing of gaze direction, rather than appreciating its value as a social signal.

In a same–different task, Kylliäinen et al. (2006) examined neural responses to faces expressing direct gaze, closed eyes, or left/right averted gaze, and motorbikes (control stimulus), in 7- to 12-year-old TD children ($n = 10$) and ASD children ($n = 10$). Early in perceptual processing (100 ms), increased activation for faces compared with motorbikes were found in both groups. At 140 ms, however, the TD group demonstrated comparable amplitudes for faces and motorbikes, but with a delayed latency for motorbikes over right inferior occipitotemporal areas. In contrast, a greater and nondelayed response to motorbikes was found in children with ASD over the same brain areas. Additionally, differences in gaze processing were observed in controls and children with ASD at 240 ms. In the TD group, enhanced activation to averted gaze relative to direct gaze or closed eyes was observed, while children with ASD demonstrated an increased response to direct gaze. These findings were interpreted to reflect increased physiological arousal elicited by direct versus averted gaze in children with ASD. Overall, neural mechanisms involved in different stages of face and gaze processing demonstrate some similarities in amplitude strength, latency, and topography in both TD and ASD, yet atypicalities are apparent in children with the disorder (Kylliäinen et al., 2006).

Lajiness-O'Neill et al. (2014) reported that adolescents with ASD ($n = 10$) demonstrated atypical neural coherence to faces expressing averted gaze in low-frequency (delta, theta, alpha) and high-frequency (beta, gamma) bands compared with controls ($n = 8$). In particular, elevated coherence was seen in ASD, primarily among temporoparietal-occipital regions, which was most prominent in the low-frequency bands, but reduced synchrony in frontal and frontotemporal-parietal areas, in the low frequencies. In controls, increased coherence was observed among frontal, frontotemporal, and frontoparietal regions across frequency bands compared with adolescents with ASD. Furthermore, to averted gaze, more synchronous interhemispheric connections were found in adolescents with ASD compared with controls in the low frequencies, as well as a lack of intrahemispheric connections in the beta band. These altered patterns of synchronous neural activity were suggested to affect functional circuitry underpinning atypical sensitivity to eye gaze following and related social difficulties in ASD.

21.3.4. Magnetoencephalography Investigations of Emotional Face Processing in Autism Spectrum Disorder

A few MEG studies have also highlighted evoked neural activity in brain regions critical for the perception of emotional faces in ASD. Using MEG and spatial filtering, Leung et al. (2018) examined activity during an implicit emotional faces task in adults with and without ASD ($n = 26$/group). Participants saw an emotional face (happy or angry) paired simultaneously with a corresponding scrambled pattern (target) on either side of a central fixation cross; they were instructed to fixate on the cross and rapidly respond left or right to the location of the target; the emotional faces were irrelevant. Between-group differences were found starting 100 ms after presentation of angry and happy faces in occipitotemporal and limbic brain areas. To both happy and angry faces, adults with ASD showed hyperactivity in key emotional face processing areas, such as the inferior temporal and fusiform gyri, amygdala and anterior insula, and ACC and hypoactivity in occipital and parietal areas and ACC compared with typical controls. In addition, no effect of emotion was found in ASD, while angry faces elicited greater activity in in posterior regions in controls. The authors suggested that individuals with ASD may lack neural specificity to angry versus happy faces. Although individuals with ASD engage traditional emotional face processing regions, overactivation and underactivation may contribute to impairment in evaluating salience and deriving social reward from emotional faces.

Leung et al. (2015) completed the same protocol in adolescents with ($n = 24$) and without ($n = 24$) ASD. Similar to adults, adolescents with ASD showed patterns of both hyperactivation and hypoactivation compared with controls in established brain areas for emotional face processing, including frontal, temporal, tempoparietal, and limbic brain areas. Of particular interest, the adolescents with ASD demonstrated reduced activity in the orbital frontal, temporal, and limbic areas, suggesting atypical recruitment of these regions during emotional face processing. The authors suggested that atypical involvement of these regions may contribute to insensitivity to angry faces related to poor associative learning and prediction of potential aversive outcomes.

Also using a beamforming approach, Wright et al. (2012) investigated induced and evoked gamma-band activation in children with ASD ($n = 13$) and TD controls ($n = 13$) during the passive viewing of emotional faces (happy, sad, fearful, angry, disgust). Between-group differences revealed reduced gamma-band (30–80 Hz) responses in ASD in lateral occipital areas, peaking in the lateral occipital cortex between 250 and 450 ms, compared with controls. The TD children showed an increase in gamma activation in visual areas, an effect that was not observed in those with ASD. In addition, a time–frequency virtual electrode analysis revealed atypical induced gamma-band power in the occipital and fusiform areas in children with ASD, while evoked gamma-band power was intact. Because induced gamma activation is thought to be important for global feature processing, abnormal induced gamma responses to emotional faces in children with ASD were suggested to underpin impairments in the early stages of holistic face processing.

21.3.5. Magnetoencephalography Functional Connectivity and Emotional Face Processing in Autism Spectrum Disorder

An increasing body of research has now conceptualized ASD as a neural network disorder (see Just et al., 2012, for a review). Thus, recent MEG studies have focused on examining the functional connections underlying important aspects of socioemotional functioning, such as emotional face processing in this disorder (Khan et al., 2013; Leung et al., 2014; Mamashli et al., 2017; Mennella et al., 2017; Safar et al., 2018). Khan et al. (2013) investigated phase–amplitude coupling (PAC) in the right fusiform gyrus, and long-range functional connectivity, as indexed by event-related normalized coherence, between the right fusiform gyrus and the whole brain to emotional faces (i.e., neutral, angry, fearful) and houses in adolescents and young adults with ($n = 17$) and without ($n = 20$) ASD. In the TD group, greater PAC between alpha phase and gamma amplitude in the right fusiform was increased in response to faces, but not to houses; this effect was absent in ASD. Moreover, in ASD, decreased long-range functional connectivity was found in the alpha frequency band between the right fusiform gyrus and left precuneus, left inferior frontal gyrus, and left ACC to emotional faces compared with houses. These results suggest reduced local and long-range connections in ASD to faces. More recently, using the emotional faces task described previously, Mennella et al. (2017) also found reduced whole-brain beta-band functional connectivity, measured using phase synchrony, in adults with ASD versus TD controls ($n = 22$/group) to angry faces. In particular, this network of reduced phase synchrony was observed at approximately 300 ms after angry face onset, involving primarily frontal–limbic connections, as well as connections to occipital areas. Of particular interest, this hypoconnected network included the left amygdala, left insula, and lingual gyrus—important areas of the social brain. Similarly, reduced whole-brain beta-band phase synchrony has been reported 0 to 400 ms following implicit angry face presentation in adolescents with ASD (n = 22) compared with TD controls (n = 17; Leung et al., 2014). This hypoconnected network involved widespread connections, importantly involving the right fusiform gyrus and right insula, with the right insula serving as a hub of reduced connectivity strength within the network. Leung et al. (2014) suggested that reduced functional connectivity to angry faces may reflect disrupted long-range neural communication among a network implicated in the rapid perception of angry faces, including the right insula, which may contribute to difficulty evaluating the emotional salience of angry faces.

Similar to adults and adolescents with ASD, atypical functional connectivity in children with ASD versus TD controls has been highlighted in recent MEG research (Safar et al., 2018). Using the emotional faces task as described previously, Safar et al. (2018) examined whole-brain functional connectivity of eight a priori regions of interest, including bilateral amygdalae, fusiform gyri, insulae, and ACC, during the implicit processing of happy and angry faces in 7- to 12-year-old children with ASD (n = 20) and TD controls (n = 22). A network of increased phase synchrony in the alpha frequency band

was revealed during the first 400 ms of implicit happy face processing in children with ASD compared with controls. This hyperconnected network involved connections among the left fusiform and right inferior frontal gyrus, and left superior frontal gyrus, as well as the right insula and right superior temporal gyrus, and bilateral orbitofrontal regions. From this network, the left fusiform gyrus and right insula showed greater connectivity strength in children with ASD compared with TD controls (85–208 ms and 73–270 ms, respectively). The authors suggested that this hyperconnected network reflects atypical communication among occipitotemporal brain areas critically implicated in the perception of happy faces, as well as frontal and limbic areas necessary for evaluation and conceptualization. Taking into account atypical patterns of functional connectivity in adolescents and adults with ASD, these results provide further evidence for an altered neurodevelopmental trajectory of emotional face processing. Unlike adolescents and adults with ASD, children with ASD in this study demonstrated the converse pattern (hyperconnectivity vs. hypoconnectivity) of functional connectivity compared with adults and adolescents with the disorder (Figure 21.5).

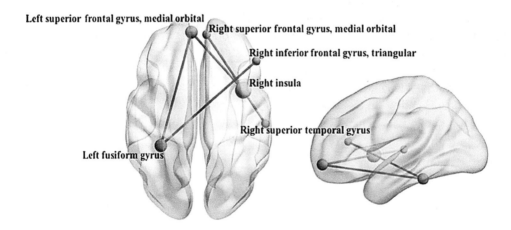

FIGURE 21.5   Network of increased alpha-band phase synchronization (0–400 ms) following happy face perception in children with autism spectrum disorder compared with typically developing controls. Node size is scaled by the mean group difference in connectivity strength. (Adapted from Safar, K., Wong, S. M., Leung, R. C., Dunkley, B. T., & Taylor, M. J. [2018]. Increased functional connectivity during emotional face processing in children with autism spectrum disorder. *Frontiers in Human Neuroscience, 12*, 408.)

It has been recently proposed that the reported discrepancies of age-related changes in the direction of connectivity in ASD may be reconciled by taking developmental stages into account (Uddin et al., 2013). Using MEG, Mamashli et al. (2018) examined the developmental trajectory of local and long-range functional connectivity both in children (7–13 years of age) and adolescents and young adults (14–21 years of age) with ASD and TD controls, while presented with emotional faces and houses. This work was an extension of that by Khan et al. (2013) described previously, with some overlap in the cohort of older participants. As in the study by Khan et al. (2013), local and long-range connectivity was assessed by PAC in the right fusiform gyrus, and normalized coherence (with respect to houses) was assessed between the right fusiform gyrus and precuneus, inferior frontal gyrus, and ACC. Although findings indicated no group differences in both metrics of local and long-range connectivity in children with ASD to emotional faces relative to houses, when combining the two age cohorts, both metrics of functional connectivity were negatively correlated with age in ASD, while positively correlated with age in TD controls. In ASD only, a multivariate linear regression analysis revealed that alpha-gamma PAC primarily contributed to predicting age, suggesting that the developmental trajectory of local connectivity during emotional face processing might be particularly disrupted in this group. These results support the hypothesis that differences in patterns of functional connectivity may evolve with age in ASD, possibly initiated by the onset of adolescence (Picci et al., 2015, 2016; Uddin et al., 2013).

21.3.6. Summary of Face Processing Studies

MEG research has mapped the temporal and spatial dynamics of neural mechanisms underlying face and emotional face processing, advancing our understanding of the neurobiology underlying social deficits characteristic of the disorder. These studies have highlighted an atypical neurodevelopmental trajectory of face processing from child to adulthood.

Adults with ASD demonstrate key differences in the strength and cortical location of neural responses to faces versus other types of visual stimuli (temporally corresponding to the N170 face-sensitive component) compared with typical controls, suggesting that in ASD, face and nonface stimuli may be processed similarly. Differences in neural activation in very early stages of face processing are also demonstrated in ASD, which may support the use of alternate face processing strategies, influencing later stages of processing (e.g., N170; Bailey et al., 2005). Abnormal gamma-band activity may also play an important role in the perception of faces in ASD, evident by the recruitment of different neural circuitry, particularly posterior brain areas versus a frontoparietal network, during the perceptual organization of faces (Sun et al., 2012). Like adults with ASD, children with the disorder may also lack face-specific sensitivity because key differences in strength and latency of neural responses to faces versus nonface stimuli at a latency presumed to correspond to the N170 are observed (Kyliäinen et al., 2006). Furthermore, both children and adults with ASD demonstrate atypical patterns of neural activation to eye gaze direction compared with controls (Hasegawa et al., 2013; Kyliäinen et al., 2006).

Young adults and adolescents with ASD demonstrate patterns of both hyperactivation and hypoactivation to emotional faces beginning in early stages of perceptual processing, suggesting abnormal recruitment of established of social brain areas (Leung et al., 2015, 2018). Atypical engagement of these regions may contribute to difficulties such as evaluating the social reward, deriving salience of emotional expressions, and immature/delayed threat processing (Leung et al., 2015, 2018). Abnormal gamma-band power also plays an important role in atypical emotion processing in children and adolescents with ASD, particularly in visual areas, thought to suggest impaired global perception of emotional faces (Wright et al., 2012).

Finally, MEG research has highlighted an atypical developmental trajectory of functional neural circuitry to emotional faces in ASD (Khan et al., 2013; Leung et al., 2014; Mamashli et al., 2017; Mennella et al., 2017; Safar et al., 2018). Differences in the direction (i.e., increased vs. decreased) of functional connectivity from children through to adults with the disorder have been observed, which may be reconciled by accounting for developmental stage, particularly adolescence, which is a period of considerable structural and functional neural maturation (Mamashli et al., 2018; Uddin et al., 2013).

21.4. VISUAL MAGNETOENCEPHALOGRAPHY STUDIES IN AUTISM SPECTRUM DISORDER

Several studies have examined functional responses in ASD in relation to visual tasks that tap both perceptual and cognitive processes using visual stimuli, other than studies using face stimuli (detailed previously). There is a significant literature indicating that those with ASD have perceptual atypicalities—sometimes improved abilities and sometimes poorer abilities compared with their TD peers (Dakin & Frith, 2005)—and atypicalities across sensory modalities are considered as core symptoms of autism (APA, 2013; Marco et al., 2011). An important question in the literature is the impact of early perceptual differences on higher level visual processing. With its temporal sensitivity, MEG is particularly valuable in examining this issue.

Falter et al. (2013) found support for enhanced early MEG responses in a visual discrimination task in 16- to 38-year-olds with ASD ($n = 16$) compared with matched controls ($n = 18$). The ASD group performed better on the task and had larger occipital responses that correlated with performance. Using the same perceptual simultaneity task, Menassa et al. (2018) measured evoked gamma phase locking in young adults with ($n = 16$) and without

($n = 17$) ASD; they found that gamma-band (~70 Hz) activity in the left frontal region correlated with responses in the ASD group only; the controls showed greater gamma activity in the parieto-occipital areas.

A number of reports have used visual motion stimuli to also assess gamma-band power or modulation because gamma is sensitive to excitatory–inhibitory balance, which has been shown to be altered in ASD. Peiker et al. (2015b) presented adults (ASD = 13, controls = 14) with a motion detection task using random dot stimuli, and analyzed data from occipital and parietal sensors. Polynomial regression analyses showed greater increases in gamma-band power with increasing motion intensity that was stronger in the ASD than control group. As response gain is controlled by excitatory–inhibitory interactions, the authors suggested that the MEG data confirmed that this balance was disturbed in ASD. Similarly, Stroganova et al. (2015) analyzed the modulation of high gamma oscillations (50–120 Hz) by the speed of moving visual gratings in boys 7 to 15 years old, with ($n = 21$) and without ($n = 26$) ASD. The frequency of the oscillatory response in gamma, which generally increased with the speed of the visual stimuli, was reduced in a subset of boys with ASD. Also, the gamma modulation was related to visual perceptual ability in the ASD group only. These findings were related to other studies by the same group showing reduced visual perceptual abilities behaviorally in ASD (Sysoeva et al., 2016, 2017).

With a more complex perceptual integration task, Peiker et al. (2015a) found evidence of poor interhemispheric integration in ASD adults compared with the matched controls ($n = 20$/group). The MEG data showed an absence of enhanced interhemispheric gamma coherence in the ASD group as well as local reductions posteriorly in beta band power that were associated with performance. They suggested that the local and global disturbances in synchronization may affect object recognition in ASD. In contrast,

Takesaki et al. (2016) found that increases in imaginary coherence in the gamma band in 4.5- to 10-year-old children with ASD and TD (n = 18/group) was associated with higher performance in the matrix analogies task, a test of nonverbal visual reasoning. This increase was anchored in visual areas in the children. Kikuchi et al. (2013) used this same task in young children (5–7 years of age) to determine whether the MEG reflected preserved abilities in those with and without ASD—26 per group. Measuring from five sensors per hemisphere overlying language-related areas, the authors reported that right lateralized connectivity in gamma increased with reading ability in the young children with ASD. Moreover, Ogawa et al. (2019) examined cortical activation patterns in adolescents with ASD (11–15 years, n = 14) during silent Japanese word-reading. The authors reported that abnormal cortical activation of the right central sulcus correlated significantly with lower visual word comprehension scores, suggesting that atypical cortical activation in the temporal-frontal area, which is associated with higher order language processing functions, such as semantic analysis, may play a crucial role in visual word comprehension in adolescents with ASD.

21.5. MAGNETOENCEPHALO-GRAPHY STUDIES OF SENSORIMOTOR ASPECTS OF AUTISM SPECTRUM DISORDER

Recently, Gaetz et al. showed deficits in the somatosensory P50m evoked response amplitude in ASD (n = 15) compared with age-matched controls (n = 15) (Gaetz et al., 2017). This component is widely taken as reflecting inhibitory processing and as such provides some level of converging support for the E/I imbalance hypothesis. Interestingly, while no latency differences were found in this component (in contradistinction to the auditory sensory responses), the diminished response amplitude was similar to that in an age-matched cohort of children with epilepsy (n = 17), also known to have imbalances of excitatory and inhibitory processes. This initial foray certainly supports the trans-disorder commonalities at a biological level, and in part provides support for the high rates of clinical diagnosis comorbidity.

Furthermore, An et al. (2018) focused on the gamma oscillations during motor control in ASD. MEG signals were recorded from children with ASD (5–7 years, n = 14) and TD children (n = 15) during a motor task. The authors observed that the ASD group exhibited a low peak frequency of motor-related gamma oscillations from the contralateral primary motor cortex, and these were associated with the severity of autism symptoms. A linear discriminant analysis using the button response time and gamma oscillations showed a high classification performance (86.2% accuracy). The findings also suggested the alterations of the gamma oscillations in ASD might reflect the cortical excitatory and inhibitory imbalance.

21.6. MAGNETOENCEPHALO-GRAPHY APPROACHES TO HIGHER COGNITIVE FUNCTIONS

With a simple picture-naming task, Buard et al. (2013) focused on classic language areas. Following MEG source analyses, they found reduced gamma activity in the right STS and left inferior frontal gyrus (IFG) at long latencies in 12 young adults with ASD compared with 35 controls, while increased beta and gamma connectivity was seen in the LH in the ASD group. None of these effects correlated with behavioral metrics, perhaps owing to the small number in the ASD group. In a similarly powered study, Braeutigam et al. (2008) examined semantic violations in adults with ASD versus controls (n = 11 in each group) using the classic N4 paradigm (Kutas & Hillyard, 1980). The authors measured evoked responses (N4) as well as phase locking of low gamma. The ASD group had smaller N4s to the incongruous words but stronger long-latency gamma in central and frontal areas to the congruous words. Only those with ASD showed an increase in gamma (>40 Hz) to the incongruous words. The authors suggested atypical but successful strategies in the ASD group because there were no behavioral differences, and further pointed out the presence of long-range connectivity in ASD.

A few studies have also examined executive functions in youth with ASD, using visual protocols. Inhibition in a go/no-go task was examined in adolescents with and without ASD (15/group), where the control condition did not require inhibition, and no-go trials could be contrasted without the confound of a speeded motor response (Vara et al., 2014). The adolescents with ASD recruited a series of frontal regions to perform the task, whereas the controls recruited frontal, temporal, and then parietal regions for equivalent task performance. The authors argued that the ASD group had a restricted inhibitory network, with inefficient longer range interactions seen in the typical population.

Another key executive function is working memory. Urbain et al. (2015), using an abstract patterns n-back task, compared MEG sources and time courses in 7- to 13-year-old children with and without ASD (20 in each group). The TD children activated the right hippocampus and ACC for correct 1-back recognition, while the ASD group showed activity in the left insula. The hippocampal strength correlated positively with performance only for the TD group, while the ACC activity was stronger in the ASD children with lower ADOS scores. Connectivity measures with the 2-back task (Urbain et al., 2016) revealed reduced alpha synchronization in the ASD group, including the insula and ACC, and reduced connectivity in a network anchored in the right fusiform correlated with symptom severity. Alpha has been strongly associated with mnemonic processes (Sauseng et al., 2005; Palva et al., 2010); this study showed its importance in school-aged children, with reductions seen in those with ASD, who are often reported to have memory impairments (e.g., Steele et al., 2007).

Some people with ASD have, however, exceptional memories for some categories of items, such as timetables—considered "savants." Neumann et al. (2010) completed an n-back task with pseudowords and shapes, with an average of nine intervening items between repeats. The ASD savant group and TD group (seven per group) did not differ on performance, but this was likely because the task did not match the abilities of the savants. Source analyses found that the ASD group activated occipital areas, while the controls activated parietal areas, which the authors suggested was related to the visual processing style commonly reported in ASD in fMRI studies (e.g., Koshino et al., 2005; Simard et al., 2015; Vogan et al., 2014). In a similar vein, Meaux et al. (2014) examined numerosity (number) estimation in adults with and without ASD ($n = 14$/group) because this is often reported as an exceptional ability. As stimuli, they used 80 to 150 dots arranged in the shape of an animal or randomly (nonanimal), and participants had to estimate the number of dots present. Group differences in performance were seen at larger numerosities, and the ASD group were not affected by the gestalt of the dot arrangement (animal vs. nonanimal), whereas the controls were. The source-analyzed MEG results showed a cascade of effects starting with reduced amplitude responses occipitally and parietally in the ASD (Figure 21.6A) and an absence of frontal activity (see Figure 21.6B). The authors suggested overlapping atypical processing in perceptual and number-related aspects of the task. When connectivity analyses were completed on these data, reduced early (70–145 ms) long-range beta synchronization was seen in ASD, which was considered to contribute to the difficulties the ASD group had with the integrative processes required with this task (Bangel et al., 2014).

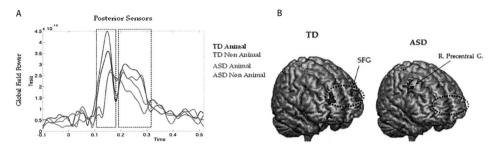

FIGURE 21.6   (A) During numerosity estimation, global field power for posterior sensors to animal and nonanimal stimuli in autism spectrum disorder (ASD) and typically developing (TD) groups, showing that differences between the stimuli appear around 120 ms (NA > A) and 200–290ms (A > NA) in TD participants. In ASD participants, differences (NA > A) were observed only in the second time window. (B) At 450 to 500 ms, bilateral superior frontal gyrus (SFG) activity was seen in TD subjects, while only right precentral gyrus activity was found for the ASD group. (Adapted from Meaux, E., Taylor, M. J., Pang, E. W., Vara, A. S., & Batty, M. [2014]. Neural substrates of numerosity estimation in autism. *Human Brain Mapping, 35*[9], 4362–4385.)

21.7. MAGNETOENCEPHALO- GRAPHY RESTING-STATE ANALYSES

Because resting-state scans are task-free, they are generally easier to complete across a wider range of ages and abilities. Resting-state analyses also allow one to probe intrinsic networks in the brain and how these may differ with typical or atypical development. Neuroimaging studies that have examined resting state have proposed that ASD is a disorder of brain connectivity that includes both or either hyperconnectivity and hypoconnectivity. A recent paradigm shift suggested that disparate age-related connectivity differences reported in ASD may be reconciled by taking developmental stages into account (Uddin et al., 2013). In particular, resting-state fMRI studies focusing on child populations demonstrate hyperconnectivity in ASD (Di Martino et al., 2011; Keown et al., 2013; Uddin et al., 2013), while reports on adolescents and adults with ASD more often report hypoconnectivity in the ASD group (Cherkassky et al., 2006; Kennedy & Courchesne, 2008; Monk et al., 2009). Most of the research has been with fMRI; hence, critical features of functional connectivity at fast frequencies in ASD have not been fully explored. Establishing the connectivity patterns linked with disrupted neurophysiological brain connectivity in ASD has important

implications for establishing a coherent model of the pathophysiology of ASD.

In young children with ASD (3–7 years old) and matched controls (35/group), Kikuchi et al. (2013) recorded resting state while the children watched and listened to a video of their choice. On average, 140 s of data were analyzed, but the authors analyzed data from only five sensors per hemisphere. They reported right-sided lateralization in low gamma (30–59 Hz), but this did not correlate with behavioral measures. In a later study with the same protocol, but a larger number of children (50/group; mean age, 5 years) analyzed theta band connectivity from a circle of 26 sensors over frontal, temporal, and parietal areas. Some reduction in long-range coherence was seen in the children with ASD, which was linked to clinical severity in a subgroup.

In smaller groups of participants (15/group) that spanned a wide age range (6–21 years), Kitzbichler et al. (2015) mapped group differences in sensory space and onto cortical surface space, and reported differences between the ASD and TD. Graph theory metric differences were also reported, but given the small numbers and wide age range, these results are in need of replication, before assigning them certainty. In the largest resting-state MEG study to date, Vakorin et al. (2017) showed that youth with ASD aged 7 to 16 years ($n = 61$)

did not show group differences compared with controls ($n = 73$) but instead exhibited altered maturational curvature in a frequency- and region-specific manner that distinguished the two groups. The ASD group demonstrated a more disordered developmental pattern than the TD youth. The most marked differences were seen in frontal areas and the cerebellum, consistent with other studies reporting these brain areas particularly implicated in ASD (e.g., Fatemi et al., 2012; Margari et al., 2018; Taylor et al., 2014).

Given the relative ease with which resting state can be acquired, and given that a wider range of participants can be included, there is much that can be learned from this approach to understanding the neurophysiological underpinnings of ASD, with greater expectations of delving into possible subgroupings of the disorder and of having a means of monitoring neural changes with interventions.

21.8. SYNTHESIS AND PERSPECTIVE

Overall, it appears that the spectro-spatiotemporal properties of MEG offer considerable promise in the study of ASD. The disorder is characterized by phenotypic heterogeneity, and thus MEG investigations of multiple brain systems are emerging, with the principal foci to date on the core areas of social impairment and language dysfunction. Two emerging hypotheses of ASD in terms of atypical connectivity and an imbalance of excitation and inhibition are increasingly being evaluated using MEG-based approaches, contributing to our mechanistic understanding of the disorder as well as providing a biological basis for stratification of ASD into subtypes of more common biological basis. As these MEG measures develop, their utility will likely evolve from providing supporting evidence for mechanistic hypotheses through biomarkers for stratification, clinical trial enrichment, and treatment selection to full clinical indicators of diagnosis, prognosis, and treatment response.

REFERENCES

Adams Jr., R. B., & Kleck, R. E. (2003). Perceived gaze direction and the processing of facial displays of emotion. *Psychological Science*, 14(6), 644–647.

Adams Jr., R. B., & Kleck, R. E. (2005). Effects of direct and averted gaze on the perception of facially communicated emotion. *Emotion*, 5(1), 3–11.

Adrien, J. L., Faure, M., Perrot, A., Hameury, L., Garreau, B., Barthelemy, C., & Sauvage, D. (1991). Autism and family home movies: Preliminary findings. *Journal of Autism and Developmental Disorders*, 21(1), 43–49.

Adrien, J. L., Lenoir, P., Martineau, J., Perrot, A., Hameury, L., Larmande, C., & Sauvage, D. (1993). Blind ratings of early symptoms of autism based upon family home movies. *Journal of the American Academy of Child & Adolescent Psychiatry*, 32(3), 617–626.

American Psychiatric Association. (2013). *Diagnostic and statistical manual of mental disorders (DSM-5)*. Washington, DC: American Psychiatric Association.

An, K., Ikeda, T., Yoshimura, Y., Hasegawa, C., Saito, D.N., Kumazaki, H., . . . Kikuchi, M. (2018). *Altered gamma oscillations during motor control in children with autism spectrum disorder. Journal of Neuroscience, 38(36)*,7878–7886.

Apicella, F., Sicca, F., Federico, R. R., Campatelli, G., & Muratori, F. (2013). Fusiform gyrus responses to neutral and emotional faces in children with autism spectrum disorders: A high density ERP study. *Behavioural Brain Research, 251*, 155–162.

Ashwin, C., Baron-Cohen, S., Wheelwright, S., O'Riordan, M., & Bullmore, E. T. (2007). Differential activation of the amygdala and the "social brain" during fearful face-processing in Asperger syndrome. *Neuropsychologia, 45*(1), 2–14.

Bailey, A. J., Braeutigam, S., Jousmäki, V., & Swithenby, S. J. (2005). Abnormal activation of face processing systems at early and intermediate latency in individuals with autism spectrum disorder: A magnetoencephalographic study. *European Journal of Neuroscience, 21*(9), 2575–2585.

Bangel, K., Batty, M., Ye, A. X., Meaux, E., Taylor, M. J., & Doesburg, S.M. (2014). Reduced beta band connectivity during number estimation in autism. *NeuroImage: Clinical, 6*, 202–213.

Baron-Cohen, S., Ring, H. A., Wheelwright S., Bullmore, E. T., Brammer, M. J., Simmons, A., & Williams, S. C. (1999). Social intelligence in the normal and autistic brain: an fMRI study. *European Journal of Neuroscience, 11*(6), 1891–1898.

Batty, M., Meaux, E., Wittemeyer, K., Rogé, B., & Taylor, M. J. (2011). Early processing of emotional faces in children with autism: An event-related potential study. *Journal of Experimental Child Psychology, 109*(4), 430–444.

Batty, M., & Taylor, M. J. (2006). The development of emotional face processing during childhood. *Developmental Science, 9*(2), 207–220.

Berman, J. I., Edgar, J. C., Blaskey, L., Kuschner, E. S., Levy, S. E., Ku, M., . . . Roberts, T. P. L. (2016). Multimodal diffusion-MRI and MEG assessment of auditory and language system development in autism spectrum disorder. *Frontiers in Neuroanatomy,10*(30).

Bernabei, P., Camaioni, L., & Levi, G. (1998). An evaluation of early development in children with autism and pervasive developmental disorders from home movies: Preliminary findings. *Autism, 2,* 243–258.

Berry-Kravis, E., Hagerman, R., Visootsak, J., Budimirovic, D., Kaufmann, W. E., Cherubini, M., . . .Carpenter, R. L. (2017). Arbaclofen in fragile X syndrome: Results of phase 3 trials. *Journal of Neurodevelopmental Disorders, 12*(9), 3.

Berry-Kravis, E. M., Hessl, D., Rathmell, B., Zarevics, P., Cherubini, M., Walton-Bowen K., . . . Hagerman, R. J. (2012). Effects of STX209 (arbaclofen) on neurobehavioral function in children and adults with fragile X syndrome: A randomized, controlled, phase 2 trial. *Science Translational Medicine, 4*(152), 127.

Braeutigam, S., Swithenby, S. J., & Bailey, A. J. (2008). Contextual integration the unusual way: A magnetoencephalographic study of responses to semantic violation in individuals with autism spectrum disorders. *European Journal of Neuroscience, 27*(4), 1026–1036.

Brandwein, A. B., Foxe, J. J., Butler, J. S., Russo, N. N., Altschuler, T. S., Gomes, H., & Molholm, S. (2013). The development of multisensory integration in high-functioning autism: High-density electrical mapping and psychophysical measures reveal impairments in the processing of audiovisual inputs. *Cerebral Cortex, 23,*1329–1341.

Bruce, V., & Young, A. (1998). *In the eye of the beholder: The science of face perception.* Oxford, UK: Oxford University Press.

Buard, I., Rogers, S. J., Hepburn, S., Kronberg, E., & Rojas, D. (2013). Altered oscillation patterns and connectivity during picture naming in autism. *Frontiers in Human Neuroscience, 7,* 742.

Bushnell, I. W. R. (2001). Mother's face recognition in newborn infants: Learning and memory. *Infant and Child Development, 10*(1–2), 67–74.

Carey, S., Diamond, R., & Woods, B. (1980). Development of face recognition: A maturational component? *Developmental Psychology, 16*(4), 257.

Casanova, M. F., van Kooten, I. A. J., Switala, A. E., van Engeland, H., Heinsen, H., Steinbusch, H. W. M., . . . Schmitz, C. (2006). Minicolumnar abnormalities in autism. *Acta Neuropathologica, 12,* 287–303.

Cherkassky, V. L., Kana, R. K., Keller, T. A., & Just, M. A. (2006). Functional connectivity in a baseline resting-state network in autism. *Neuroreport, 17*(16), 1687–1690.

Clifford, S., Young, R., & Williamson, P. (2007). Assessing the early characteristics of autistic disorder using video analysis. *Journal of Autism and Developmental Disorders, 37*(2), 301–313.

Corbett, B. A., Carmean, V., Ravizza, S., Wendelken, C., Henry, M. L., Carter, C., & Rivera, S. M. (2009). A functional and structural study of emotion and face processing in children with autism. *Psychiatry Research: Neuroimaging, 173*(3), 196–205.

Critchley, H. D., Daly, E. M., Bullmore, E. T., Williams, S. C., Van Amelsvoort, T., Robertson, D. M., . . . Murphy, D. G. (2000). The functional neuroanatomy of social behaviour: Changes in cerebral blood flow when people with autistic disorder process facial expressions. *Brain, 123*(11), 2203–2212.

Crookes, K., & McKone, E. (2009). Early maturity of face recognition: No childhood development of holistic processing, novel face encoding, or facespace. *Cognition, 111*(2), 219–247.

Dakin, S., & Frith, U. (2005). Vagaries of visual perception in autism. *Neuron, 48*(3), 497–507.

Dalton, K. M., Nacewicz, B. M., Johnstone, T., Schaefer, H. S., Gernsbacher, M. A., Goldsmith, H. H., . . . Davidson, R. J. (2005). Gaze fixation and the neural circuitry of face processing in autism. *Nature Neuroscience, 8*(4), 519.

Dapretto, M., Davies, M. S., Pfeifer, J. H., Scott, A. A., Sigman, M., Bookheimer, S. Y., & Iacoboni, M. (2006). Understanding emotions in others: Mirror neuron dysfunction in children with autism spectrum disorders. *Nature Neuroscience, 9*(1), 28.

Deeley, Q., Daly, E. M., Surguladze, S., Page, L., Toal, F., Robertson, D., . . . Andrew, C. (2007). An event related functional magnetic resonance imaging study of facial emotion processing in Asperger syndrome. *Biological Psychiatry, 62*(3), 207–217.

Demopoulos, C., Yu, N., Tripp, J., Mota, N., Brandes-Aitken, A. N., Desai, S. S., . . . Marco, E. J. (2017). Magnetoencephalographic imaging of auditory and somatosensory cortical responses in children with autism and sensory processing dysfunction. *Frontiers in Human Neuroscience, 11*(259).

De Sonneville, L. M. J., Verschoor, C. A., Njiokiktjien, C., Op het Veld, V., Toorenaar, N., & Vranken, M. (2002). Facial identity and facial emotions: Speed, accuracy, and processing strategies in children and adults. *Journal of Clinical and Experimental Neuropsychology, 24*(2), 200–213.

Diamond, R., & Carey, S. (1977). Developmental changes in the representation of faces. *Journal of Experimental Child Psychology, 23*(1), 1–22.

Di Martino, A., Kelly, C., Grzadzinski, R., Zuo, X. N., Mennes, M., Mairena, M. A., . . . Milham, M. P. (2011). Aberrant striatal functional connectivity in children with autism. *Biological Psychiatry, 69*(9), 847–856.

Di Martino, A., Ross, K., Uddin, L. Q., Sklar, A. B., Castellanos, F. X., & Milham, M. P. (2009). Functional brain correlates of social and nonsocial processes in autism spectrum disorders: An activation likelihood estimation meta-analysis. *Biological Psychiatry, 65*(1), 63–74.

Edgar, J. C., Fisk Iv, C. L., Berman, J. I., Chudnovskaya, D., Liu, S., Pandey, J., . . . Roberts, T. P. L. (2015). Auditory encoding abnormalities in children with autism spectrum disorder suggest delayed development of auditory cortex. *Molecular Autism, 6*(69).

Edgar, J. C., Murray, R., Kuschner, E. S., Pratt, K., Paulson, D. N., Dell, J., . . . Roberts, T. P. L. (2015). The maturation of auditory responses in infants and young children: A cross-sectional study from 6 to 59 months. *Frontiers in Neuroanatomy, 9*(131).

Eimer, M. (2000). The face-specific N170 component reflects late stages in the structural encoding of faces. *Neuroreport, 11*(10), 2319–2324.

Erickson, C. A., Veenstra-Vanderweele, J. M., Melmed, R. D., McCracken, J. T., Ginsberg, L. D., Sikich, L., . . . King BH. (2014). STX209 (arbaclofen) for autism spectrum disorders: An 8-week open-label study. *Journal of Autism and Developmental Disorders, 44*(4), 958–964.

Falter, C. M., Braeutigam, S., Nathan, R., Carrington, S., & Bailey, A. J. (2013). Enhanced access to early visual processing of perceptual simultaneity in autism spectrum disorders. *Journal of Autism and Developmental Disorders, 43*(8), 1857–1866.

Farroni, T., Massaccesi, S., Pividori, D., & Johnson, M. H. (2004). Gaze following in newborns. *Infancy, 5*(1), 39–60.

Farroni, T., Menon, E., Rigato, S., & Johnson, M. H. (2007). The perception of facial expressions in newborns. *European Journal of Developmental Psychology, 4*(1), 2–13.

Fatemi, S. H., Aldinger, K. A., Ashwood, P., Bauman, M. L., Blaha, C. D., Blatt, G. J., . . . Estes, A. M. (2012). Consensus paper: Pathological role of the cerebellum in autism. *Cerebellum, 11*(3), 777–807.

Field, T. M., Woodson, R., Cohen, D., Greenberg, R., Garcia, R., & Collins, K. (1983). Discrimination and imitation of facial expressions by term and preterm neonates. *Infant Behavior and Development, 6*, 485–489.

Flagg, E. J., Oram Cardy, J. E., Roberts, W., & Roberts, T. P. L. (2005). Language lateralization development in children with autism: Insights from the late field magnetoencephalogram. *Neuroscience Letters, 386*, 82–87.

Flin, R. H. (1980). Age effects in children's memory for unfamiliar faces. *Developmental Psychology, 16*(4), 373.

Flin, R. H. (1985). Development of face recognition: An encoding switch?. *British Journal of Psychology, 76*(1), 123–134.

Fox, S. E., Wagner, J., Shrock, C. L., Flusberg, H. T., & Nelson, C. A. (2013). Neural processing of facial identity and emotion in infants at high-risk for autism spectrum disorders. *Frontiers in Human Neuroscience, 7*, 89.

Fries, P. (2009). Neuronal gamma-band synchronization as a fundamental process in cortical computation. *Annual Review of Neuroscience, 32*, 209–224.

Gaetz, W., Bloy, L., Wang, D. J., Port, R. G., Blaskey, L., Levy, S. E., & Roberts, T. P. L. (2014). GABA estimation in the brains of children on the autism spectrum: Measurement precision and regional cortical variation. *NeuroImage, 86*, 1–9.

Gaetz, W., Jurkiewicz, M. T., Kessler, S. K., Blaskey, L., Schwarts, E. S., & Roberts, T. P. L. (2017). Neuromagnetic responses to tactile stimulation of the fingers: Evidence for reduced cortical inhibition for children with autism spectrum disorder and children with epilepsy. *Neuroimage: Clinical, 16*, 624–633.

Gage, N. M., Siegel, B., Callen, M., & Roberts, T. P. L. (2003b). Cortical sound processing in children with autism disorder: An MEG investigation. *Neuroreport, 14*(16).

Gage, N. M., Siegel, B., & Roberts, T. P. L. (2003a). Cortical auditory system maturational abnormalities in children with autism disorder: An MEG investigation. *Developmental Brain Research, 144*, 201–209.

Gandal, M. J., Edgar, J. C., Ehrlichman, R. S., Mehta, M., Roberts, T. P. L., & Siegel, S. J. (2010). Validating γ oscillations and delayed auditory responses as translational biomarkers of autism. *Biological Psychiatry, 68*, 1100–1106.

Goren, C. C., Sarty, M., & Wu, P. Y. (1975). Visual following and pattern discrimination of face-like stimuli by newborn infants. *Pediatrics, 56*(4), 544–549.

Halit, H., de Haan, M., & Johnson, M. H. (2000). Modulation of event-related potentials by prototypical and atypical faces. *Neuroreport, 11*(9), 1871–1875.

Hansen, P., Kringelbach, M., & Salmelin, R. (Eds.). (2010). *MEG: An introduction to methods.* Oxford, UK: Oxford University Press.

Hari, R., & Puce, A. (2017). *MEG-EEG primer.* Oxford, UK: Oxford University Press.

Harms, M. B., Martin, A., & Wallace, G. L. (2010). Facial emotion recognition in autism spectrum disorders: A review of behavioral and neuroimaging studies. *Neuropsychology Review, 20*(3), 290–322.

Hasegawa, N., Kitamura, H., Murakami, H., Kameyama, S., Sasagawa, M., Egawa, J., . . . Someya, T. (2013). Altered activity of the primary visual area during gaze processing in individuals with high-functioning autistic spectrum disorder: A magnetoencephalography study. *Neuropsychobiology, 68*(3), 181–188.

Haxby, J. V., Hoffman, E. A., & Gobbini, M. I. (2000). The distributed human neural system for face perception. *Trends in Cognitive Sciences, 4*(6), 223–233.

Haxby, J. V., Hoffman, E. A., & Gobbini, M. I. (2002). Human neural systems for face recognition and social communication. *Biological Psychiatry, 51*(1), 59–67.

Hobson, R. P., & Lee, A. (1998). Hello and goodbye: A study of social engagement in autism. *Journal of Autism and Developmental Disorders, 28*(2), 117–127.

Hood, B. M., Macrae, C. N., Cole-Davies, V., & Dias, M. (2003). Eye remember you: The effects of gaze direction on face recognition in children and adults. *Developmental Science, 6*(1), 67–71.

Hubl, D., Bölte, S., Feineis–Matthews, S., Lanfermann, H., Federspiel, A., Strik, W., . . . Dierks, T. (2003). Functional imbalance of visual pathways indicates alternative face processing strategies in autism. *Neurology, 61*(9), 1232–1237.

Insel, T., Cuthbert, B., Garvey, M., Heinssen, R., Pine, D. S., Quinn, K., Sanislow, C., & Wang, P. (2010). Research domain criteria (RDoC): Toward a new classification framework for research on mental disorders. *American Journal of Psychiatry, 167*(7), 748–751.

Jansen, L. M. C., Gispen-De Wied, C. C., Wiegant, V. M., Westenberg, H. G. M., Lahuis, B. E., & Van Engeland, H. (2006). Autonomic and neuroendocrine responses to a psychosocial stressor in adults with autistic spectrum disorder. *Journal of Autism and Developmental Disorders, 36*, 891–899.

Johnson, B. W., Crain, S., Thornton, R., Tesan, G., & Reid, M. (2010). Measurement of brain function in pre-school children using a custom sized whole-head MEG sensor array. *Clinical Neurophysiology, 121*(3), 340–349.

Just, M. A., Keller, T. A., Malave, V. L., Kana, R. K., & Varma, S. (2012). Autism as a neural systems disorder: A theory of frontal-posterior underconnectivity. *Neuroscience & Biobehavioral Reviews, 36*(4), 1292–1313.

Kasai, K., Hashimoto, O., Kawakubo, Y., Yumoto, M., Kamio, S., Itoh, K., . . . Kato, N. (2005). Delayed automatic detection of change in speech sounds in adults with autism: A magnetoencephalographic study. *Clinical Neurophysiology, 116*, 1655–1664.

Kennedy, D. P., & Courchesne, E. (2008). The intrinsic functional organization of the brain is altered in autism. *NeuroImage, 39*(4), 1877–1885.

Keown, C. L., Shih, P., Nair, A., Peterson, N., Mulvey, M. E., & Müller, R. A. (2013). Local functional overconnectivity in posterior brain regions is associated with symptom severity in autism spectrum disorders. *Cell Reports, 5*(3), 567–572.

Khan, S., Gramfort, A., Shetty, N. R., Kitzbichler, M. G., Ganesan, S., Moran, J. M., . . . Herbert, M. R. (2013). Local and long-range functional connectivity is reduced in concert in autism spectrum disorders. *Proceedings of the National Academy of Sciences, 110*(8), 3107–3112.

Kikuchi, M., Shitamichi, K., Ueno, S., Yoshimura, Y., Remijn, G. B., Nagao, K., . . . Minabe, Y. (2010). Neurovascular coupling in the human somatosensory cortex: A single trial study. *NeuroReport, 21*, 1106–1110.

Kikuchi, M., Shitamichi, K., Yoshimura, Y., Ueno, S., Hiraishi, H., Hirosawa, T., . . . Oi, M. (2013). Altered brain connectivity in 3-to 7-year-old children with autism spectrum disorder. *NeuroImage: Clinical, 2*, 394–401.

Kitzbichler, M. G., Khan, S., Ganesan, S., Vangel, M. G., Herbert, M. R., Hämäläinen, M. S., & Kenet, T. (2015). Altered development and multifaceted band-specific abnormalities of resting state networks in autism. *Biological Psychiatry, 77*(9), 794–804.

Kolb, B., Wilson, B., & Taylor, L. (1992). Developmental changes in the recognition and comprehension of facial expression: Implications for frontal lobe function. *Brain and Cognition, 20*(1), 74–84.

Koshino, H., Carpenter, P. A., Minshew, N. J., Cherkassky, V. L., Keller, T. A., & Just, M. A. (2005). Functional connectivity in an fMRI working memory task in high-functioning autism. *NeuroImage, 24*(3), 810–821.

Kurita, T., Kikuchi, M., Yoshimura, Y., Hiraishi, H., Hasegawa, C., Takahashi, T., . . . Minabe, Y. (2016). Atypical bilateral brain synchronization in the early stage of human voice auditory processing in young children with autism. *PLoS One, 1*(4).

Kutas, M., & Hillyard, S. A. (1980). Reading senseless sentences: Brain potentials reflect semantic incongruity. *Science, 207*(4427), 203–205.

Kylliäinen, A., Braeutigam, S., Hietanen, J. K., Swithenby, S. J., & Bailey, A. J. (2006). Face-and gaze-sensitive neural responses in children with autism: A magnetoencephalographic study. *European Journal of Neuroscience, 24*(9), 2679–2690.

Lajiness-O'Neill, R., Richard, A. E., Moran, J. E., Olszewski, A., Pawluk, L., Jacobson, D., . . . Bowyer, S. M. (2014). Neural synchrony examined with magnetoencephalography (MEG) during eye gaze processing in autism spectrum disorders: Preliminary findings. *Journal of Neurodevelopmental Disorders, 6*(1), 15.

Leung, R. C., Pang, E. W., Anagnostou, E., & Taylor, M. J. (2018). Young adults with autism spectrum disorder show early atypical neural activity during emotional face processing. *Frontiers in Human Neuroscience, 12,* 57.

Leung, R. C., Pang, E. W., Cassel, D., Brian, J. A., Smith, M. L., & Taylor, M. J. (2015). Early neural activation during facial affect processing in adolescents with autism spectrum disorder. *NeuroImage: Clinical, 7,* 203–212.

Leung, R. C., Ye, A. X., Wong, S. M., Taylor, M. J., & Doesburg, S. M. (2014). Reduced beta connectivity during emotional face processing in adolescents with autism. *Molecular Autism, 5*(1), 51.

Luo, Q., Holroyd, T., Jones, M., Hendler, T., & Blair, J. (2007). Neural dynamics for facial threat processing as revealed by gamma band synchronization using MEG. *NeuroImage, 34*(2), 839–847.

Marco, E. J., Hinkley, L. B., Hill, S. S., & Nagarajan, S. S. (2011). Sensory processing in autism: A review of neurophysiologic findings. *Pediatric Research, 69*(5 Pt 2), 48R–54R.

Margari, L., De Giacomo, A., Craig, F., Palumbi, R., Peschechera, A., Margari, M., . . . Dicuonzo, F. (2018). Frontal lobe metabolic alterations in autism spectrum disorder: A 1h-magnetic resonance spectroscopy study. *Neuropsychiatric Disease and Treatment, 14,* 1871.

Matsuzaki, J., Kagitani-Shimono, K., Goto, T., Sanefuji, W., Yamamoto, T., Sakai, S., . . . Taniike, M. (2012). Differential responses of primary auditory cortex in autistic spectrum disorder with auditory hypersensitivity. *NeuroReport, 23*(2).

Matsuzaki, J., Kagitani-Shimono, K., Sugata, H., Hanaie, R., Nagatani, F., Yamamoto, T., . . . Taniike, M. (2017). Delayed mismatch field latencies in autism spectrum disorder with abnormal auditory sensitivity: A magnetoencephalographic study. *Frontiers in Human Neuroscience, 11*(446).

Matsuzaki, J., Kagitani-Shimono, K., Sugata, H., Hirata, M., Hanaie, R., Nagatani, F., . . . Taniike, M. (2014). Progressively increased M50 responses to repeated sounds in autism spectrum disorder with auditory hypersensitivity: A magnetoencephalographic study. *PLoS One, 9*(7).

Matsuzaki, J., Ku, M., Berman, J. I., Blaskey, L., Bloy, L., Chen, Y.-H., . . . Roberts, T. P. L. (2019). Abnormal auditory mismatch fields in adults with autism spectrum disorder. *Neuroscience Letters, 698,* 140–145.

McFadden, K. L., Hepburn, S., Winterrowd, E., Schmidt, G. L., & Rojas, D. C. (2012). Abnormalities in gamma-band responses to language stimuli in first-degree relatives of children with autism spectrum disorder: An MEG study. *BMC Psychiatry, 12*(213).

McPartland, J., Dawson, G., Webb, S. J., Panagiotides, H., & Carver, L. J. (2004). Event-related brain potentials reveal anomalies in temporal processing of faces in autism spectrum disorder. *Journal of Child Psychology and Psychiatry, 45*(7), 1235–1245.

Meaux, E., Taylor, M. J., Pang, E. W., Vara, A. S., & Batty, M. (2014). Neural substrates of numerosity estimation in autism. *Human Brain Mapping, 35*(9), 4362–4385.

Menassa, D. A., Braeutigam, S., Bailey, A., & Falter-Wagner, C. M. (2018). Frontal evoked γ activity modulates behavioural performance in autism spectrum disorders in a perceptual simultaneity task. *Neuroscience Letters, 665,* 86–91.

Mennella, R., Leung, R. C., Taylor, M. J., & Dunkley, B. T. (2017). Disconnection from others in autism is more than just a feeling: Whole-brain neural synchrony in adults during implicit processing of emotional faces. *Molecular Autism, 8*(1), 7.

Mondloch, C. J., Maurer, D., & Ahola, S. (2006). Becoming a face expert. *Psychological Science, 17*(11), 930–934.

Monk, C. S., Peltier, S. J., Wiggins, J. L., Weng, S. J., Carrasco, M., Risi, S., & Lord, C. (2009). Abnormalities of intrinsic functional connectivity in autism spectrum disorders. *NeuroImage, 47*(2), 764–772.

Näätänen, R., Gaillard, A. W. K., Mantysalo, S., & Gaillard, W. K. (1978). Early selective-attention effect on evoked potential reinterpreted. *Acta Psychologica, 42,* 313–329.

Näätänen, R., Paavilainen, P., Rinne, T., & Alho, K. (2007). The mismatch negativity (MMN) in basic research of central auditory processing: A review. *Clinical Neurophysiology, 118,* 2544–2590.

Näätänen, R., & Picton, T. (1987). The B1 wave of the human electric and magnetic response to sound: A review and an analysis of the component structure. *Psychophysiology, 24*(4), 375–425.

Nomi, J. S., & Uddin, L. Q. (2015). Face processing in autism spectrum disorders: From brain regions to brain networks. *Neuropsychologia, 71,* 201–216.

O'Connor, K., Hamm, J. P., & Kirk, I. J. (2007). Neurophysiological responses to face, facial regions and objects in adults with Asperger's syndrome: An ERP investigation. *International Journal of Psychophysiology, 63*(3), 283–293.

Ogai, M., Matsumoto, H., Suzuki, K., Ozawa, F., Fukuda, R., Uchiyama, I., . . . Takei, N. (2003). fMRI study of recognition of facial expressions in high-functioning autistic patients. *NeuroReport, 14*(4), 559–563.

Ogawa, R., Kagitani-Shimono, K., Matsuzaki, J., Tanigawa, J., Hanaie, R., Yamamoto, T., . . . Taniike, M. (2019). Abnormal cortical activation during silent reading in adolescents with autism spectrum disorder. *Brain and Development, 41*(3), 234–244.

Okada, Y., Hämäläinen, M., Pratt, K., Mascarenas, A., Miller, P., Han, M., . . . Paulson, D. (2016). BabyMEG: A whole-head pediatric magnetoencephalography system for human brain development research. *Review of Scientific Instruments, 87,* 094301.

Okada, Y., Pratt, K., Atwood, C., Mascarenas, A., Reineman, R., Nurminen, J., & Paulson, D. (2006). BabySQUID: A mobile, high-resolution multichannel magnetoencephalography system for neonatal brain assessment. *Review of Scientific Instruments, 77,* 024301.

Oram Cardy, J. E., Ferrari, P., Flagg, E. J., Roberts, W., & Roberts, T. P. L. (2004). Prominence of M50 auditory evoked response over M100 in childhood and autism. *NeuroReport, 15*(12).

Oram Cardy, J. E., Flagg, E. J., Roberts, W., & Roberts, T. P. L. (2005). Delayed mismatch field for speech and non-speech sounds in children with autism. *NeuroReport, 16*(5).

Oram Cardy, J. E., Flagg, E. J., Roberts, W., & Roberts, T. P. L. (2008). Auditory evoked fields predict language ability and impairment in children. *International Journal of Psychophysiology, 68,* 170–175.

Orekhova, E. V., Tsetlin, M. M., Butorina, A. V., Novikova, S. I., Gratchev, V. V., Sokolov, P. A., . . . Stroganova, T. A. (2012). Auditory cortex responses to clicks and sensory modulation difficulties in children with autism spectrum disorders (ASD). *PLoS One, 7*(6).

Osterling, J., & Dawson, G. (1994). Early recognition of children with autism: A study of first birthday home videotapes. *Journal of Autism and Developmental Disorders, 24*(3), 247–257.

Paetau, R., Ahonen, A., Salonen, O., & Sams, M. (1995). Auditory evoked magnetic fields to tones and pseudowords in healthy children and adults. *Journal of Clinical Neurophysiology, 12*(2),177–185.

Palva, J. M., Monto, S., Kulashekhar, S., & Palva, S. (2010). Neuronal synchrony reveals working memory networks and predicts individual memory capacity. *Proceedings of the National Academy of Sciences, 107*(16), 7580–7585.

Peiker, I., David, N., Schneider, T. R., Nolte, G., Schöttle, D., & Engel, A. K. (2015a). Perceptual integration deficits in autism spectrum disorders are associated with reduced interhemispheric gamma-band coherence. *Journal of Neuroscience, 35*(50), 16352–16361.

Peiker, I., Schneider, T. R., Milne, E., Schöttle, D., Vogeley, K., Münchau, A., . . . David, N. (2015b). Stronger neural modulation by visual motion intensity in autism spectrum disorders. *PLoS One, 10*(7), e0132531.

Pelphrey, K. A., Morris, J. P., & McCarthy, G. (2005). Neural basis of eye gaze processing deficits in autism. *Brain, 128*(5), 1038–1048.

Pelphrey, K. A., Morris, J. P., McCarthy, G., & LaBar, K. S. (2007). Perception of dynamic changes in facial affect and identity in autism. *Social Cognitive and Affective Neuroscience, 2*(2), 140–149.

Picci, G., Gotts, S. J., & Scherf, K. S. (2016). A theoretical rut: Revisiting and critically evaluating the generalized under/over-connectivity hypothesis of autism. *Developmental Science, 19*(4), 524–549.

Picci, G., & Scherf, K. S. (2015). A two-hit model of autism: Adolescence as the second hit. *Clinical Psychological Science, 3*(3), 349–371.

Pierce, K., Haist, F., Sedaghat, F., & Courchesne, E. (2004). The brain response to personally familiar faces in autism: Findings of fusiform activity and beyond. *Brain, 127*(12), 2703–2716.

Pierce, K., Müller, R. A., Ambrose, J., Allen, G., & Courchesne, E. (2001). Face processing occurs outside the fusiform "face area" in autism: Evidence from functional MRI. *Brain, 124*(10), 2059–2073.

Pierce, K., & Redcay, E. (2008). Fusiform function in children with an autism spectrum disorder is a matter of "who." *Biological Psychiatry, 64*(7), 552–560.

Port, R. G., Anwar, A. R., Ku, M., Carlson, G. C., Siegel, S. J., & Roberts, T. P. L. (2015). Prospective MEG biomarkers in ASD: Pre-clinical evidence and clinical promise of electrophysiological signatures. *Yale Journal of Biology and Medicine, 88,* 25–36.

Port, R. G., Edgar, J. C., Ku, M., Bloy, L., Murray, R., Blaskey, L., . . . Roberts, T. P. L. (2016). Maturation of auditory neural processes in autism spectrum disorder—A longitudinal MEG study. *NeuroImage: Clinical, 11,* 566–577.

Port, R. G., Gaetz, W., Bloy, L., Wang, D. J., Blaskey, L., Kuschner, E. S., . . . Roberts, T. P. L. (2017). Exploring the relationship between cortical GABA concentrations, auditory gamma-band responses and development in ASD: Evidence for an altered maturational trajectory in ASD. *Autism Research, 10,* 593–607.

Rinne, T., Alho, K., Ilmoniemi, R. J., Virtanen, J., & Näätänen, R. (2000). Separate time behaviors of the temporal and frontal mismatch negativity sources. *NeuroImage, 12,* 14–19.

Rinne, T., Särkkä, A., Degerman, A., Schröger, E., & Alho, K. (2006). Two separate mechanisms underlie auditory change detection and involuntary control of attention. *Brain Research, 1077,* 135–143.

Roberts, T. P. L., Cannon, K. M., Tavabi, K., Blaskey, L., Khan, S. Y., Monroe, J. F., . . . Edgar, J. C. (2011). Auditory magnetic mismatch field latency: A biomarker for language impairment in autism. *Biological Psychiatry, 70,* 263–269.

Roberts, T. P. L., Heiken, K., Kahn, S. Y., Qasmieh, S., Blaskey, L., Solot, C., . . . Edgar, J. C. (2012). Delayed magnetic mismatch negativity field, but not auditory M100 response, in specific language impairment. *NeuroReport, 23*(8), 463–468.

Roberts, T. P. L., Khan, S. Y., Blaskey, L., Dell, J., Levy, S. E., Zarnow, D. M., & Edgar, J. C. (2009). Developmental correlation of diffusion anisotropy with auditory-evoked response. *NeuroReport, 20,* 1586–1591.

Roberts, T. P. L., Khan, S. Y., Rey, M., Monroe, J. F., Cannon, K., Blaskey, L., . . . Edgar, J. C. (2010). MEG detection of delayed auditory evoked responses in autism spectrum disorders: Towards an imaging biomarker for autism. *Autism Research, 3,* 8–18.

Roberts, T. P. L., Lanza, M. R., Dell, J., Qasmieh, S., Hines, K., Blaskey, L., . . . Berman, J. I. (2013). Maturational differences in thalamocortical white matter microstructure and auditory evoked response latencies in autism spectrum disorders. *Brain Research, 1537,* 79–85.

Roberts, T. P. L., Paulson, D. N., Hirschkoff, E., Pratt, K., Mascarenas, A., Miller, P., . . . & Edgar, J. C. (2014). Artemis 123: Development of a whole-head infant and young child MEG system. *Frontiers in Human Neuroscience, 8*(99).

Rojas, D. C., Maharajh, K., Teale, P. D., Kleman, M. R., Benkers, T. L., Carlson, J. P., & Reite, M. L. (2006). Development of the 40 Hz steady state auditory evoked magnetic field from ages 5 to 52. *Clinical Neurophysiology, 117,* 110–117.

Rojas, D. C., Maharajh, K., Teale, P., & Rogers, S. J. (2008). Reduced neural synchronization of gamma-band MEG oscillations in first-degree relatives of children with autism. *BMC Psychiatry, 8,* 66.

Rudin, M., & Sauter, A. (1992). In-vivo magnetic resonance spectroscopy II. *Magnetic Resonance Imaging, 10*(5), 723–731.

Safar, K., Wong, S. M., Leung, R. C., Dunkley, B. T., & Taylor, M. J. (2018). Increased functional connectivity during emotional face processing in children with autism spectrum disorder. *Frontiers in Human Neuroscience, 12,* 408.

Sauseng, P., Klimesch, W., Doppelmayr, M., Pecherstorfer, T., Freunberger, R., & Hanslmayr, S. (2005). EEG alpha synchronization and functional coupling during top-down processing in a working memory task. *Human Brain Mapping, 26*(2), 148–155.

Schmidt, G. L., Rey, M. M., Oram Cardy, J. E., & Roberts, T. P. L. (2009). Absence of M100 source asymmetry in autism associated with language functioning. *NeuroReport, 20*(11),1037–1041.

Schultz, R. T., Gauthier, I., Klin, A., Fulbright, R. K., Anderson, A. W., Volkmar, F., . . . Gore, J. C. (2000). Abnormal ventral temporal cortical activity during face discrimination among individuals with autism and Asperger syndrome. *Archives of General Psychiatry, 57*(4), 331–340.

Simard, I., Luck, D., Mottron, L., Zeffiro, T. A., & Soulières, I. (2015). Autistic fluid intelligence: Increased reliance on visual functional connectivity with diminished modulation of coupling by task difficulty. *NeuroImage: Clinical, 9,* 467–478.

Smith, A. D., Hood, B. M., & Hector, K. (2006). Eye remember you two: Gaze direction modulates face recognition in a developmental study. *Developmental Science, 9*(5), 465–472.

Steele, S. D., Minshew, N. J., Luna, B., & Sweeney, J. A. (2007). Spatial working memory deficits in autism. *Journal of Autism and Developmental Disorders, 37,* 605–612.

Stroganova, T. A., Butorina, A. V., Sysoeva, O. V., Prokofyev, A. O., Nikolaeva, A. Y., Tsetlin, M. M., & Orekhova, E. V. (2015). Altered modulation of gamma oscillation frequency by speed of visual motion in children with autism spectrum disorders. *Journal of Neurodevelopmental Disorders, 7*(1), 21.

Sun, L., Grützner, C., Bölte, S., Wibral, M., Tozman, T., Schlitt, S., . . . Uhlhaas, P. J. (2012). Impaired gamma-band activity during perceptual organization in adults with autism spectrum disorders: Evidence for dysfunctional network activity in frontal-posterior cortices. *Journal of Neuroscience, 32*(28), 9563–9573.

Sysoeva, O. V., Davletshina, M. A., Orekhova, E. V., Galuta, I. A., & Stroganova, T. A. (2016). Reduced oblique effect in children with autism spectrum disorders (ASD). *Frontiers in Neuroscience, 9,* 512.

Sysoeva, O. V., Galuta, I. A., Davletshina, M. S., Orekhova, E. V., & Stroganova, T. A. (2017). Abnormal size-dependent modulation of motion perception in children with autism spectrum disorder (ASD). *Frontiers in Neuroscience, 11,* 164.

Takahashi, H., Kamio, Y., & Tobimatsu, S. (2016). Autism spectrum disorder. In S. Tobimatsu

& R. Kakigi (Eds.), *Clinical applications of magnetoencephalography* (pp. 247–274). Tokyo, Japan: Springer.

Takesaki, N., Kikuchi, M., Yoshimura, Y., Hiraishi, H., Hasegawa, C., Kaneda, R., . . . Minabe, Y. (2016). The contribution of increased gamma band connectivity to visual non-verbal reasoning in autistic children: A MEG study. *PloS One, 11*(9), e0163133.

Tang, J., Falkmer, M., Horlin, C., Tan, T., Vaz, S., & Falkmer, T. (2015). Face recognition and visual search strategies in autism spectrum disorders: Amending and extending a recent review by Weigelt et al. *PloS One,* 10(8), e0134439.

Tanigawa, J., Kagitani-Shimono, K., Matsuzaki, J., Ogawa, R., Hanaie, R., Yamamoto, T., . . . Ozono, K. (2018). Atypical auditory language processing in adolescents with autism spectrum disorder. *Clinical Neurophysiology, 129,* 2029–2037.

Taylor, M. J., Batty, M., & Itier, R. J. (2004). The faces of development: A review of early face processing over childhood. *Journal of Cognitive Neuroscience, 16*(8), 1426–1442.

Taylor, M. J., Doesburg, S. M., & Pang, E. W. (2014). Neuromagnetic vistas into typical and atypical development of frontal lobe functions. *Frontiers in Human Neuroscience, 8,* 453.

Tecchio, F., Benassi, F., Zappasodi, F., Gialloreti, L. E., Palermo, M., Seri, S., & Rossini, P. M. (2003). Auditory sensory processing in autism: A magnetoencephalographic study. *Biological Psychiatry, 54,* 647–654.

Thomas, L. A., De Bellis, M. D., Graham, R., & LaBar, K. S. (2007). Development of emotional facial recognition in late childhood and adolescence. *Developmental Science, 10*(5), 547–558.

Tonks, J., Williams, W. H., Frampton, I., Yates, P., & Slater, A. (2007). Assessing emotion recognition in 9–15-years olds: Preliminary analysis of abilities in reading emotion from faces, voices and eyes. *Brain Injury, 21*(6), 623–629.

Uddin, L. Q., Supekar, K., Lynch, C. J., Khouzam, A., Phillips, J., Feinstein, C., . . . Menon, V. (2013). Salience network–based classification and prediction of symptom severity in children with autism. *JAMA Psychiatry, 70*(8), 869–879.

Uddin, L. Q., Supekar, K., & Menon, V. (2013). Reconceptualizing functional brain connectivity in autism from a developmental perspective. *Frontiers in Human Neuroscience, 7,* 458.

Uljarevic, M., & Hamilton, A. (2013). Recognition of emotions in autism: A formal meta-analysis. *Journal of Autism and Developmental Disorders, 43*(7), 1517–1526.

Urbain, C. M., Pang, E. W., & Taylor, M. J. (2015). Atypical spatiotemporal signatures of working memory brain processes in autism. *Translational Psychiatry, 5*(8), e617.

Urbain, C., Vogan, V. M., Ye, A. X., Pang, E. W., Doesburg, S. M., & Taylor, M. J. (2016). Desynchronization of fronto-temporal networks during working memory processing in autism. *Human Brain Mapping, 37*(1), 153–164.

Vara, A. S., Pang, E. W., Doyle-Thomas, K. A., Vidal, J., Taylor, M. J., & Anagnostou, E. (2014). Is inhibitory control a "no-go" in adolescents with autism spectrum disorder? *Molecular Autism, 5*(1), 6.

Vakorin, V. A., Doesburg, S. M., Leung, R. C., Vogan, V. M., Anagnostou, E., & Taylor, M. J. (2017). Developmental changes in neuromagnetic rhythms and network synchrony in autism. *Annals of Neurology, 81*(2), 199–211.

Vogan, V. M., Morgan, B. R., Lee, W., Powell, T. L., Smith, M. L., & Taylor, M. J. (2014). The neural correlates of visuo-spatial working memory in children with autism spectrum disorder: Effects of cognitive load. *Journal of Neurodevelopmental Disorders, 6*(1), 19.

Wagner, J. B., Hirsch, S. B., Vogel-Farley, V. K., Redcay, E., & Nelson, C. A. (2013). Eye-tracking, autonomic, and electrophysiological correlates of emotional face processing in adolescents with autism spectrum disorder. *Journal of Autism and Developmental Disorders, 43*(1), 188–199.

Wallace, S., Coleman, M., Pascalis, O., & Bailey, A. (2006). A study of impaired judgment of eye-gaze direction and related face-processing deficits in autism spectrum disorders. *Perception, 35*(12), 1651–1664.

Webb, S. J., Dawson, G., Bernier, R., & Panagiotides, H. (2006). ERP evidence of atypical face processing in young children with autism. *Journal of Autism and Developmental Disorders, 36*(7), 881.

Webb, S. J., Merkle, K., Murias, M., Richards, T., Aylward, E., & Dawson, G. (2009). ERP responses differentiate inverted but not upright face processing in adults with ASD. *Social Cognitive and Affective Neuroscience, 7*(5), 578–587.

Werner, E., Dawson, G., Osterling, J., & Dinno, N. (2000). Brief report. Recognition of autism spectrum disorder before one year of age: A retrospective study based on home videotapes. *Journal of Autism and Developmental Disorders, 30*(2), 157–162.

Wilson, T. W., Rojas, D. C., Reite, M. L., Teale, P. D., & Rogers, S. J. (2007). Children and adolescents with autism exhibit reduced MEG steady-state gamma responses. *Biological Psychiatry, 62,*192–197.

Wolff, C., & Schroèger, E. (2001). Human pre-attentive auditory change-detection with single, double, and triple deviations as revealed by mismatch negativity additivity. *Neuroscience Letters, 311,* 37–40.

Wright, B., Alderson-Day, B., Prendergast, G., Bennett, S., Jordan, J., Whitton, C., . . . Green, G. (2012). Gamma activation in young people with autism spectrum disorders and typically-developing controls when viewing emotions on faces. *PLoS One, 7*(7), e41326.

Yoshimura, Y., Kikuchi, M., Hayashi, N., Hiraishi, H., Hasegawa, C., Takahashi, T., . . . Minabe, Y. (2017). Altered human voice processing in the frontal cortex and a developmental language delay in 3- to 5-year-old children with autism spectrum disorder. *Scientific Reports, 7*, 17116.

Yoshimura, Y., Kikuchi, M., Shitamichi, K., Ueno, S., Munesue, T., Ono, Y., . . . Minabe, Y. (2013). Atypical brain lateralisation in the auditory cortex and language performance in 3- to 7-year-old children with high-functioning autism spectrum disorder: A child-customised magnetoencephalography (MEG) study. *Molecular Autism, 4*(38).

Veenstra-Vander Weele, J., Cook, E.H., King, B. H., Zarevics, P., Cherubini, M., Walton-Bowen, K., . . . Carpenter, R. L. (2017). Arbaclofen in children and adolescents with autism spectrum disorder: A randomized, controlled, phase 2 trial. *Neuropsychopharmacology, 42*(7), 1390–1398.

Zwaigenbaum, L., Bryson, S., Rogers, T., Roberts, W., Brian, J., & Szatmari, P. (2005). Behavioral manifestations of autism in the first year of life. *International Journal of Developmental Neuroscience, 23*(2–3), 143–152.

22

FUNCTIONAL WOUNDS OF AN INVISIBLE INJURY

VISUALIZING COGNITION IN POST-TRAUMATIC STRESS DISORDER

Benjamin T. Dunkley and Margot J. Taylor

22.1. EMERGENCE OF POST-TRAUMATIC STRESS DISORDER AS A CLINICAL DIAGNOSIS

Post-traumatic stress disorder (PTSD) has, in some form or another, existed for millennia—survivors of violence, be it from war, assault, natural disasters, or abuse, and the psychological impact these experiences impart, have been described since antiquity. Much of the historical descriptors come from the chroniclers of war; since ancient encounters of swords and spears through to the modern-day battlefields of machine guns and artillery, what we would consider today to be PTSD has variously been called "soldier's heart," "shell shock," "war neuroses," and "battle fatigue" (Abdul-Hamid & Hughes, 2014). Of course, anyone can suffer from the disorder, but it seems to have been documented in the past usually within the context of war. Thus, it appears to be a ubiquitous phenomenon suffered in times of trauma.

Its modern definition was formalized in 1980 with the publication of the *Diagnostic and Statistical Manual of Mental Disorders,* third edition (DSM-III), where it was classified as an Anxiety-Related Disorder, up until the DSM-IV-TR (American Psychatric Association, 2000). Recently, PTSD was redefined in the DSM-5 as a Trauma- and Stressor-Related Disorder, arising from transient or chronic exposure to a traumatic or stressful event (American Psychiatric Association, 2013). It is widely recognized as a serious and debilitating chronic illness that also brings with it a number of primary symptoms, as well as functional impairments and secondary deficits in cognition, emotion, and physiological well-being. This can have a huge impact on an individual's quality of life, as well as placing an enormous

Benjamin T. Dunkley and Margot J. Taylor, *Functional Wounds of an Invisible Injury: Visualizing Cognition in Post-traumatic Stress Disorder* In: *Fifty Years of Magnetoencephalography.* Edited by: Andrew C. Papanicolaou, Timothy P. L. Roberts, and James W. Wheless, Oxford University Press (2020). © Oxford University Press. DOI: 10.1093/oso/9780190935689.003.0022.

burden on healthcare systems and damaging economic productivity. The primary diagnosis is often compounded by comorbid conditions, such as anxiety and depression, which require their own treatment regimens.

Most people will experience first-hand a deeply traumatic event during their lifetime (such as conflict, terrorism, natural disasters, assaults, accidents, or childhood abuse), and the lifetime prevalence of PTSD is estimated to be about 7% to 8% in the United States (US Department of Veterans Affairs, 2015)—however, the condition is very likely to be underdiagnosed, especially in less economically developed countries, where a much higher lifetime prevalence is probable. Overwhelmingly, PTSD is most commonly associated with and seen in war veterans (van Zyl, Oosthuizen, & Seedat, 2008), and while rates depend on the conflict, country, and population studied, the general presence of PTSD in combat veterans is estimated to be more than 20%, and even up to 60% (Ramchand et al., 2010).

PTSD is comprised of a four-cluster symptom constellation that includes (a) persistent re-experiencing of the traumatic episode (e.g., nightmares, flashbacks, and rumination on the memory); (b) persistent hypervigilance/hyperarousal (e.g., the feeling of always "being on edge," irritability and aggression, heightened reflexive startle), (c) avoidance (e.g., deliberately avoiding reminders of the traumatic event); and (d) emotional numbing and withdrawal (e.g., negative thoughts and affect, decreased interest in activities, feelings of isolation). With the latest DSM-5 revision, a "dissociative" subtype has been identified, and this includes feelings of depersonalization and disconnection from others, and sometimes derealization (i.e., a break in the sense of reality and surroundings).

Increasingly, as with other psychiatric illness, PTSD is framed within the context of *dysfunctional neurobiological networks and circuitry,* in addition to the classical segregative view of atypical, isolated, regional changes in functional physiology. Noninvasive neuroimaging has played a fundamental role in uncovering the neurobiological circuitry correlates of psychiatric disease, and this has increased since the advent of commonplace magnetic resonance imaging (MRI) machines, including both functional and structural measures of large-scale circuits. The evolution in thought and application specifically to PTSD was first proposed by Rauch, Shin, and Phelps (2006), who formalized the "neurocircuitry model of PTSD," which posited that the emergent behavior and cognitive phenotypes of PTSD primarily arise from the interactions among three key neurobiological structures: the amygdalae, the prefrontal cortex (PFC), and the hippocampi. This theory states that (a) exaggerated amygdalae activity underlies maladaptive fear responses and conditioned associations with traumatic stimuli; (b) decreased top-down control mediated by frontal cortices fails to sufficiently suppress/extinguish fear, in addition to dysfunctional attention and orienting responses; and (c) atypical hippocampal functioning subserves episodic memory consolidation and recollection that underlie traumatic re-experiencing and nightmares. Crucially, they proposed that it is not just the maladaptive functioning of these areas in isolation that cause the symptoms of PTSD but also how they connect and communicate with one another, particularly with regard to fronto-amygdalae and amygdalae-hippocampi circuits and interactions. This theory was formalized by earlier animal models that used behavioral assays of fear acquisition, conditioning, and extinction, and by human neuroimaging studies that have similarly examined threat perception, emotion, memory, and executive function.

While the underlying neurobiological abnormalities of the disorder have been informed by neuroimaging, the "holy grail" of psychiatry would be the identification of noninvasive imaging measures that can objectively distinguish those with a disorder from those without—essentially, a black-box scenario in which pattern classification delineates a sufferer from those unaffected, on an individual basis.

Despite the long-standing promise that imaging would revolutionize this field, however, there currently exist no reliable biomarkers/biological fingerprints of mental illness. In the case of PTSD, neuroimaging findings have often produced conflicting results, particularly with regard to structural measures, where volumetric and morphological alterations can be subtle or inconsistent or show substantial overlap with other conditions.

On the other hand, functional imaging, driven by explosion in the use of functional magnetic resonance imaging (fMRI), has shown a degree of promise—in PTSD at least, these measures seem to consistently identify reduced PFC functioning and elevated amygdala responses (Fenster, Lebois, Ressler, & Suh, 2018). This technique has revealed changes in functional circuitry in PTSD, and advances in data science, statistics, and pattern classification have shown that it might be possible to identify individuals with PTSD with these types of data (Zhang, Chen, Long, Cui, & Chen, 2016).

However, fMRI is essentially blind to neural measures that change quickly, and it lacks the ability to capture fast rhythmic changes in neural activity that occur at cognitively and behaviorally relevant timescales. This is needed to characterize the temporal evolution of responses that play out over the course of fast-acting and real-time behavior. Moreover, research into the underlying pathophysiology of psychiatric conditions has been impeded by the fact that these imaging techniques allow only indirect links to cellular and physiological mechanisms underlying observed signal changes and thus only limited relations to preclinical research.

The important point is that the emergent properties of high-level cognition and behavior are generated by the dynamic and coordinated interaction of functionally specialized areas that generate behavior and scaffold on structural architecture. There are now substantial data showing that dynamic fluctuations in regional and interregional neurophysiological interactions support core psychological processes (Fries, 2005), and linking precise measures of brain activity with behavior and cognition will allow for more effective treatment programs.

Thus, magnetoencephalography (MEG) has played an increasingly pivotal role in elucidating the areas and networks, as well as their timing and frequency-specific dynamics that underlie symptoms in PTSD and the maladaptive cognition and behavior sequelae seen in the disorder. This has been driven by a paradigm shift in neuroscience that has historically sought to explain psychological processes as being tied to a specific brain region, and that is now moving to an integrative approach. This approach aims to explain the emergent phenomenon of cognition and behavior by the interaction among areas and has gained considerable traction within the context of PTSD and psychiatry more generally. In line with these developments, there has been a reorientation to explaining disease by imaging "invisible" phenomena, such as electromagnetic activity, and the increased temporal sensitivity to capture dynamic neural activity at behaviorally relevant timescales pertinent to dysfunctional behavior and cognition. In line with a shifting consensus in psychiatry, that pathology comes about by maladaptive brain circuits and connectomics, MEG represents a potent tool for imaging brain circuit function and dysfunction in PTSD.

22.2. MAGNETOENCEPHALO-GRAPHY STUDIES OF POST-TRAUMATIC STRESS DISORDER

22.2.1. Task-Related Evoked Response

A variety of studies have examined functional responses in PTSD in relation to tasks that tap into the cognitive difficulties experienced by those with PTSD—this approach allows the examination of transient, time locked, and phase locked physiological responses that can capture millisecond-by-millisecond fluctuations in brain activity. This method is also powerful because the studies can be compared with electroencephalography (EEG) studies using similar tasks.

A core component of PTSD is impairment of traumatic reminders and threat processing, with elevated vigilance and attentional biases to threat—which can be adaptive in theaters of war, on the lookout for enemy combatants and surprise attack, but are maladaptive in everyday life. One study found *reduced* evoked responses in occipital cortices for the perception of aversive stimuli in those with PTSD and traumatic exposure (Catani, Adenauer, Keil, Aichinger, & Neuner, 2009) and PTSD hyperactivity in parietal cortices related to aversive pictures—these measures directly correlated with PTSD symptom subscores, suggesting a neurobiological cause for attentional biases and aversive reactions to traumatic reminders. A more recent study by Todd et al. (2015) examined responses to word threat cues in an attentional blink protocol in soldiers with and without PTSD, using words related to the military campaign in which they had served. The control soldiers showed midline frontal activity, between 90 and 340 ms, in regions associated with emotion regulation, whereas the soldiers with PTSD did not, and instead had enhanced visual cortex activation, interpreted to index greater priority given over to the processing of the trauma stimuli. A similar group of soldiers with and without PTSD were presented with photographs that included ones from the war zone, within the context a working memory task (Dunkley et al., 2018). In the immediate recognition aspect of the task, soldiers with PTSD showed rapid and sustained increased activity in the left temporal pole and superior frontal gyrus for war-related imagery, as well as enhanced visual processing. In contrast, soldiers without PTSD had greater activity in the left temporal-parietal junction and right inferior frontal gyrus for war imagery, the latter again suggesting intact emotional regulation. In the delayed recognition task, both groups of soldiers showed greater

occipital activity for war compared with neutral images, but the PTSD group also showed elevated, sustained activation compared with controls for the war images in limbic areas. This pattern was stable over a 2-year testing interval, suggesting long-term changes in the neural processing of traumatic reminders.

Although most studies have included soldiers, Adenauer et al. (2010) assessed visual processing of threat cues in refugees with and without PTSD compared with controls. Using sensor space and dipole analyses of MEG responses to IAP affective pictures, the authors found increased dipole strength in the right frontal areas to aversive pictures from 130 to 160 ms in those with PTSD. In contrast, the control groups showed greater activity to emotional pictures in a later time window (205–256 ms) in parietal occipital areas. The authors argued that this indexed increased vigilance followed by avoidance in the PTSD group (Adenauer et al., 2010).

While PTSD is thought to result in part from a dysregulation of emotional neurocircuitry, and hence sufferers are sensitive to trauma-related stimuli, it also affects other cognitive functions in more subtle ways. One domain of dysfunction is that of mental flexibility, a core executive function that involves the ability to shift perspectives or behaviors when presented with new information. It is essential for appropriate social-cognitive interactions. Soldiers with and without PTSD completed a mental flexibility (set-shifting) task while MEG data were recorded (Pang et al., 2014). Between-group differences showed significant activations in paralimbic cortex (i.e., cingulate and parahippocampal gyrus) in the soldiers with PTSD. These areas are not typically recruited for set-shifting but are implicated in the neurocircuitry of PTSD, suggesting that dysfunctional activity may be driven by increased responses in limbic areas, which are not adequately modulated by prefrontal cortical regions. They also found reduced activity in the right insula, reported to be a key region for resilience against PTSD (Simmons et al.,

2012). The authors suggested that the early paralimbic response affects downstream cognitive function in those with PTSD.

Only one study has looked at auditory responses in a small group of soldiers with PTSD compared with civilian controls (Hunter et al., 2011). They examined the sensory gating potential at 50 ms, as it is believed to be preattentive and to reflect impairment in filtering redundant stimuli. The M50 was localized to the superior temporal gyrus, and the soldiers had significantly reduced responses in the right hemisphere, which correlated with hyperarousal, as well as a composite PTSD symptom severity score. The correlations were not in the expected direction, however, suggesting that a larger study is needed to verify the findings, as well as the asymmetrical findings that could not be explained. However, the authors suggested that the abnormal inhibitory response has a protective effect and may ameliorate the PTSD symptoms.

22.2.2. Task-Related Local Induced Oscillations

In addition to transient evoked responses, a number of MEG studies of PTSD have examined induced oscillatory (i.e., time locked, but not *phase locked*) responses in relation to task-dependent processing. These types of analyses offer a window into dysfunction not afforded by the trial-averaged evoked-type analyses—they can reveal mechanistic insights into the underlying microcircuitry that is responsible for functional impairment in psychiatric disorders, across a variety of frequency ranges that are thought to play functionally specialized roles. While oscillatory activity and synchronization are inherently smeared in terms of their temporal characteristics (to which an evoked analysis would be more ideally suited), they do reveal frequency-specific interactions that can provide information about specific pathophysiology.

The majority of studies analyzing task-related band-limited oscillations in PTSD have

shown relatively low-frequency atypicalities (beta frequency and below) rhythms related to local inhibition (Jensen & Mazaheri, 2010) and the ongoing cognitive state (Engel & Fries, 2010). For example, a recurring theme seems to be reduced theta and alpha oscillatory activity, particularly in right frontotemporal and parietal brain regions (Badura-Brack et al., 2015; Khanna et al., 2017; McDermott et al., 2016). Specifically, these studies include evidence of elevated frontotemporal theta oscillations that were observed in a task of combat-related words, suggesting deficits at the intersection of attention and emotion regulation (Khanna et al., 2017). Others have found evidence of altered attentional resource allocation in the processing of sensory information, where reduced alpha activity in motor, parietal, and frontal cortices has been reported in a task of nonthreatening tactile perception and found to be directly related to increased PTSD severity (Badura-Brack et al., 2015). Other studies have found working memory and alpha oscillatory dysfunction related to encoding and maintenance, with a bilateral frontoparietal network engaged to a greater degree during a task of verbal memory (McDermott et al., 2016). Together, these studies suggest localized regional deficits in pulsed inhibition, indexed by low-frequency oscillations that explain cognitive deficits.

A number of studies have used tasks that incorporated emotionally relevant or threatening stimuli (Badura-Brack, McDermott, Heinrichs-Graham, et al., 2018; Catani, Adenauer, Keil, et al., 2009; Khanna et al., 2017) in examining local oscillatory power changes. Perception of combat-related pictures has been show to yield increased theta in the left hippocampus and amygdala and concomitant decreases in the PFC in the PTSD group (Khanna et al., 2017), while over a broad frequency range (0.1–10 Hz), there was an increase in superior parietal cortex oscillatory activity in response to unpleasant images (Catani, Adenauer, Haas, et al., 2009). Elevated amygdala activity has been observed in soldiers with PTSD for the processing of threatening faces that was not exhibited during the perception of neutral expressions, suggesting that rapid and sustained amygdala oscillations subserve treat assessment (Badura-Brack, McDermott, Heinrichs-Graham, et al., 2018).

In other studies, attention training has been shown to directly reduce PTSD symptom severity and modulate associated oscillatory responses in a number of tasks that tap key deficits in PTSD. One study has shown that attention control and bias modification treatment can lead to increases in theta oscillations in working memory networks that were associated with a reduction of symptom presence, suggesting the importance of dysfunctional theta oscillations in explaining some core PTSD symptoms (McDermott et al., 2016). Another study has shown that such intervention also leads to modulating neurophysiological dynamics in visual pathways and threat-processing regions—and that these dysfunctional oscillations are plastic and amenable to behavioral intervention techniques.

22.2.3. Task-Related Large-Scale Circuits and Synchrony

Building on those reports that have examined regional oscillatory power, other studies have increasingly turned to interregional synchrony to define functional connectivity. By exploiting the phenomenon of oscillations and quantifying the degree to which multiple regions align their ongoing phases, researchers have been able to capture task-related connectivity at the timescale at which the data were recorded. In this way, it is possible to image the dynamic fluctuations in cross-regional communication and see how large-scale circuitry plays a role in the primary symptoms and cognitive sequelae of PTSD.

For example, facets of executive function are known to be compromised in PTSD, such as cognitive flexibility—this refers to the ability to switch one's mental train of thought between differing concepts. Using a task-switching paradigm (i.e., implicit flexibility), it has been shown that soldiers with PTSD show a comparable ability to deal with easy task shifts, but a reduced ability to deal with difficult rule changes. However, correct responses seem to be mediated by theta oscillations, and this compensatory behavior is anchored in the right superior parietal region, a polysensory hub critical for spatial perception and sustained attention (Dunkley, Sedge, et al., 2015).

In another study, soldiers with PTSD showed an affective memory bias, where they exhibited a reduced ability to correctly identify neutral stimuli after a delay period, but a comparable ability to recall affective stimuli (war-related), compared with combat-matched non-PTSD peers, in a visual working memory and delayed recognition task. Underlying multiple facets of this behavior (including encoding, recall, recognition, and correctly identifying novel stimuli) was heightened alpha synchrony among frontotemporal and limbic regions (Dunkley, Pang, Sedge, Jetly, & Taylor, 2016). Previous work has shown that alpha synchrony plays a key functional role in maintaining memory representations (Palva, Monto, Kulashekhar, & Palva, 2010). This suggests greater mnemonic processing of these war reminders in the soldiers who developed PTSD.

Recently, an implicit threat-perception paradigm embedded in a go/no-go task examined implicit threat-processing and network responses in soldiers with PTSD. When shown neutral facial expressions, there was no difference in synchrony in relation to trauma-exposed peers, but there was broadband hypersynchrony among regions such as the amygdalae and orbitofrontal cortex when exposed to threatening "angry" faces (Dunkley et al., 2016). This revealed an implicit threat perception bias and a tuned fear network for processing such emotional expressions in others. This study was recently supplemented with a longitudinal component that examined the stability of these responses over time—crucially, these hypersynchronous signatures remained elevated 2 years later in the PTSD group, in line with little symptom remission (Dunkley et al 2018), suggesting that this response again indexes a long-term alteration in cognitive processes.

22.2.4. Resting-State Regional Power Changes

Early studies using resting-state designs have examined localized changes in the power spectrum and rather inconsistently report differential changes in power across canonical frequency ranges. However, these studies have been consistent in the location of oscillatory changes, with differences between PTSD and controls noted in regions concordant with previous human imaging and analogous to regions in rodent models. These areas include the medial temporal regions, ventral medial prefrontal cortex (vmPFC), hippocampi, parahippocampal areas, insulae, and amygdalae (Badura-Brack et al., 2017; Kolassa et al., 2007; Rutledge, 2015; Schalinski, Moran, Elbert, Reindl, & Wienbruch, 2017).

In addition, decreases in power were found in the PTSD population in the medial frontal regions, including delta changes in the frontal pole and vmPFC (Rutledge, 2015) and in the precuneus (Kolassa et al., 2007). Several other studies reported increased power bilaterally in frontal regions in the delta, theta, and alpha frequencies (Badura-Brack et al., 2017; Ray et al., 2006; Schalinski et al., 2017). The increases in delta oscillations in two of these studies were associated with a greater number of dissociative experiences, suggesting a particular link between the delta frequency range and PTSD symptomology (Ray et al., 2006; Schalinski et al., 2017). Because delta is close to the noise floor in MEG, caution is needed in interpreting these findings.

Recent studies have also shown changes in regional power spectrum that were related to treatment effects (Badura-Brack, McDermott, Becker, et al., 2018). Attention control training (ACT) and attention bias modification treatment (ABMT) have been shown to reduce symptoms of PTSD and to modulate occipital and medial temporal intrinsic activity, respectively, showing that brain oscillations can be modified and normalized with targeted behavioral therapy and intervention that aim to rectify the attentional biases inherent in PTSD.

22.2.5. Resting-State Neurophysiological Connectivity

Again exploiting the fact that disparate groups of neurons oscillate and synchronize to facilitate communication, recent studies of PTSD resting state have examined phase–phase interactions to define functional connectivity. This was first studied by Georgopoulos et al. (2010), who looked at sensor–space synchronization and found that subjects with PTSD could be distinguished from civilian controls (2010) and that, generally, there was an increase in sensor-level synchrony in the temporal and parietal regions in the PTSD group and a decrease in large-scale level synchronization (Engdahl et al., 2010; James et al., 2013). Building on this work examining sensor-level synchronization, James et al. (2015) applied predictive modeling and classification algorithms to resting MEG data, which could delineate PTSD not only from a control cohort but also from a PTSD plus comorbid disorder cohort, with accuracy rates of more than 90% in males and more than 80% in females.

More recently, source–space analyses allowed for a description of specific regions showing interregional oscillations and synchrony that was associated with PTSD. High-frequency oscillations anchored in the left hippocampus distinguished a group with PTSD from trauma-exposed controls, and this was related to PTSD symptom severity. Other key regions, such as the medical frontal areas, were associated with severity of depression and anxiety (Dunkley et al., 2014). It was found that triggering stimuli, comprised of photographs taken from the war zone in which the soldiers had served, could induce synchrony in the trauma-exposed controls that resembled the PTSD group. This exposure to trauma-related stimuli led to increases in low and high gamma connectivity in brain regions and networks associated with fear conditioning and memory (e.g., amygdalae, hippocampi), resembling the pattern seen in the PTSD group. Network analyses revealed that the PTSD group elicited hyperconnectivity in the low and high gamma ranges in frontal and temporal regions and between or within networks (i.e., default mode network (DMN) to other networks such as salience (SAL), visual [VIS], and dorsal attention network [DAN]) before exposure to triggering stimuli (Dunkley, Doesburg, et al., 2015).

A further analysis of the data using partial regression methods also showed that low-frequency alpha oscillations were reduced in PTSD and that these patterns of connectivity could differentiate those with PTSD not only from a trauma-exposed control group but also from those with mild traumatic brain injury (mTBI) and a civilian control group (Misic et al., 2016). However, these increases were attenuated in comparison to combat-exposed controls due to the general hyperconnectivity at resting state (Misic et al., 2016). Further analyses revealed that increased connectivity in the low and high gamma range occurred with simultaneous decrease in signal variability in temporal regions.

Along these lines, network metrics revealed a general decrease in clustering coefficient and modularity in the alpha frequencies that is indicative of a departure from local connectivity (Rowland et al., 2017). In another study, the shift away from local network connectivity to internetwork connectivity (i.e., DMN–SAL) was associated with greater PTSD symptom severity and lower resiliency, specifically in the alpha and beta ranges (Brunetti et al., 2017).

22.2.6. Distinguishing Post-traumatic Stress Disorder From Mild Traumatic Brain Injury

In the military population in particular, mTBI or concussion and PTSD are often reported to co-occur, and the two conditions can have overlapping symptoms, for example, attentional, emotional, and memory difficulties. Disentangling the neural underpinnings of the cognitive and emotional effect of PTSD and mTBI is challenging (Wilde et al., 2015) but important clinically because therapy and potential interventions vary. Recent papers have also examined the relations between PTSD and mTBI (Rowlands et al., 2018), suggesting that advanced MEG analyses may be particularly valuable to determine the overlapping and distinct neural mechanisms (Spadoni et al., 2018).

In mTBI, the most frequently reported abnormality is an increase in slowing, often in delta (Huang et al., 2009), although the full delta frequency range is difficult to measure in MEG because of the system noise floor. Nevertheless, low frequency shifts in the spectrum have been reported in discrete brain areas, such as the frontal and temporal lobes (Swan et al., 2015).

Others have also analyzed the resting state using connectivity to image circuit dysfunction in mTBI. One study investigated amplitude envelope correlations and showed increased connectivity in mTBI for delta, theta, and alpha ranges across widespread areas of the temporal, parietal, and subcortical brain areas that correlated with symptoms (Dunkley et al., 2015), particularly those of impulsivity and attentional difficulties. The authors argued that multiple networks and frequency bands were affected by mTBI and that the cognitive sequelae could be related to these large-scale alterations in brain connectivity, in particular an inability for regions to segregate coupled activity. Recently, it was also noted that specific intrinsic networks are affected by injury, including the default mode and motor network (Dunkley et al., 2018), where internal coupling within these circuits was directly related to symptom presence; however, when regressing out comorbid symptoms, motor coupling associations with concussion symptoms disappeared, while DMN coupling was directly related to deficits. This suggests that the DMN is particularly susceptible to mTBI injury.

In task-based studies using the same protocols, distinct patterns of results are seen in the two groups. For example, da Costa et al. (2014) assessed those with mTBI compared with controls with the same mental flexibility task that Pang et al. (2014) used with PTSD participants. In contrast to the PTSD group, those with mTBI had delayed response behaviorally and in the MEG responses in areas related to executive function, as well as more disorganized activity. In a working memory task (as used in Dunkley et al., 2018, in PTSD), Shah-Basak et al. (2018) reported that those with concussion showed early reduced parietal activity, related to concussion symptom severity, which was interpreted as evidence of impaired top-down attention processes. While soldiers with PTSD had increased activation in the left temporal pole, those with concussion had increased activity in right medial temporal regions consistent with inefficient visual and mnemonic processing.

These types of comparisons suggest that although there is symptom overlap in concussion (mTBI) and PTSD, the underlying neural origins differ significantly. MEG is the most appropriate technology to elucidate these differences.

22.3. FUTURE DIRECTIONS AND APPLICATIONS

Rapid developments in MEG technology also promise an increasing use in the field of PTSD research and in psychiatric conditions more generally. With the advent of machine learning and pattern classification algorithms, MEG data hold potential to aid in the objective diagnosis of PTSD, prognosticate outcome, and guide individualized treatment strategies. Already, studies using MEG connectomics data, like those described here, are able to reliably identify with about 80% accuracy those with mTBI (Vakorin et al., 2016), and preliminary data using a similar approach show

a robust and reliable way to different those with PTSD from those who were exposed to trauma. Crucially, those with traumatic exposure showed subthreshold PTSD symptoms, showing that MEG data could potentially elucidate subtle neurophysiological differences in those with similar experiential episodes.

Examined longitudinally, measurement of those with PTSD and applying similar analyses will allow us to prognosticate with regard to treatment outcome and will allow clinicians to be able to determine when it is appropriate to "return to work/play/deployment." Potentially, it could be used as a screening tool for preexisting neurophysiological risk factors for the development of PTSD following traumatic exposure; for example, soldiers might be scanned during training and before deployment in much the same way eyesight or physical fitness is assessed—of course, there are a number of important ethical considerations with regard to that application. Similarly, exciting developments in cryogen-free systems using optically pumped magnetometers (OPMs) also have potential in first responders or during battlefield deployment (Boto et al., 2018).

Finally, as is evident from this chapter, much of the work and what we know about the neurophysiological underpinnings of PTSD derive from military populations, particularly those that have seen combat—little research has been conducted on PTSD caused by other types of trauma, or in younger groups, for instance, and there is a growing realization of the need to understand PTSD in these nonmilitary groups because they may have distinct subtypes.

22.4. CONCLUSION

MEG has played a significant part in our understanding of the neurobiology and pathophysiology of PTSD. Not only has its ability to examine dynamic functional circuitry provided powerful explanations for the core behavioral phenotypes of PTSD, it has also proved to be a particularly potent tool in understanding the often subtle neurophysiological abnormalities that contribute to peripheral and comorbid cognitive sequelae. Furthermore, in combination with progress in analytics, such as machine learning for diagnostics, treatment strategies like targeted neuromodulation and rehabilitation, and advances in cryogen-free, room-temperature sensors, MEG will continue to contribute to our understanding of PTSD and aid in the development of individualized medicine.

REFERENCES

Abdul-Hamid, W. K., & Hughes, J. H. (2014). Nothing new under the sun: Post-traumatic stress disorders in the ancient world? *Early Science and Medicine, 19*(6), 549–557.

Adenauer, H., Pinösch, S., Catani, C., Gola, H., Keil, J., Kißler, J., & Neuner, F. (2010). Early processing of threat cues in posttraumatic stress disorder-evidence for a cortical vigilance-avoidance reaction. *Biological Psychiatry, 68*(5), 451–458.

American Psychiatric Association. (2000). *Diagnostic and statistical manual of mental disorders* (4th ed.). Arlington, VA: American Psychiatric Association.

American Psychiatric Association. (2013). *Diagnostic and statistical manual of mental disorders* (5th ed.). Arlington, VA: American Psychiatric Association.

Badura-Brack, A. S., Becker, K. M., McDermott, T. J., Ryan, T. J., Becker, M. M., Hearley, A. R., . . . Wilson, T. W. (2015). Decreased somatosensory activity to non-threatening touch in combat veterans with posttraumatic stress disorder. *Psychiatry Research, 233*(2), 194–200.

Badura-Brack, A. S., Heinrichs-Graham, E., McDermott, T. J., Becker, K. M., Ryan, T. J., Khanna, M. M., & Wilson, T. W. (2017). Resting-state neurophysiological abnormalities in posttraumatic stress disorder: A magnetoencephalography study. *Frontiers in Human Neuroscience, 11*, 205.

Badura-Brack, A. S., McDermott, T. J., Becker, K. M., Ryan, T. J., Khanna, M. M., Pine, D. S., . . . Wilson, T. W. (2018). Attention training modulates resting-state neurophysiological abnormalities in posttraumatic stress disorder. *Psychiatry Research—Neuroimaging, 271*, 135–141.

Badura-Brack, A. S., McDermott, T. J., Heinrichs-Graham, E., Ryan, T. J., Khanna, M. M., Pine, D. S., . . . Wilson, T. W. (2018). Veterans with PTSD demonstrate amygdala hyperactivity while viewing threatening faces: A MEG study. *Biological Psychology, 132*, 228–232.

Boto, E., Holmes, N., Leggett, J., Roberts, G., Shah, V., Meyer, S. S., . . . Brookes, M. J. (2018). Moving magnetoencephalography towards real-world applications with a wearable system. *Nature. 555*, 657–661.

Brunetti, M., Marzetti, L., Sepede, G., Zappasodi, F., Pizzella, V., Sarchione, F., . . . Di Giannantonio, M. (2017). Resilience and cross-network connectivity: A neural model for post-trauma survival. *Progress in Neuro-Psychopharmacology and Biological Psychiatry, 77*, 110–119.

Catani, C., Adenauer, H., Haas, S., Pinoesch, S., Keil, J., Aichinger, H., . . . Neuner, F. (2009). Early cortical activation towards aversive stimuli in patients with PTSD and comorbid depression compared to patients with major depression. *Psychophysiology, 46*, S157.

Catani, C., Adenauer, H., Keil, J., Aichinger, H., & Neuner, F. (2009). Pattern of cortical activation during processing of aversive stimuli in traumatized survivors of war and torture. *European Archives of Psychiatry and Clinical Neuroscience, 259*(6), 340–351.

Dunkley, B. T., Doesburg, S. M., Jetly, R., Sedge, P. A., Pang, E. W., & Taylor, M. J. (2015). Characterising intra- and inter-intrinsic network synchrony in combat-related post-traumatic stress disorder. *Psychiatry Research—Neuroimaging, 234*(2), 172–181.

Dunkley, B. T., Doesburg, S. M. S. M., Sedge, P. A. P. A., Grodecki, R. J. J., Shek, P. N. N., Pang, E. W. E. W. E. W., & Taylor, M. J. M. J. (2014). Resting-state hippocampal connectivity correlates with symptom severity in post-traumatic stress disorder. *NeuroImage: Clinical, 5*, 377–384.

Dunkley, B. T., Pang, E. W., Sedge, P. A., Jetly, R., & Taylor, M. J. (2016). Alpha hypersynchrony and atypical memory processes in soldiers with post-traumatic stress disorder. *Journal of Neuroimaging in Psychiatry & Neurology, 1*(2), 54–63.

Dunkley, B. T., Sedge, P. A., Doesburg, S. M., Grodecki, R. J., Jetly, R., Shek, P. N., . . . Pang, E. W. (2015). Theta, mental flexibility, and post-traumatic stress disorder: Connecting in the parietal cortex. *PLoS One, 10*(4), e0123541.

Dunkley, B. T., Urban, K., Da Costa, L., Wong, S. M., Pang, E. W., & Taylor, M. J. (2018). Default mode network oscillatory coupling is increased following concussion. *Frontiers in Neurology, 9*, 280.

Engdahl, B., Leuthold, A. C., Tan, H.-R. M., Lewis, S. M., Winskowski, A. M., Dikel, T. N., & Georgopoulos, A. P. (2010). Post-traumatic stress disorder: A right temporal lobe syndrome? *Journal of Neural Engineering, 7*(6), 066005.

Engel, A. K., & Fries, P. (2010). Beta-band oscillations-signalling the status quo? *Current Opinion in Neurobiology, 20*(2), 156–165.

Fenster, R. J., Lebois, L. A. M., Ressler, K. J., & Suh, J. (2018). Brain circuit dysfunction in post-traumatic stress disorder: From mouse to man. *Nature Reviews Neuroscience, 19*, 535–551.

Fries, P. (2005). A mechanism for cognitive dynamics: Neuronal communication through neuronal coherence. *Trends in Cognitive Sciences, 9*(10), 474–480.

Georgopoulos, A. P., Tan, H.-R. M., Lewis, S. M., Leuthold, A. C., Winskowski, A. M., Lynch, J. K., & Engdahl, B. (2010). The synchronous neural interactions test as a functional neuromarker for post-traumatic stress disorder (PTSD): A robust classification method based on the bootstrap. *Journal of Neural Engineering, 7*(1), 16011.

Huang, M.-X., Theilmann, R. J., Robb, A., Angeles, A., Nichols, S., Drake, A., . . . Lee, R. R. (2009). Integrated imaging approach with MEG and DTI to detect mild traumatic brain injury in military and civilian patients. *Journal of Neurotrauma, 26*(8), 1213–1226.

Hunter, M., Villarreal, G., McHaffie, G. R., Jimenez, B., Smith, A. K., Calais, L. A., . . . Cañive, J. M. (2011). Lateralized abnormalities in auditory M50 sensory gating and cortical thickness of the superior temporal gyrus in post-traumatic stress disorder: Preliminary results. *Psychiatry Research—Neuroimaging, 191*(2), 138–144.

James, L. M., Belitskaya-Lévy, I., Lu, Y., Wang, H., Engdahl, B. E., Leuthold, A. C., & Georgopoulos, A. P. (2015). Development and application of a diagnostic algorithm for posttraumatic stress disorder. *Psychiatry Research—Neuroimaging, 231*(1), 1–7.

James, L. M., Engdahl, B. E., Leuthold, A. C., Lewis, S. M., Van Kampen, E., & Georgopoulos, A. P. (2013). Neural network modulation by trauma as a marker of resilience: Differences between veterans with posttraumatic stress disorder and resilient controls. *JAMA Psychiatry, 70*(4), 410–418.

Jensen, O., & Mazaheri, A. (2010). Shaping functional architecture by oscillatory alpha activity: Gating by inhibition. *Frontiers in Human Neuroscience, 4*, 186.

Khanna, M. M., Badura-Brack, A. S., McDermott, T. J., Embury, C. M., Wiesman, A. I., Shepherd, A., . . . Wilson, T. W. (2017). Veterans with post-traumatic stress disorder exhibit altered emotional processing and attentional control during an emotional Stroop task. *Psychological Medicine, 47*(11), 2017–2027.

Kolassa, I.-T., Wienbruch, C., Neuner, F., Schauer, M., Ruf, M., Odenwald, M., & Elbert, T. (2007). Altered oscillatory brain dynamics after repeated traumatic stress. *BMC Psychiatry, 7*, 56.

McDermott, T. J., Badura-Brack, A. S., Becker, K. M., Ryan, T. J., Bar-Haim, Y., Pine, D. S., . . . Wilson, T. W. (2016). Attention training improves aberrant neural dynamics during working memory processing in veterans with PTSD. *Cognitive, Affective and Behavioral Neuroscience, 16*(6), 1140–1149.

Misic, B., Dunkley, B. T., Sedge, P. A., Costa, L. Da, Fatima, Z., Berman, M. G., . . . Taylor, M. J. (2016). Post-Traumatic Stress Constrains the Dynamic Repertoire of Neural Activity. *Journal of Neuroscience, 36*(2), 419–431.

Palva, J. M., Monto, S., Kulashekhar, S., & Palva, S. (2010). Neuronal synchrony reveals working memory networks and predicts individual memory capacity. *Proceedings of the National Academy of Sciences of the United States of America, 107*(16), 7580–7585.

Pang, E. W., Sedge, P., Grodecki, R., Robertson, A., MacDonald, M. J., Jetly, R., . . . Taylor, M. J. (2014). Colour or shape: Examination of neural processes underlying mental flexibility in posttraumatic stress disorder. *Translational Psychiatry, 4*(8), e421.

Ramchand, R., Schell, T. L., Karney, B. R., Osilla, K. C., Burns, R. M., & Caldarone, L. B. (2010). Disparate prevalence estimates of PTSD among service members who served in Iraq and Afghanistan: Possible explanations. *Journal of Traumatic Stress, 23*, 59–68.

Rauch, S. L., Shin, L. M., & Phelps, E. A. (2006). Neurocircuitry models of posttraumatic stress disorder and extinction: Human neuroimaging research-past, present, and future. *Biological Psychiatry, 60*, 376–382.

Ray, W. J., Odenwald, M., Neuner, F., Schauer, M., Ruf, M., Wienbruch, C., . . . Elbert, T. (2006). Decoupling neural networks from reality: Dissociative experiences in torture victims are reflected in abnormal brain waves in left frontal cortex. *Psychological Science, 17*(10), 825–829.

Rowland, J. A., Stapleton-Kotloski, J. R., Alberto, G. E., Rawley, J. A., Kotloski, R. J., Taber, K. H., & Godwin, D. W. (2017). Contrasting effects of posttraumatic stress disorder and mild traumatic brain injury on the whole-brain resting-state network: A magnetoencephalography study. *Brain Connectivity, 7*(1), 45–57.

Rutledge, O. (2015). Characterization of combat-induced PTSD in OEF/OIF veterans using MEG-based imaging. *ProQuest Dissertations and Theses.* Retrieved from http://easyaccess.lib.cuhk.edu.hk/login?url=http://search.proquest.com/docview/1722488943?accountid=10371%5Chttp://findit.lib.cuhk.edu.hk/852cuhk/?url_ver=Z39.88-2004&rft_val_fmt=info:ofi/fmt:kev:mtx:disserta

tion&genre=dissertations+%26+theses&sid=Pro Q:P

Schalinski, I., Moran, J. K., Elbert, T., Reindl, V., & Wienbruch, C. (2017). Oscillatory magnetic brain activity is related to dissociative symptoms and childhood adversities: A study in women with multiple trauma. *Journal of Affective Disorders, 218,* 428–436.

Shah-Basak, P. P., Urbain, C., Wong, S., da Costa, L., Pang, E. W., Dunkley, B. T., & Taylor, M. J. (2018). Concussion Alters the Functional Brain Processes of Visual Attention and Working Memory. *Journal of Neurotrauma, 35*(2). Published Online 15 Jan 2018.

Simmons, A. N., Fitzpatrick, S., Strigo, I. A., Potterat, E. G., Johnson, D. C., Matthews, S. C., . . . Paulus, M. P. (2012). Altered insula activation in anticipation of changing emotional states: Neural mechanisms underlying cognitive flexibility in special operations forces personnel. *NeuroReport, 23,* 234–239.

Swan, A. R., Nichols, S., Drake, A., Angeles, A., Diwakar, M., Song, T., . . . Huang, M. (2015). MEG Slow-wave detection in patients with mild traumatic brain injury and ongoing symptoms correlated with long-term neuropsychological outcome. *Journal of Neurotrauma, 32,* 1510–1521.Todd, R. M., MacDonald, M. J., Sedge, P., Robertsone A., Jetly, R., Taylor, M. J., & Pang, E. W. (2015). Soldiers with Posttraumatic Stress Disorder See a World Full of Threat: Magnetoencephalography Reveals Enhanced Tuning to Combat-Related Cues. *Biological Psychiatry.*

US Department of Veterans Affairs. (2015). How common is PTSD?—PTSD: National Center for PTSD. Retrieved from https://www.ptsd.va.gov/understand/common/common_veterans.asp

Vakorin, V. A., Doesburg, S. M., da Costa, L., Jetly, R., Pang, E. W., & Taylor, M. J. (2016). Detecting mild traumatic brain injury using resting state magnetoencephalographic connectivity. *PLoS Computational Biology, 12*(12), e1004914.

van Zyl, M., Oosthuizen, P. P., & Seedat, S. (2008). Post traumatic stress disorder: Undiagnosed cases in a tertiary inpatient setting. *African Journal of Psychiatry, 11*(2), 119–122.

Wilde, E. A., Bouix, S., Tate, D. F., Lin, A. P., Newsome, M. R., Taylor, B. A., . . . York, G. (2015). Advanced neuroimaging applied to veterans and service personnel with traumatic brain injury: state of the art and potential benefits. *Brain Imaging and Behavior, 9,* 367–402. Published 08 September 2015.

Zhang, Y., Chen, H., Long, Z., Cui, Q., & Chen, H. (2016). Altered effective connectivity network of the thalamus in post-traumatic stress disorder: A resting-state FMRI study with Granger causality method. *Applied Informatics, 3*(8).

23

IDENTIFYING NEURAL ABNORMALITIES IN SCHIZOPHRENIA

J. Christopher Edgar and Gregory A. Miller

23.1. INTRODUCTION

This chapter considers the use of magnetoencephalography (MEG) in understanding brain dysfunction in schizophrenia (Sz). As detailed in introductory chapters of this book, MEG has been considered for clinical purposes since the 1980s, with clinical indications currently approved for epilepsy and presurgical localization. MEG studies of Sz first appeared in 1989. Specifically, Reite Teale, Goldstein, Whalen, and Linnville (1989) published in the *Archives of General Psychiatry* a study reporting abnormal left–right hemisphere lateralization of the auditory cortex neural generators in adults with Sz (a study completed using a single-channel axial second-order gradiometer). In a Comment in the same issue, Reeve, Rose, and Weinberger (1989) provided an overview of MEG, noting that since MEG measures are not distorted by differences in brain, cerebrospinal fluid (CSF), skull, or scalp resistivity, MEG has the potential to localize sources in three dimensions more accurately than electroencephalography (EEG). Reeve et al. went on to note that, although MEG research in psychiatric populations is of interest, work in this area was limited by expensive MEG systems with small sensor arrays (at that time ~$1 million for a seven-channel system and shielded room). Reeve concluded that, "Even if the theoretical and practical limitations can be overcome, the value of the data provided by MEG for understanding and/or treating psychiatric disorders is uncertain" (p. 576).

As detailed later, much has been learned about brain function in Sz through the use of MEG, and the number of MEG studies of Sz increases year to year. A clinical MEG exam for Sz, however, is still far in the future. This

J. Christopher Edgar and Gregory A. Miller, *Identifying Neural Abnormalities in Schizophrenia* In: *Fifty Years of Magnetoencephalography*. Edited by: Andrew C. Papanicolaou, Timothy P. L. Roberts, and James W. Wheless, Oxford University Press (2020). © Oxford University Press.
DOI: 10.1093/oso/9780190935689.003.0023.

is, in part, because more research is needed to identify neural measures that reliably and robustly predict risk and/or conversion to, or to identify neural measures that are clear treatment targets (e.g., used to evaluate response to therapy). The high cost of obtaining and operating a MEG system also remains an obstacle. Rather than providing a comprehensive review of the MEG Sz literature, this chapter focuses on MEG brain measures that have received the most attention: resting-state studies and studies examining auditory encoding processes. As detailed later, these studies indicate that continued research in this area is of interest, with findings suggesting a focus on resting-state and task-related low-frequency activity. Studies examining changes in brain activity in response to therapy (psychological or pharmacological) are also of interest. (Although not reviewed here, readers with interest in Sz are encouraged to read, among others, studies examining the somatosensory system (Edgar et al., 2005; Wilson et al., 2007, 2011), visual system (Grent-'t-Jong et al., 2016; Silverstein et al., 2006), multisystem processing (Robson et al., 2016; Sanfratello, Aine, & Stephen, 2018), as well as recent MEG studies examining whole-brain functional connectivity in Sz (Alamian et al., 2017; Brookes et al., 2015; Hirvonen et al., 2017).

23.2. RESTING-STATE BRAIN ACTIVITY IN SCHIZOPHRENIA

Early MEG studies examined resting-state oscillatory activity in Sz. A few early studies examining resting-state alpha activity found decreased alpha frequency and power in adults with Sz (Canive et al., 1998; Canive et al., 1996), with these findings replicating EEG studies reporting diminished resting-state alpha-band power in Sz, both untreated/neuroleptic-naïve (Miyauchi, Endo, Kajiwara, Ishii, & Okajima, 1996; Miyauchi et al., 1990; Nagase, Okubo, & Toru, 1996) and treated (Fenton, Fenwick, Dollimore, Dunn, & Hirsch, 1980; Saletu et al., 1994; Sponheim, Clementz, Iacono, & Beiser,

1994), as well as across different *Diagnostic and Statistical Manual of Mental Disorders* (DSM) subtypes (Miyauchi et al., 1996; Sponheim et al., 1994). A very recent resting-state study found that patients high in positive symptoms showed decreased alpha power, indicating that decreased alpha was clinically significant (Zeev-Wolf et al., 2018).

Compared with resting-state alpha studies, assessment of resting-state low-frequency (delta and theta) oscillatory activity has received greater attention in MEG studies. These studies have built on EEG studies reporting more delta (1–4 Hz) and theta (4–8 Hz) resting-state activity in Sz than controls (Canive et al., 1998; Fehr et al., 2001; Pascual-Marqui et al., 1999; B. Rockstroh et al., 1997; Sponheim et al., 1994; Weinberger, 1988; Wienbruch et al., 2003; Winterer, Ziller, Dorn, Frick, Mulert, Wuebben, & Herrmann, 2000), with a meta-analysis concluding that enhanced low-frequency activity in Sz is a robust finding (Galderisi, Mucci, Volpe, & Boutros, 2009). Although delta and theta oscillatory activity is common in stages 3 and 4 of slow wave sleep (Iramina & Ueno, 1996; Llinas, Urbano, Leznik, Ramirez, & van Marle, 2005; Rechtschaffen & Kales, 1968), such activity during awake states is pathological in adults, associated with traumatic brain injury (Huang et al., 2012), Alzheimer disease (Fernandez et al., 2002), and brain lesions (Vieth, Kober, & Grummich, 1996). Given increased low-frequency activity during the waking state in Sz and given that individuals with Sz typically do not show frank pathology on structural magnetic resonance imaging (MRI), it has been suggested that portions of the brain in Sz might be in an inactive "sleep-like state" (Lisman, 2012; Llinas et al., 2005) or that slowing in Sz reflects subtle brain pathology.

With regard to MEG research, using whole-brain MEG source–space measures, Wienbruch et al. (2003) described a method to apply a z-score-based analysis for single subjects and noted that, after a normative database is established, comparison of individual data against scores from a demographically matched control group allows fine distinctions and comparisons unattainable by clinical observation or traditional neuroimaging alone. Using this normative approach, B. S. Rockstroh, Wienbruch, Ray, and Elbert (2007) reported that the spatial topography of low-frequency activity distinguishes individuals with Sz from individuals with neurotic/affective diagnoses. Two recent MEG studies have examined low-frequency activity at rest throughout the brain in Sz. Using L2-minimum norm estimate localization, Fehr et al. (2001) observed higher frontotemporal and posterior delta/theta activity in Sz patients than adult controls. Using frequency-domain vector-based spatio-temporal analysis using L1-minimum norm (VESTAL), Huang et al. (2009, 2012) and as shown in Figure 23.1, Chen et al. (2016) observed abnormal low-frequency activity in frontal and temporoparietal regions in adults with Sz. The Fehr et al. (2001) and Chen et al. (2016) studies thus both indicate frontal as well as posterior low-frequency abnormalities in Sz.

There is increasing evidence that the resting-state low-frequency abnormalities observed in Sz are associated with negative symptoms and poor cognitive ability. Fehr et al. (2003) reported that temporal delta dipole density positively correlated with negative symptoms, and B. S. Rockstroh et al. (2007) observed that individuals with Sz with more affective flattening and less depression displayed more frontocentral slowing. Similar associations between delta and theta slow wave activity and negative symptoms have been reported in EEG studies (Gattaz, Mayer, Ziegler, Platz, & Gasser, 1992). Recently, Chen et al. (2016) found that increased right-frontal delta slowing was associated with negative symptom, attention, and functional capacity impairments. The Chen et al. findings support previous findings (Ferrarelli et al., 2012; Narayanan et al., 2013; Sponheim, Clementz, Iacono, & Beiser, 2000), as well as the meta-analysis by Boutros et al. (2008), suggesting that abnormally elevated resting-state frontal delta is a strong Sz biological correlate, predicting cognitive performance and occupational function in Sz.

The overall pattern of low-frequency findings in Sz is consistent with the notion of frontal

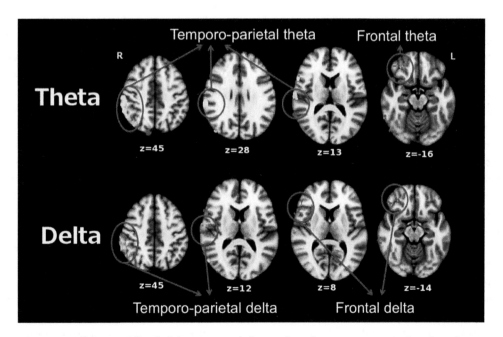

FIGURE 23.1 Clusters in *yellow/red* show more right hemisphere slow wave activity in the schizophrenia group ($N = 37$) than in the control group ($N = 41$) ($p < 0.05$, family-wise corrected).

lobe pathology in Sz affecting multiple domains. For example, symptoms such as poor initiative, social withdrawal, and impaired attention are similar to the symptoms observed in patients with frontal-lobe disease (Weinberger, 1988). Lisman (2012) hypothesized that an abnormal balance between excitatory and inhibitory synapses in the frontal lobe could cause cognitive deficits and negative symptoms in Sz. In this context, increased frontal delta activity may contribute to neural network dysfunction and thus to negative symptoms and cognitive impairment in Sz. Low-frequency abnormalities may also be a risk factor for an endophenotype because studies have shown low-frequency abnormalities in Sz patients and their relatives (Hong, Summerfelt, Mitchell, O'Donnell, & Thaker, 2012; Venables, Bernat, & Sponheim, 2009), leading to the conclusion that abnormal low-frequency neural oscillations appear to be a heritable risk factor/trait for Sz (Boutros et al., 2008; Hong et al., 2012; Venables et al., 2009).

As discussed in the following section, low-frequency abnormalities in Sz are not specific to the resting state. For example, EEG studies have shown that early auditory encoding abnormalities in Sz are best characterized by decreased low-frequency phase locking (Blumenfeld & Clementz, 2001; Clementz & Blumenfeld, 2001; Edgar et al., 2008; Jansen, Hegde, & Boutros, 2004; Johannesen et al., 2005; Popov, Jordanov, Weisz, et al., 2011). Using MEG, Edgar et al. (2014) observed greater left superior temporal gyrus (STG) prestimulus power (~4–20 Hz) in Sz than in HC. These and other studies indicate that low-frequency oscillatory abnormalities appear to be a primary abnormality in Sz, observed at rest as well as during tasks.

23.3. AUDITORY STUDIES

Taking advantage of the ability to localize the generators of neural activity, the earliest MEG studies examining the auditory system in Sz focused on the location of the auditory 100-ms (M100) neural generators. Using a seven-channel MEG system, Reite et al. (1989) noted

more posterior and more vertical orientations of the left than right auditory M100 neural generators in controls ($N = 6$) and a lack of this asymmetry in adults with paranoid Sz ($N = 6$). The Reite et al. findings mirrored prior findings of atypical asymmetries of primary/secondary auditory cortex in individuals with Sz in structural studies, such as atypical planum temporale and STG structural asymmetries (for reviews, see Shapleske, Rossell, Woodruff, & David, 1999; Sommer, Ramsey, & Kahn, 2001).

The significance of atypical STG asymmetries in Sz is unclear. Heim, Kissler, Elbert, and Rockstroh (2004) suggested that the abnormal functional STG asymmetry they observed in a study examining the position of the auditory M100 response in Sz and dyslexia might be linked to abnormal language development, and they hypothesized that developmental dyslexia with its altered hemisphere asymmetry might be a precursor for Sz. Teale, Carlson, Rojas, and Reite (2003) observed reduced hemisphere asymmetry of STG 40-Hz steady-state auditory response in patients with Sz and noted that the findings "seem to be consonant with the suggestion of Crow and colleagues, who have advanced theories relating Sz to disturbances in language function, especially involving the temporal lobe" (p. 1152). Finally, Petty et al. (1995) suggested that the atypical PT asymmetries might be "linked conceptually to two key symptoms of Sz—auditory hallucinations and thought disorder" (p. 6).

Although intriguing, especially given the excess of individuals with dyslexia found in the relatives of Sz patients (Fish, 1987; Richardson, 1994), MEG studies have shown atypical patterns of STG asymmetry for other patient populations (e.g., schizoaffective subjects [Teale, Reite, Rojas, Sheeder, & Arciniegas, 2000] and patients with fragile X syndrome [Rojas et al., 2001]), so their contributory role in Sz symptoms and language problems has yet to be firmly established. Indeed, the significance of atypical brain asymmetries must come to be understood in the context of its frequent appearance in individuals with no psychopathology (Geschwind & Levitsky, 1968). Using MEG, Edgar et al. (2006) found the expected right–left M100 anterior–posterior positional asymmetry for normal control subjects, and the reduction of this asymmetry for individuals with Sz or dyslexia. In the same study, Edgar et al. found that the Sz and dyslexia subjects also had higher minor physical anomaly scores than normal controls, and analyses of individual minor physical anomaly items revealed a relationship between high palate and M100 asymmetry. Edgar et al. concluded that the findings indicated that M100 positional asymmetry is not a diagnostically specific feature and that atypical hemisphere asymmetries may instead be simply epiphenomenal, indicating a disturbance in brain development common to many neurodevelopmental disorders (e.g., slow fetal development).

Although providing an impetus for the use of MEG to understand brain dysfunction in Sz (and other neurodevelopmental disorders), the line of research examining hemisphere asymmetry abnormalities in Sz has not been pursued, with a literature search suggesting the most recent MEG publications on this topic in 2013 (Wang et al., 2013) and 2014 (Wang et al., 2014). Although studies examining the location of the M100 neural generators are not now common, MEG studies examining auditory cortex neural generators in Sz have increased throughout the first two decades of this century. These studies have examined activity of primary/secondary auditory neural generators to pure tone and steady-state stimuli (e.g., Blumenfeld & Clementz, 2001; Hamm, Gilmore, Picchetti, Sponheim, & Clementz, 2011; Popov, Jordanov, Weisz, et al., 2011; Shin et al., 2012; Smith et al., 2010), as well as examination of auditory system change detection responses such as the mismatch field response and the oddball response (Boutros, Gjini, Wang, & Bowyer, 2018; Braeutigam, Dima, Frangou, & James, 2018; Gaebler et al., 2015; Jordanov et al., 2011; Naatanen & Kahkonen, 2009; Sauer et al., 2017; Thonnessen et al.,

2008). These studies demonstrate auditory encoding abnormalities in individuals with Sz. For example, using pure-tone stimuli and applying time–frequency analyses to examine poststimulus activity and left and right auditory cortex neural generators, Edgar et al. (2008) showed poststimulus low-frequency abnormalities in adults with Sz (total power and intertrial coherence), findings consistent with other studies showing decreased low-frequency poststimulus activity in adults with Sz (Gilmore, Clementz, & Buckley, 2004; Winterer, Ziller, Dorn, Frick, Mulert, Wuebben, Herrmann, et al., 2000). To the extent that early auditory evoked responses such as the M50 and M100 responses are generated by a reorganization of ongoing oscillations in the MEG (Basar, 1980; Brandt, 1997; David, Harrison, & Friston, 2005; Sayers, Beagley, & Henshall, 1974), these findings indicate a deficit in individuals with Sz in synchronizing the phase of ongoing low-frequency oscillatory activity (see also Jansen et al., 2004). Thus, a second body of research has implicated low-frequency activity in Sz.

Perhaps the most extensive and intensive use of MEG in the Sz literature has been investigations of neural mechanisms contributing to the so-called sensory gating deficit. The measure is typically a ratio between the amplitude of the response to the second of two clicks separated by 500 ms to the amplitude of the response to the first click. Patients with Sz have often been reported to show a higher ratio, due either to a smaller first response or less suppression of the second response. More than three decades of EEG studies have had little success in clarifying the nature of deficit or identifying relevant neural mechanisms. MEG source analysis has reliably pointed to generators in Heschl's gyrus, but controversy remains about mechanisms. For example, a MEG study with unusually large patient and control samples replicated the ratio deficit but pointed more to S1 than to S2 as driving the ratio effects (Smith et al., 2010). Methods-oriented studies have noted substantial individual differences in source strength and orientation(e.g., Edgar et al., 2003) and potentially complex relationships among diverse measures of sensory gating (e.g., Hanlon et al., 2005; Schubring, Popov, Miller, & Rockstroh, 2018), complicating interpretations about Sz.

More recently, there has been interest in studying auditory driving responses in Sz. Researchers have used 40-Hz auditory driving stimuli to examine dysfunction in the 40-Hz neural circuit networks in Sz, given hypothesized abnormalities in pyramidal cells and inhibitory interneuron networks in the superficial cortical layers in Sz (for a review, see Gandal, Edgar, Klook, & Siegel, 2012). Many EEG studies have observed 40-Hz steady-state abnormalities in Sz (Brenner, Sporns, Lysaker, & O'Donnell, 2003; Hall et al., 2011; Hamm, Gilmore, & Clementz, 2012; Hong et al., 2004; Koenig, van Swam, Dierks, & Hubl, 2012; Krishnan et al., 2009; Kwon et al., 1999; Lenz, Fischer, Schadow, Bogerts, & Herrmann, 2011; Light et al., 2006; Rass et al., 2012; Spencer, Niznikiewicz, Nestor, Shenton, & McCarley, 2009; Spencer, Salisbury, Shenton, & McCarley, 2008). MEG steady-state studies applying source localization also show 40-Hz abnormalities in Sz. For example, Teale et al. (2008) observed decreased STG 40-Hz driving intertrial coherence and evoked activity bilaterally in patients with Sz.

The use of 40-Hz auditory steady-state stimuli and relatively long interstimulus intervals (ISI; e.g., greater than 1 s) allows examination of both early transient responses (such as the 50-ms and 100-ms auditory responses) and steady-state activity (Jacobson & Fitzgerald, 1997; Pantev et al., 1993). Because left and right STG regions are the primary generators of the early transient responses (Hari, 1990; Hari, Aittoniemi, Jarvinen, Katila, & Varpula, 1980; Makela, Hamalainen, Hari, & McEvoy, 1994; Naatanen & Picton, 1987; Pelizzone et al., 1987; Reite, Teale, Zimmerman, Davis, & Whalen, 1988; Yvert, Crouzeix, Bertrand, Seither-Preisler, & Pantev, 2001), as well as the 40-Hz steady-state

response (Herdman et al., 2003; Ross, Picton, & Pantev, 2002), some studies have used source localization to directly assess the left and right STG cortical microcircuits involved in auditory encoding. As an example, using a 40-Hz steady-state task with a relatively long ISI, Edgar et al. (2014) showed multiple disruptions in STG auditory areas in Sz, including STG poststimulus low-frequency abnormalities (4–16 Hz) as well as 40-Hz steady-state abnormalities.

Recent research has sought to examine the methods used to obtain auditory encoding measures. Examining the construct validity of 40-Hz steady-state MEG and EEG measures, Edgar et al. (2017) demonstrated limitations examining 40-Hz steady-state activity in EEG sensor space (e.g., inability to assess hemisphere differences in the strength of the 40-Hz steady-state response) and thus advantages of directly assessing 40-Hz steady-state source–space activity in left and right STG. Examining a variety of head models (spherical and realistic) and a variety of dipole source modeling strategies (dipole source localization and dipoles fixed to Heschl's gyrus), Edgar et al. demonstrated generality in results across head and source modeling strategies and concluded that the use of a MEG or EEG spherical head model with sources manually fixed to left and right Heschl's gyrus is an effective and efficient method for measuring the left and right STG 40-Hz steady-state response.

Building on and extending this 40-Hz steady-state methods study, Edgar et al. (2018) used MEG and EEG spherical head models with sources manually fixed to left and right Heschl's gyri to compare MEG and EEG in identifying control and Sz group differences in poststimulus low-frequency (4–16 Hz) and 40-Hz steady-state processes. Also of interest was comparing source modeling results to EEG sensor results, with the hypothesis of better group differentiation for EEG source and MEG source than EEG sensor measures given greater predictive utility for source measures. The Edgar et al. (2018) results indicated that, whereas controls and Sz auditory encoding low-frequency group-difference effects were generally comparable across modality and analysis strategies, 40-Hz steady-state difference findings were much more dependent on modality and analysis strategy. In particular, low-frequency analyses did not support the hypothesis of better group differentiation for source than sensor measures, with poststimulus low-frequency group differences observed across all recording strategies (source and sensor), indicating that the detection of low-frequency group differences is generally not reliant on recording or analysis strategy. In contrast, the 40-Hz steady-state analyses supported the study hypothesis, although in the context of an age-related decrease in left STG 40-Hz steady-state activity in the adults controls, the expected control > Sz 40-Hz steady-state group differences were evident only in the younger participants' source–space measures. For EEG, given strong age-related 40-Hz steady-state changes in the adult controls, 40-Hz steady-state group differences were in the unexpected direction in older participants.

These results help make sense of the 40-Hz steady-state inconsistencies in the literature—in some studies, 40-Hz steady-state activity is greater in controls than individuals with Sz (Brenner et al., 2003; Krishnan et al., 2009; Kwon et al., 1999; Light et al., 2006; Spencer et al., 2008; Teale et al., 2008; Tsuchimoto et al., 2011; Vierling-Claassen, Siekmeier, Stufflebeam, & Kopell, 2008), in some the reverse (Hamm et al., 2012), and in some studies no group differences are observed (Hong et al., 2004; Rass et al., 2012). The Edgar et al. (2018) findings, as well as the 40-Hz meta-analysis by Thune, Recasens, and Uhlhaas (2016), thus indicate that auditory cortex 40-Hz deficits are more robustly observed in younger patient populations. Although there is currently great interest in using tasks that activate gamma neural circuits in first-episode and prodromal and at-risk populations to better understand gamma deficits at the onset and preceding the onset of Sz, previous MEG and EEG studies suggest caution because a 40-Hz

steady-state response is less often observed in younger populations (Cho et al., 2015; Edgar et al., 2016; Rojas et al., 2006).

Recent MEG studies of auditory encoding processes in Sz have sought to examine auditory encoding processes throughout the brain rather than focusing on left and right auditory cortex neural generators. As an example, Chen et al. (2018) showed weaker poststimulus auditory encoding activity in controls than patients with Sz in right frontal areas as well as STG regions, indicating that auditory encoding abnormalities in Sz are not specific to STG. As shown in Figure 23.2, Chen et al. also recruited unaffected relatives of the patients with Sz and showed that auditory encoding abnormalities in the patients and relatives were shared only in left STG, thus indicating that the identification of endophenotypes in Sz must consider specific brain region rather than a composite MEG or EEG sensor measure (see Edgar et al., 2003, for an extended discussion). Further work examining auditory processes throughout the brain is of interest.

23.4. ASSESSING THE EFFECT OF PSYCHOLOGICAL AND PHARMACOLOGICAL TREATMENT

Despite growing evidence of auditory encoding abnormalities in Sz and greater specification of auditory encoding abnormalities through source time–frequency analyses, little is known about whether these abnormalities can be normalized. Reviewing EEG N100 studies, Rosburg, Boutros, and Ford (2008) noted that most studies find that N100 amplitude is not normalized by treatment with antipsychotic medications. As an example, Ford et al. (1994) did not observe any change in N100 amplitude deficit in a sample of patients with Sz tested before and then 4 weeks after treatment with antipsychotic medication. As N100 abnormalities are observed in unmedicated chronic patients (Brockhaus-Dumke et al., 2008; Laurent et al., 1999), as well as in unmedicated first-episode patients and in individuals at-risk for

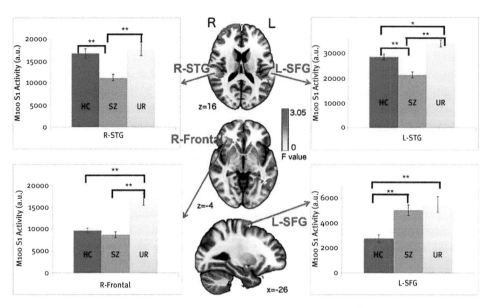

FIGURE 23.2   M100 analysis of variance M100 group differences for controls ($N = 70$), adults with schizophrenia ($N = 69$), and unaffected relatives (UR).

Sz (Brockhaus-Dumke et al., 2008), N100 abnormalities may reflect a trait unaffected by treatment.

Although findings to date have been discouraging, a lack of medication findings in studies examining EEG scalp activity may reflect the fact that analyses examining the relationship between EEG scalp activity and medication and/or clinical measures are inherently limited because spatially aggregated scalp measures can mask specific relationships and may not provide information about hemisphere differences, owing to the superposition of activity from multiple brain regions at the scalp sensors (Edgar et al., 2003, 2017). In addition, since time–frequency measures may more directly reflect discrete neurobiological mechanisms, such measures may more strongly associate with clinical measures than a composite time–domain evoked response. Furthermore, studies examining associations between clinical measures and time–frequency activity at specific brain regions may reveal relationships masked at scalp sensors.

Studies examining the effect of medication are, however, often difficult to conduct and/or interpret. As an example, in an unpublished study,

Edgar and Miller examined associations between auditory encoding low-frequency phase locking and medication status. In particular, MEG from 45 controls and 45 patients with Sz administered a standard paired-click task produced left and right hemisphere 100-ms STG phase locking measures. As shown in Figure 23.3, patients on typical antipsychotics ($N = 12$; haloperidol and fluphenazine) showed less STG theta-band phase locking than controls and patients on atypical antipsychotics ($N = 25$; aripiprazole, olanzapine, risperidone, quetiapine). Although these findings suggested that atypical antipsychotics may normalize STG theta-band activity and that normalization of theta-band phase locking would be a promising target of treatment in patients, such findings are inherently confounded. Specifically, since patients were not randomly assigned to a medication group, it is difficult to interpret typical and atypical medication effects, with group differences also potentially due to susceptibility to extrapyramidal side effects or signs of tardive dyskinesia (and thus patients nonrandomly assigned by their clinician to an atypical antipsychotic), medication compliance differences between groups, cognitive differences between groups, and so on. As an example, as shown in

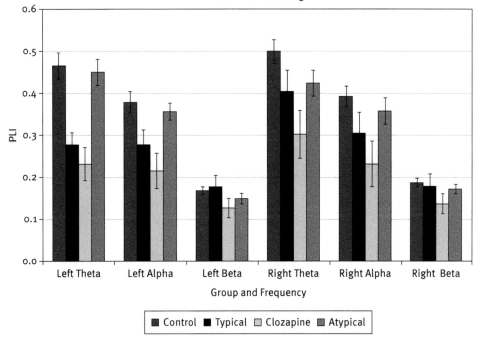

FIGURE 23.3   Group (control, typical, clozapine, atypical) M100 S1 superior temporal gyrus phase locking index (PLI) mean values are shown as a function of frequency (theta, alpha, beta) and hemisphere. The PLI quantifies trial-to-trial phase variability. Standard error of the mean bars are shown. Less theta-band phase locking was observed in patients on typical antipsychotics and patients on clozapine than in controls and patients on atypical antipsychotics.

Figure 23.3, the patients on clozapine had less theta-band STG phase locking than controls and patients on atypicals, with patients on clozapine appearing as a somewhat distinct subgroup. To the extent that patients on clozapine represent a distinct genetic subtype of Sz, the present STG phase locking findings may reflect genetic differences, with mice and human studies showing strain (genetic) differences on the effect of pharmacological compounds on auditory responses (e.g., Lu et al., 2007; Maxwell et al., 2006).

To more directly examine such issues, studies randomly assigning patients to medication groups, dose-response studies, and longitudinal studies are needed. For example, the observation of reduced N100 amplitude in patients on high doses of antipsychotics compared with patients with low doses of antipsychotics may indicate a dose-dependent relationship (Baribeau-Braun, Picton, &

Gosselin, 1983). Examination of STG phase locking activity in patients with early-onset Sz, as well as in family members, would also be of interest to determine the extent to which STG phase locking dysfunction is associated with the onset of the disorder as well as whether STG phase locking abnormalities are a risk factor. There is reason to think that STG phase locking abnormalities would be observed in both groups. Brockhaus-Dumke et al. (2008) observed small N100 S1 in unmedicated patients with chronic Sz, in unmedicated first-episode patients, and in prodromal subjects who later developed Sz. Decreased N100 was not observed in at-risk subjects who did not go on to develop Sz (within a 24-month follow-up period). They concluded that their findings support the hypothesis that reduced N100 amplitude reflects a stable trait and a risk indicator of Sz already present in prodromal and early stages of Sz.

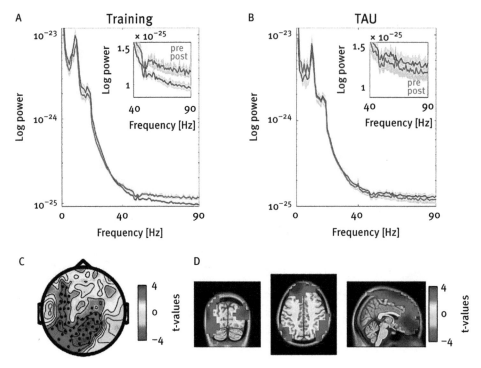

FIGURE 23.4 (A) Power spectrum of the training group for pretraining (*blue*) and post-training (*red*) assessments. The *inset* illustrates high-frequency gamma activity (40–90 Hz). (B) Same as part A but for the treatment-as-usual (TAU) group. (C) Topography of the change in gamma activity from pretraining to post-training in the training group (cluster permutation test, $p < 0.05$). *Black dots* show normalized locations of sensors included in the cluster (same for both groups). (D) Source localization of the effect in part C, masked according to significance (cluster permutation test, $p < 0.05$). The *color bar* in parts C and D indicates the distribution of t values. The *shading* indicates standard error of the mean. a.u. = arbitrary units; HC = Healthy Control; SFG = superior frontal gyrus; STG = superior temporal gyrus; SZ = schizophrenia; UR = Unaffected Relative.

Another promising line of MEG research in the Sz literature is the identification of neural mechanisms associated with targeted sensory and cognitive training. After replicating the sensory gating deficit (Popov, Jordanov, Weisz, et al., 2011) and establishing a similar deficit in chronic and first-admission Sz (Carolus et al., 2014), Popov, Rockstroh, and colleagues showed that targeted training improved both gating and neuropsychological test performance (Popov, Jordanov, Rockstroh, et al., 2011) and normalized alpha power, as well as improving clinical symptoms (Popov, Rockstroh, Weisz, Elbert, & Miller, 2012). As shown in Figure 23.4, this training also normalized resting-state gamma, which correlated with neuropsychological test performance (Popova et al., 2018). When this approach to training was extended to recognition of facial emotion, MEG showed that the training specifically improved alpha and that this improvement predicted improved emotion-recognition performance and neuropsychological test performance (Popov et al., 2015; Popova et al., 2014).

23.5. CONCLUSION

MEG resting-state and auditory-response studies indicate that a focus of future research should be the identification of neural network processes associated with the generation of low-frequency activity as well as multimodal studies examining association between brain structure (e.g., diffusion measures) and function to better understand low-frequency activity. As detailed previously, although the use of single-channel EEG can robustly differentiate controls and individuals with Sz with respect to low-frequency activity, electromagnetic neuroimaging is needed to examine the specific generators. To identify optimal clinical procedures (reliable, robust, and fast), EEG/MEG studies are needed to help identify the data collection and analysis methods that robustly discriminate groups, with current findings indicating that construct-valid measures may not always distinguish groups better than methods we might consider suboptimal.

REFERENCES

Alamian, G., Hincapie, A. S., Pascarella, A., Thiery, T., Combrisson, E., Saive, A. L., . . . Jerbi, K. (2017). Measuring alterations in oscillatory brain networks in schizophrenia with resting-state MEG: State-of-the-art and methodological challenges. *Clinical Neurophysiology, 128*(9), 1719–1736.

Baribeau-Braun, J., Picton, T. W., & Gosselin, J. Y. (1983). Schizophrenia: A neurophysiological evaluation of abnormal information processing. *Science, 219*(4586), 874–876.

Basar, E. (1980). *EEG-brain dynamics: Relation between EEG and brain evoked potentials.* New York, NY: Elsevier.

Blumenfeld, L. D., & Clementz, B. A. (2001). Response to the first stimulus determines reduced auditory evoked response suppression in schizophrenia: Single trials analysis using MEG. *Clinical Neurophysiology, 112*(9), 1650–1659.

Boutros, N. N., Arfken, C., Galderisi, S., Warrick, J., Pratt, G., & Iacono, W. (2008). The status of spectral EEG abnormality as a diagnostic test for schizophrenia. *Schizophrenia Research, 99*(1-3), 225–237.

Boutros, N. N., Gjini, K., Wang, F., & Bowyer, S. M. (2018). Evoked potentials investigations of deficit versus nondeficit schizophrenia: EEG-MEG preliminary data. *Clinical EEG and Neuroscience, 50*(2).

Braeutigam, S., Dima, D., Frangou, S., & James, A. (2018). Dissociable auditory mismatch response and connectivity patterns in adolescents with schizophrenia and adolescents with bipolar disorder with psychosis: A magnetoencephalography study. *Schizophrenia Research, 193,* 313–318.

Brandt, M. E. (1997). Visual and auditory evoked phase resetting of the alpha EEG. *Internation Journal of Psychophysiology, 26*(1–3), 285–298.

Brenner, C. A., Sporns, O., Lysaker, P. H., & O'Donnell, B. F. (2003). EEG synchronization to modulated auditory tones in schizophrenia, schizoaffective disorder, and schizotypal personality disorder. *American Journal of Psychiatry, 160*(12), 2238–2240.

Brockhaus-Dumke, A., Schultze-Lutter, F., Mueller, R., Tendolkar, I., Bechdolf, A., Pukrop, R., . . . Ruhrmann, S. (2008). Sensory gating in schizophrenia: P50 and N100 gating in antipsychotic-free subjects at risk, first-episode, and chronic patients. *Biological Psychiatry, 64*(5), 376–384.

Brookes, M. J., Hall, E. L., Robson, S. E., Price, D., Palaniyappan, L., Liddle, E. B., . . . Morris, P. G. (2015). Complexity measures in magnetoencephalography: Measuring "disorder" in schizophrenia. *PLoS One, 10*(4), e0120991.

Canive, J. M., Lewine, J. D., Edgar, J. C., Davis, J. T., Miller, G. A., Torres, F., & Tuason, V. B. (1998). Spontaneous brain magnetic activity in schizophrenia patients treated with aripiprazole. *Psychopharmacology Bulletin, 34*(1), 101–105.

Canive, J. M., Lewine, J. D., Edgar, J. C., Davis, J. T., Torres, F., Roberts, B., . . . Tuason, V. B. (1996). Magnetoencephalographic assessment of spontaneous brain activity in schizophrenia. *Psychopharmacology Bulletin, 32*(4), 741–750.

Carolus, A. M., Schubring, D., Popov, T. G., Popova, P., Miller, G. A., & Rockstroh, B. S. (2014). Functional cognitive and cortical abnormalities in chronic and first-admission schizophrenia. *Schizophrenia Research, 157*(1-3), 40–47.

Chen, Y. H., Howell, B., Edgar, J. C., Huang, M., Kochunov, P., Hunter, M. A., . . . Canive, J. M. (2018). Associations and heritability of auditory encoding, gray matter, and attention in schizophrenia. *Schizophrenia Bulletin, 45*(4), 859–870.

Chen, Y. H., Stone-Howell, B., Edgar, J. C., Huang, M., Wootton, C., Hunter, M. A., . . . Canive, J. M. (2016). Frontal slow-wave activity as a predictor of negative symptoms, cognition and functional capacity in schizophrenia. *British Journal of Psychiatry, 208*(2), 160–167.

Cho, R. Y., Walker, C. P., Polizzotto, N. R., Wozny, T. A., Fissell, C., Chen, C. M., & Lewis, D. A. (2015). Development of sensory gamma oscillations and cross-frequency coupling from childhood to early adulthood. *Cerebral Cortex, 25*(6), 1509–1518.

Clementz, B. A., & Blumenfeld, L. D. (2001). Multichannel electroencephalographic assessment of auditory evoked response suppression in schizophrenia. *Experimental Brain Research, 139*(4), 377–390.

David, O., Harrison, L., & Friston, K. J. (2005). Modelling event-related responses in the brain. *Neuroimage, 25*(3), 756–770.

Edgar, J. C., Chen, Y.-H., Lanza, M., Howell, B., Chow, V. Y., Heiken, K., . . . Canive, J. M. (2014). Cortical thickness as a contributor to abnormal oscillations in schizophrenia? *Neuroimage: Clinical, 4*, 122–129.

Edgar, J. C., Fisk, C. L., Chen, Y. H., Stone-Howell, B., Liu, S., Hunter, M. A., . . . Miller, G. A. (2018). Identifying auditory cortex encoding abnormalities in schizophrenia: The utility of low-frequency versus 40 Hz steady-state measures. *Psychophysiology, 55*(8), e13074.

Edgar, J. C., Fisk, C. L., Liu, S., Pandey, J., Herrington, J. D., Schultz, R. T., & Roberts, T. P. (2016). Translating adult electrophysiology findings to younger patient populations: Difficulty measuring 40-hz auditory steady-state responses in typically developing children and children with autism spectrum disorder. *Developmental Neuroscience, 38*(1), 1–14.

Edgar, J. C., Fisk Iv, C. L., Chen, Y. H., Stone-Howell, B., Hunter, M. A., Huang, M., . . . Miller, G. A. (2017). By our bootstraps: Comparing methods for measuring auditory 40 Hz steady-state neural activity. *Psychophysiology, 54*(8), 1110–1127.

Edgar, J. C., Hanlon, F. M., Huang, M. X., Weisend, M. P., Thoma, R. J., Carpenter, B., . . . Miller, G. A. (2008). Superior temporal gyrus spectral abnormalities in schizophrenia. *Psychophysiology, 45*(5), 812–824.

Edgar, J. C., Huang, M. X., Weisend, M. P., Sherwood, A., Miller, G. A., Adler, L. E., & Canive, J. M. (2003). Interpreting abnormality: An EEG and MEG study of P50 and the auditory paired-stimulus paradigm. *Biological Psychology, 65*(1), 1–20.

Edgar, J. C., Miller, G. A., Moses, S. N., Thoma, R. J., Huang, M. X., Hanlon, F. M., . . . Canive, J. M. (2005). Cross-modal generality of the gating deficit. *Psychophysiology, 42*(3), 318–327.

Edgar, J. C., Yeo, R. A., Gangestad, S. W., Blake, M. B., Davis, J. T., Lewine, J. D., & Canive, J. M. (2006). Reduced auditory M100 asymmetry in schizophrenia and dyslexia: Applying a developmental instability approach to assess atypical brain asymmetry. *Neuropsychologia, 44*(2), 289–299.

Fehr, T., Kissler, J., Moratti, S., Wienbruch, C., Rockstroh, B., & Elbert, T. (2001). Source distribution of neuromagnetic slow waves and MEG-delta activity in schizophrenic patients. *Biological Psychiatry, 50*(2), 108–116.

Fehr, T., Kissler, J., Wienbruch, C., Moratti, S., Elbert, T., Watzl, H., & Rockstroh, B. (2003). Source distribution of neuromagnetic slow-wave activity in schizophrenic patients--effects of activation. *Schizophrenia Research, 63*(1–2), 63–71.

Fenton, G. W., Fenwick, P. B., Dollimore, J., Dunn, T. L., & Hirsch, S. R. (1980). EEG spectral analysis in schizophrenia. *British Journal of Psychiatry, 136*, 445–455.

Fernandez, A., Maestu, F., Amo, C., Gil, P., Fehr, T., Wienbruch, C., . . . Ortiz, T. (2002). Focal temporoparietal slow activity in Alzheimer's disease revealed by magnetoencephalography. *Biological Psychiatry, 52*(7), 764–770.

Ferrarelli, F., Sarasso, S., Guller, Y., Riedner, B. A., Peterson, M. J., Bellesi, M., . . . Tononi, G. (2012). Reduced natural oscillatory frequency of frontal thalamocortical circuits in schizophrenia. *Archives of General Psychiatry, 69*(8), 766–774.

Fish, B. (1987). Infant predictors of the longitudinal course of schizophrenic development. *Schizophrenia Bulletin, 13*(3), 395–409.

Gaebler, A. J., Mathiak, K., Koten, J. W., Jr., Konig, A. A., Koush, Y., Weyer, D., . . . Zvyagintsev, M. (2015). Auditory mismatch impairments are characterized by core neural dysfunctions in schizophrenia. *Brain, 138*(Pt 5), 1410–1423.

Galderisi, S., Mucci, A., Volpe, U., Boutros, N. (2009). Evidence-based medicine and electrophysiology in schizophrenia. *Clinical EEG and Neuroscience, 40*, 62–77.

Gandal, M. J., Edgar, J. C., Klook, K., & Siegel, S. J. (2012). Gamma synchrony: Towards a translational biomarker for the treatment-resistant symptoms of schizophrenia. *Neuropharmacology, 62*(3), 1504–1518.

Gattaz, W. F., Mayer, S., Ziegler, P., Platz, M., & Gasser, T. (1992). Hypofrontality on topographic EEG in schizophrenia: Correlations with neuropsychological and psychopathological parameters. *European Archives of Psychiatry and Clinical Neuroscience, 241*(6), 328–332.

Geschwind, N., & Levitsky, W. (1968). Human brain: Left-right asymmetries in temporal speech region. *Science, 161*(3837), 186–187.

Gilmore, C. S., Clementz, B. A., & Buckley, P. F. (2004). Rate of stimulation affects schizophrenia-normal differences on the N1 auditory-evoked potential. *Neuroreport, 15*(18), 2713–2717.

Grent-'t-Jong, T., Rivolta, D., Sauer, A., Grube, M., Singer, W., Wibral, M., & Uhlhaas, P. J. (2016). MEG-measured visually induced gamma-band oscillations in chronic schizophrenia: Evidence for impaired generation of rhythmic activity in ventral stream regions. *Schizophrenia Research, 176*(2–3), 177–185.

Hall, M. H., Taylor, G., Sham, P., Schulze, K., Rijsdijk, F., Picchioni, M., . . . Salisbury, D. F. (2011). The early auditory gamma-band response is heritable and a putative endophenotype of schizophrenia. *Schizophrenia Bulletin, 37*(4), 778–787.

Hamm, J. P., Gilmore, C. S., & Clementz, B. A. (2012). Augmented gamma band auditory steady-state responses: Support for NMDA hypofunction in schizophrenia. *Schizophrenia Research, 138*(1), 1–7.

Hamm, J. P., Gilmore, C. S., Picchetti, N. A., Sponheim, S. R., & Clementz, B. A. (2011). Abnormalities of neuronal oscillations and temporal integration to low- and high-frequency auditory stimulation in schizophrenia. *Biological Psychiatry, 69*(10), 989–996.

Hanlon, F. M., Miller, G. A., Thoma, R. J., Irwin, J., Jones, A., Moses, S. N., . . . Canive, J. M. (2005). Distinct M50 and M100 auditory gating deficits in schizophrenia. *Psychophysiology, 42*(4), 417–427.

Hari, R. (1990). The neuromagnetic method in the study of the human auditory cortex. In M. H. F. Grandori & G. Romani (Eds.), *Auditory evoked magnetic fields and potentials advances in audiology.* Basel, Switzerland: Karger.

Hari, R., Aittoniemi, K., Jarvinen, M. L., Katila, T., & Varpula, T. (1980). Auditory evoked transient and sustained magnetic fields of the human brain: Localization of neural generators. *Experiments of Brain Research, 40*(2), 237–240.

Heim, S., Kissler, J., Elbert, T., & Rockstroh, B. (2004). Cerebral lateralization in schizophrenia and dyslexia: Neuromagnetic responses to auditory stimuli. *Neuropsychologia, 42*(5), 692–697.

Herdman, A. T., Wollbrink, A., Chau, W., Ishii, R., Ross, B., & Pantev, C. (2003). Determination of activation areas in the human auditory cortex by means of synthetic aperture magnetometry. *Neuroimage, 20*(2), 995–1005.

Hirvonen, J., Wibral, M., Palva, J. M., Singer, W., Uhlhaas, P., & Palva, S. (2017). Whole-brain source-reconstructed MEG-data reveal reduced long-range synchronization in chronic schizophrenia. *eNeuro, 4*(5).

Hong, L. E., Summerfelt, A., McMahon, R., Adami, H., Francis, G., Elliott, A., . . . Thaker, G. K. (2004). Evoked gamma band synchronization and the liability for schizophrenia. *Schizophrenia Research, 70*(2–3), 293–302.

Hong, L. E., Summerfelt, A., Mitchell, B. D., O'Donnell, P., & Thaker, G. K. (2012). A shared low-frequency oscillatory rhythm abnormality in resting and sensory gating in schizophrenia. *Clinical Neurophysiology, 123*(2), 285–292.

Huang, M. X., Nichols, S., Robb, A., Angeles, A., Drake, A., Holland, M., . . . Lee, R. R. (2012). An automatic MEG low-frequency source imaging approach for detecting injuries in mild and moderate TBI patients with blast and non-blast causes. *Neuroimage, 61*(4), 1067–1082.

Huang, M. X., Theilmann, R. J., Robb, A., Angeles, A., Nichols, S., Drake, A., . . . Lee, R. R. (2009). Integrated imaging approach with MEG and DTI to detect mild traumatic brain injury in military and civilian patients. *Journal of Neurotrauma, 26*(8), 1213–1226.

Iramina, K., & Ueno, S. (1996). Source estimation of spontaneous MEG activity and auditory evoked responses in normal subjects during sleep. *Brain Topography, 8*(3), 297–301.

Jacobson, G. P., & Fitzgerald, M. B. (1997). Auditory evoked gamma band potential in normal subjects. *Journal of the American Academy of Audiology, 8*(1), 44–52.

Jansen, B. H., Hegde, A., & Boutros, N. N. (2004). Contribution of different EEG frequencies to auditory evoked potential abnormalities in schizophrenia. *Clinical Neurophysiology, 115*(3), 523–533.

Johannesen, J. K., Kieffaber, P. D., O'Donnell, B. F., Shekhar, A., Evans, J. D., & Hetrick, W. P. (2005). Contributions of subtype and spectral frequency analyses to the study of P50 ERP amplitude and suppression in schizophrenia. *Schizophrenia Research, 78*(2–3), 269–284.

Jordanov, T., Popov, T., Weisz, N., Elbert, T., Paul-Jordanov, I., & Rockstroh, B. (2011). Reduced mismatch negativity and increased variability of brain activity in schizophrenia. *Clinical Neurophysiology, 122*(12), 2365–2374.

Koenig, T., van Swam, C., Dierks, T., & Hubl, D. (2012). Is gamma band EEG synchronization reduced during auditory driving in schizophrenia patients with auditory verbal hallucinations? *Schizophrenia Research, 141*(2–3), 266–270.

Krishnan, G. P., Hetrick, W. P., Brenner, C. A., Shekhar, A., Steffen, A. N., & O'Donnell, B. F. (2009). Steady state and induced auditory gamma deficits in schizophrenia. *Neuroimage, 47*(4), 1711–1719.

Kwon, J. S., O'Donnell, B. F., Wallenstein, G. V., Greene, R. W., Hirayasu, Y., Nestor, P. G., . . . McCarley, R. W. (1999). Gamma frequency-range abnormalities to auditory stimulation in schizophrenia. *Archives of General Psychiatry, 56*(11), 1001–1005.

Laurent, A., Garcia-Larrea, L., d'Amato, T., Bosson, J. L., Saoud, M., Marie-Cardine, M., . . . Dalery, J. (1999). Auditory event-related potentials and clinical scores in unmedicated schizophrenic patients. *Psychiatry Research, 86*(3), 229–238.

Lenz, D., Fischer, S., Schadow, J., Bogerts, B., & Herrmann, C. S. (2011). Altered evoked gamma-band responses as a neurophysiological marker of schizophrenia? *International Journal of Psychophysiology, 79*(1), 25–31.

Light, G. A., Hsu, J. L., Hsieh, M. H., Meyer-Gomes, K., Sprock, J., Swerdlow, N. R., & Braff, D. L. (2006). Gamma band oscillations reveal neural network cortical coherence dysfunction in schizophrenia patients. *Biological Psychiatry, 60*(11), 1231–1240.

Lisman, J. (2012). Excitation, inhibition, local oscillations, or large-scale loops: What causes the symptoms of schizophrenia? *Current Opinions in Neurobiology, 22*(3), 537–544.

Llinas, R., Urbano, F. J., Leznik, E., Ramirez, R. R., & van Marle, H. J. (2005). Rhythmic and dysrhythmic thalamocortical dynamics: GABA systems and the edge effect. *Trends in Neuroscience, 28*(6), 325–333.

Lu, B. Y., Martin, K. E., Edgar, J. C., Smith, A. K., Lewis, S. F., Escamilla, M. A., . . . Canive, J. M. (2007). Effect of catechol O-methyltransferase val(158)met polymorphism on the p50 gating endophenotype in schizophrenia. *Biological Psychiatry, 62*(7), 822–825.

Makela, J. P., Hamalainen, M., Hari, R., & McEvoy, L. (1994). Whole-head mapping of middle-latency auditory evoked magnetic fields. *Electroencephalography and Clinical Neurophysiology, 92*(5), 414–421.

Maxwell, C. R., Liang, Y., Kelly, M. P., Kanes, S. J., Abel, T., & Siegel, S. J. (2006). Mice expressing constitutively active Gsalpha exhibit stimulus encoding deficits similar to those observed in schizophrenia patients. *Neuroscience, 141*(3), 1257–1264.

Miyauchi, T., Endo, S., Kajiwara, S., Ishii, M., & Okajima, J. (1996). Computerized electroencephalogram in untreated schizophrenics: A comparison between disorganized and paranoid types. *Psychiatry and Clinical Neurosciences, 50*(2), 71–78.

Miyauchi, T., Tanaka, K., Hagimoto, H., Miura, T., Kishimoto, H., & Matsushita, M. (1990). Computerized EEG in schizophrenic patients. *Biological Psychiatry, 28*(6), 488–494.

Naatanen, R., & Kahkonen, S. (2009). Central auditory dysfunction in schizophrenia as revealed by the mismatch negativity (MMN) and its magnetic equivalent MMNm: A review. *International Journal of Neuropsychopharmacology, 12*(1), 125–135.

Naatanen, R., & Picton, T. (1987). The N1 wave of the human electric and magnetic response to sound: A review and an analysis of the component structure. *Psychophysiology, 24*(4), 375–425.

Nagase, Y., Okubo, Y., & Toru, M. (1996). Electroencephalography in schizophrenic patients: Comparison between neuroleptic-naive state and after treatment. *Biological Psychiatry, 40*(6), 452–456.

Narayanan, B., O'Neil, K., Berwise, C., Stevens, M. C., Calhoun, V. D., Clementz, B. A., . . . Pearlson, G. D.

(2013). Resting state electroencephalogram oscillatory abnormalities in schizophrenia and psychotic bipolar patients and their relatives from the Bipolar and Schizophrenia Network on Intermediate Phenotypes Study. *Biological Psychiatry. 76*(6), 456–465.

Pantev, C., Elbert, T., Makeig, S., Hampson, S., Eulitz, C., & Hoke, M. (1993). Relationship of transient and steady-state auditory evoked fields. *Electroencephalography and Clinical Neurophysiology, 88*(5), 389–396.

Pascual-Marqui, R. D., Lehmann, D., Koenig, T., Kochi, K., Merlo, M. C., Hell, D., & Koukkou, M. (1999). Low resolution brain electromagnetic tomography (LORETA) functional imaging in acute, neuroleptic-naive, first-episode, productive schizophrenia. *Psychiatry Research, 90*(3), 169–179.

Pelizzone, M., Hari, R., Makela, J. P., Huttunen, J., Ahlfors, S., & Hamalainen, M. (1987). Cortical origin of middle-latency auditory evoked responses in man. *Neuroscience Letters, 82*(3), 303–307.

Petty, R. G., Barta, P. E., Pearlson, G. D., McGilchrist, I. K., Lewis, R. W., Tien, A. Y., . . . Powers, R. E. (1995). Reversal of asymmetry of the planum temporale in schizophrenia. *American Journal of Psychiatry, 152*(5), 715–721.

Popov, T., Jordanov, T., Rockstroh, B., Elbert, T., Merzenich, M. M., & Miller, G. A. (2011). Specific cognitive training normalizes auditory sensory gating in schizophrenia: A randomized trial. *Biological Psychiatry, 69*(5), 465–471.

Popov, T., Jordanov, T., Weisz, N., Elbert, T., Rockstroh, B., & Miller, G. A. (2011). Evoked and induced oscillatory activity contributes to abnormal auditory sensory gating in schizophrenia. *Neuroimage, 56*(1), 307–314.

Popov, T., Rockstroh, B., Weisz, N., Elbert, T., & Miller, G. A. (2012). Adjusting brain dynamics in schizophrenia by means of perceptual and cognitive training. *PLoS One, 7*(7), e39051.

Popov, T. G., Carolus, A., Schubring, D., Popova, P., Miller, G. A., & Rockstroh, B. S. (2015). Targeted training modifies oscillatory brain activity in schizophrenia patients. *Neuroimage: Clinical, 7,* 807–814.

Popova, P., Popov, T. G., Wienbruch, C., Carolus, A. M., Miller, G. A., & Rockstroh, B. S. (2014). Changing facial affect recognition in schizophrenia: Effects of training on brain dynamics. *Neuroimage: Clinical, 6,* 156–165.

Popova, P., Rockstroh, B., Miller, G. A., Wienbruch, C., Carolus, A. M., & Popov, T. (2018). The impact of cognitive training on spontaneous gamma oscillations in schizophrenia. *Psychophysiology, 55*(8), e13083.

Rass, O., Forsyth, J. K., Krishnan, G. P., Hetrick, W. P., Klaunig, M. J., Breier, A., . . . Brenner, C. A. (2012). Auditory steady state response in the schizophrenia, first-degree relatives, and schizotypal personality disorder. *Schizophrenia Research, 136*(1–3), 143–149.

Rechtschaffen, A., Kales, A. (1968). *A manual of standardized terminology, techniques and scoring system for sleep stages of human subjects.* Bethesda, MD: US Department of Health, Education and Welfare.

Reeve, A., Rose, D. F., & Weinberger, D. R. (1989). Magnetoencephalography: Applications in psychiatry. *Archives of General Psychiatry, 46*(6), 573–576.

Reite, M., Teale, P., Goldstein, L., Whalen, J., & Linnville, S. (1989). Late auditory magnetic sources may differ in the left hemisphere of schizophrenic patients: A preliminary report. *Archives of General Psychiatry, 46*(6), 565–572.

Reite, M., Teale, P., Zimmerman, J., Davis, K., & Whalen, J. (1988). Source location of a 50 msec latency auditory evoked field component. *Electroencephalography and Clinical Neurophysiology, 70*(6), 490–498.

Richardson, A. J. (1994). Dyslexia, handedness and syndromes of psychosis-proneness. *International Journal of Psychophysiology, 18*(3), 251–263.

Robson, S. E., Brookes, M. J., Hall, E. L., Palaniyappan, L., Kumar, J., Skelton, M., . . . Morris, P. G. (2016). Abnormal visuomotor processing in schizophrenia. *Neuroimage: Clinical, 12*, 869–878.

Rockstroh, B., Watzl, H., Kowalik, Z. J., Cohen, R., Sterr, A., Muller, M., & Elbert, T. (1997). Dynamical aspects of the EEG in different psychopathological states in an interview situation: A pilot study. *Schizophrenia Research, 28*(1), 77–85.

Rockstroh, B. S., Wienbruch, C., Ray, W. J., & Elbert, T. (2007). Abnormal oscillatory brain dynamics in schizophrenia: A sign of deviant communication in neural network? *BMC Psychiatry, 7*, 44.

Rojas, D. C., Benkers, T. L., Rogers, S. J., Teale, P. D., Reite, M. L., & Hagerman, R. J. (2001). Auditory evoked magnetic fields in adults with fragile X syndrome. *Neuroreport, 12*(11), 2573–2576.

Rojas, D. C., Maharajh, K., Teale, P. D., Kleman, M. R., Benkers, T. L., Carlson, J. P., & Reite, M. L. (2006). Development of the 40Hz steady state auditory evoked magnetic field from ages 5 to 52. *Clinical Neurophysiology, 117*(1), 110–117.

Rosburg, T., Boutros, N. N., & Ford, J. M. (2008). Reduced auditory evoked potential component N100 in schizophrenia: A critical review. *Psychiatry Research, 161*(3), 259–274.

Ross, B., Picton, T. W., & Pantev, C. (2002). Temporal integration in the human auditory cortex as represented by the development of the steady-state magnetic field. *Hearing Research, 165*(1–2), 68–84.

Saletu, B., Kufferle, B., Grunberger, J., Foldes, P., Topitz, A., & Anderer, P. (1994). Clinical, EEG mapping and psychometric studies in negative schizophrenia: Comparative trials with amisulpride and fluphenazine. *Neuropsychobiology, 29*(3), 125–135.

Sanfratello, L., Aine, C., & Stephen, J. (2018). Neuroimaging investigations of dorsal stream processing and effects of stimulus synchrony in schizophrenia. *Psychiatry Research: Neuroimaging, 278*, 56–64.

Sauer, A., Zeev-Wolf, M., Grent-'t-Jong, T., Recasens, M., Wacongne, C., Wibral, M., . . . Uhlhaas, P. J. (2017). Impairment in predictive processes during auditory mismatch negativity in ScZ: Evidence from event-related fields. *Human Brain Mapping, 38*(10), 5082–5093.

Sayers, B. M., Beagley, H. A., & Henshall, W. R. (1974). The mechanism of auditory evoked EEG responses. *Nature, 247*(5441), 481–483.

Schubring, D., Popov, T., Miller, G. A., & Rockstroh, B. (2018). Consistency of abnormal sensory gating in first-admission and chronic schizophrenia across quantification methods. *Psychophysiology, 55*(4).

Shapleske, J., Rossell, S. L., Woodruff, P. W., & David, A. S. (1999). The planum temporale: A systematic, quantitative review of its structural, functional and clinical significance. *Brain Research: Brain Research Reviews, 29*(1), 26–49.

Shin, K. S., Jung, W. H., Kim, J. S., Jang, J. H., Hwang, J. Y., Chung, C. K., & Kwon, J. S. (2012). Neuromagnetic auditory response and its relation to cortical thickness in ultra-high-risk for psychosis. *Schizophrenia Research, 140*(1-3), 93–98.

Silverstein, S., Uhlhaas, P. J., Essex, B., Halpin, S., Schall, U., & Carr, V. (2006). Perceptual organization in first episode schizophrenia and ultra-high-risk states. *Schizophrenia Research, 83*(1), 41–52.

Smith, A. K., Edgar, J. C., Huang, M., Lu, B. Y., Thoma, R. J., Hanlon, F. M., . . . Canive, J. M. (2010). Cognitive abilities and 50- and 100-msec paired-click processes in schizophrenia. *American Journal of Psychiatry, 167*(10), 1264–1275.

Sommer, I. E., Ramsey, N. F., & Kahn, R. S. (2001). Language lateralization in schizophrenia, an fMRI study. *Schizophrenia Research, 52*(1–2), 57–67.

Spencer, K. M., Niznikiewicz, M. A., Nestor, P. G., Shenton, M. E., & McCarley, R. W. (2009). Left auditory cortex gamma synchronization and auditory hallucination symptoms in schizophrenia. *BMC Neuroscience, 10*, 85.

Spencer, K. M., Salisbury, D. F., Shenton, M. E., & McCarley, R. W. (2008). Gamma-band auditory steady-state responses are impaired in first episode psychosis. *Biological Psychiatry, 64*(5), 369–375.

Sponheim, S. R., Clementz, B. A., Iacono, W. G., & Beiser, M. (1994). Resting EEG in first-episode and chronic schizophrenia. *Psychophysiology, 31*(1), 37–43.

Sponheim, S. R., Clementz, B. A., Iacono, W. G., & Beiser, M. (2000). Clinical and biological concomitants of resting state EEG power abnormalities in schizophrenia. *Biological Psychiatry, 48*(11), 1088–1097.

Teale, P., Carlson, J., Rojas, D., & Reite, M. (2003). Reduced laterality of the source locations for generators of the auditory steady-state field in schizophrenia. *Biological Psychiatry, 54*(11), 1149–1153.

Teale, P., Collins, D., Maharajh, K., Rojas, D. C., Kronberg, E., & Reite, M. (2008). Cortical source estimates of gamma band amplitude and phase are different in schizophrenia. *Neuroimage, 42*(4), 1481–1489.

Teale, P., Reite, M., Rojas, D. C., Sheeder, J., & Arciniegas, D. (2000). Fine structure of the auditory M100 in schizophrenia and schizoaffective disorder. *Biological Psychiatry, 48*(11), 1109–1112.

Thonnessen, H., Zvyagintsev, M., Harke, K. C., Boers, F., Dammers, J., Norra, C., & Mathiak, K. (2008). Optimized mismatch negativity paradigm reflects deficits in schizophrenia patients: A combined EEG and MEG study. *Biological Psychology, 77*(2), 205–216.

Thune, H., Recasens, M., & Uhlhaas, P. J. (2016). The 40-Hz auditory steady-state response in patients with schizophrenia: A meta-analysis. *JAMA Psychiatry, 73*(11), 1145–1153.

Tsuchimoto, R., Kanba, S., Hirano, S., Oribe, N., Ueno, T., Hirano, Y., . . . Onitsuka, T. (2011). Reduced high and low frequency gamma synchronization in patients with chronic schizophrenia. *Schizophrenia Research, 133*(1–3), 99–105.

Venables, N. C., Bernat, E. M., & Sponheim, S. R. (2009). Genetic and disorder-specific aspects of resting state EEG abnormalities in schizophrenia. *Schizophrenia Bulletin, 35*(4), 826–839.

Vierling-Claassen, D., Siekmeier, P., Stufflebeam, S., & Kopell, N. (2008). Modeling GABA alterations in schizophrenia: A link between impaired inhibition and altered gamma and beta range auditory entrainment. *Journal of Neurophysiology, 99*(5), 2656–2671.

Vieth, J. B., Kober, H., & Grummich, P. (1996). Sources of spontaneous slow waves associated with brain lesions, localized by using the MEG. *Brain Topography, 8*(3), 215–221.

Wang, Y., Feng, Y., Jia, Y., Xie, Y., Wang, W., Guan, Y., . . . Huang, L. (2013). Absence of auditory M100 source asymmetry in schizophrenia and bipolar disorder: A MEG study. *PLoS One, 8*(12), e82682.

Wang, Y., Jia, Y., Feng, Y., Zhong, S., Xie, Y., Wang, W., . . . Huang, L. (2014). Overlapping auditory M100 and M200 abnormalities in schizophrenia and bipolar disorder: A MEG study. *Schizophrenia Research, 160*(1–3), 201–207.

Weinberger, D. R. (1988). Schizophrenia and the frontal lobe. *Trends in Neuroscience, 11*(8), 367–370.

Wienbruch, C., Moratti, S., Elbert, T., Vogel, U., Fehr, T., Kissler, J., . . . Rockstroh, B. (2003). Source distribution of neuromagnetic slow wave activity in schizophrenic and depressive patients. *Clinical Neurophysiology, 114*(11), 2052–2060.

Wilson, T. W., Rojas, D. C., Teale, P. D., Hernandez, O. O., Asherin, R. M., & Reite, M. L. (2007). Aberrant functional organization and maturation in early-onset psychosis: Evidence from magnetoencephalography. *Psychiatry Research, 156*(1), 59–67.

Wilson, T. W., Slason, E., Asherin, R., Kronberg, E., Teale, P. D., Reite, M. L., & Rojas, D. C. (2011). Abnormal gamma and beta MEG activity during finger movements in early-onset psychosis. *Developmental Neuropsychology, 36*(5), 596–613.

Winterer, G., Ziller, M., Dorn, H., Frick, K., Mulert, C., Wuebben, Y., & Herrmann, W. M. (2000). Frontal dysfunction in schizophrenia: A new electrophysiological classifier for research and clinical applications. *European Archives of Psychiatry and Clinical Neuroscience, 250*(4), 207–214.

Winterer, G., Ziller, M., Dorn, H., Frick, K., Mulert, C., Wuebben, Y., . . . Coppola, R. (2000). Schizophrenia: Reduced signal-to-noise ratio and impaired phase-locking during information processing. *Clinical Neurophysiology, 111*(5), 837–849.

Yvert, B., Crouzeix, A., Bertrand, O., Seither-Preisler, A., & Pantev, C. (2001). Multiple supratemporal sources of magnetic and electric auditory evoked middle latency components in humans. *Cerebral Cortex, 11*(5), 411–423.

Zeev-Wolf, M., Levy, J., Jahshan, C., Peled, A., Levkovitz, Y., Grinshpoon, A., & Goldstein, A. (2018). MEG resting-state oscillations and their relationship to clinical symptoms in schizophrenia. *Neuroimage: Clinical, 20*, 753–761.

24

BIOMARKERS IN PEDIATRIC MAGNETOENCEPHALOGRAPHY

Julia M. Stephen, Isabel Solis, John F. L. Pinner,
and Felicha T. Candelaria-Cook

24.1. INTRODUCTION

Children have been examined with magnetoencephalography (MEG) since the inception of the technique for clinical assessment for epilepsy and presurgical mapping. However, clinical research in pediatric populations, with the goal of identifying new clinical applications for MEG, has emerged primarily over the past two decades. Through these efforts, a number of recent studies indicate that MEG may be a useful tool for informing us about the biological underpinnings of developmental disorders and providing potential biomarkers for atypical brain development before an age at which behavioral measures differentiate these children from individuals with normal development and other overlapping developmental disorders. MEG is of particular relevance to pediatric populations because of the child-friendly atmosphere and noninvasiveness of the technique (Ciesielski & Stephen, 2014). Unlike electroencephalography (EEG), which requires that sensors be directly attached to the child's head with low impedance, MEG only requires that the head be placed near the sensors. Therefore, preparation time, including placing head position indicator coils, can be as short as 10 minutes and does not scale with the number of sensors used. MEG is also a more child-friendly study than magnetic resonance imaging (MRI), with a silent environment for data collection and the option of either seated or supine position. The open design of MEG systems allows the child to see around the room and reduces the chance of claustrophobia. Recent advances in current sensor technology (Borna et al., 2017; Tierney et al., 2018) may also lead to additional flexibility in subject movement and experimental paradigms and are of particular interest for the

Julia M. Stephen, Isabel Solis, John F. L. Pinner, and Felicha T. Candelaria-Cook, *Biomarkers in Pediatric Magnetoencephalography* In: *Fifty Years of Magnetoencephalography*. Edited by: Andrew C. Papanicolaou, Timothy P. L. Roberts, and James W. Wheless, Oxford University Press (2020).
© Oxford University Press. DOI: 10.1093/oso/9780190935689.003.0024.

application of MEG to pediatric populations based on the opportunity to have personalized sensor placement to optimize signal strength for each participant.

Based on the known developmental changes in the neurophysiology of the brain (de Graaf-Peters & Hadders-Algra, 2006), there are specific markers that may emerge in children with atypical brain development. One of the most robust findings in normal development is that the latency of stimulus-evoked brain responses (e.g., response to sensory input) decreases over childhood and then gradually increases again into old age (Allison et al., 1984). These changes in latency during childhood occur in parallel with changes in myelination (de Graaf-Peters & Hadders-Algra, 2006; Lyall et al., 2016), which is known to speed the transfer of information along axons within the brain. MEG has reliably replicated this change in evoked sensory response latency through a series of studies in normally developing individuals (Lutter et al., 2006; Paetau et al., 1995; Pihko et al., 2009; Taylor et al., 2011). These normative studies have laid the groundwork for examining changes in response latencies as a potential biomarker in developmental psychopathology. For example, if a particular disorder interrupts the development of myelination, an expected result would be delayed development of these sensory responses, which may be reflected in delayed response latencies (Cardy et al., 2008; Coffman et al., 2013; Oram Cardy et al., 2005a; Wakai et al., 2007).

MEG also provides a sensitive measure of neural oscillations. Neural oscillations have been studied using preclinical studies (e.g., Gray & Singer, 1989), invasive neurophysiological recordings in humans during surgery, and noninvasively using EEG and MEG. These studies have led to the conclusion that neural oscillations are integral to brain function across species and reflect population responses that result from the complex excitatory/inhibitory balance within gray matter (Basar et al., 2001; Singer, 2011; Uhlhaas et al., 2008). Neural oscillations are also sensitive to developmental changes demonstrated by a shift in the distribution of spectral power across childhood (Clarke et al., 2001) and changes in frequency (Berchicci et al., 2011) and spectral power (Heinrichs-Graham et al., 2018) of the resting brain rhythms with increasing age. Neural oscillations have also been shown to be altered with imbalances between inhibitory and excitatory neurons, providing additional targets for biomarker development with MEG.

This chapter is designed to briefly review pediatric MEG research with an emphasis on results that support development of future biomarkers that can support new clinical indications for MEG. One of the challenges in identification of developmental disorders is that cognitive development and complex social interactions emerge slowly over childhood. Therefore, current approaches for identifying long-term developmental delays must wait for certain abilities to emerge to confirm that higher cognitive functioning is impaired in these children. For example, despite the autism diagnostic criteria requiring evidence for atypical development before 3 years of age, the average age of diagnosis remains at approximately 4 years of age (Baio et al., 2018). A primary challenge for identifying developmental disorders is the variability in biological age at which both behavioral and cognitive milestones are met across children (Siegler, 1994; Vereijken, 2010). This variability in the emergence of behavioral and cognitive functioning has led to a wait-and-see approach by many pediatricians (Raspa et al., 2015). However, at the same time, long-term outcome studies have indicated that early intervention leads to the best outcomes across developmental disorders (Fricke et al., 2013; Landsem et al., 2015; Wallace & Rogers, 2010). Therefore, a primary goal of the use of neuroimaging studies for developmental disorders is to identify early markers of atypical brain development to allow for early intervention to improve outcomes (Sullivan et al., 2014). That is, identification of neural biomarkers that provide higher sensitivity and specificity to altered brain function relative to cognitive and behavioral assessments is a primary aim of using neuroimaging measures for developmental disorders. We will review the work of others in using MEG to assess atypical brain development in children in the search for neural biomarkers. We will then describe our work to identify atypical brain development in children with fetal alcohol spectrum disorder (FASD) as a future application for the use of MEG. The chapter concludes with an overview of future directions and gaps in the literature to support the use of MEG for pediatric disorders.

24.2. APPLICATION OF MAGNETOENCEPHALOGRAPHY TO AUTISM SPECTRUM DISORDER

Coincident with the reports of increased prevalence of autism spectrum disorder (ASD) (Boat et al., 2015), some of the earliest pediatric studies indicated that MEG may be sensitive to alterations in brain development in children with ASD (Gage et al., 2003a, 2003b; Roberts et al., 2008). Roberts and colleagues reported changes in basic auditory processing in children with ASD, including delays in the right hemisphere M100 response (Gage et al., 2003a) and associations between auditory responses and language processing measures (Flagg et al., 2005). In contrast, Yoshimura et al. (2013) did not find a latency delay in the M50 response in children with ASD relative to HC, although M50 latency predicted language performance in controls showing partial consistency with Flagg et al. (2005). Additional studies described in detail in the comprehensive review by Kikuchi et al. (2016) report differences in children with ASD with more complex stimuli including language stimuli and alterations in the mismatch field, with some variability in hemispheric effects. The variations in results are likely related to a number of factors, including variations in experimental design, differences in ages studied, and heterogeneity within the ASD population. For example, the interstimulus interval between auditory tones

has a direct influence on the evoked response, which also changes rapidly over development (Lutter et al., 2006; Paetau et al., 1995; Stephen et al., 2017).

Roberts et al. (2008) expanded on their early finding with a series of studies replicating the results in a larger sample, indicating that genotype influences M100 latency (Jenkins et al., 2016), providing complementary findings in white matter microstructure using diffusion tensor imaging (Roberts et al., 2013) and performing longitudinal studies demonstrating that earlier M100 latency delays were predictive of M100 delays at later time points and were also predictive of cognitive performance at an older age (Port et al., 2016). These results provide considerable support for the use of MEG to identify a biomarker of ASD in children. Our cross-sectional study (Stephen et al., 2017) partially replicated the reports of a delayed M100 response in children with ASD described previously. However, the delay in the M100 response appeared to emerge only in children older than 24 months. The small sample size of the study indicates the need for additional studies examining auditory processing at this younger age, but the results provide supporting evidence that M100 latencies in children with ASD are delayed in children 2 to 5 years of age and may provide a more reliable measure of disability than behavioral/observational measures alone. These results provide support for MEG being sensitive to atypical brain developmental measures in children with ASD.

An additional question when developing a biomarker is whether the measure is specific to the disorder of interest. A study by Demopolous (2017) indicates that children with sensory processing disorder (SPD) also differ from children with ASD, despite the behavioral overlap in sensory sensitivity between ASD and SPD populations. They examined both auditory and somatosensory delays in the M200 in children with ASD and SPD, and despite ASD having delayed responses in both modalities, the sensory delays did not correlate with each other, suggesting that the sensory deficits were not a generalized deficit in individual patients. This result indicates some specificity for latency measures obtained with MEG and may also help to explain some of the variability within the ASD diagnostic category. Additional work by Roberts and colleagues indicates specificity of the M100 delay relative to children with specific language impairment (SLI). However, other results from our lab indicate that children with FASD experience a similar delay in the M100 latency at preschool age (Stephen et al., 2012). Interestingly, this M100 delay was not present in adolescents with FASD (Coffman et al., submitted). Combined, these results may indicate that the persistence of the M100 delay across ages may be specific to individuals with ASD. Importantly, the behavioral phenotype of children with ASD and FASD are quite distinct, supporting the utility of a combined brain/behavioral marker to determine diagnostic category in this case.

Based on a general hypothesis of dysconnectivity in ASD, recent MEG studies have also examined neural oscillations and frequency-based connectivity to test this hypothesis. Despite no group differences in regional connectivity based on phase lag index (PLI), Takahashi et al. (2018) identified differences in global measures of connectivity in delta and gamma bands, supporting the broader hypothesis of altered connectivity in ASD. Interestingly, delta band indicated decreased small-worldness, whereas gamma band showed the opposite pattern, which is also consistent with a more refined hypothesis in ASD—poor long-range connectivity and increased local connectivity. These results are only partially supported by the study of Lajiness-O'Neill and colleagues (2018), which indicated reduced connectivity in gamma band. These results may or may not conflict based on differences in their methodology; For example, Lajiness-O'Neill performed connectivity analysis on source-based time courses, whereas Takahashi et al. performed analysis at the sensor level. Takesaki et al. (2016) also

reported increased gamma band connectivity in ASD; however, this study examined connectivity during performance of a nonverbal spatial task. Results further indicate that this increase in gamma connectivity within occipital lobe in children with ASD is related to their improved nonverbal spatial abilities. Urbain et al. (2016) provide additional support for the task-related group differences demonstrating again decreased gamma connectivity in children with ASD relative to controls during performance of a working memory task. While a number of studies have reported alterations in neural oscillations, replication studies related to specific alterations in neural oscillations have not been performed. Therefore, we consider neural oscillations to be an emerging measure for clinical use, but it is premature to point to any of these individual studies for an indication of a biomarker.

24.3. IDENTIFYING NEUROLOGICAL EFFECTS OF PREMATURITY

Multiple groups have also used MEG to examine brain development in children born preterm. Prematurity is a risk factor for poorer cognitive performance into adulthood experienced by up to 40 to 50% of preterm infants (Neubauer et al., 2008; Voss et al., 2007). Prematurity is associated with increased risk for neurological complications, including cerebral palsy, asphyxiation during birth, and intraventricular hemorrhage; however, poorer cognitive performance in individuals born preterm is not directly associated with these risk factors (Broitman et al., 2007). Instead, risk is primarily conferred based on level of prematurity, with the youngest infants having the highest risk (Alexander et al., 2019). Therefore, multiple questions motivate research in preterm infants, including identifying which children are at the highest risk for persistent cognitive impairments and understanding what changes in cortical functioning have occurred as a result of preterm birth to better guide interventions. Consistent with behavioral measures demonstrating impaired executive functioning in preterm children, Mossad and colleagues (2017) identified reduced activation in regions activated during a Theory of Mind Task (right inferior frontal gyrus, left inferior temporal gyrus, and right fusiform gyrus) in 7- to 12-year-old children born very preterm relative to term-born controls. This reduced activation was associated with less differentiation between true and false beliefs in the preterm children, with more group differences evident in left than right hemisphere. Furthermore, Pihko et al. (2016) identified changes in response inhibition during a somatosensory go/no-go task in extremely preterm children at age 6 years. Consistent with a role of alpha in suppressing irrelevant information, alpha power following a nontarget stimulus was larger in full-term children relative to preterm children. Suppression of alpha following the stimulus was also decreased in preterm children, suggesting an inability to shift attention toward relevant stimuli.

Doesburg et al. (2011a, 20111b, 2013) completed a series of studies of school-aged children born prematurely. Consistent with Llinas et al.'s (1999) thalamocortical dysrhythmia framework of developmental disorders, children born very prematurely (<32 weeks gestational age) demonstrated altered alpha oscillations with reduced alpha power (Doesburg et al., 2011a), reduced long-range synchronization (Doesburg et al., 2010, 2011a), and reduced peak frequency (Doesburg et al., 2011b). While the reduced peak frequency is explained in terms of the thalamocortical dysrhythmia, this may also be consistent with delayed cortical development based on the reports of increasing alpha frequency with increasing age. In further studies of children born extremely prematurely, Ye et al. (2016) reported that overall brain network connectivity was reduced in children born preterm relative to term children at school age. In addition to showing increased frontal gamma/alpha ratios in extremely low gestational age

(ELGA) infants, Doesburg et al. (2013) also demonstrated that this ratio is correlated with visual-spatial abilities in ELGA infants only, perhaps indicating that these altered neural oscillations represent activity responsible for successful completion of spatial–working memory tasks. This ratio provides a summary of resting networks represented by alpha power, in contrast to task-related networks represented by gamma power. Alterations in this ratio are expected to represent networks that may be less responsive to task initiation or completion. Further, gamma/alpha ratio is related to an estimate of cumulative neonatal pain experienced by the infants during care in the neonatal intensive care unit (Doesburg et al., 2013). This is important because neonatal pain, while not avoidable, may be further minimized when caring for preterm children in the neonatal intensive care unit, and this strong association between neonatal pain and brain development in the preterm infants may indicate a causal relationship supporting these alterations in care. Finally, our study in preterm infants indicated that brain development in children at 6 months of age is influenced by maternal post-traumatic stress disorder symptoms, emphasizing the important role maternal health may play in brain development (Sanjuan et al., 2016).

A recent systematic review of the auditory event-related potential (ERP) literature (Depoorter et al., 2018) suggests that a number of evoked potential measures provide associations with neurodevelopmental outcome, with prospective longitudinal studies providing the strongest evidence. Between the MEG studies reviewed here and the associated ERP measures, MEG may provide an important tool for identifying early markers of long-term cognitive impairments in children born preterm. However, the small number of studies ($N = 13$) that met review criteria indicates that more research is needed to identify a reliable, clinically informative biomarker of risk for cognitive impairments in children born preterm.

24.4. FURTHERING OUR UNDERSTANDING OF NORMAL BRAIN DEVELOPMENT

Within the context of developing biomarkers for atypical brain development, it is important to understand the development of normal brain function across the age spectrum. The frontoparietal network (FPN) has been identified as a set of regions that are associated with higher order cognition in both adults and children. This network is responsible for completing three distinct tasks: the initiation of a task, the set maintenance of task priorities, and error processing or adjustment of behavior due to task feedback (Fair et al., 2007). The cortical network connectivity of the FPN is mature in adulthood but appears less connected during development based on functional magnetic resonance imaging (fMRI) studies (Fair et al., 2007). Recent studies have identified overlapping functional and structural connectivity networks using fMRI and MEG in adults and children (Barnes et al., 2016; Boersma et al., 2011; Brookes et al., 2011; de Pasquale et al., 2010; Liu et al., 2010). Brain networks have been examined using graph theoretical approaches (Bullmore & Sporns, 2009), independent component analysis, and power spectral density (PSD) of the physiological frequency bands (Figure 24.1). The alpha and theta frequency bands are of particular interest because they are related to cognitive functioning and FPN functioning (Klimesch, 1999). Neural oscillations in the alpha frequency range are closely associated with attention, which is an integral component of higher cognitive functioning and is also the dominant frequency during resting state. Furthermore, alpha oscillations are the first to develop (Basar, 2012; Klimesch, 1999). Alpha power increases with age as theta power decreases (Klimesch, 1999; Somsen et al., 1997).

We are currently collecting resting-state data in normally developing children to better understand neural oscillations across the pediatric age range. We obtained resting data collected during eyes-open and eyes-closed states for 10 minutes in 73 healthy children 9 to 14 years of age (mean = 11.72 years; standard deviation = 1.85; 34 female). We hypothesized that older children would have higher parietal alpha power and higher frontal theta power relative to younger children. Participants completed the Dimensional Change Card Sort Test (DCCS) from the National Institutes of Health Toolbox to assess task-switching or set-shifting ability. Source analysis was performed using the MNE dSPM inverse modeling approach. DCCS performance scores were correlated with theta (4–7 Hz) and alpha (8–12 Hz) spectral power for four frontoparietal regions

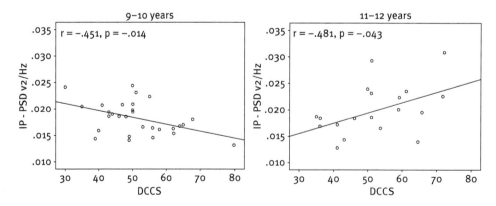

FIGURE 24.1   Correlation between power spectral density (PSD) and Dimensional Change Card Sort Test (DCCS) scores in theta band for inferior parietal (IP) region in the 9- to 10-year age group (*left*) and the 11- to 12-year age group (*right*).

(rostral middle frontal [RMF] and caudal anterior cingulate [CAC] and two posterior regions (inferior parietal [IP] and precuneus [PC] defined by the *Desikan-Killiany-Tourville Atlas*) using Pearson correlations. We found a significant negative correlation in theta power in young children (i.e., 9–10 years) between all FPN regions and DCCS performance (RMF: $r = -0.451$, $p = 0.014$; CAC: $r = -0.425$, $p = 0.021$; IP: $r = -0.451$, $p = 0.014$; and PC: $r = -0.435$, $p = 0.018$). Thus, indicating lower theta power across FPN was related to higher performance scores on DCCS. The opposite was seen in older children (i.e., 11–12 years), who had a positive association between DCCS performance and inferior parietal region in theta ($r = 0.481$, $p = 0.043$). The oldest group did not show any significant correlations in either alpha or theta with DCCS performance.

These results provide support for the role of resting neural oscillations as a marker of cognitive development in normally developing children and provide additional evidence for systematic changes in neural oscillations throughout childhood that need to be taken into consideration when establishing biomarkers for developmental psychopathology.

24.5. EMERGING APPLICATION OF MAGNETOENCEPHALOGRAPHY: EXAMINING BRAIN DEVELOPMENT IN CHILDREN WITH PRENATAL ALCOHOL EXPOSURE

A broad literature of both animal and human studies has confirmed that prenatal alcohol exposure (PAE) affects both structural and functional brain development (Coffman et al., 2013; Green et al., 2013; Lebel et al., 2008; Savage et al., 2002; Sowell et al., 2008b; Stephen et al., 2018; Valenzuela et al., 2012; Zucca & Valenzuela, 2010). High doses of PAE lead to structural changes in the brain with alterations in the corpus callosum, basal ganglia, and cerebellum noted in individuals with fetal alcohol syndrome (FAS) (Mattson et al.,

1992, 1996; Sowell et al., 1996). Additional effects on the gamma-aminobutyric acid type A (GABA-A) inhibitory interneurons have been reported by investigators examining low-dose rodent models of PAE (Valenzuela et al., 2012; Zucca & Valenzuela, 2010). These low-dose effects may still have considerable impact on brain function based on the role that inhibitory interneurons that are thought to play in the generation of gamma oscillations (Uhlhaas & Singer, 2006). Despite considerable evidence of dose effects and broad-ranging changes in brain structure and function, only children with FAS can be identified through an objective biomarker based on dysmorphic facial features (Jones & Smith, 1973). The FASD spectrum (with disabilities ranging from minor to severe) includes children with FAS, a term coined by Jones and Smith (1973), partial fetal alcohol syndrome (pFAS), and alcohol-related neurodevelopmental disorder (ARND). Recent studies indicate that, conservatively, 2 to 5% of children in the United States experience behavioral or cognitive effects due to prenatal alcohol exposure (May et al., 2018), in contrast to the 0.1% worldwide prevalence of FAS (Popova et al., 2017). With no visible structural abnormalities in this broader FASD category, identifying sensitive and specific biomarkers is imperative (Kodituwakku et al., 2007, 2011; Mattson et al., 1997, 2013).

Over the past 10 years, there has been a series of studies to facilitate the use of MEG as a tool to identify children at risk for cognitive and behavioral effects associated with PAE. In a cohort of preschool-aged children, 3 to 6 years, we presented results of a passive listening task, in which young children with FASD had significant delays in auditory M100 and M200 response latencies (Stephen et al., 2012). We suggested that auditory responses may be a useful marker of alcohol-related damage given that this delay was found across the FASD spectrum. Then, in a separate study in an older FASD cohort, adolescents aged 12 to 21 years, the visual M100 response latency was also delayed in adolescents with FASD (Coffman et al., 2013). The visual M100 latency delay corresponded to increased gamma power over right central cortex in FASD participants (Stephen et al., 2013). Delayed visual M100 in adolescents with FASD further supports the finding of basic sensory deficits following PAE. Other deficits related to FASD have also been described in visual perception (Bjuland et al., 2013), visual construction (Johnson, 2007), feature processing (Koenen et al., 2007), general sensory processing in each of the five senses (Ohls et al., 2016), and performance of an auditory oddball task (Tesche et al., 2015). However, Tesche et al. (2015) did not report a delay in auditory processing in older children with FASD, consistent with our findings in the same adolescent cohort (Coffman et al., submitted). These results support MEG as a tool to measure PAE effects on brain processing speed through latency measures, but age-related changes in these measures need to be taken into account.

Other studies indicate that children with FASD have impaired corticocortical connectivity due to a variety of structural differences, including microstructural abnormalities (Honey et al., 2012). Aside from abnormalities in the corpus callosum, widespread decreases in white matter integrity were reported in children 5 to 13 years of age (Lebel et al., 2008; Sowell et al., 2008a). Structural abnormalities often translate into altered function as reported in fMRI resting-state functional connectivity studies in children with FASD (Wozniak et al., 2011). Taken together, the structural deficits found in children with FASD are expected to impede both intrahemispheric and interhemispheric transfer of information. In a few recent fMRI studies, children with FASD were found to have reduced functional connectivity compared with healthy controls, along with impaired interhemispheric connectivity attributed to impaired white matter connectivity. Li, Santhanam and colleagues (2011) reported reduced default mode network functional connectivity in children with FASD. Wozniak and colleagues (2011) reported

impaired interhemispheric connectivity in children with PAE, which corresponded with impaired white matter connectivity and reduction in global efficiency (2013). MEG studies have added to FASD literature by highlighting the importance of neural oscillations in coordinating local and global connectivity. Recently, MEG has been useful for identifying differences in task-based neural oscillations in adolescent children with FASD (Bolanos et al., 2017; Stephen et al., 2013).

We recently conducted a resting-state study in children 8 to 12 years of age with FASD (26 FASD, 21 healthy controls; for detailed methods, see Bolanos et al., 2017; Coffman et al., 2013). Using 2 minutes of eyes-open and eyes-closed resting-state data, sensor and source power spectral density was compared between groups. We found that children with FASD had reduced theta (4–7 Hz) and alpha (8–12 Hz) power during resting-state conditions, along with increased theta and alpha reactivity (Figure 24.2). When sources were localized, children with FASD revealed greater reduction in alpha power and reactivity within the right superior parietal region, as well as greater reduction in theta power and theta reactivity within the left medial orbitofrontal cortex and pars triangularis frontal regions. Our results were consistent with the fMRI literature and suggest reduced corpus callosum connectivity in children with FASD. Results from our lab and others have found similar hemisphere-specific deficits in FASD, ranging from reduced gamma-band oscillations with differences primarily identified in right hemisphere (Stephen et al., 2013) to decreased white matter integrity in right hemisphere (Green et al., 2013). However, most FASD studies show bilateral deficits within the FASD spectrum.

In another study from our lab, adolescents with FASD and healthy controls, aged 12 to 21 years, performed a 2-minute, eyes-open rest task (for details, see Coffman et al., 2013). When frequency bands were examined by cortical region at the sensor level, adolescents with FASD were found to have decreased theta

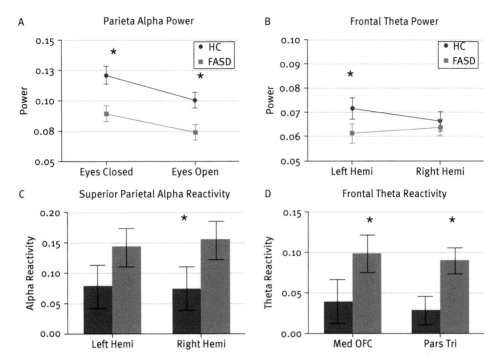

FIGURE 24.2 Sensor and source spectral power group mean differences in children 8 to 12 years old. FASD = fetal alcohol spectrum disorder; HC = healthy controls; MedOFC = medial orbitofrontal cortex; ParsTri = pars triangularis.

and alpha band power compared with healthy controls, similar to what was reported in the 8- to 12-year-olds. However, the regions of significance shifted for our adolescent group. Adolescents with FASD showed decreased theta band activity in both the right parietal and right occipital regions, but no significant differences in the frontal regions survived false discovery rate correction for multiple comparisons. Additionally, the FASD group had reduced alpha band activity in the left occipital region, but no differences in the parietal region. A primary limitation of these results is that the analysis was performed at the sensor level. Additional studies are needed to directly compare source-based spectral power across the age ranges to better determine FASD-specific alterations in the theta and alpha bands.

In summary, our lab has reported multiple effects of PAE assessed with MEG. However, different effects are reported across these measures across the age spectrum. For example, our recent publication (Stephen et al., 2018)

reported "hypersynchrony," or broadband *increases* in spectral power, in 6-month-old infants with PAE, in contrast to the *decreases* in spectral power in children with FASD reported in the 8- to 12-year-old and 12- to 21-year-old cohorts described previously. The measures of hypersynchrony in infants with PAE may provide an early indicator of PAE even in the absence of maternal acknowledgment of alcohol consumption during pregnancy and are consistent with prior EEG studies (Chernick et al., 1983; Havlicek et al., 1977). However, executive function deficits, a core deficit in children with FASD, do not emerge until after 3 years of age. Therefore, it is unclear which of the children with PAE are at risk for long-term cognitive and behavioral deficits due to PAE, indicating a need for additional longitudinal studies to pinpoint which early markers are most predictive of long-term outcomes in children with PAE. As evidenced in the literature (Bolanos et al., 2017; Stephen et al., 2013), alterations in neural oscillations in older children with FASD may provide biomarkers for guiding intervention approaches.

24.6. SUMMARY AND FUTURE DIRECTIONS

The current literature describing MEG clinical research in pediatric populations includes a number of studies that indicate that MEG is sensitive to small changes in brain developmental patterns across neurological and developmental disorders. The large number of underlying physiological mechanisms that lead to altered brain development, in conjunction with the sensitivity of MEG to both latency changes and neural oscillations, provides strong evidence that MEG may provide sensitive and specific markers for developmental disorders. However, the current state of the field points to the need for replication studies originating in independent laboratories to establish the reliability and robustness of candidate biomarkers. Furthermore, additional normative studies are needed to parse out the role of neural oscillations in brain function and establish the test–retest reliability of neural oscillations across the developmental spectrum. This chapter has focused on results in three neurological/developmental disorders that have the largest literature in the pediatric age range for the field of MEG. Also, each of the indications described (autism spectrum disorder, prematurity, and fetal alcohol spectrum disorder) affect more than 1% of the population, with only partial to minimal overlap.

However, there is continued concern regarding how expensive neuroimaging studies are and how they will be able to directly address human health needs (Ahmed et al., 2013). Therefore, it is imperative to convert neuroimaging research studies into clinically useful tools. One of the primary aims of pediatric MEG studies over the next 10 years should be to conduct multisite studies to establish replicability of biomarkers, sensitivity to the disorder of interest, and specificity relative to other disorders. Additional developmental disorders may be explored in the context of these larger studies to establish specificity as well as to better understand the role of neural biomarkers in influencing behavior.

Finally, prior MEG studies in adults and children have indicated that brain measures are malleable through various intervention techniques (e.g., music training and auditory training). Therefore, future approaches of MEG may also provide the opportunity to identify targets for neurostimulation techniques (e.g., transcranial direct current stimulation [tDCS], transcranial magnetic stimulation [TMS], and transcranial alternating current stimulation [tACS]) or behavioral interventions. One of the considerable challenges in developmental disorders is understanding what type of intervention will be most beneficial for children. Objective measures of normalized brain function may provide a means to categorize intervention techniques into effective versus ineffective tools. Additional studies may also indicate certain interventions based on the individual subject response, in line with the dimensional approach to understanding mental illness (Insel et al., 2010). Evaluation of performance at young ages remains challenging because of the slow cognitive developmental trajectory and the subjectivity of parent-report measures. Therefore, objective measures of brain development in health and disease are expected to inform our understanding of both typical and atypical brain development to support treatment across pediatric disorders.

ACKNOWLEDGMENTS

We would like to thank the parents and children who participated in each of the studies. The research was supported in part by grants from the National Institutes of Health (R01AA021771 and P50AA022534) and the National Science Foundation (1539067).

REFERENCES

Ahmed, A. O., Buckley, P. F., & Hanna, M. (2013), Neuroimaging schizophrenia: A picture is worth a thousand words, but is it saying anything important? *Current Psychiatry Reports, 15,* 345.

Alexander, B., Kelly, C. E., Adamson, C., Beare, R., Zannino, D., Chen, J., ... Thompson, D. K. (2019). Changes in neonatal regional brain volume associated with preterm birth and perinatal factors. *Neuroimage, 185,* 654–663.

Allison, T., Hume, A. L., Wood, C. C., & Goff, W. R. (1984). Developmental and aging changes in somatosensory, auditory and visual evoked potentials. *Electroencephalography and Clinical Neurophysiology, 58,* 14–24.

Baio, J., Wiggins, L., Christensen, D. L., Maenner, M. J., Daniels, J., Warren, Z., ... Dowling, N. F. (2018), Prevalence of autism spectrum disorder among children aged 8 years—Autism and developmental disabilities monitoring network, 11 sites, United States, 2014. *MMWR Surveillance Summary, 67,* 1–23.

Barnes, J. J., Nobre, A. C., Woolrich, M. W., Baker, K., & Astle, D. E. (2016). Training working memory in childhood enhances coupling between frontoparietal control network and task-related regions. *Journal of Neuroscience, 36,* 9001–9011.

Basar, E. (2012), A review of alpha activity in integrative brain function: Fundamental physiology, sensory coding, cognition and pathology. *International Journal of Psychophysiology, 86,* 1–24.

Basar, E., Basar-Eroglu, C., Karakas, S., & Schurmann, M. (2001). Gamma, alpha, delta, and theta oscillations govern cognitive processes. *International Journal of Psychophysiology, 39,* 241–248.

Berchicci, M., Zhang, T., Romero, L., Peters, A., Annett, R., Teuscher, U., ... Comani, S. (2011). Development of mu rhythm in infants and preschool children. *Developmental Neuroscience, 33,* 130–143.

Bjuland, K. J., Lohaugen, G. C., Martinussen, M., & Skranes, J. (2013). Cortical thickness and cognition in very-low-birth-weight late teenagers. *Early Human Development, 89,* 371–380.

Boat, T., Bell, C., Buka, S., Costello, E. J., Durkin, M., Edwall, G., ... Zima, B. (2015). Prevalence of autism spectrum disorders. In T. Boat & J. Wu (Eds.), *Mental disorders and disabilities among low-income children.* Washington, DC: National Academy Press.

Boersma, M., Smit, D. J., De Bie, H. M., Van Baal, G. C., Boomsma, D. I., De Geus, E. J., ... Stam, C. J. (2011). Network analysis of resting state EEG in the developing young brain: Structure comes with maturation. *Human Brain Mapping, 32,* 413–425.

Bolanos, A. D., Coffman, B. A., Candelaria-Cook, F. T., Kodituwakku, P., & Stephen, J. M. (2017). Altered neural oscillations during multisensory integration in adolescents with fetal alcohol spectrum disorder. *Alcoholism: Clinical and Experimental Research, 41,* 2173–2184.

Borna, A., Carter, T. R., Goldberg, J. D., Colombo, A. P., Jau, Y. Y., Berry, C., ... Schwindt, P. D. D. (2017). A 20-channel magnetoencephalography system based on optically pumped magnetometers. *Physics in Medicine and Biology, 62,* 8909–8923.

Broitman, E., Ambalavanan, N., Higgins, R. D., Vohr, B. R., Das, A., Bhaskar, B., ... Carlo, W. A. (2007). Clinical data predict neurodevelopmental outcome better than head ultrasound in extremely low birth weight infants. *Journal of Pediatrics, 151,* 500–505.

Brookes, M. J., Woolrich, M., Luckhoo, H., Price, D., Hale, J. R., Stephenson, M. C., ... Morris, P. G. (2011). Investigating the electrophysiological basis of resting state networks using magnetoencephalography. *Proceedings of the National Academy of Science U S A, 108,* 16783–16788.

Bullmore, E., & Sporns, O. (2009), Complex brain networks: Graph theoretical analysis of structural and functional systems. *Nature Reviews Neuroscience, 10,* 186–198.

Cardy, J. E. O., Flagg, E. J., Roberts, W., & Roberts, T. P. L. (2008). Auditory evoked fields predict language ability and impairment in children. *International Journal of Psychophysiology, 68,* 170–175.

Chernick, V., Childiaeva, R., & Ioffe, S. (1983). Effects of maternal alcohol intake and smoking on neonatal electroencephalogram and anthropometric measurements. *American Journal of Obstetrics and Gynecology, 146,* 41–47.

Ciesielski, K., & Stephen, J. (2014). Pediatric MEG: Investigating spatio-temporal connectivity of developing networks. In S. Supek & C. Aine (Eds.), *Magnetoencephalography: From signals to dynamic cortical networks.* Heidelberg, Germany: Springer Verlag.

Clarke, A. R., Barry, R. J., McCarthy, R., & Selikowitz, M. (2001). Age and sex effects in the EEG: Development of the normal child. *Clinical Neurophysiology, 112,* 806–814.

Coffman, B. A., Kodituwakku, P., Kodituwakku, E. L., Romero, L., Sharadamma, N. M., Stone, D., & Stephen, J. M. (2013). Primary visual response (M100) delays in adolescents with FASD as measured with MEG. *Human Brain Mapping, 34,* 2852–2862.

De Graaf-Peters, V. B., & Hadders-Algra, M. (2006). Ontogeny of the human central nervous system: What is happening when? *Early Human Development, 82,* 257–266.

De Pasquale, F., Della Penna, S., Snyder, A. Z., Lewis, C., Mantini, D., Marzetti, L., ... Corbetta, M. (2010). Temporal dynamics of spontaneous

MEG activity in brain networks. *Proceedings of the National Academy of Science U S A, 107*, 6040–6045.

Depoorter, A., Fruh, J., Herrmann, K., Zanchi, D., & Weber, P. (2018). Predicting neurodevelopmental outcome in preterm born infants using auditory event-related potentials: A systematic review. *Neuroscience and Biobehavioral Reviews, 89*, 99–110.

Doesburg, S. M., Chau, C. M., Cheung, T. P., Moiseev, A., Ribary, U., Herdman, A. T., . . . Grunau, R. E. (2013). Neonatal pain-related stress, functional cortical activity and visual-perceptual abilities in school-age children born at extremely low gestational age. *Pain, 154*, 1946–1952.

Doesburg, S. M., Ribary, U., Herdman, A. T., Cheung, T., Moiseev, A., Weinberg, H., . . . Grunau, R. E. (2010). Altered long-range phase synchronization and cortical activation in children born very preterm. *IFMBE Proceedings, 29*, 250–253.

Doesburg, S. M., Ribary, U., Herdman, A. T., Miller, S. P., Poskitt, K. J., Moiseev, A., . . . Grunau, R. E. (2011a). Altered long-range alpha-band synchronization during visual short-term memory retention in children born very preterm. *Neuroimage, 54*, 2330–2339.

Doesburg, S. M., Ribary, U., Herdman, A. T., Moiseev, A., Cheung, T., Miller, S. P., . . . Grunau, R. E. (2011b). Magnetoencephalography reveals slowing of resting peak oscillatory frequency in children born very preterm. *Pediatric Research, 70*, 171–175.

Fair, D. A., Dosenbach, N. U., Church, J. A., Cohen, A. L., Brahmbhatt, S., Miezin, F. M., . . . Schlaggar, B. L. (2007). Development of distinct control networks through segregation and integration. *Proceedings of the National Academy of Science of the United States of America, 104*, 13507–13512.

Flagg, E. J., Cardy, J. E., Roberts, W., & Roberts, T. P. (2005). Language lateralization development in children with autism: Insights from the late field magnetoencephalogram. *Neuroscience Letters, 386*, 82–87.

Fricke, S., Bowyer-Crane, C., Haley, A. J., Hulme, C., & Snowling, M. J. (2013). Efficacy of language intervention in the early years. *Journal of Child Psychology and Psychiatry, 54*, 280–290.

Gage, N. M., Siegel, B., Callen, M., & Roberts, T. P. (2003a). Cortical sound processing in children with autism disorder: An MEG investigation. *NeuroReport, 14*, 2047–2051.

Gage, N. M., Siegel, B., & Roberts, T. P. (2003b). Cortical auditory system maturational abnormalities in children with autism disorder: An MEG investigation. *Brain Research: Developmental Brain Research, 144*, 201–209.

Gray, C. M., & Singer, W. (1989). Stimulus-specific neuronal oscillations in orientation columns of cat visual cortex. *Proceedings of the National Academy of Science U S A, 86*, 1698–1702.

Green, C. R., Lebel, C., Rasmussen, C., Beaulieu, C., & Reynolds, J. N. (2013). Diffusion tensor imaging correlates of saccadic reaction time in children with fetal alcohol spectrum disorder. *Alcoholism: Clinical and Experimental Research, 1*, 161–172 .

Havlicek, V., Childiaeva, R., & Chernick, V. (1977). EEG frequency spectrum characteristics of sleep states in infants of alcoholic mothers. *Neuropadiatrie, 8*, 360–373.

Heinrichs-Graham, E., McDermott, T. J., Mills, M. S., Wiesman, A. I., Wang, Y. P., Stephen, J. M., . . . Wilson, T. W. (2018). The lifespan trajectory of neural oscillatory activity in the motor system. *Developments in Cognitive Neuroscience, 30*, 159–168.

Honey, C. J., Thesen, T., Donner, T. H., Silbert, L. J., Carlson, C. E., Devinsky, O., . . . Hasson, U. (2012). Slow cortical dynamics and the accumulation of information over long timescales. *Neuron, 76*, 423–434.

Insel, T., Cuthbert, B., Garvey, M., Heinssen, R., Pine, D. S., Quinn, K., . . . Wang, P. (2010). Research domain criteria (RDoC): Toward a new classification framework for research on mental disorders. *American Journal of Psychiatry, 167*, 748–751.

Jenkins, J., 3rd., Chow, V., Blaskey, L., Kuschner, E., Qasmieh, S., Gaetz, L., . . . Roberts, T. P. (2016). Auditory evoked M100 response latency is delayed in children with 16p11.2 deletion but not 16p11.2 duplication. *Cerebral Cortex, 26*, 1957–1964.

Johnson, S. (2007). Cognitive and behavioural outcomes following very preterm birth. *Seminars in Fetal Neonatal Medicine, 12*, 363–373.

Jones, K. L., & Smith, D. W. (1973). Recognition of the fetal alcohol syndrome in early infancy. *Lancet, 302*, 999–1001.

Kikuchi, M., Yoshimura, Y., Mutou, K., & Minabe, Y. (2016). Magnetoencephalography in the study of children with autism spectrum disorder. *Psychiatry Clinical: Neuroscience, 70*, 74–88.

Klimesch, W. (1999). EEG alpha and theta oscillations reflect cognitive and memory performance: A review and analysis. *Brain Research: Brain Research Review, 29*, 169–195.

Kodituwakku, P., Segall, J. M., & Beatty, G. K. (2011). Cognitive and behavioral effects of prenatal alcohol exposure. *Future Neurology, 6*, 237–259.

Kodituwakku, P. W. (2007). Defining the behavioral phenotype in children with fetal alcohol spectrum disorders: A review. *Neuroscience and Biobehavioral Reviews, 31*, 192–201.

Koenen, K. C., Moffitt, T. E., Poulton, R., Martin, J., & Caspi, A. (2007). Early childhood factors associated with the development of post-traumatic stress disorder: Results from a longitudinal birth cohort. *Psychological Medicine, 37*, 181–192.

Lajiness-O'Neill, R., Brennan, J. R., Moran, J. E., Richard, A. E., Flores, A. M., Swick, C., & Bowyer, S. M. (2018). Patterns of altered neural synchrony in the default mode network in autism spectrum disorder revealed with magnetoencephalography (MEG): Relationship to clinical symptomatology. *Autism Research, 11*, 434–449.

Landsem, I. P., Handegard, B. H., Ulvund, S. E., Kaaresen, P. I., & Ronning, J. A. (2015). Early intervention influences positively quality of life as reported by prematurely born children at age nine and their parents; a randomized clinical trial. *Health and Quality of Life Outcomes, 13*, 25.

Lebel, C., Rasmussen, C., Wyper, K., Walker, L., Andrew, G., Yager, J., & Beaulieu, C. (2008). Brain diffusion abnormalities in children with fetal alcohol spectrum disorder. *Alcoholism: Clinical and Experimental Research, 32*, 1732–1740.

Li, Z., Santhanam, P., Coles, C. D., Lynch, M. E., Hamann, S., Peltier, S., & Hu, X. (2011). Increased "default mode" activity in adolescents prenatally exposed to cocaine. *Human Brain Mapping, 32*(5), 759–770.

Liu, Z., Fukunaga, M., De Zwart, J. A., & Duyn, J. H. (2010). Large-scale spontaneous fluctuations and correlations in brain electrical activity observed with magnetoencephalography. *Neuroimage, 51*, 102–111.

Llinas, R. R., Ribary, U., Jeanmonod, D., Kronberg, E., & Mitra, P. P. (1999). Thalamocortical dysrhythmia: A neurological and neuropsychiatric syndrome characterized by magnetoencephalography. *Proceedings of the National Academy of Science U S A, 96*, 15222–15227.

Lutter, W. J., Maier, M., & Wakai, R. T. (2006). Development of MEG sleep patterns and magnetic auditory evoked responses during early infancy. *Clinical Neurophysiology, 117*, 522–530.

Lyall, A. E., Savadjiev, P., Shenton, M. E., & Kubicki, M. (2016), Insights into the brain: Neuroimaging of brain development and maturation. *Journal of Neuroimaging in Psychiatry & Neurology, 1*, 10–19.

Mattson, S. N., Riley, E. P., Gramling, L., Delis, D. C., & Jones, K. L. (1997), Heavy prenatal alcohol exposure with or without physical features of fetal alcohol syndrome leads to IQ deficits. *Journal of Pediatrics, 131*, 718–721.

Mattson, S. N., Riley, E. P., Jernigan, T. L., Ehlers, C. L., Delis, D. C., Jones, K. L., . . . Bellugi, U. (1992). Fetal alcohol syndrome: A case report of neuropsychological, MRI and EEG assessment of two children. *Alcoholism: Clinical and Experimental Research, 16*, 1001–1003

Mattson, S. N., Riley, E. P., Sowell, E. R., Jernigan, T. L., Sobel, D. F., & Jones, K. L. (1996). A decrease in the size of the basal ganglia in children with fetal alcohol syndrome. *Alcoholism: Clinical and Experimental Research, 20*, 1088–1093.

Mattson, S. N., Roesch, S. C., Glass, L., Deweese, B. N., Coles, C. D., Kable, J. A., . . . Riley EP; CIFASD (2013). Further development of a neurobehavioral profile of fetal alcohol spectrum disorders. *Alcoholism: Clinical and Experimental Research, 37*, 517–528.

May, P. A., Chambers, C. D., Kalberg, W. O., Zellner, J., Feldman, H., Buckley, D., . . . Hoyme, H. E. (2018). Prevalence of fetal alcohol spectrum disorders in 4 us communities. *JAMA, 319*, 474–482.

Mossad, S. I., Smith, M. L., Pang, E. W., & Taylor, M. J. (2017). Neural correlates of "Theory of Mind" in very preterm born children. *Human Brain Mapping, 38*, 5577–5589.

Neubauer, A. P., Voss, W., & Kattner, E. (2008). Outcome of extremely low birth weight survivors at school age: The influence of perinatal parameters on neurodevelopment. *European Journal of Pediatrics, 167*, 87–95.

Ohls, R. K., Cannon, D. C., Phillips, J., Caprihan, A., Patel, S., Winter, S., . . . Lowe, J. (2016). Preschool assessment of preterm infants treated with darbepoetin and erythropoietin. *Pediatrics, 137*, 1–9.

Oram Cardy, J. E., Flagg, E. J., Roberts, W., & Roberts, T. P. (2005a). Delayed mismatch field for speech and non-speech sounds in children with autism. *Neuroreport, 16*, 521–525.

Paetau, R., Ahonen, A., Salonen, O., & Sams, M. (1995). Auditory evoked magnetic fields to tones and pseudowords in healthy children and adults. *Journal of Clinical Neurophysiology, 12*, 177–185.

Pihko, E., Lonnberg, P., Lauronen, L., Wolford, E., Andersson, S., Lano, A., . . . Nevalainen, P. (2016). Lack of cortical correlates of response inhibition in 6-year-olds born extremely preterm: Evidence from a go/nogo task in magnetoencephalographic recordings. *Frontiers in Human Neuroscience, 10*, 666.

Pihko, E., Nevalainen, P., Stephen, J., Okada, Y., & Lauronen, L. (2009). Maturation of somatosensory cortical processing from birth to adulthood revealed by magnetoencephalography. *Clinical Neurophysiology, 120*, 1552–1561.

Popova, S., Lange, S., Probst, C., Gmel, G., & Rehm, J. (2017). Estimation of national, regional, and global prevalence of alcohol use during pregnancy and fetal alcohol syndrome: A systematic review and meta-analysis. *Lancet: Global Health, 5,* e290–e299.

Port, R. G., Edgar, J. C., Ku, M., Bloy, L., Murray, R., Blaskey, L., . . . Roberts, T. P. (2016). Maturation of auditory neural processes in autism spectrum disorder—A longitudinal MEG study. *NeuroImage: Clinical, 11,* 566–577.

Raspa, M., Levis, D. M., Kish-Doto, J., Wallace, I., Rice, C., Barger, B., . . . Wolf, R. B. (2015). Examining parents' experiences and information needs regarding early identification of developmental delays: Qualitative research to inform a public health campaign. *Journal of Developmental and Behavioral Pediatrics, 36,* 575–585.

Roberts, T. P., Lanza, M. R., Dell, J., Qasmieh, S., Hines, K., Blaskey, L., . . . Berman, J. I. (2013). Maturational differences in thalamocortical white matter microstructure and auditory evoked response latencies in autism spectrum disorders. *Brain Research, 1537,* 79–85.

Roberts, T. P., Schmidt, G. L., Egeth, M., Blaskey, L., Rey, M. M., Edgar, J. C., & Levy, S. E. (2008). Electrophysiological signatures: Magnetoencephalographic studies of the neural correlates of language impairment in autism spectrum disorders. *International Journal of Psychophysiology, 68,* 149–160.

Sanjuan, P. M., Poremba, C., Flynn, L. R., Savich, R., Annett, R. D., & Stephen, J. (2016). Association between theta power in 6-month old infants at rest and maternal PTSD severity: A pilot study. *Neuroscience Letters, 630,* 120–126.

Savage, D. D., Becher, M., De La Torre, A. J., & Sutherland, R. J. (2002). Dose-dependent effects of prenatal ethanol exposure on synaptic plasticity and learning in mature offspring. *Alcoholism: Clinical and Experimental Research, 26,* 1752–1758.

Siegler, R. S. (1994). Cognitive variability: A key to understanding cognitive-development. *Current Directions in Psychological Science, 3,* 1–5.

Singer, W. (2011). Dynamic formation of functional networks by synchronization. *Neuron, 69,* 191–193.

Somsen, R. J., Van't Klooster, B. J., Van Der Molen, M. W., Van Leeuwen, H. M., & Licht, R. (1997). Growth spurts in brain maturation during middle childhood as indexed by EEG power spectra. *Biological Psychology, 44,* 187–209.

Sowell, E. R., Jernigan, T. L., Mattson, S. N., Riley, E. P., Sobel, D. F., & Jones, K. L. (1996). Abnormal development of the cerebellar vermis in children prenatally exposed to alcohol: Size reduction in lobules I-V. *Alcoholism: Clinical and Experimental Research, 20,* 31–34.

Sowell, E. R., Johnson, A., Kan, E., Lu, L. H., Van Horn, J. D., Toga, A. W., . . . Bookheimer, S. Y. (2008a).

Mapping white matter integrity and neurobehavioral correlates in children with fetal alcohol spectrum disorders. *Journal of Neuroscience, 28,* 1313–1319.

Sowell, E. R., Mattson, S. N., Kan, E., Thompson, P. M., Riley, E. P., & Toga, A. W. (2008b). Abnormal cortical thickness and brain-behavior correlation patterns in individuals with heavy prenatal alcohol exposure. *Cerebral Cortex, 18,* 136–144.

Stephen, J., Kodituwakku, P., Kodituwakku, E. L., Romero, L., Peters, A. M., Sharadamma, N. M., . . . Coffman, B. A. (2012). Delays in auditory processing identified in preschool children with FASD. *Alcoholism: Clinical and Experimental Research, 36,* 1720–1727.

Stephen, J. M., Coffman, B. A., Stone, D. B., & Kodituwakku, P. (2013). Differences in MEG gamma oscillatory power during performance of a prosaccade task in adolescents with FASD. *Frontiers in Human Neuroscience, 7,* 900.

Stephen, J. M., Flynn, L., Kabella, D., Schendel, M., Cano, S., Savage, D. D., . . . Bakhireva, L. N. (2018). Hypersynchrony in MEG spectral amplitude in prospectively-identified 6-month-old infants prenatally exposed to alcohol. *NeuroImage: Clinical, 17,* 826–834.

Stephen, J. M., Hill, D. E., Peters, A., Flynn, L., Zhang, T., & Okada, Y. (2017). Development of auditory evoked responses in normally developing preschool children and children with autism spectrum disorder. *Developmental Neuroscience, 39,* 430–441.

Sullivan, K., Stone, W. L., & Dawson, G. (2014). Potential neural mechanisms underlying the effectiveness of early intervention for children with autism spectrum disorder. *Research in Development Disability, 35,* 2921–2932.

Takahashi, H., Nakahachi, T., Stickley, A., Ishitobi, M., & Kamio, Y. (2018). Relationship between physiological and parent-observed auditory over-responsiveness in children with typical development and those with autism spectrum disorders. *Autism, 22,* 291–298.

Takesaki, N., Kikuchi, M., Yoshimura, Y., Hiraishi, H., Hasegawa, C., Kaneda, R., . . . Minabe, Y. (2016). The contribution of increased gamma band connectivity to visual non-verbal reasoning in autistic children: A MEG study. *PLoS One, 11,* e0163133.

Taylor, M. J., Mills, T., & Pang, E. W. (2011). The development of face recognition: Hippocampal and frontal lobe contributions determined with MEG. *Brain Topography, 24,* 261–270.

Tesche, C. D., Kodituwakku, P. W., Garcia, C. M., & Houck, J. M. (2015). Sex-related differences in auditory processing in adolescents with fetal alcohol spectrum disorder: A magnetoencephalographic study. *NeuroImage: Clinical, 7,* 571–587.

Tierney, T. M., Holmes, N., Meyer, S. S., Boto, E., Roberts, G., Leggett, J., . . . Barnes, G. R. (2018). Cognitive neuroscience using wearable magnetometer arrays: Non-invasive assessment of language function. *Neuroimage, 181*, 513–520.

Uhlhaas, P. J., Haenschel, C., Nikolic, D., & Singer, W. (2008). The role of oscillations and synchrony in cortical networks and their putative relevance for the pathophysiology of schizophrenia. *Schizophrenia Bulletin, 34*, 927–943.

Uhlhaas, P. J., & Singer, W. (2006). Neural synchrony in brain disorders: Relevance for cognitive dysfunctions and pathophysiology. *Neuron, 52*, 155–168.

Urbain, C., Vogan, V. M., Ye, A. X., Pang, E. W., Doesburg, S. M., & Taylor, M. J. (2016). Desynchronization of fronto-temporal networks during working memory processing in autism. *Human Brain Mapping, 37*, 153–164.

Valenzuela, C. F., Morton, R. A., Diaz, M. R., & Topper, L. (2012). Does moderate drinking harm the fetal brain? Insights from animal models. *Trends in Neuroscience, 35*, 284–292.

Vereijken, B. (2010). The complexity of childhood development: Variability in perspective. Physical Therapy, 90, 1850–1859.

Voss, W., Neubauer, A. P., Wachtendorf, M., Verhey, J. F., & Kattner, E. (2007). Neurodevelopmental outcome in extremely low birth weight infants: What is the minimum age for reliable developmental prognosis? *Acta Paediatrica, 96*, 342–347.

Wakai, R. T., Lutter, W. J., Chen, M., & Maier, M. M. (2007). On and off magnetic auditory evoked responses in early infancy: A possible marker of brain immaturity. *Clinical Neurophysiology, 118*, 1480–1487.

Wallace, K. S., & Rogers, S. J. (2010). Intervening in infancy: Implications for autism spectrum disorders. *Journal of Child Psychology and Psychiatry, 51*, 1300–1320.

Wozniak, J. R., Mueller, B. A., Muetzel, R. L., Bell, C. J., Hoecker, H. L., Nelson, M. L., . . . Lim, K. O. (2011). Inter-hemispheric functional connectivity disruption in children with prenatal alcohol exposure. *Alcoholism: Clinical and Experimental Research, 35*, 845–861.

Ye, A. X., Aucoin-Power, M., Taylor, M. J., & Doesburg, S. M. (2016). Disconnected neuromagnetic networks in children born very preterm: Disconnected MEG networks in preterm children. *NeuroImage: Clinical, 11*, 376–384.

Yoshimura, Y., Kikuchi, M., Shitamichi, K., Ueno, S., Munesue, T., Ono, Y., . . . Minabe, Y. (2013). Atypical brain lateralisation in the auditory cortex and language performance in 3- to 7-year-old children with high-functioning autism spectrum disorder: A child-customised magnetoencephalography (MEG) study. *Molecular Autism, 4*, 38.

Zucca, S., & Valenzuela, C. F. (2010). Low concentrations of alcohol inhibit BDNF-dependent GABAergic plasticity via L-type Ca2+ channel inhibition in developing CA3 hippocampal pyramidal neurons. *Journal of Neuroscience, 30*, 6776–6781.

25

MAGNETOENCEPHALOGRAPHY IN ALZHEIMER DISEASE

CORRELATION WITH CURRENT BIOMARKERS

David López-Sanz,* Jaisalmer de Frutos-Lucas,* Gianluca Susi,
and Fernando Maestú

25.1. AGING AND DEMENTIA

The number of people older than 60 years is rapidly growing in our society, and the proportion of older people in the population is expected to increase even more in the near future. This aging pattern can be explained by two main factors: first, the significant increase in life expectancy that modern societies are experiencing, and second, a marked birth rate reduction that, in most countries, is currently near or below replacement level (Harper, 2014). It is expected that by 2050, the number people older than 60 years will equal the number of people younger than 15 years.

This aging pattern represents one of the biggest challenges that financial and health institutions have to deal with today. The numbers of those with ill health and disability will inevitably rise during the next decades, and so will the associated economical costs.

Dementia is a condition characterized by a progressive decline of cognitive abilities that limits independence in daily living activity. Importantly, it is highly associated with aging, which is considered the main risk factor for its development. The number of patients affected is also expected to grow, and by 2050 well in excess of 100 million people will have developed dementia worldwide according to the Alzheimer's Disease International (2015) report. Dementia is not a disease itself, but rather a group of symptoms that may be caused by

*These authors have contributed equally to this chapter and share first authorship.

David López-Sanz, Jaisalmer de Frutos-Lucas, Gianluca Susi, and Fernando Maestú, *Magnetoencephalography in Alzheimer Disease: Correlation With Current Biomarkers* In: *Fifty Years of Magnetoencephalography*. Edited by: Andrew C. Papanicolaou, Timothy P. L. Roberts, and James W. Wheless, Oxford University Press (2020). © Oxford University Press. DOI: 10.1093/oso/9780190935689.003.0025.

several different diseases producing different types of dementia, such as vascular dementia, frontotemporal dementia, or dementia with Lewy bodies, among others. However, the most common cause of dementia is Alzheimer disease (AD), which accounts for about 60 to 80% of the cases. AD is particularly characterized by the presence of episodic memory decline, initially with anterograde deficits (i.e., inability to form new memories), and affecting almost every cognitive domain in more advanced stages. The study of dementia, and in particular AD considering its prevalence, is crucial given the high burden of disability and years of life lost that this condition accounts for.

AD-related pathology tends to accumulate in the brain very slowly and insidiously before any cognitive symptoms become evident. In fact, several studies have shown that even 20 years before the onset of cognitive decline, AD pathology could be detected in the brain (Jack et al., 2011). The main signatures of AD pathology characterized to date are (a) the accumulation of extracellular amyloid-beta protein (Aβ) in the form of plaques, and (b) the phosphorylation of the microtubule-associated protein tau forming paired helical filaments or neurofibrillary tangles. Several other factors such as neuroinflammation (Heneka et al., 2015) or vascular pathology (Miyakawa, 2010) are also implicated in the pathogenesis and progression of AD and are receiving increasing attention in recent literature.

Although dementia and AD have been classically detected mainly through neuropsychological assessment, in recent years neuroimaging techniques are increasing their relevance in the diagnosis of dementia. Cortical shrinkage measured through volumetric magnetic resonance imaging (MRI), particularly over medial temporal regions (Busatto et al., 2003), has been long used as an imaging biomarker for the identification of AD, along with glucose hypometabolism as measured by fluorodeoxyglucose positron emission tomography (FDG-PET) in

clinical practice. However, more recently, newer PET radiotracers reflecting accumulation of tau and Aβ have been incorporated into this process (Jack et al., 2011). Up to this date, magnetoencephalography (MEG) has not provided biomarkers for AD diagnosis, although very significant advances have been made in this direction. All the previously mentioned pathophysiological alterations have implications in synaptic transmission at a very early stage of the disease, making MEG a suitable technique for a biomarker identification in dementia. In this chapter, we will briefly summarize the most relevant findings in MEG literature in the field of dementia due to AD and also in its preclinical stages by reviewing different types of analyses typically employed in the literature. Furthermore, the relationship between MEG findings and their substrate at the neuronal level is also summarized to provide a basis for relating them with other biomarkers.

AD can be considered as a long-lasting neuropathological process with different stages, providing different neurophysiological profiles. Typically, the AD continuum can be divided in three main stages: preclinical, prodromal, and dementia. In the preclinical stage, the insidious neuropathological process starts with the accumulation of the amyloid protein and the phosphorylation of the tau protein, although cognitive impairment is not evidenced in neuropsychological assessment. However, older adult subjects can start noticing cognitive disabilities in daily living activities, developing what has been called subjective cognitive decline (SCD). SCD is characterized by a cognitive performance within the normal range on neuropsychological testing with a subjective feeling of worsening of cognitive functions at a higher rate than expected. At the prodromal stage, cognitive impairment can be evidenced by neuropsychological tests, although it is not sufficiently severe to be considered dementia and was therefore termed mild cognitive impairment (MCI). The increased accumulation of amyloid and phosphorylation of the tau protein at the MCI stage can predict which patients could develop dementia.

25.2. MAGNETOENCEPHALO-GRAPHY PROFILES AT THE DEMENTIA STAGE

As mentioned previously, MEG is a useful technique to approach the pathogenesis and progression of AD because its combined high temporal and sufficient spatial resolution may enable the detection of those very first physiological changes that alter neural communication and inevitably lead to the clinical symptomatology that characterizes the disease. Ultimately, MEG is able to capture the modulation of the neuronal rhythms and the reorganization of the brain networks that take place as the neuropathological process advances— and given its noninvasiveness, it allows the monitoring of such changes over time.

A growing body of literature is emerging trying to describe the neurophysiological hallmarks of AD employing MEG. There are different metrics that can be applied to address this challenge, from single-channel analyses to connectivity analyses, both at rest and during the execution of a task in which performance is expected to be affected by the disease. One thing to keep in mind during MEG recording of AD patients in the resting state is that somnolence is more likely to happen, so it is important to make sure that the participant is awake (Verdoorn et al., 2011).

25.2.1. Single-Channel Analysis

Regarding single-channel analyses, a reduction in absolute and relative power in high-frequency bands, together with a power increase in low-frequency bands, has been observed in several brain regions, mainly involving left temporal, left parietal, and left occipital cortices (Engels et al., 2017; Fernández et al., 2002, 2003, 2006, 2013). Similarly, one of the most replicated findings is a shift to the left in the frequency of the alpha peak, mean frequency, and median frequency of the power spectrum of AD patients compared with healthy controls (HCs) (Gómez, Hornero, Abásolo, Fernández, & Escudero, 2007; Montez et al., 2009; Van Cappellen Van Walsum et al., 2003). The scientific community has devoted special attention to this reduction in alpha power. Such decrease could be better understood considering the functional roles ascribed to the alpha rhythm, which is said to be involved in supporting and modulating attentional states and facilitating communication between separate groups of neurons (Hari & Puce, 2017). In this vein, AD patients exhibit decreased alpha band reactivity (i.e., the reduction of the signal amplitude at eyes open compared with eyes closed in the resting state) than older adult HCs (Franciotti et al., 2006). Alpha sources have also been found to be distinct between HCs and patients suffering from AD. In this regard, Osipova, Ahveninen, Jensen, Ylikoski, and Pekkonen (2005) described robust alpha sources in the parieto-occipital sulcus in HCs, whereas this signal emerged predominantly from temporal sources in AD patients. Ishii et al. (2010) also found an increase in alpha sources in frontal regions in early AD, which negatively correlated with cognitive performance.

Employing a different approach, several studies describe lower complexity in the MEG signal from AD recordings (Gómez, Hornero, Abásolo, Fernández, & Escudero, 2009; Gomez, Hornero, Abasolo, Fernandez, & Poza, 2009; Hornero, Abásolo, Escudero, & Gómez, 2009) as well as lower entropy (Bruña et al., 2012; Hornero et al., 2009; Poza, Hornero, Escudero, Fernández, & Sánchez, 2008) and in general more predictable dynamics (Gómez et al., 2007). The repeated finding of lower complexity values in AD patients is generally interpreted as a trend toward simpler brain activity and could imply a loss of independent oscillators underlying brain activity.

As can be gathered from the previously cited studies, a general slowing of the power spectrum is the most relevant characteristic of AD pathology at the single-channel analysis level. MEG is very sensitive to such changes, although unfortunately they are not specific biomarkers of AD because a similar slowing has been described in several other neurological and psychiatric diseases (Dickinson, DiStefano, Senturk, & Jeste, 2018; Petrovic et al., 2017). In addition, the MEG signal is less complex, more regular, and more predictable in the presence of AD (Engels et al., 2017).

25.2.2. Functional Connectivity and Graph Theory

With regard to connectivity analyses, once again different methodologies can be applied, which, in general, depict the coordinated dynamics of distant brain areas, because a statistical relationship is expected between time series of functionally connected brain regions. Such brain synchronization is thought to underlie successful brain processing and normal cognitive functioning, which enables the assessment of the reorganization of such functional systems under pathological conditions, and particularly the study of AD neurophysiological changes at the network level.

Functional connectivity (FC) outlines the temporal synchronization of the activity in remote brain regions, while effective connectivity (EC) captures the influence of one region over another, providing information about directionality of the interaction. Employing coherence measures to estimate FC, an increase in connectivity in the delta band, as well as a decrease in connectivity in high-frequency bands, has been described in AD (Alonso et al., 2011; Escudero, Sanei, Jarchi, Abásolo, & Hornero, 2011; Franciotti et al., 2006), although some authors have failed to find a significant difference in coherence between AD patients and HCs (Stam et al., 2002). On the other hand, Ranasinghe et al. (2014) found that reduced coherence in alpha band at rest in AD patients robustly correlated with cognitive deficits in executive function, episodic memory, and visuospatial abilities. Another way to estimate

FC is through synchronization likelihood. Using this method, AD patients exhibited lower FC in alpha, beta, and gamma bands, but increased FC in delta (Stam et al., 2002, 2006). Decreased FC in the alpha and beta bands was also reported using virtual electrodes, especially in parieto-temporal regions (Koelewijn et al., 2017), and the phase lag index (Stam et al., 2008). Increased connectivity in low-frequency bands has been reported more seldomly in AD patients and mainly affects posterior areas of the brain (Alonso et al., 2011; Escudero et al., 2011; Stam et al., 2006). As for EC, when utilizing Granger causality, theta, beta, and gamma bands exhibited decreases in connectivity, while increases in delta were also reported (Juan-Cruz, Gómez, Poza, Fernández, & Hornero, 2017). Considering all MEG-based connectivity studies, a recent review on this topic (Mandal, Banerjee, Tripathi, & Sharma, 2018) concluded that the most prominent feature of AD recordings is a reduction in connectivity in high-frequency bands, particularly alpha and beta bands. Furthermore, FC increases, particularly between temporoparietal and parieto-occipital regions, have also been reported in some studies.

Finally, graph theory has been used to shed light to the study of brain networks, enabling the analysis of the modular and hierarchical dynamics of brain hub regions. These sorts of analyses have shown, for example, that individuals suffering from AD present a reduction of hub regions' relevance in the network (de Haan, van der Flier, Wang, et al., 2012; Yu et al., 2017) and also a decreased connectivity between different brain modules (de Haan, van der Flier, Koene, et al., 2012; de Haan, van der Flier, Wang, et al., 2012; de Haan, Mott, van Straaten, Scheltens, & Stam, 2012), which could indeed explain why they also exhibit lower FC. As a matter of fact, these network abnormalities correlated with worse cognitive performance in several domains. Beyond that, a more random organization of brain networks characterizes AD, in terms of lower clustering coefficient and shorter characteristic path length (Stam et al., 2008), as well as reduced neural complexity in lower frequencies (Van Cappellen Van Walsum et al., 2003).

25.3. MAGNETOENCEPHALO-GRAPHY IN PRECLINICAL AND PRODROMAL ALZHEIMER DISEASE

The MEG research in AD patients has resulted in considerable knowledge of the clinical stage of AD and has described possible electrophysiological markers of the disease that may underlie the characteristic cognitive impairments found in dementia. However, recent research efforts are being devoted to earlier stages of the disease, the so-called prodromal or even earlier preclinical or asymptomatic phases of AD. As briefly mentioned, AD pathology accumulates at a very slow rate in the brain. As a consequence, after cognitive symptoms are fully detectable by standard neuropsychological assessment, it seems to be already too late for currently available drugs to produce any significant improvement or even slowing of disease progression, as reflected in the absence of a relevant success in pharmaceutical clinical trials thus far (Anderson, Hadjichrysanthou, Evans, & Wong, 2017). Synaptic disruption is expected to occur relatively early in the progression of AD, according to the cascade of events underlying AD pathogenesis formulated by Jack et al. (2013). Thus, MEG should be able to capture relevant alterations in those subjects known to have an increased risk for developing AD before dementia is clinically observable.

25.3.1. Single-Channel Analysis

MCI was described as an intermediate stage to fill the gap between healthy aging and clinical dementia. It is characterized by a significant cognitive worsening in one or more domains that does not limit subjects' independence (Petersen et al., 1999). Furthermore, MCI patients are known to have an increased risk for dementia,

with an annual conversion rate of about 8 to 15% (Petersen, 2016). In fact, the literature involving the power spectral properties of MEG signals in MCI patients is highly consistent in reporting a similar pattern to that found in AD, characterized by a shift to the left of the power spectrum with a relative increase of lower frequency bands power (delta and theta) with respect to faster brain rhythms (alpha and beta) (López, Cuesta, et al., 2014). Interestingly, this study showed that the pattern of changes evidenced in MCI participants was more accentuated in those patients with more than one cognitive domain affected (the so-called multidomain MCI) compared with those with single-domain MCI. This finding reinforces the idea that early synaptic alterations underlying pathophysiology of AD may be the basis of cognitive deterioration in dementia. Furthermore, the main frequency of alpha rhythm, which is typically known as the individual alpha peak, is known to be slowed in AD and is already present in the MCI stage (Garcés et al., 2013).

Power spectral alterations have been observed at even earlier stages, in healthy older adults with SCD. The SCD stage is characterized by the presence of a subjective feeling of cognitive worsening in the absence of objective impairment in standardized neuropsychological assessment (Jessen et al., 2014). Remarkably, older adults with SCD present an increased risk for dementia between two- and five-fold depending on the study setting (Buckley et al., 2016; Wolfsgruber et al., 2016). A significant decrease in alpha power has also been found in this population, affecting broad brain regions, showing largest disruption over similar areas to that shown by MCI (López-Sanz et al., 2016). Interestingly, alpha peak frequency was still not affected in SCD as it was in MCI participants, leading to the hypothesis that synaptic alterations throughout the preclinical stages progress gradually during the successive stages.

Some studies have shown that power spectral properties as measured by MEG in the preclinical stages of AD are closely tied with some of the current biomarkers employed in

AD detection. Gray matter atrophy has been largely associated with MEG power alterations. For instance, alpha peak slowing and amplitude reduction over broad brain regions have been associated with gray matter loss in the hippocampus in different studies (Garcés et al., 2013; López-Sanz et al., 2016) in MCI and SCD participants. Furthermore, alpha power reduction along the AD continuum was also linked to occipital cortical shrinkage (Babiloni et al., 2015). Lastly, increases in delta and theta power have been related to a reduced entorhinal and hippocampal volumes, respectively, in Aβ-positive MCI patients (Nakamura et al., 2018). Although very scarcely, power alterations have also been studied in relation to PET biomarkers. In the previously cited study by Nakamura et al., an increase in delta power was shown to be associated with glucose hypometabolism over posterior cingulate cortex (a classical marker of AD) as measured by FDG-PET. Furthermore, despite a significant alpha power decrease in the MCI group, Aβ accumulation over orbitofrontal regions was associated with a specific power increase in those regions, interpreted as a toxic effect produced by Aβ over surrounding inhibitory neurons, leading to local hyperexcitability.

25.3.2. Functional Connectivity and Graph Theory

Synchronization between distant brain regions is a fundamental aspect for cognitive performance affected in AD patients. However, a detailed description of the course of FC alterations during the preclinical stages of the disease could be important in the search for an early biomarker of the disease. Some signs of the prevailing disconnection reported in AD have been already documented in MCI patients during resting state with MEG. For instance, Gómez, Stam, Hornero, Fernandez, and Maestu (2009) reported a significant mean FC decrease in the beta band, which, in a subsequent study, was shown to affect mainly the connection between supramarginal gyrus, temporal regions, and right precentral gyrus in

that frequency range (Cuesta et al., 2015). This same study also reported a significant disconnection in the alpha band between bilateral inferior parietal regions and the hippocampus, classically AD-related regions already at the MCI stage. Interestingly, alpha band synchronization seems to be sensitive to AD progression, correctly distinguishing the different stages along the continuum (Ranasinghe et al., 2014). Default mode network, the most critical resting-state network in AD progression, also shows early alterations in the MCI stage and even in SCD older adults, with decreased synchronization values in the alpha band (López-Sanz et al., 2017). Furthermore, this functional decoupling seems to be related to structural deterioration of white matter tracts as shown by a MEG study in combination with diffusion tensor imaging (Garcés et al., 2014). This finding was interpreted as a sign of the widely known relationship between tau accumulation and axonal damage (Kowall & Kosik, 1987), which reinforces the relationship between MEG findings and multimodal biomarkers for the detection of AD.

Despite the body of literature supporting the presence of functional desynchronization in the preclinical stages of AD, there are a number of studies reporting an increase in synchronization over certain brain regions in the early stages of the disease. MCI and SCD older adults were recently shown to share a common pattern of alterations involving two different subnetworks with opposed alterations. A significant hyposynchronization over posterior brain regions, including parietal, medial temporal, and occipital areas, was found along with a marked hypersynchronization over more anterior areas (López-Sanz et al., 2017). Importantly, these increased FC levels have proved useful in predicting conversion from MCI to AD in a 2-year follow-up study (López, Bruña, et al., 2014) and were able to correctly distinguish MCI from healthy older adults in the first multicenter blind study conducted to date with MEG (Maestú et al., 2015). Moreover, the fact that increased FC has also been observed in healthy older adult carriers of the APOE ε4 allele has led to the hypothesis that the ubiquitous finding of the disconnection in AD patients is preceded by a phase of hypersynchronization, which is eventually followed by a collapse of the connectivity, leading to network breakdown in later stages (López-Sanz et al., 2017) and corroborated by computational neuroscience models (de Haan, van Straaten, Gouw, & Stam, 2017).

FC analyses have been employed for a shorter period of time in the context of dementia research, which limits the amount of works studying its relationship with current AD biomarkers. Nevertheless, some promising findings point out the relevance of FC in this field and support the previously mentioned hypothesis of FC trajectory along the AD continuum. A recent study by Nakamura et al. (2017) showed that healthy older adults with increased Aβ levels show enhanced synchronization between precuneus and bilateral inferior parietal regions. A possible interpretation of these findings was shown by previous work, indicating that soluble Aβ oligomers and early plaques may lead to a disruption in the excitatory/inhibitory balance of the networks, which could be the initial event triggering the cascade of alterations leading to AD (Busche & Konnerth, 2016). According to this hypothesis, hyposynchronization may appear at later stages, after the initial connectivity increase, and therefore can be interpreted as a result of neurodegeneration, which seems to be supported by its relationship to hippocampal atrophy (López-Sanz et al., 2017). Another study trying to associate MEG profiles with current biomarkers evaluated the correlation between the levels of the phosphorylated tau and FC values. This study found an increased FC between the medial temporal lobe and the anterior cingulate cortex with increased levels of p-tau, supporting the idea of the transneuronal degeneration (Canuet et al., 2015).

25.4. NEURAL UNDERPINNINGS OF MAGNETOENCEPHALOGRAPHY FINDINGS IN ALZHEIMER DISEASE

As mentioned in the previous sections, the degenerative mechanisms resulting from multimodal monitoring of AD involve synapse disturbances and neuronal loss, which take place progressively along the disease continuum and are characterized by distinctive temporal, spectral, and spatial evolution. The literature offers various hypotheses regarding causal relations among the phenomena that compose the pathophysiological cascade of AD. Since MEG directly measures postsynaptic activity of pyramidal neurons (Hansen, Kringelbach, & Salmelin, 2010; Susi et al., 2019), it represents a useful tool for assessing such hypotheses.

A recently proposed framework of coordination of MEG oscillations is based on the mechanism of "dynamical relaying" (Baillet, 2017), that is, a star-like network motif characterized by a symmetric relay that a central area provides for the indirect communication between outer areas (Vicente, Gollo, Mirasso, Fischer, & Pipa, 2008), which would explain synchrony and organization of brain rhythms among different cortical regions (both within and between different bands (see Florin & Baillet, 2015), mediated by the thalamus or other hub regions. Among other things, the thalamus is known to be responsible for communication between the cortical surface and subcortical nuclei (Sanz-Leon, Knock, Spiegler, & Jirsa, 2015). The dynamic relaying mechanism, which in its basic formulation is shown using generic neuronal pools (Gollo, Mirasso, Sporns, & Breakspear, 2014; Vicente et al., 2008), when contextualized to brain networks reveals that the slower delta-to-alpha rhythms mark the net excitability of outer cell assemblies (Baillet, 2017), playing a key role on the network's FC. With the nuclei and the white matter tracts of the corticothalamic network affected differently in AD (Sanz-Leon et al., 2015; Zarei et al., 2010), this framework allows us to interpret the progressive modification of within-band and cross-frequency FC between cortical areas (Engels et al., 2016; Florin & Baillet, 2015), as well as the disruption of the power spectrum noticeable with MEG.

Considering many studies that confirm that the alpha rhythm emerges from the reciprocal connections between cortex and thalamus (Freyer et al., 2011; Maier & Hindriks, 2011), computational models based on the same mechanism seem to increasingly unveil the substrate of the power disruption observed in AD. Using a thalamocortical network model that oscillates within the alpha frequency band, with connection ratios and distances derived from the mammalian thalamocortical system, Abuhassan et al. (2014) showed that the dynamics of the thalamic and cortical oscillations are significantly influenced by corticocortical synaptic loss and suggest that thalamic atrophy is a secondary pathology to cortical shrinkage in AD. Interestingly, Bhattacharya, Coyle, and Maguire (2011) show that an AD-like variation of synaptic connectivity parameters in the thalamic cell populations produces an electrophysiological correlate of slowing of alpha rhythms and a simultaneous decrease of alpha band power in the brain. It is possible that the thalamus is not the origin of all neurophysiological dysfunctions described previously. However, the altered signals at the cortical level could affect the thalamus's ability to synchronize long-distance regions and as a consequence provoke an inadequate network functioning. Taking a look at the whole picture, the starting point seems to reside in the hyperactivity and disinhibition process induced by the amyloid deposits (described by Nakamura et al., 2017, 2018; de Haan, van Straaten, Gouw, & Stam, 2017; and Palop & Mucke, 2010), which seems to trigger a positive feedback loop involving the neurotoxic amyloid deposits at the cortical level, assuming a causal role in pathophysiological cascade (Bero et al., 2011; Cirrito et al., 2005).

25.5. CONCLUSION

MEG is a useful tool in the study of the pathogenesis of AD, both in preclinical and advanced stages of the disease. Its high spatial and temporal resolution give rise to a wide range of metrics and analysis techniques that allow us to explore the neurophysiological changes in which AD pathology results from different perspectives. Accordingly, we are starting to unveil how AD induces a series of functional changes in the brain. One of the most robust findings is a general slowing of the power spectrum starting in the preclinical stages. Similarly, a reorganization of brain networks takes place even at the asymptomatic stages, following a pattern that is hypothesized to begin with an increase in FC as a consequence of neuronal hyperexcitability produced by Aβ, followed by an FC decrease in the later stages. Such connectivity decrement is thought to become even more intense throughout the course of the disease. Finally, in individuals who have fully developed AD pathology, an overall network desynchronization can be observed, which has led researchers to consider AD as a disconnection syndrome.

Since AD neuropathology occurs in the brain up to 20 years before the first clinical symptoms arise, these findings are particularly relevant given the fact that early biomarkers are urgently needed in order to identify potential candidates for future interventional studies, as well as indicators of disease progression. In this regard, more research is needed that combines MEG technology with other classical methods for deriving AD biomarkers, such as cerebrospinal fluid, PET, or MRI. Also, the next step in AD research employing MEG should be the development and validation of diagnostic biomarkers that can be applied at the individual level. Such tools would enable the classification of healthy older adults according to their chances of evolving to a clinical AD pattern. A successful attempt to develop such biomarkers at the MCI stage was carried out in a multicenter study (Maestú et al., 2015), in which an interhemispheric and frontoparietal hypersynchronization was identified as the best discriminator between MCI patients and healthy controls.

The earlier in the disease process that are able to detect individuals at high risk for developing AD, the more likely it will be that different kinds of interventions result in successful outcomes. Such a scenario would require the monitoring of participants in long-term longitudinal studies. Given that MEG is a completely noninvasive technique that can be applied multiple times at no risk to the individual, we conclude that a greater effort should be made in order to fully characterize AD pathology through different MEG signal markers. Also, more research is needed with respect to different protection and risk factors that could modulate or alter the typical disease progression (as defined by MEG), from lifestyle variables (e.g., educational level, exercise, diet, smoking) to genetic risk factors.

REFERENCES

Abuhassan, K., Coyle, D., Belatreche, A., & Maguire, L. (2014). Compensating for synaptic loss in Alzheimer's disease. *Journal of Computational Neuroscience, 36*(1), 19–37.

Alonso, J. F., Poza, J., Mañanas, M. A., Romero, S., Fernández, A., & Hornero, R. (2011). MEG connectivity analysis in patients with Alzheimer's disease using cross mutual information and spectral coherence. *Annals of Biomedical Engineering, 39*(1), 524–536.

Alzheimer's Disease International. (2015). *World Alzheimer report 2015: The global impact of dementia, an analysis of prevalence, incidence, cost and trends.* Retrieved from https://www.alz.co.uk/research/world-report-2015

Anderson, R. M., Hadjichrysanthou, C., Evans, S., & Wong, M. M. (2017). Why do so many clinical trials of therapies for Alzheimer's disease fail? *Lancet, 390*(10110), 2327–2329.

Babiloni, C., Del Percio, C., Boccardi, M., Lizio, R., Lopez, S., Carducci, F., . . . Frisoni, G. B. (2015). Occipital sources of resting-state alpha rhythms are related to local gray matter density in subjects with amnesic mild cognitive impairment and Alzheimer's disease. *Neurobiology of Aging, 36*(2), 556–570.

Baillet, S. (2017). Magnetoencephalography for brain electrophysiology and imaging. *Nature Neuroscience, 20*(3), 327–339.

Bero, A. W., Yan, P., Roh, J. H., Cirrito, J. R., Stewart, F. R., Raichle, M. E., . . . Holtzman, D. M. (2011). Neuronal activity regulates the regional vulnerability to amyloid-beta deposition. *Nature Neuroscience, 14*(6), 750–756.

Bhattacharya, B. S., Coyle, D., & Maguire, L. P. (2011). A thalamo-cortico-thalamic neural mass model to study alpha rhythms in Alzheimer's disease. *Neural Networks, 24*(6), 631–645.

Bruña, R., Poza, J., Gómez, C., García, M., Fernández, A., & Hornero, R. (2012). Analysis of spontaneous MEG activity in mild cognitive impairment and Alzheimer's disease using spectral entropies and statistical complexity measures. *Journal of Neural Engineering, 9*(3), 036007.

Buckley, R., Maruff, P., Ames, D., Bourgeat, P., Martins, R. N., Masters, C. L., . . . Ellis, K. A. (2016). Subjective memory decline predicts greater rates of clinical progression in preclinical Alzheimer's disease. *Alzheimer's and Dementia, 12*(7), 796–804.

Busatto, G. F., Garrido, G. E. ., Almeida, O. P., Castro, C. C., Camargo, C. H. ., Cid, C. G., . . . Bottino, C. M. (2003). A voxel-based morphometry study of temporal lobe gray matter reductions in Alzheimer's disease. *Neurobiology of Aging, 24*(2), 221–231.

Busche, M. A., & Konnerth, A. (2016). Impairments of neural circuit function in Alzheimer's disease. *Philosophical Transactions of the Royal Society of London. Series B, Biological Sciences, 371*(1700), 20150429.

Canuet, L., Pusil, S., López, M. E., Bajo, R., Pineda-Pardo, J. Á., Cuesta, P., . . . Maestú, F. (2015). Network disruption and cerebrospinal fluid amyloid-beta and phospho-tau levels in mild cognitive impairment. *Journal of Neuroscience, 35*(28), 10325–10330.

Cirrito, J. R., Yamada, K. A., Finn, M. B., Sloviter, R. S., Bales, K. R., May, P. C., . . . Holtzman, D. M. (2005). Synaptic activity regulates interstitial fluid amyloid-β levels in vivo. *Neuron, 48*(6), 913–922.

Cuesta, P., Garcés, P., Castellanos, N. P., López, M. E., Aurtenetxe, S., Bajo, R., . . . Maestú, F. (2015). Influence of the APOE ε4 allele and mild cognitive impairment diagnosis in the disruption of the MEG resting state functional connectivity in sources space. *Journal of Alzheimer's Disease, 44*(2), 493–505.

de Haan, W., Mott, K., van Straaten, E. C. W., Scheltens, P., & Stam, C. J. (2012). Activity dependent degeneration explains hub vulnerability in Alzheimer's disease. *PLoS Computational Biology, 8*(8), e1002582.

de Haan, W., van der Flier, W. M., Koene, T., Smits, L. L., Scheltens, P., & Stam, C. J. (2012). Disrupted modular brain dynamics reflect cognitive dysfunction in Alzheimer's disease. *NeuroImage, 59*(4), 3085–3093.

de Haan, W., van der Flier, W. M., Wang, H., Van Mieghem, P. F. A., Scheltens, P., & Stam, C. J. (2012). Disruption of functional brain networks in Alzheimer's disease: What can we learn from graph spectral analysis of resting-state magnetoencephalography? *Brain Connectivity*, 2(2), 45–55.

de Haan, W., van Straaten, E. C. W., Gouw, A. A., & Stam, C. J. (2017). Altering neuronal excitability to preserve network connectivity in a computational model of Alzheimer's disease. *PLOS Computational Biology*, 13(9), e1005707.

Dickinson, A., DiStefano, C., Senturk, D., & Jeste, S. S. (2018). Peak alpha frequency is a neural marker of cognitive function across the autism spectrum. *European Journal of Neuroscience*, 47(6), 643–651.

Engels, M. M. A., van der Flier, W. M., Stam, C. J., Hillebrand, A., Scheltens, P., & van Straaten, E. C. W. (2017). Alzheimer's disease: The state of the art in resting-state magnetoencephalography. *Clinical Neurophysiology*, 128(8), 1426–1437.

Engels, M. M. A., Yu, M., Arjan, H., Scheltens, P., van der Flier, W. M., van Straaten, E. C. W., & Stam, C. J. (2016). MEG cross-frequency analysis in patients with Alzheimer´s Disease. *Alzheimer's & Dementia*, 12(7), P1087–P1088.

Escudero, J., Sanei, S., Jarchi, D., Abásolo, D., & Hornero, R. (2011). Regional coherence evaluation in mild cognitive impairment and Alzheimer's disease based on adaptively extracted magnetoencephalogram rhythms. *Physiological Measurement*, 32(8), 1163–1180.

Fernández, A., Arrazola, J., Maestú, F., Amo, C., Gil-Gregorio, P., Wienbruch, C., & Ortiz, T. (2003). Correlations of hippocampal atrophy and focal low-frequency magnetic activity in Alzheimer disease: Volumetric MR imaging-magnetoencephalographic study. *AJNR: American Journal of Neuroradiology*, 24(3), 481–487.

Fernández, A., Maestú, F., Amo, C., Gil, P., Fehr, T., Wienbruch, C., . . . Ortiz, T. (2002). Focal temporoparietal slow activity in Alzheimer's disease revealed by magnetoencephalography. *Biological Psychiatry*, 52(7), 764–770.

Fernández, A., Turrero, A., Zuluaga, P., Gil-Gregorio, P., del Pozo, F., Maestu, F., & Moratti, S. (2013). MEG delta mapping along the healthy aging–Alzheimer's disease continuum: Diagnostic implications. *Journal of Alzheimer's Disease*, 35(3), 495–507.

Fernández, A., Turrero, A., Zuluaga, P., Gil, P., Maestú, F., Campo, P., & Ortiz, T. (2006). Magnetoencephalographic parietal δ dipole density in mild cognitive impairment. *Archives of Neurology*, 63(3), 427.

Florin, E., & Baillet, S. (2015). The brain's resting-state activity is shaped by synchronized cross-frequency coupling of neural oscillations. *NeuroImage*, 111, 26–35.

Franciotti, R., Iacono, D., Penna, S. D., Pizzella, V., Torquati, K., Onofrj, M., & Romani, G. L. (2006). Cortical rhythms reactivity in AD, LBD and normal subjects: A quantitative MEG study. *Neurobiology of Aging*, 27(8), 1100–1109.

Freyer, F., Roberts, J. A., Becker, R., Robinson, P. A., Ritter, P., & Breakspear, M. (2011). Biophysical mechanisms of multistability in resting-state cortical rhythms. *Journal of Neuroscience*, 31(17), 6353–6361.

Garcés, P., Angel Pineda-Pardo, J., Canuet, L., Aurtenetxe, S., López, M. E., Marcos, A., . . . Maestú, F. (2014). The Default Mode Network is functionally and structurally disrupted in amnestic mild cognitive impairment: A bimodal MEG-DTI study. *NeuroImage: Clinical*, 6, 214–221.

Garcés, P., Vicente, R., Wibral, M., Pineda-Pardo, J. Á., López, M. E., Aurtenetxe, S., . . . Fernández, A. (2013). Brain-wide slowing of spontaneous alpha rhythms in mild cognitive impairment. *Frontiers in Aging Neuroscience*, 5(DEC), 1–7.

Gollo, L. L., Mirasso, C., Sporns, O., & Breakspear, M. (2014). Mechanisms of zero-lag synchronization in cortical motifs. *PLoS Computational Biology*, 10(4), e1003548.

Gómez, C., Hornero, R., Abásolo, D., Fernández, A., & Escudero, J. (2007). Analysis of the magnetoencephalogram background activity in Alzheimer's disease patients with auto-mutual information. *Computer Methods and Programs in Biomedicine*, 87(3), 239–247.

Gómez, C., Hornero, R., Abásolo, D., Fernández, A., & Escudero, J. (2009). Analysis of MEG background activity in Alzheimer's disease using non-linear methods and ANFIS. *Annals of Biomedical Engineering*, 37(3), 586–594.

Gomez, C., Hornero, R., Abasolo, D., Fernandez, A., & Poza, J. (2009). Study of the MEG background activity in Alzheimer's disease patients with scaling analysis methods. In *2009 Annual International Conference of the IEEE Engineering in Medicine and Biology Society* (pp. 3485–3488). Piscataway, NJ: IEEE.

Gomez, C., Stam, C. J., Hornero, R., Fernandez, A., & Maestu, F. (2009). Disturbed beta band functional connectivity in patients with mild cognitive impairment: An MEG study. *IEEE Transactions on Biomedical Engineering*, 56(6), 1683–1690.

Hansen, P., Kringelbach, M., & Salmelin, R. (Eds.). (2010). *MEG: An introduction to methods*. Oxford, UK: Oxford University Press.

Hari, R., & Puce, A. (2017). *MEG-EEG primer*. Oxford, UK: Oxford University Press.

Harper, S. (2014). Economic and social implications of aging societies. *Science (New York), 346*(6209), 587–591.

Heneka, M. T., Carson, M. J., Khoury, J. E., Landreth, G. E., Brosseron, F., Feinstein, D. L., . . . Kummer, M. P. (2015). Neuroinflammation in Alzheimer's disease. *Lancet: Neurology, 14*(4), 388–405.

Hornero, R., Abásolo, D., Escudero, J., & Gómez, C. (2009). Nonlinear analysis of electroencephalogram and magnetoencephalogram recordings in patients with Alzheimer's disease. *Philosophical Transactions of the Royal Society A: Mathematical, Physical and Engineering Sciences, 367*(1887), 317–336.

Ishii, R., Canuet, L., Kurimoto, R., Ikezawa, K., Aoki, Y., Azechi, M., . . . Takeda, M. (2010). Frontal shift of posterior alpha activity is correlated with cognitive impairment in early Alzheimer's disease: A magnetoencephalography-beamformer study. *Psychogeriatrics, 10*(3), 138–143.

Jack, C. R., Albert, M. S., Knopman, D. S., McKhann, G. M., Sperling, R. A., Carrillo, M. C., . . . Phelps, C. H. (2011). Introduction to the recommendations from the National Institute on Aging-Alzheimer's Association workgroups on diagnostic guidelines for Alzheimer's disease. *Alzheimer's and Dementia, 7*(3), 257–262.

Jack, C. R., Knopman, D. S., Jagust, W. J., Petersen, R. C., Weiner, M. W., Aisen, P. S., . . . Trojanowski, J. Q. (2013). Tracking pathophysiological processes in Alzheimer's disease: An updated hypothetical model of dynamic biomarkers. *Lancet: Neurology, 12*(2), 207–216.

Jessen, F., Amariglio, R. E., van Boxtel, M., Breteler, M., Ceccaldi, M., Chételat, G., . . . Wagner, M. (2014). A conceptual framework for research on subjective cognitive decline in preclinical Alzheimer's disease. *Alzheimer's and Dementia, 10*(6), 844–852.

Juan-Cruz, C., Gómez, C., Poza, J., Fernández, A., & Hornero, R. (2017). Assessment of effective connectivity in Alzheimer's disease using Granger causality. In J. Ibáñez, J. González-Vargas, J. Azorín, M. Akay, & J. Pons (Eds.), *Converging Clinical and Engineering Research on Neurorehabilitation II. Biosystems and Biorobotics* (Vol. 15, pp. 763–767). New York, NY: Springer, Cham.

Koelewijn, L., Bompas, A., Tales, A., Brookes, M. J., Muthukumaraswamy, S. D., Bayer, A., & Singh, K. D. (2017). Alzheimer's disease disrupts alpha and beta-band resting-state oscillatory network connectivity. *Clinical Neurophysiology, 128*(11), 2347–2357.

Kowall, N. W., & Kosik, K. S. (1987). Axonal disruption and aberrant localization of tau protein characterize the neuropil pathology of Alzheimer's disease. *Annals of Neurology, 22*(5), 639–643.

López-Sanz, D., Brunã, R., Garcés, P., Camara, C., Serrano, N., Rodríguez-Rojo, I. C., . . . Maestú, F. (2016). Alpha band disruption in the AD-continuum starts in the Subjective Cognitive Decline stage: A MEG study. *Scientific Reports, 6*, 37685.

López-Sanz, D., Bruña, R., Garcés, P., Martín-Buro, M. C., Walter, S., Delgado, M. L., . . . Maestú, F. (2017). Functional connectivity disruption in subjective cognitive decline and mild cognitive impairment: A common pattern of alterations. *Frontiers in Aging Neuroscience, 9*, 109.

López-Sanz, D., Garcés, P., Álvarez, B., Delgado-Losada, M. L., López-Higes, R., & Maestú, F. (2017). Network disruption in the preclinical stages of Alzheimer's disease: From subjective cognitive decline to mild cognitive impairment. *International Journal of Neural Systems, 27*(8), 1750041.

López, M. E., Bruña, R., Aurtenetxe, S., Pineda-Pardo, J. A., Marcos, A., Arrazola, J., . . . Maestú, F. (2014). Alpha-band hypersynchronization in progressive mild cognitive impairment: A magnetoencephalography study. *Journal of Neuroscience, 34*(44), 14551–14559.

López, M. E., Cuesta, P., Garcés, P., Castellanos, P. N., Aurtenetxe, S., Bajo, R., . . . Fernandez, A. (2014). MEG spectral analysis in subtypes of mild cognitive impairment. *Age (Dordrecht, Netherlands), 36*(3), 9624.

Maestú, F., Peña, J.-M., Garcés, P., González, S., Bajo, R., Bagic, A., . . . Magnetoencephalography International Consortium of Alzheimer's Disease. (2015). A multicenter study of the early detection of synaptic dysfunction in Mild Cognitive Impairment using Magnetoencephalography-derived functional connectivity. *NeuroImage: Clinical, 9*, 103–109.

Maier, J. X., & Hindriks, R. (2011). Modeling the physiological mechanisms of multistability in spontaneous corticothalamic dynamics. *Journal of Neuroscience, 31*(32), 11423–11424.

Mandal, P. K., Banerjee, A., Tripathi, M., & Sharma, A. (2018). A comprehensive review of magnetoencephalography (MEG) studies for brain functionality in healthy aging and Alzheimer's disease (AD). *Frontiers in Computational Neuroscience, 12*, 60.

Miyakawa, T. (2010). Vascular pathology in Alzheimer's disease. *Psychogeriatrics, 10*(1), 39–44.

Montez, T., Poil, S.-S., Jones, B. F., Manshanden, I., Verbunt, J. P. A., van Dijk, B. W., . . . Linkenkaer-Hansen, K. (2009). Altered temporal correlations in parietal alpha and prefrontal theta oscillations in early-stage Alzheimer disease. *Proceedings of the*

National Academy of Sciences of the United States of America, 106(5), 1614–1619.

Nakamura, A., Cuesta, P., Fernández, A., Arahata, Y., Iwata, K., Kuratsubo, I., . . . Kato, T. (2018). Electromagnetic signatures of the preclinical and prodromal stages of Alzheimer's disease. Brain, 141(5), 1470–1485.

Nakamura, A., Cuesta, P., Kato, T., Arahata, Y., Iwata, K., Yamagishi, M., . . . Ito, K. (2017). Early functional network alterations in asymptomatic elders at risk for Alzheimer's disease. Scientific Reports, 7(1), 6517.

Osipova, D., Ahveninen, J., Jensen, O., Ylikoski, A., & Pekkonen, E. (2005). Altered generation of spontaneous oscillations in Alzheimer's disease. NeuroImage, 27(4), 835–841.

Palop, J. J., & Mucke, L. (2010). Amyloid-B-induced neuronal dysfunction in Alzheimer's disease: From synapses toward neural networks. Nature Neuroscience, 13(7), 812–818.

Petersen, R. C. (2016). Mild cognitive impairment. Continuum (Minneapolis, MN), 22(2 Dementia), 404–418.

Petersen, R. C., Smith, G. E., Waring, S. C., Ivnik, R. J., Tangalos, E. G., & Kokmen, E. (1999). Mild cognitive impairment: Clinical characterization and outcome. Archives of Neurology, 56(3), 303–308.

Petrovic, J., Milosevic, V., Zivkovic, M., Stojanov, D., Milojkovic, O., Kalauzi, A., & Saponjic, J. (2017). Slower EEG alpha generation, synchronization and "flow": Possible biomarkers of cognitive impairment and neuropathology of minor stroke. PeerJ, 5, e3839.

Poza, J., Hornero, R., Escudero, J., Fernández, A., & Sánchez, C. I. (2008). Regional analysis of spontaneous MEG rhythms in patients with Alzheimer's disease using spectral entropies. Annals of Biomedical Engineering, 36(1), 141–152.

Ranasinghe, K. G., Hinkley, L. B., Beagle, A. J., Mizuiri, D., Dowling, A. F., Honma, S. M., . . . Vossel, K. A. (2014). Regional functional connectivity predicts distinct cognitive impairments in Alzheimer's disease spectrum. NeuroImage: Clinical, 5, 385–395.

Sanz-Leon, P., Knock, S. A., Spiegler, A., & Jirsa, V. K. (2015). Mathematical framework for large-scale brain network modeling in The Virtual Brain. NeuroImage, 111, 385–430.

Stam, C. J., de Haan, W., Daffertshofer, A., Jones, B. F., Manshanden, I., van Cappellen van Walsum, A. M., . . . Scheltens, P. (2008). Graph theoretical analysis of magnetoencephalographic functional connectivity in Alzheimer's disease. Brain, 132(1), 213–224.

Stam, C. J., Jones, B. F., Manshanden, I., van Cappellen van Walsum, A. M., Montez, T., Verbunt, J. P. A., . . . Scheltens, P. (2006). Magnetoencephalographic evaluation of resting-state functional connectivity in Alzheimer's disease. NeuroImage, 32(3), 1335–1344.

Stam, C. J., van Cappellen van Walsum, A. M., Pijnenburg, Y. A. L., Berendse, H. W., de Munck, J. C., Scheltens, P., & van Dijk, B. W. (2002). Generalized synchronization of MEG recordings in Alzheimer's disease: Evidence for involvement of the gamma band. Journal of Clinical Neurophysiology, 19(6), 562–574.

Susi, G., de Frutos-Lucas, J., Niso, G., Ye-Chen, S. M., Toro, L. A., Chino Vilca, B. N., & Maestú, F. (2019). Healthy and pathological neurocognitive aging: Spectral and functional connectivity analyses using magnetoencephalography. In B. G. Oxford Research Encyclopedia of Psychology. Oxford, UK: Oxford University Press.

Van Cappellen Van Walsum, A. M., Pijnenburg, Y. A. L., Berendse, H. W., Van Dijk, B. W., Knol, D. L., Scheltens, P., & Stam, C. J. (2003). A neural complexity measure applied to MEG data in Alzheimer's disease. Clinical Neurophysiology, 114(6), 1034–1040.

Verdoorn, T. A., McCarten, J. R., Arciniegas, D. B., Golden, R., Moldauer, L., Georgopoulos, A., . . . Rojas, D. C. (2011). Evaluation and tracking of Alzheimer's disease severity using resting-state magnetoencephalography. Journal of Alzheimer's Disease, 26(Suppl 3), 239–255.

Vicente, R., Gollo, L. L., Mirasso, C. R., Fischer, I., & Pipa, G. (2008). Dynamical relaying can yield zero time lag neuronal synchrony despite long conduction delays. Proceedings of the National Academy of Sciences of the United States of America, 105(44), 17157–17162.

Wolfsgruber, S., Kleineidam, L., Wagner, M., Mösch, E., Bickel, H., Lühmann, D., . . . AgeCoDe Study Group. (2016). Differential Risk of Incident Alzheimer's Disease Dementia in Stable Versus Unstable Patterns of Subjective Cognitive Decline. Journal of Alzheimer's Disease, 54(3), 1135–1146.

Yu, M., Engels, M. M. A., Hillebrand, A., van Straaten, E. C. W., Gouw, A. A., Teunissen, C., . . . Stam, C. J. (2017). Selective impairment of hippocampus and posterior hub areas in Alzheimer's disease: An MEG-based multiplex network study. Brain, 140(5), 1466–1485.

Zarei, M., Patenaude, B., Damoiseaux, J., Morgese, C., Smith, S., Matthews, P. M., . . . Jenkinson, M. (2010). Combining shape and connectivity analysis: An MRI study of thalamic degeneration in Alzheimer's disease. NeuroImage, 49(1), 1–8.

POSTSCRIPT

FIFTY YEARS OF MAGNETOENCEPHALOGRAPHY— AN "INTERIM" EPILOGUE

Timothy P. L. Roberts, James W. Wheless, and
Andrew C. Papanicolaou

AS IS evident from the scientific chapters of this book, the technology of magnetoencephalography offers a combination of spatial, temporal, and spectral resolution, unique among neuroimaging technologies. While functional magnetic resonance imaging (fMRI) accommodates spatial resolution, it lacks the millisecond resolution (because of the reliance on a slow hemodynamic response) to identify subtle latency shifts, or the specificity to distinguish theta- versus alpha- versus gamma-band oscillatory activity. While electroencephalography (EEG) offers the needed temporal resolution, it fails to adequately localize brain sources, owing to the physics of inverse modeling and the dependence of scalp electric potentials on tissue electrical conductivity. Thus, although fMRI may see "activity," it cannot characterize important attributes of its nature. Conversely, EEG may detect "anomalies" but not be able to attribute them to a particular spatial source.

Over the 50-year history of magnetoencephalography (MEG), technical progress has been achieved in realizing the potential described previously—new methods harness spatial, spectral, and temporal specificity. Initial applications capitalized on the exquisite temporal resolution to detect anomalous brain activity and used simple "instantaneous" models to localize the source. Immediate clinical application was found in the study of epilepsy and seizure disorders (in which spontaneous electrographic anomalies are characteristic, and for which surgical treatment mandates "source localization"). Thus, the early clinical application of MEG has been focused on the field of epilepsy, with significant and profound contributions being made, such that MEG is widely used as part of the presurgical workup of epilepsy patients, worldwide. The adoption of MEG into the standard of care for epilepsy must be regarded as a testament to the validity of the technology.

Timothy P. L. Roberts, James W. Wheless, and Andrew C. Papanicolaou, *Postscript: Fifty Years of Magnetoencephalography—An "Interim" Epilogue* In: *Fifty Years of Magnetoencephalography*. Edited by: Andrew C. Papanicolaou, Timothy P. L. Roberts, and James W. Wheless, Oxford University Press (2020). © Oxford University Press. DOI: 10.1093/oso/9780190935689.003.0026.

However, the source modeling of instantaneous anomalous activity represents only one aspect of the capabilities of MEG. Technical consideration of the unique attributes and capabilities of MEG have spurred advances toward other clinical applications, currently poorly served by conventional radiological and neurological techniques. In particular, consideration of neural signal transmission (e.g., response latencies), or spectral balance (e.g., theta/gamma), or dynamic connectivity metrics offers promise in an array of psychiatric conditions such as autism spectrum disorder (ASD), attention-deficit hyperactivity disorder (ADHD), and post-traumatic stress disorder (PTSD), currently not well diagnosed or characterized by MRI or computed tomography (CT). Harnessing the intrinsic technical strengths of MEG promises to yield advances in these disorders of brain function and network dynamics where structural methods alone may be lacking.

That said, evidence suggests that the integration of multimodal imaging capabilities may ultimately not only yield diagnostic advances but also point toward mechanistic bases. Whether these are used to form "converging evidence" for diagnosis or to distinguish subpopulations across heterogeneous diagnoses (or to identify common neurophysiological mechanisms across clinical diagnoses), the combination of structural and microstructural findings from MRI, neurochemistry from advanced magnetic resonance spectroscopy (MRS), and in vivo electrophysiology from MEG offers a tantalizing armory for research and clinical advances over the next 50 years. Matching technical capabilities to clinical needs remains the priority of the field and the most promising avenue for progress.

INDEX

Tables and figures are indicated by *t* and *f* following the page number. Numbers followed by n indicate notes.